Pharmacologic Principles of CANCER TREATMENT

Bruce Chabner, M.D.

Associate Director
Clinical Oncology Program
Division of Cancer Treatment
National Cancer Institute
Bethesda, Maryland

1982 **W. B. Saunders Company**

Philadelphia London Toronto Mexico City Rio de Janeiro Sydney Tokyo

W. B. Saunders Company: West Washington Square
Philadelphia, PA 19105

1 St. Anne's Road
Eastbourne, East Sussex BN21 3UN, England

1 Goldthorne Avenue
Toronto, Ontario M8Z 5T9, Canada

Apartado 26370—Cedro 512
Mexico 4, D.F., Mexico

Rua Coronel Cabrita, 8
Sao Cristovao Caixa Postal 21176
Rio de Janeiro, Brazil

9 Waltham Street
Artarmon, N.S.W. 2064, Australia

Ichibancho, Central Bldg., 22-1 Ichibancho
Chiyoda-Ku, Tokyo 102, Japan

Library of Congress Cataloging in Publication Data

Main entry under title:

Pharmacologic principles of cancer treatment.

1. Cancer—Chemotherapy. 2. Antineoplastic agents.
I. Chabner, Bruce. [DNLM: 1. Neoplasms—Drug therapy.
AZ 267 C427p]

RC271.C5P48 616.99'4061 81-40737

ISBN 0-7216-2477-4 AACR2

Pharmacologic Principles of Cancer Treatment ISBN 0-7216-2477-4

Last digit is the print number: 9 8 7 6 5 4 3 2 1

DEDICATION

This book represents the culmination of a personal interest in medicine and pharmacology that was awakened during my teenage years in Shelbyville, Illinois. My father, Louis Chabner, was a family practitioner, an unusual person with many cultural and scientific interests apart from the daily practice of medicine. He had a particular fascination with therapeutics and pharmacology, and had the good fortune to practice during the years of initial development of antibiotics and corticosteroids. His first experiences with new drugs became a regular topic of family conversation. He remains in my mind a most compassionate and tenacious physician, a person unwilling to accept the *status quo*. In different times he would have been a fine oncologist and, I suspect, would have enjoyed this book, which is dedicated to him.

CONTRIBUTORS

RICHARD A. BENDER, M.D.

Assistant Member II, Department of Biochemistry, Scripps Clinic and Research Foundation, La Jolla, CA. Clinical Assistant Professor of Medicine, University of California, San Diego, CA.

JERRY M. COLLINS, Ph.D.

Chemical Engineering Section, Biomedical Engineering and Instrumentation Branch, Division of Research Services, National Institutes of Health, Bethesda, MD.

MICHAEL COLVIN, M.D.

Associate Professor of Oncology and Medicine, Johns Hopkins University School of Medicine, Baltimore, MD. Active Staff, The Johns Hopkins Hospital, Baltimore, MD.

ROBERT L. DEDRICK, Ph.D.

Chief, Chemical Engineering Section, Biomedical Engineering and Instrumentation Branch, Division of Research Services, National Institutes of Health, Bethesda, MD.

ROSS C. DONEHOWER, M.D.

Assistant Professor of Oncology and Medicine, Johns Hopkins University School of Medicine, Baltimore, MD. Attending Physician, The Johns Hopkins Hospital and The Johns Hopkins Oncology Center, Baltimore, MD.

CHARLES EIL, M.D., Ph.D.

Assistant Professor of Medicine, Uniformed Services University of The Health Sciences, Bethesda, MD. Staff Endocrinologist, Endocrinology and Metabolism Branch—Dept. of Medicine, National Naval Medical Center, Bethesda, MD.

CHARLES ERLICHMAN, M.D., F.R.C.P.(C)

Assistant Professor, University of Toronto School of Medicine, Toronto, Ontario, Canada. Staff Physician, Princess Margaret Hospital, Toronto, Ontario, Canada.

DANIEL GLAUBIGER, M.D., Ph.D.

Senior Investigator, Pediatric Oncology Branch, Division of Cancer Treatment, National Cancer Institute, Bethesda, MD.

I. DAVID GOLDMAN, M.D.

Professor of Medicine and Pharmacology; Chairman, Divisions of Medical Oncology and Biochemical Pharmacology, Medical College of Virginia, Richmond, VA.

KENNETH R. HANDE, M.D.

Assistant Professor of Medicine and Pharmacology, Vanderbilt University School of Medicine, Nashville, TN. Research Associate, Nashville VA Medical Center, Nashville, TN.

DAVID G. JOHNS, M.D., Ph.D.

Chief, Laboratory of Medicinal Chemistry and Biology, Developmental Therapeutics Program, Division of Cancer Treatment, National Cancer Institute, Bethesda, MD.

KURT W. KOHN, M.D., Ph.D.

Chief, Laboratory of Molecular Pharmacology, Division of Cancer Treatment, National Cancer Institute, Bethesda, MD.

MARC E. LIPPMAN, M.D.

Head, Medical Breast Cancer Section, Medicine Branch, National Cancer Institute, Bethesda, MD. Clinical Associate Professor of Medicine and Pharmacology, Uniformed Services University of The Health Sciences, Bethesda, MD.

YUNG-PIN LIU, Ph.D.

Clinical Pharmacology Branch, National Cancer Institute, Bethesda, MD.

JOHN J. McCORMACK, Ph.D.

Professor of Pharmacology, College of Medicine, University of Vermont, Burlington, VT.

CHARLES E. MYERS, M.D.

Attending Physician, Medicine Branch; Chief, Clinical Pharmacology Branch; National Cancer Institute, Bethesda, MD.

ARNER RAMU, M.D.

Lecturer in Experimental Oncology, Department of Radiation and Clinical Oncology, Hadassah University Hospital, Jerusalem, Israel.

PAUL S. RITCH, M.D.

Assistant Professor of Medicine, Medical College of Wisconsin, Milwaukee, WI. Attending Physician; Consultant; Milwaukee County Medical Complex, Milwaukee, WI.

RICHARD L. SCHILSKY, M.D.

Assistant Professor of Medicine, University of Missouri School of Medicine, Columbia, MO. Attending Physician, University Hospital; Chief, Hematology/Medical Oncology, Harry S. Truman Memorial VA Hospital, Columbia, MO.

STANLEY E. SHACKNEY, M.D.

Head, Section of Cell Kinetics, Clinical Pharmacology Branch, Division of Cancer Treatment, National Cancer Institute, Bethesda, MD.

DAVID H. SHIBA, Ph.D.

Postdoctoral Associate, Dept. of Pharmacology, Yale University School of Medicine, New Haven, CT.

ROBERT J. WEINKAM, Ph.D.

Associate Professor of Medicinal Chemistry, School of Pharmacy, Purdue University, West Lafayette, IN.

LEONARD A. ZWELLING, M.D.

Cancer Expert, Laboratory of Molecular Pharmacology, Developmental Therapeutics Program, Division of Cancer Treatment, National Cancer Institute, Bethesda, MD.

PREFACE

The development and successful use of drugs for treating cancer in the past three decades have provided the basis for a new subspecialty in internal medicine—medical oncology. No other field of medicine is more closely tied to a laboratory discipline than this. The interdependence between medical oncology and antineoplastic pharmacology is evident in every phase of cancer treatment from protocol planning to dose modification, drug level monitoring, and new drug evaluation.

This new book was undertaken in recognition of the importance of antineoplastic pharmacology in cancer treatment. It attempts to provide a comprehensive and detailed examination of the preclinical and clinical pharmacology of antineoplastic drugs. Given the rapid growth of knowledge in this field, this objective is beyond the capabilities of any one author. For this reason I sought the help of a number of knowledgeable contributors, chosen for their grasp of both the laboratory and the clinical aspects of these drugs. These co-authors deserve my most sincere appreciation for their patience during the tedious process of revising, editing, and proofreading their manuscripts. Equally deserving of my thanks are Mary Cowell and her staff at W. B. Saunders, and my editorial assistant Kathleen Moore.

We all hope that the final product will serve to enlighten, inspire, and encourage those committed to the belief that cancer will ultimately yield to drug therapy.

BRUCE A. CHABNER, M.D.

ACKNOWLEDGMENTS

This book has come into being through the efforts of a number of key individuals who are not recognized elsewhere in the text but deserve equal credit for the final product. Foremost has been Kathleen Moore, my able secretary and editorial assistant, whose tireless efforts to produce perfect copy made the job of writing and editing easier for all of us. My editor at Saunders, Mary Cowell, and my copy editor, David Harvey, ably molded the diverse individual contributions into a coherent whole. To my clinical colleagues at the National Cancer Institute, to my dedicated co-workers in the laboratory, and especially to my fellow pharmacologists Drs. Charles Myers, David Johns, and Joseph Bertino I owe particular gratitude for stimulating my personal interest in this field and suggesting the seemingly limitless applications of pharmacology to the problem of cancer treatment. And finally I want to thank my family for their patience and understanding during my years of occupation, and preoccupation, with this work; their indulgence of my interest in cancer pharmacology gave me the time and encouragement to finish this book.

CONTENTS

INTRODUCTION

In the past 30 years, since the discovery of antifolates and their introduction as effective antileukemic agents, drug therapy has truly revolutionized the treatment of malignant disease. Curative treatments have been discovered for many of the cancers that afflict children and young adults, including acute lymphocytic leukemia, Hodgkin's disease, testicular carcinoma, and others. These advances have generated great interest in every phase of drug research, leading to the development of a body of knowledge known formally as antineoplastic pharmacology. This field of research deals with the isolation, chemical and biochemical characterization, and experimental and clinical use of drugs for treatment of cancer.

Additional research efforts have been directed toward identifying new classes of active agents, chemically modifying known active drugs for the purpose of eliminating unwanted side effects, and determining the biochemical basis for selectivity of drug action against malignant cells. The resulting body of knowledge not only is useful to the experimental pharmacologist, but has a direct bearing on the design of clinical regimens and the understanding of drug effects, both toxic and therapeutic, in man. It is our purpose in this book to present a comprehensive examination of the experimental and clinical properties of antineoplastic agents in a form understandable to both experimentalists and clinicians.

The introductory chapters provide a background of general principles of drug action and usage. Thus, topics such as drug transport, cellular pharmacology, cell kinetics, pharmacokinetics, and principles of drug level monitoring are considered in detail. These topics are essential to the understanding of subsequent chapters, which deal with specific classes of clinically effective antineoplastic agents. Compounds of unproved value and those that have failed to show activity in clinical trial receive attention only to the extent that their experience has relevance to the use of active agents. The scope of this work does not include immunotherapeutic compounds. The level of presentation for each of these subjects is rigorous, but the text is intended for both a laboratory and a clinical audience.

It is with some hesitation that I and my co-authors have undertaken this project in view of the explosive pace of research in the cancer drug field. Nevertheless, we feel that a synthesis of both principles and facts, as found in this text, can serve as an important landmark in the cancer research effort in much the same way that a conference serves as both an ingathering and a point of departure. Thus, we hope that this book will stand as a measure of dramatic recent progress in our young field as well as a signpost to indicate the direction of future research.

Section I

THE ROLE OF DRUGS IN CANCER TREATMENT

I

Bruce A. Chabner

The treatment of cancer, more than that of any other disease, requires the cooperative efforts of widely divergent medical specialties. Although cancer has been for centuries the concern of the surgeon, new treatment approaches have created important roles for the radiotherapist and internist in the management of cancer patients, and have placed the decision-making process in the hands of these new specialists. Steps in the treatment decision-making process are discussed in this chapter in order to provide the reader with an understanding of the overall role of drugs in cancer therapy.

DETERMINANTS OF TREATMENT PLANNING

The primary determinant of treatment is the histologic diagnosis. Malignant neoplasms occur in over 100 different pathologic forms, each with a characteristic natural history, pattern of progression, and responsiveness to treatment. Thus, the *histologic diagnosis*, usually made by surgical excision of a primary tumor or metastasis, is of critical importance as a first step in treatment planning. The clinical oncologist must be alert to the possibility of atypical presentation of treatable and even curable tumors, such as germ cell tumors of the testis. For example, germ cell tumors on occasion may arise in the thoracic or abdominal cavity in the absence of a primary testicular tumor, but these unusual presentations retain the same excellent response to appropriate chemotherapy.[1] In certain cases — as, for example, bronchogenic carcinoma or the non-Hodgkin's lymphomas — accurate histologic *subtyping* of tumors is important, since the subtypes of these diseases have different patterns of clinical response to treatment. Subtyping may require the characterization of cell surface immunologic markers, for example, to distinguish T- and B-cell lymphomas, or the identification of specific intracellular secretory granules or enzymatic markers such as dopa decarboxylase in small cell carcinoma of the lung. The essential point is that the precise histologic identity of a tumor is the single most important determinant of treatment choice and patient management. Blind treatment, in cases lacking a histologic diagnosis, is rarely successful.[2]

The next step in treatment planning is to determine the extent of disease, and specifically to determine whether the tumor is curable by local treatment measures such as surgery or radiation therapy. The process of determining the extent of disease is termed *staging*, and plays an important role in making therapeutic choices for diseases that are responsive to multiple types of treatment. For example, malignant lymphomas are curable with radiotherapy in most cases if the tumor is confined to one lymph node region (Stage I). More extensive lymph node involvement or dissemination to extranodal sites necessitates treatment with more intensive and broadly applied therapies, usually chemotherapy. The specific combination of therapies used depends on a number of factors, including the susceptibility of the particular type of neoplasm to drug or radiation therapy, and the patient's probable tolerance of the side effects and complications of the various possible treatments. Thus, while curative chemotherapy regimens exist for a substantial fraction of patients with diffuse histiocytic lymphoma, not all patients with this diagnosis are suitable candidates for intensive treatment. Those with underlying medical problems — e.g., heart disease, diabetes, or chronic pulmonary disease — might well suffer severely disabling or fatal complications from potentially curative regimens, as indicated in Table 1–1. In such cases the physician must weigh the chances of successful treatment against the probability of serious side effects from each of the therapeutic alternatives. The ultimate decision must be based on a thorough understanding of the *basic* and *clinical* pharmacology of the drugs in question, as well as an appreciation of the potential benefits and risks of alternative forms of treatment, such as radiotherapy and surgery.

DRUGS IN CANCER TREATMENT

Although drugs represent a relatively recent addition to the complement of weapons available for treating cancer, they are now employed at some time during the course of the illness of most cancer patients. Patients who have metastatic disease at the time of diagnosis usually undergo a surgical biopsy to establish the diagnosis. They may also undergo resection or irradiation of the primary tumor if the mass is producing incapacitating or potentially lethal local complications, such as obstruction of the bile duct, gastrointestinal tract, or respiratory tract. At this point, if malignant disease remains, drug treatment becomes the primary mode of treatment, offering either palliation, as in the case of most adenocarcinomas, or possible cure for lymphomas, testicular cancer, and other neoplasms (see Table 1–2).

Drug treatment regimens are based on a number of considerations. These include cell kinetic, pharmacokinetic, and biochemical-pharmacologic considerations; predictive *in vitro* tests; and, most important, prior empirical knowledge of the responsiveness of the pathologic category of tumor to specific drugs. These topics are considered in detail in succeeding chapters, but are reviewed briefly at this juncture in order to illustrate the broad range of factors that influence the planning of drug treatment regimens.

The Kinetic Basis of Drug Therapy

The objective of cancer treatment is to reduce the tumor cell population to zero cells. Chemotherapy experiments employing rapidly growing transplanted tumors in mice have established the validity of the *fractional cell kill hypothesis*. This states that a given drug concentration applied for a defined time interval will kill a constant fraction of the cell population, independent of the absolute number of cells. Thus, each treatment cycle kills a specific fraction of the remaining cells. The results of treatment are a direct function of (1) the dose of drug administered and (2) the frequency of repetition of treatment.

Most current chemotherapy regimens are

TABLE 1–1. Toxicity of BACOP Regimen for Treating Diffuse Histiocytic Lymphoma[33]*

Drugs	*Toxicity*	*Patients at Increased Risk*
Bleomycin	Pulmonary fibrosis	Chronic pulmonary disease; elderly
Doxorubicin (Adriamycin)	Cardiomyopathy; myelosuppression	History of heart disease; elderly
Cyclophosphamide	Hair loss; cystitis; myelosuppression	None
Vincristine (Oncovin)	Motor-sensory neuropathy	Elderly
Prednisone	Decreased glucose tolerance	Diabetic

*Risk of drug toxicity will also be increased in patients with compromised ability to eliminate a drug owing to renal (bleomycin) or hepatic (doxorubicin, vincristine) dysfunction. In general, elderly patients are at increased risk of toxicity because of underlying medical problems and possibly lower rates of drug elimination.

TABLE 1–2. Curability of Cancer with Drugs

Disease	*Therapy*	*Probable Cure Rate*
ADULTS		
Diffuse histiocytic lymphoma (stages III and IV)	Combination chemotherapy	40% or greater
Hodgkin's disease (Stage III or IV)	Combination chemotherapy	50% or greater
Testicular carcinoma (Stage III)	Combination chemotherapy ± surgery	50% or greater
Gestational choriocarcinoma	Methotrexate ± actinomycin D	90%
Ovarian carcinoma	Alkylating agents or combination chemotherapy	10%
Acute myelocytic leukemia	Combination chemotherapy	10%
CHILDREN		
Acute lymphocytic leukemia	Combination chemotherapy and cranial irradiation	50% or greater
Burkitt's lymphoma	Cyclophosphamide or combination chemotherapy	50% or greater
Wilms' tumor	Surgery, chemotherapy, and irradiation	50% or greater

based on these considerations and employ cycles of intensive therapy repeated as frequently as allowed by the tolerance of dose-limiting tissues such as bone marrow or gastrointestinal tract. The object of these cycles is to reduce the absolute number of remaining tumor cells to zero (or less than one) through the multiplicative effect of successive fractional cell kills [(10^{11} cells) $\times$ 0.01 $\times$ 0.01 $\times$ 0.01. . . .]. In treating the large and kinetically heterogeneous tumors found in man, the fractional cell kill hypothesis probably does not apply as well as in the animal tumor models. Most clinical neoplasms are recognized at a stage of decelerating growth that is due to poor vascularity, competition for nutrients, and other unidentified factors. These tumors contain a high fraction of slowly dividing or nondividing cells (termed G_0 cells). Since many antineoplastic agents are most effective against rapidly dividing cells, the initial kinetic situation is unfavorable for drug treatment. However, an initial reduction in cell numbers produced by surgery, radiotherapy, or cell cycle–nonspecific drugs (alkylating agents, doxorubicin [Adriamycin]) stimulates the slowly dividing cells into more rapid cell division where they become increasingly susceptible to therapy with cell cycle–specific agents (methotrexate, cytosine arabinoside, bleomycin). Thus, an initially slowly responding tumor may actually become more responsive to therapy with continued treatment. The fractional cell kill may actually increase with sequential courses of treatment.

On the other hand, the fractional cell kill hypothesis must be modified in a negative sense to take into account the biochemical heterogeneity of human tumors, an unfavorable property with respect to treatment response. Isoenzyme typing of tumor cells has indicated that most human tumors studied thus far have evolved from a single clone of malignant cells.[3] However, newly developed techniques for *in vitro* cloning of solid tumors have shown this original homogeneity does not persist during later stages of tumor growth. It has been clearly demonstrated that both experimental and human tumors are composed of cell types with differing biochemical, morphologic, and drug-response characteristics.[4] This heterogeneity likely results from somatic mutation of the original tumor line and probably accounts for outgrowth of resistant tumor cells during relapse of formerly sensitive tumors. When subjected to the selective pressure of drug treatment, sensitive tumor cells are destroyed, but the subpopulation of resistant cells survives and proliferates. This process of selecting out resistant cells has been amply demonstrated in cell culture as well as *in vivo*.[5] Thus, cell kill tends to decrease with subsequent courses of treatment, as resistant cell types are selected out, and single-agent treatment is rarely curative. With the possible exceptions of (1) treatment of gestational choriocarcinoma with methotrexate and (2) cyclophosphamide treatment of Burkitt's lymphoma, single-agent chemotherapy has not produced longterm survival or cure of advanced malignancies. The most successful drug treatment regimens have combined two or more agents, each of which has a different mechanism of action and each of which has antitumor activity when used individually.

Prediction of Drug Response

The selection of drugs for treating specific diseases is based largely on past experience as reflected in the results of previous clinical trials. However, it would be desirable to predict sensitivity for the specific tumor and patient at hand, and thus avoid the needless toxicity of ineffective agents. Various experimental systems have been studied intensively in the hope of their ultimate use for this purpose. Human tumor fragments can be grown in immunologically incompetent mice[6] (athymic, or nude, mice or thymectomized and irradiated mice) or under the renal capsule of mice.[7] Neither of these systems is entirely satisfactory for routine clinical use; certain tumor types, such as breast carcinomas, do not grow reliably in the immunodeprived mice, while the intact immune system of recipient animals in the subcapsular assay causes tumor regression after the first week of growth. Both systems have the advantage of exposing tumor to drug in the intact animal, allowing the test to be conducted in a pharmacokinetic setting relevant to clinical treatment. All systems require technical expertise and extensive animal facilities beyond the scope of most clinical institutions. Finally, neither the immunodeprived mouse nor the subcapsular assay has been validated as a predictor of response in man.

The *in vitro* culture of human tumors in semisolid media poses a more promising means of pretreatment selection of agents. The technique described by Hamburger and Salmon[8] allows reliable culture of human ovarian cancers, renal cell carcinomas, malignant melanomas, soft tissue sarcomas, and multiple myeloma cells, but less consistent growth of other forms of malignancy. Predictive tests for drug sensitivity are performed by preliminary incubation of a single cell suspension with a range of drug concentrations; after one hour the drug is removed and cells are plated in the semisolid medium. A retrospective analysis of *in vitro* sensitivity and treatment results in 66 patients with ovarian carcinoma, myeloma, and melanoma indicated that the *in vitro* test correctly predicts drug resistance (96 per cent true negative) but has a lower true positive rate of 62 per cent, as only 26 of 42 tumors sensitive *in vitro* responded *in vivo* to the indicated drug.[9] Thus, the assay has considerable value for predicting drug *resistance* for at least these three tumors; it has less value for predicting sensitivity, although the apparent failures may have been due to inadequate drug dosage, pharmacokinetic variability (as discussed below), or other factors that affect drug concentration and duration of exposure in the clinical setting. This assay has some clear disadvantages, including the inconsistent growth of important solid tumors such as breast, lung, and colon carcinoma; the low cloning efficiency of most human tumors (less than 1 per cent); the time required to obtain results (two to three weeks); the problem of testing drugs such as cyclophosphamide, hexamethylmelamine, and procarbazine, which require metabolic activation; and the failure of testing conditions to simulate the drug concentration and duration of exposure that occur *in vivo*. Initial assay conditions were formulated to allow tumor cell exposure to one tenth the maximal drug concentration achieved *in vivo* for one hour, but these conditions are unsuitable for duplicating the *in vivo* cytotoxicity of agents that act in the DNA synthetic phase of the cell cycle. Thus, drugs such as methotrexate and cytosine arabinoside have little effect on cell populations exposed for brief periods; their cytotoxicity is highly dependent on prolonged periods of tumor cell exposure, as revealed in clinical treatment regimens. Even for those tumors that grow in the *in vitro* system, the number of colonies formed is usually less than 50 per plate and thus inadequate to evaluate drug response in one half of tumors tested, and the test system is able to detect cell kill over a narrow range of one log cell kill or less. Despite this long list of limitations, the *in vitro* assay system, with technical improvements, may well become an important aid in choosing antineoplastic therapy.

Biochemical tests based on a knowledge of

the mechanism of action of specific drugs have provided helpful predictions of response in animal tumor systems, but few have been carefully evaluated in man. Test systems have focused on one or several specific determinants, such as the concentration of a key enzyme (deoxycytidine kinase for cytosine arabinoside)[10] or the presence of a specific cytoplasmic receptor (estrogen receptor for estradiol).[11] A few of these tests — most notably, the test for estrogen receptor in breast cancer — have become a cornerstone for making therapeutic decisions; other tests offer considerable promise. The duration of complete remission in acute myelocytic leukemia correlates with the ability of leukemic cells to activate cytosine arabinoside to the active triphosphate form *in vitro*.[12] (Ara-CTP is an inhibitor of DNA synthesis, and is also incorporated into DNA.) High concentrations of alkaline phosphatase, a nucleotide degrading enzyme, are predictive of resistance to 6-mercaptopurine in man.[13] Similarly, high concentrations of dihydrofolate reductase have been associated with resistance to methotrexate.[14] However, these biochemical tests have not been studied prospectively in a sizable patient population to prove their value in routine treatment of leukemia. Each of these examples is considered in greater detail in subsequent chapters.

Pharmacokinetic Determinants of Response

Although the outcome of cancer chemotherapy may depend in large part on the inherent sensitivity of the tumor under treatment, pharmacokinetic factors such as drug absorption, metabolism, and elimination are extremely important in determining the dose, schedule, and route of drug administration. The actual process of planning therapy based on pharmacokinetic considerations is dealt with in Chapter 2.

Pharmacokinetic factors are important not only in protocol design, but also in determining toxicity and response in individual patients. Pharmacokinetics are known to be extremely variable from one patient to the next and may account for the inconsistent responses of tumors that are "sensitive" *in vitro*. Since this interindividual variation is not always predictable on the basis of differences in renal or hepatic function, direct measurement of plasma drug concentrations provides a better guide for dosage adjustment to ensure adequate and safe drug exposure. The interindividual variability in oral absorption of a number of agents, including hexamethylmelamine, methotrexate (in doses over 15 mg/m^2), 5-fluorouracil, and phenylalanine mustard, has been documented by pharmacokinetic studies and must be taken into consideration in planning the route of therapy. In addition, drug monitoring may provide a valuable guide to delayed elimination of agents such as methotrexate, thus allowing early institution of "rescue" procedures[15] and dose adjustment. Reliable assays are available for many antineoplastic agents (Table 1–3); those done by high-pressure liquid chromatography or gas-liquid chromatography require the services of specialized laboratories and usually cannot be performed on a routine basis. A few, such as the competitive binding assays for methotrexate, are available in most cancer treatment centers and have established importance as a guide to the prediction of drug toxicity in high-dose therapy. Principles employed in drug monitoring and their application to cancer treatment are discussed in detail in a subsequent chapter. The utility of various assays is also indicated in the discussion of individual agents.

TABLE 1–3. Drug Assays Useful in Cancer Chemotherapy*

Competitive Protein Binding
Methotrexate
Allopurinol
5-FdUMP (active nucleotide of 5-FU, ftorafur, FUdR)
Radioimmunoassay
Cytosine arabinoside
Bleomycin
? Doxorubicin
Vinca alkaloids
Steroidal agents
High-Pressure Liquid Chromatography
5-FU
Hexamethylmelamine
Phenylalanine mustard
6-Thiopurines
Doxorubicin

*See Pinedo HM (ed.): Clinical Pharmacology of Antineoplastic Drugs. Elsevier/North Holland Biomedical Press, Amsterdam, 1978.

STRATEGIES OF CLINICAL CHEMOTHERAPY

Combination Chemotherapy

Although the first effective drugs for treating cancer were brought to clinical trial in the mid and late 1940s, initial therapeutic results were disappointing. Although impressive regressions of acute lymphocytic leukemia and adult lymphomas were obtained with single agents such as nitrogen mustard, antifolates, corticosteroids, and the vinca alkaloids, responses were only partial and of short duration. When complete remissions were obtained, as in acute lymphocytic leukemia, they were usually less than nine months in duration and relapse was associated with resistance to the original agents used. Attempts at retreatment with new agents usually met with a less satisfactory response or frank resistance to further therapy. Increased doses could not be given because of prohibitive bone marrow or neurotoxicity (vincristine), and few patients derived lasting benefit from single-agent treatment. The introduction of cyclic combination chemotherapy for acute lymphocytic leukemia of childhood in the early 1960s marked a turning point in the effective treatment of neoplastic disease; such combinations are now a standard component of most treatment strategies for advanced cancer.

The superior results of combination chemotherapy as compared with single-agent treatment derive from the following considerations. First, initial resistance to any given single agent is frequent, even in the most responsive tumors; for example, in patients with Hodgkin's disease, the response rate to alkylating agents or procarbazine (the most active single drugs) does not exceed 50 per cent. Second, initially responsive tumors rapidly acquire resistance after drug exposure, probably owing either to selection of pre-existing resistant tumor cells from a heterogeneous tumor cell population (as mentioned previously) or to actual drug induction of resistance. The use of multiple agents, each with cytotoxic activity in the disease under consideration, but with different mechanisms of action, allows for independent cell killing by each agent. Cells resistant to one agent might still be sensitive to the other drugs in the regimen. Third, if these drugs also have non-overlapping toxicities, each can be used in full dosage and the effectiveness of each agent will be maintained in the combination. Drugs such as vincristine, prednisone, bleomycin, hexamethylmelamine, L-asparaginase, and others that lack bone marrow toxicity are particularly valuable for combination with traditional myelosuppressive agents. Based on these principles, curative combinations have been devised for diseases that were not curable with single-agent treatment, including acute lymphocytic leukemia (vincristine-prednisone ± doxorubicin and L-asparaginase), Hodgkin's disease (MOPP), histiocytic lymphoma (C-MOPP), and testicular carcinoma (bleomycin-vinblastine-*cis*-dichlorodiammineplatinum [*cis*-DDP]).

The detailed scheduling of drugs in these combinations was initially based on both practical and theoretical considerations. Intermittent cycles of treatment were used to allow for periods of recovery of host bone marrow and immune function. This strategy allowed for retreatment with full therapeutic doses as frequently as possible in keeping with the fractional cell kill hypothesis. It seems most reasonable to initiate therapy with cell cycle–nonspecific drugs such as the alkylating agents or nitrosoureas (if active against the disease in question) in order to reduce tumor bulk and recruit slowly dividing cells into active DNA synthesis. This phase of cytoreduction can then be followed within the same cycle of treatment by cell cycle–dependent agents such as methotrexate or the fluoropyrimidines. An example of a regimen in which cycle–nonspecific drugs are followed by cycle–specific agents is shown in Table 1–4. More recent combinations have incorporated non-myelosuppressive agents such as bleomycin, vincristine, prednisone, or high-dose methotrexate with leucovorin rescue in the "off-period" between doses of myelotoxic drugs, in order to provide continuous suppression of tumor growth. High-dose methotrexate with leucovorin rescue has proved to be particularly useful in this capacity in the "off-period" because of its minimal effect on white blood cell and platelet counts.

Cytokinetic considerations also influence the specific scheduling of drug combinations. S-phase (DNA synthetic phase)–specific drugs, such as cytosine arabinoside and methotrexate, tend to block cells during the period of DNA synthesis. Repeat courses of these agents are most effective if administered during the period of rapid recovery of

TABLE 1–4. Drug Sequences in Combination Chemotherapy

CAMF Protocol for Breast Cancer (under evaluation at National Cancer Institute)

		Day	
	(mg/m²)	1	9
Cyclophosphamide	750	x	
Doxorubicin	30	x	
Methotrexate	40		x
5-Fluorouracil	500		x

Repeat every 21 days until progressive disease

NOTABLE FEATURES
1. Cytoreduction with cycle–nonspecific agents on day 1
2. Cycle–specific drugs on day 8
3. Methotrexate given before 5-fluorouracil to enhance 5-FdUMP and 5-FUTP formation

DNA synthesis that follows the period of suppression of DNA synthesis. Burke and co-workers have found evidence for periods of increased DNA synthetic activity and increased susceptibility to cytosine arabinoside approximately ten days after the first treatment.[16] Although it is difficult to monitor cytokinetic parameters during routine clinical treatment, new instruments such as the fluorescence-activated cell sorter and microfluorometer are capable of providing such information on patients with leukemia.

Specific drug interactions, both favorable and unfavorable, must be considered in developing combination regimens. These interactions may take the form of pharmacokinetic, cytokinetic, or biochemical effects that influence the effectiveness of a second component of a combination. Patterns of toxicity are a primary concern. Drugs that cause renal toxicity, such as *cis*-DDP, must be used cautiously in combination with other agents (such as methotrexate or bleomycin) that depend on renal elimination as their primary mechanism of excretion. Regimens that employ *cis*-DDP prior to methotrexate, as in the treatment of head and neck cancer, must incorporate careful monitoring of renal function, pretreatment hydration, and dose adjustment for methotrexate to ensure that altered methotrexate excretion will not lead to severe drug toxicity.

Biochemical interactions may also be important considerations in determining the choice of agents and their sequence of administration. The sequence of methotrexate and 5-fluorouracil is critical in determining the cytotoxicity of this combination in experimental systems. In cell culture, synergistic results are obtained when methotrexate precedes 5-fluorouracil by at least one hour,[17] probably because of increased activation of 5-fluorouracil to its nucleotide form. The opposite sequence (fluoropyrimidine, then methotrexate) leads to antagonistic results, owing to fluoropyrimidine block of the thymidylate synthetase pathway. This block preserves intracellular folates in their active tetrahydrofolate form and renders inconsequential the methotrexate block of dihydrofolate reductase. Several important drug interactions, shown in Table 1–5, deserve consideration in planning combination regimens. However, it should also be remembered that none of these sequences has been proved to produce results superior to those achieved by simultaneous use of the same drugs; in most cases, the appropriate clinical trials that might prove the importance of specific sequences have not been performed.

Finally, all drug combination regimens require dose adjustment scales to allow increases or decreases of dose according to

TABLE 1–5. Drug Interactions in Combination Chemotherapy*

Transport
1. *Vincristine* enhances *methotrexate* uptake

Metabolic Activation
1. *Methotrexate* increases *5-fluorouracil* activation
2. *Methotrexate* increases *cytosine arabinoside* activation
3. *Thymidine* increases *5-fluorouracil* incorporation into RNA
4. Inhibitors of *de novo* pyrimidine synthesis enhance 5-fluorouracil incorporation into RNA and formation of active nucleotides

Antagonism of Antitumor Effect
1. *5-Fluorouracil* pretreatment prevents antifolate action of *methotrexate*
2. *L-Asparaginase* pretreatment blocks antitumor effect of *methotrexate*

Reversal of Toxicity (Rescue)
1. 5-Formyl tetrahydrofolic acid (*leucovorin*) prevents *methotrexate* toxicity
2. *Deoxycytidine* prevents toxicity of *cytosine arabinoside*
3. *Allopurinol* blocks *5-fluorouracil* activation by normal tissues

*See drug-related chapters for detailed discussion and references.

toxicity. It becomes difficult to determine which of the several agents is responsible for excessive toxicity if overlapping toxicity patterns are present. In this setting, arbitrary scales of dose adjustment according to bone marrow toxicity are usually provided with protocols. Underdosing may also be a problem, particularly for drugs given by the oral route, such as hexamethylmelamine or melphalan, which display variable bioavailability. Drug level monitoring could be useful in this situation, but has not been routinely employed to date to verify bioavailability of oral agents.

Alternatives to Cyclic, Fixed Combination Therapy

In the first combination chemotherapy trials, such as MOPP chemotherapy of Hodgkin's disease,[18] the overall strategy was to deliver repetitive cycles of a fixed drug combination over a finite time period, then to restage the patient to rule out the presence of occult residual disease, and to discontinue treatment in complete remitters. The duration of unmaintained complete remission then served as an index of the completeness of response. A plateau in the disease-free survival curve indicated a "cured" fraction of the patient population. In an effort to improve the long-term disease-free survival rate associated with cyclic chemotherapy, the basic strategy has been modified in a number of ways:

1. Goldie and Coldman[22] offered a theoretical analysis of tumor cell resistance, reasoning that such resistance to individual agents develops through spontaneous mutation in the absence of drug exposure. The probability of there appearing a cell resistant to any given drug is a direct function of the spontaneous rate of mutation to resistance and the number of cells (the size of the tumor) (Fig. 1–1). The use of single agents or single specific combinations for extended periods will select and encourage the outgrowth of resistant cells. Multiple drugs with independent mechanisms of action will discourage the selection of clones resistant to any given agent. In addition, it is theoretically of benefit to use alternating combinations of drugs to discourage the outgrowth of clones resistant to multiple drugs.[19] Alternative drug combinations that do not share common mechanisms of action with primary treatment regimens have been identified by trials in patients resistant to the primary treatment. An example is the ABVD regimen for Hodgkin's disease, which incorporates four agents (*A*driamycin [doxorubicin], *b*leomycin, *v*inblastine, and *D*TIC) that have activity in patients who relapsed on MOPP (nitrogen *m*ustard, *O*ncovin [vincristine], *p*rednisone, *p*rocarbazine). ABVD can be used in alternating cycles with MOPP and appears to improve the percentage of complete remission.[19] Information is insufficient at present to draw firm conclusions regarding the effectiveness of alternating combinations in improving patient survival. This strategy has not been successful in earlier trials in breast cancer[20] and small cell carcinoma of the lung,[21] perhaps because of the limited effectiveness of individual agents in these diseases.

2. A second alternative is to use noncross-

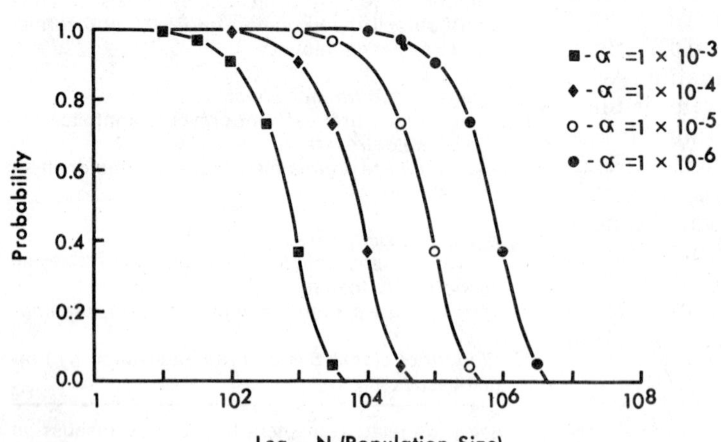

Figure 1–1. Probability of the existence of no resistant phenotypes as a function of the mutation rate (α) and tumor size (N). The almost identical profile of each curve reflects the independence of the time required for a class of tumors to proceed from the state when only 5 per cent have resistant phenotypes to that when 95 per cent have such phenotypes. (Reproduced with permission from Goldie JH, and Coldman AJ: A mathematical model for relating the drug sensitivity of tumors to their spontaneous mutation rate. Cancer Treat. Rep. 63:1727–1733, 1979.)

resistant agents for maintenance therapy, after induction of complete remission with the standard combination. This strategy has proved successful in preventing relapse in childhood acute lymphocytic leukemia, but has not improved survival in solid tumor chemotherapy.

3. A third approach is to employ hormonal agents, such as estradiol, to stimulate hormone-responsive cells into active DNA synthesis and thus render these cells increasingly vulnerable to cell cycle–specific drugs such as methotrexate and 5-fluorouracil. Such schemes are effective in experimental models, but have not been proved to increase response rates clinically.

4. A final alternative is to employ marrow-ablative doses of chemotherapy in order to increase tumor cell kill, and to rescue the host with either autologous bone marrow harvested prior to treatment or marrow from a histocompatible donor. The latter approach (rescue with marrow from a donor) has the advantage of infusing marrow that is free of malignant cells. However, marrow donated by a second person contains lymphocytes that may cause so-called "graft-versus-host" disease, a potentially lethal complication. Both autologous marrow (stored marrow from the patient, harvested prior to therapy) and allogeneic marrow are able to reconstitute bone marrow, but high-dose chemotherapy has limited utility for other reasons:

A. Dose-limiting toxicities to organs other than bone marrow, such as nitrosourea toxicity to lung, kidneys, or liver,[23, 24] may prevent dose escalation.

B. High-dose chemotherapy is difficult to employ in repeated cycles because of severe toxicity to organs and limited bone marrow available for reinfusion. A single course of therapy usually fails to eradicate a tumor.

C. Finally, it is not clear that a linear relationship exists between drug dose and tumor cell kill for all drugs and all tumors. In experimental tumor models, with most tumor cells in active phases of growth, increased cell kill does result from higher drug doses, but, in treating human tumors, cell kill may well be limited to the fraction of cells in active proliferation.

The reader is referred to reviews of ablative chemotherapy with marrow transplantation for a more complete discussion of this controversial subject.[25]

Combined Radiation and Chemotherapy

A further innovation in the use of antineoplastic drugs is to combine drugs with irradiation. The design of integrated chemotherapy–radiotherapy trials presents special problems because of the synergistic effects of the two modalities on *both normal and malignant tissue.* The normal tissue of greatest concern is the bone marrow. Radiation given to the pelvic or midline abdominal areas produces a decline in blood counts and a decrease in bone marrow reserve. Appropriate shielding of the pelvic structures and the use of megavoltage radiation with limited scatter can preserve a significant portion of this marrow-bearing tissue. The sequence of administration may be of crucial importance. Total nodal irradiation followed by combination chemotherapy has proved to be practicable for treatment of Hodgkin's disease. The "sandwiching" of irradiation between courses of chemotherapy is also well tolerated in Hodgkin's therapy. However, the alternate sequence of MOPP followed by total nodal irradiation is less well tolerated because of severe myelosuppression in the radiation phase of treatment. The primary conclusion to draw is that one must anticipate cumulative effects of both chemotherapy and irradiation on bone marrow reserve.

Some chemotherapeutic agents greatly potentiate the effects of irradiation on normal tissues and may lead to synergistic toxicity for organs usually resistant to radiation damage. Doxorubicin sensitizes both normal and malignant cells to x-ray damage, possibly because both doxorubicin and x-rays produce free radical damage to tissues. If the drug and mediastinal irradiation are given concurrently, enhanced toxicity is observed for heart, esophagus, and lung. In a similar manner, bleomycin enhances x-ray damage to pulmonary tissue. Actinomycin D and 5-fluorouracil both act as enhancing agents for radiation therapy in experimental systems; increased toxicity to normal tissue, and perhaps tumor, has been observed clinically with both agents. Methotrexate may produce recall reactions in previously irradiated skin. Prednisone suppresses the immediate reaction to pulmonary irradiation, but withdrawal of steroids may be associated with a serious flare in radiation-induced pneumonitis. Thus, drugs and irradiation can be safely interdigitated only if consideration is given to these known interactions;

reduction of radiation dose or an alteration in drug dose or schedule may be necessary to avoid untoward effects.

A final negative consideration in the combined use of radiotherapy and chemotherapy is the carcinogenicity of both modalities. As discussed in greater detail in Chapter 6, alkylating agents and procarbazine are highly carcinogenic in animals and are strongly suspected of causing tumors in man. Irradiation is also strongly mutagenic, and therefore carcinogenic. Thus, it is not surprising that the combination of alkylating agents and procarbazine with irradiation has led to an estimated 6 per cent incidence of second malignancies in patients with Hodgkin's disease.[26] Acute myelocytic leukemia is the most common type of second malignancy in patients with Hodgkin's disease and has also been reported after alkylating agent treatment (alone or in combination with x-ray) for ovarian cancer, multiple myeloma, adjuvant breast cancer, and various other types of malignancy. The exact incidence of second tumors following specific regimens is difficult to quantitate because of the brief survival of most patients undergoing such treatment and uncertainty as to the number of patients at risk in published retrospective studies. Nonetheless, there is sufficient evidence of irradiation-drug synergy to warrant caution in accepting combinations of irradiation and carcinogenic drugs, particularly for patients who have an excellent chance of cure or long-term survival by single-modality treatment.

Adjuvant Chemotherapy

Chemotherapeutic agents are clearly a logical choice for treatment of patients with disseminated malignancy. However, they may also be used to advantage in patients who exhibit little evidence of residual disease but are at high risk of relapse. For example, despite an apparent complete surgical resection of primary tumor, certain patients are at high risk of developing recurrent disease at distant sites. In this setting it is logical to consider the benefits of prophylactic or "adjuvant" chemotherapy following surgical removal of the tumor and lymph nodes. For patients with primary breast cancer and axillary lymph node involvement, adjuvant chemotherapy with melphalan or with the cyclophosphamide-methotrexate-fluorouracil combination has delayed systemic recurrence; the latter regimen has led to improved overall survival in premenopausal patients.[27] Adjuvant chemotherapy with doxorubicin, cyclophosphamide, and methotrexate has also lowered the recurrence rate in patients with soft tissue sarcomas.[28] The reader is referred to other sources for a more complete discussion of the results of adjuvant therapy in specific diseases.[29] However, a brief review of the theoretical basis for adjuvant treatment may aid in understanding the potential positive and negative results of such therapy.

The need for adjuvant therapy arises from two sources: (1) the high recurrence rate following surgery for apparently localized tumors such as breast cancer, soft tissue sarcoma, osteogenic sarcoma, Dukes B and C colon cancer, level 3–5 malignant melanoma, and various solid neoplasms of childhood; and (2) the failure of chemotherapy or combined modality treatment to cure patients after recurrence of disease. In addition, there is experimental evidence to support the hypothesis that neoplasms are most sensitive to chemotherapy at their earliest stages of growth. This increased sensitivity of subclinical tumors is believed to result from their high growth fraction (most cells are in active progression through the cell cycle), shorter cell cycle times, and therefore a greater fractional cell kill for a given dose of drug.[30] As the same tumors become clinically obvious, their growth fraction falls, the cell cycle time lengthens, and they become much less sensitive to treatment. A second important consideration is the relationship of tumor cell resistance to tumor bulk. As stressed by Goldie and Coldman,[22] the probability of a tumor population containing resistant cells is a function of total number of cells present. Therefore, subclinical tumors are more likely than metastatic tumors to be cured by a specific schedule or type of chemotherapy.[22] A final positive impetus for adjuvant chemotherapy stems from the fact that patients are able to tolerate chemotherapy with fewer complications when they are not debilitated by metastatic disease.

The disadvantages of adjuvant therapy relate to immediate patient discomfort and to the short- and long-term risks of such treatment. A fraction of patients receiving adjuvant treatment will have been cured by the primary surgical procedure, and will therefore experience needless risks and toxicity if treated with adjuvant therapy. Unfortunately, there is no way of identifying these "cured" patients at the time of surgery. The risks of immediate and late toxicities of chemotherapy must also be considered and are discussed in subsequent chapters. In the adjuvant setting, late complications such as carcinogenicity and sterility assume greater importance; neither risk has been adequately quantitated, although the alkylating agents and procarbazine appear to be the most potent in both capacities.

Additional late effects must also be weighed in making a decision for adjuvant chemotherapy. These include the cardiotoxicity of doxorubicin (a particular danger in older patients), pulmonary toxicity of bleomycin, renal toxicity of the nitrosoureas, and bone marrow hypoplasia with alkylating agents and nitrosoureas. A telling example of late toxicity is provided by the National Cancer Institute study of doxorubicin, cyclophosphamide, and methotrexate for adjuvant therapy of soft tissue sarcoma.[31] Despite a marked improvement in relapse rate, approximately 60 per cent of patients treated with these drugs were found to have decreased cardiac contractility (Fig. 1–2), and six of the first 62 patients treated developed overt congestive heart failure due to doxorubicin cardiac toxicity.

In summary, cancer chemotherapeutic agents have had a profound influence on the treatment and survival of patients with cancer. Because these agents have the potential for causing severe or disabling toxicity and yet must be used at maximal doses in order to ensure full therapeutic benefit,[32] the physician is literally walking a therapeutic tightrope and must constantly balance gain against likely toxicities. In this effort, every advantage must be sought.

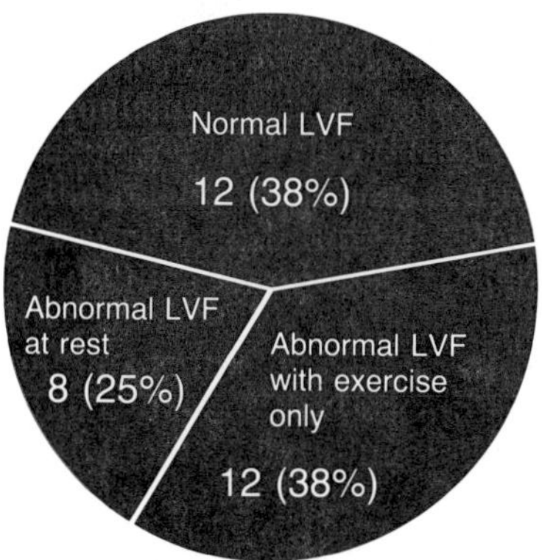

Figure 1–2. Distribution of rest and exercise left ventricular functional (LVF) abnormalities in 32 patients after doxorubicin. Exercise enhances detection of abnormal LVF in these patients. (Reproduced with permission from Gottdiener et al.: Doxorubicin cardiotoxicity: assessment of late left ventricular dysfunction by radionuclide cineangiography. Ann. Intern. Med. 94:430–435, 1981.)

ROLE OF CLINICAL PHARMACOLOGY IN CANCER TREATMENT

It should be apparent from the foregoing discussion that an intimate knowledge of drug action and disposition is essential to the design and application of effective cancer chemotherapy. Some of the more obvious roles for the clinical pharmacologist in the cancer treatment process may be summarized as follows:

1. *Design of chemotherapy regimens.* As outlined in our previous discussion, this process must take into account not only the empirical history of drug responsiveness of the tumor type in question, but also the mechanism of action of the drug, its possible biochemical and pharmacologic interaction with other potentially useful agents, and the specific biochemical and cytokinetic characteristics of the tumor.

2. *Pretreatment prediction of response in an individual patient.* This facet of the treatment decision will require *in vitro* growth of tumor cells or biochemical testing of tumor extracts for specific enzymes or response markers.

3. *Pharmacokinetic analysis.* The profile of drug concentration versus time is the primary determinant of tumor cell kill and toxicity for any given agent; it may be modified by alterations in drug distribution and elimination, and by drug interactions. The adjustment of dose to compensate for these factors is an essential step in individualizing cancer treatment, in order to prevent underdosing or excessive drug exposure, and may require drug level monitoring in individual patients.

In the following chapters, both the theoretical and practical considerations pertinent to the clinical use of antineoplastic drugs are presented in detail. It is hoped that the reader will sense not only the intellectual challenge but also the great potential of antineoplastic pharmacology as the foundation of future cancer treatment.

References

1. Richardson RL, Schumacher RA, Fen MF, et al.: The unrecognized extranodal germ cell cancer syndrome. Ann. Intern. Med. 94:181–185, 1981.
2. Woods RL, Fox RM, Tattersall MH, et al.: Metastatic adenocarcinoma of unknown primary site: a randomized study of two combination-chemotherapy regimens. N. Engl. J. Med. 303:87–89, 1980.
3. Fialkow PJ: Clonal origin of human tumors. Biochim. Biophys. Acta 458:283–321, 1976.
4. Calabresi P, Dexter DL, and Heppner GH: Clinical and pharmacological implications of cancer cell differentiation and heterogeneity. Biochem. Pharmacol. 28:1933–1941, 1979.
5. de Saint Vincent BR, Dechamps M, and Buttin G: The modulation of the thymidine triphosphate pool of Chinese hamster cells by dCMP deaminase and UDP reductase. J. Biol. Chem. 255:162–167, 1980.
6. Giovanella BC, Stehlin JS, Williams, LJ, et al.: Heterotransplantation of human cancers into nude mice — a model for human cancer chemotherapy. Cancer 42:2269–2281, 1978.
7. Bogden AE, Haskell PM, LePage DI, et al.: Growth of human tumor xenografts implanted under the renal capsule of normal immunocompetent mice. Exp. Cell. Biol. 47:281–293, 1979.
8. Hamburger AW, and Salmon SE: Primary bioassay of human tumor stem cells. Science 197:461–463, 1977.
9. Salmon SE, Alberts DS, Durie BGM, et al.: Clinical correlations of drug sensitivity in the human tumor stem cell assay. Recent Results Cancer Res. 74:300–305, 1980.
10. Tattersall MNH, Ganeshagura K, and Hoffbrand AV: Mechanisms of resistance of human acute leukaemia cells to cytosine arabinoside. Br. J. Haematol. 27:39–46, 1974.
11. McGuire WL, Carbone PP, Sears ME, et al.: Estrogen receptors in human breast cancer: an overview. *In* McGuire WL, Carbone PP, and Vollmer EP (eds.): Estrogen Receptors in Human Cancer. Raven Press, New York, 1975, pp. 1–7.
12. Rustum YM, and Preisler HD: Correlation between leukemic cell retention of 1-beta-D-arabinofuranosyl cytosine 5′-triphosphate and response to therapy. Cancer Res. 39:42–49, 1979.
13. Lee MH, Huang YM, and Sartorelli AC: Alkaline phosphatase activities of 6-thiopurine-sensitive and -resistant sublines of sarcoma 180. Cancer Res. 38:2413–2418, 1978.
14. Alt FW, Kellems RE, Bertino JR, et al.: Selective multiplication of dihydrofolate reductase genes in methotrexate-resistant variants of cultured murine cells. J. Biol. Chem. 253:1357–1370, 1978.
15. Stoller R, Hande KR, Jacobs SA, et al.: The use of plasma pharmacokinetics to predict and prevent methotrexate toxicity. N. Engl. J. Med. 297:630–634, 1977.
16. Vaughan WP, Karp JE, and Burke PE: Long chemotherapy-free remissions after single-cycle timed-sequential chemotherapy for acute myelocytic leukemia. Cancer 45:859–865, 1980.
17. Cadman E, Heimer R, and Davis L: Enhanced 5-fluorouracil nucleotide formation after methotrexate administration: explanation for drug synergism. Science 205:1135–1137, 1979.
18. DeVita VT, Simon RM, Hubbard SM, et al.: Curability of advanced Hodgkin's disease with chemotherapy. Ann. Intern. Med. 92:587–595, 1980.
19. Sartoro A, Bonadonna G, Bonfante V, et al.: Non-cross-resistant regimens (MOPP and ABVD) vs. MOPP alone in Stage IV Hodgkin's disease. Proc. Am. Soc. Clin. Oncol. 21:470, 1980.
20. Tormey DC, Falkson G, Simon RM, et al.: A randomized comparison of two sequentially administered combination regimens to a single regimen in metastatic breast cancer. Cancer Clin. Trials 2:247–256, 1979.
21. Cohen MH, Ihde DC, Bunn PA, et al.: Cyclic alternating combination chemotherapy of small cell bronchogenic carcinoma. Cancer Treat. Rep. 63:163–170, 1979.
22. Goldie JH, and Coldman AJ: A mathematic model for relating the drug sensitivity of tumors to their spontaneous mutation rate. Cancer Treat. Rep. 63:1727–1733, 1979.
23. Hundley R, and Lukens JN: Nitrosourea-associated pulmonary fibrosis. Cancer Treat. Rep. 63:2128–2130, 1979.
24. Harmon WE, Cohen HJ, Schneeberger EE, et al.: Chronic renal failure in children treated with methyl CCNU. N. Engl. J. Med. 300:1200–1203, 1979.
25. Deisseroth A, and Abrams RA: The role of autologous stem cell reconstitution and intensive therapy for resistant neoplasms. Cancer Treat. Rep. 63:461–471, 1979.
26. Coleman CN, Williams CJ, Flint A, et al.: Hematologic neoplasia in patients treated for Hodgkin's disease. N. Engl. J. Med. 297:1249–1252, 1977.
27. Bonadonna G, Brusamolino E, Valagussa P, et al.: Combination chemotherapy as an adjuvant treatment in operable breast cancer. N. Engl. J. Med. 294:405–410, 1976.
28. Rosenberg SA, Kent H, Costa J, et al.: Prospective randomized evaluation of the role of limb-sparing surgery, radiation therapy, and adjuvant chemoimmunotherapy in the treatment of adult soft-tissue sarcomas. Surgery 84:62–69, 1978.
29. Jones SE, and Salmon SE (eds.): Adjuvant Therapy of Cancer III. Grune & Stratton, New York, 1981.
30. Salmon SE: Kinetics of minimal residual disease. Recent Results Cancer Res. 67:5–15, 1979.
31. Gottdiener JS, Mathisen DJ, Borer JS, et al.: Doxorubicin cardiotoxicity: assessment of late left ventricular dysfunction by radionuclide cineangiography. Ann. Intern. Med. 94:430–435, 1981.
32. Bonadonna G, and Valagussa P: Dose response effect of adjuvant chemotherapy in breast cancer. N. Engl. J. Med. 304:10–15, 1981.
33. Schein PS, DeVita VT, Hubbard SM, et al.: Bleomcyin, adriamycin, cyclophosphamide, vincristine, and prednisone (BACOP) combination chemotherapy in the treatment of advanced diffuse histiocytic lymphoma. Ann. Intern. Med. 85:417–422, 1976.

PHARMACOKINETICS OF ANTINEOPLASTIC AGENTS AT THE CELLULAR LEVEL

2

I. David Goldman

INTRODUCTION

It is a requirement that all currently useful chemotherapeutic agents must penetrate tumor cell membranes before interacting with intracellular target sites to achieve their pharmacologic effects. Vascular perfusion of the tumor and diffusion within the tumor matrix determine the rate and extent of drug accumulation at the tumor cell membrane. However, after arrival at that critical interface, a variety of structural, electrical, and thermodynamic factors determine qualitative and quantitative properties of drug transport across the tumor cell membrane. The mechanisms by which pharmacologic agents as well as physiologic substrates and catabolites penetrate cell membranes are complex. Little is known about molecular interactions between the transported species and membrane constituents as substances traverse cell membranes. Similarly, the mechanisms by which cellular energy metabolism is coupled to membrane transport systems are, for most transported species, only superficially understood. Transport of a variety of cytotoxic agents conforms, in many respects, to processes observed for physiologic substances, but other aspects of antineoplastic drug transport are unique. Although it is difficult to relate data on basic membrane transport properties of drugs to the outcome of treatment of malignant diseases in animal and human tumor systems, nonetheless, knowledge of membrane transport and of the techniques used to study it has provided important insights into elements of the drug-cell interaction that play a critical role in drug cytotoxicity, selectivity, and resistance. Hence, it is important for experimentalists and physicians who utilize these drugs to understand factors that govern membrane transport and the relationship between transport and drug efficacy. These perspectives provide an essential element in the rational development of single and multiple drug regimens, and may explain the efficacy of some drug regimens designed empirically. Further, when membrane transport is a key determinant of cytotoxicity and selectivity, identification of the molecular basis of drug transport can suggest structural modifications of the drug that may produce agents with greater potency and selectivity.

This chapter provides an overview of membrane transport of antineoplastic agents within the context of the principles that govern transport of biologic substrates across mammalian cell membranes. When possible, drug transport is related to mechanisms of drug action in order to demonstrate how membrane transport can determine drug efficacy. The chapter does not present a comprehensive review of the drug transport literature, but rather uses selected, well-documented examples to illustrate important principles. The cellular pharmacokinetic approach is emphasized; i.e., the study of the interaction between drug and the intact cell. This encompasses membrane transport, metabolic transformations of the agent in the cell, and the interaction between the drug and/or its metabolite and its target site(s) within the intracellular compartment of the intact cell. This investigative approach seeks to identify those parameters of the drug-cell interaction that are critical determinants of cytotoxicity and selectivity, how these interactions are controlled, how they can be modified, and how they are perturbed in multidrug regimens. This is an important, only recently recognized dimension in the pharmacologic analysis of drug action that complements studies of whole animal pharmacokinetics and biochemical analyses of drug-target interactions in cell-free systems. Indeed, for some agents such as antifolates, an understanding of the consequences of the interaction between the drug and the intact cell has led to the recognition of important new elements in the mechanism of action of this class of compounds.

MECHANISMS OF MEMBRANE TRANSPORT

Membrane transport of antineoplastic agents must be considered within the context of principles of membrane transport of physiologic substances. Pharmacologic agents that are analogues of naturally occurring substrates, such as 4-amino antifolates, cytotoxic purine and pyrimidine nucleosides and bases, and phenylalanine mustard, utilize carrier-mediated transport systems that have as a primary function the translocation of their naturally occurring counterparts. Transport of drugs by passive diffusion conforms to the same physical principles that govern diffusion of physiologic substances. When studies are undertaken to explore the mechanism of transport of an antineoplastic agent, experiments must be designed within the context of the known properties of physiologically important transport systems. Accordingly, the following review of mechanisms of membrane transport in general emphasizes principles most relevant to the transport of antineoplastic agents.

Passive Diffusion

The cell membrane can be considered a barrier to the free movement of solute molecules into, and out of, the cell. Viewing the cell membrane as an inert barrier with a defined lipid and protein matrix with potential aqueous channels, factors that will determine the ability of a molecule to penetrate that membrane relate largely to size and lipid solubility.[1-3] The greater the lipid solubility and the smaller the size, the more likely it is that the molecule will pass through the cell membrane.

Figure 2–1 illustrates the time course of appearance of drug in the intracellular water determined by passive diffusion, when the drug is added to the extracellular compart-

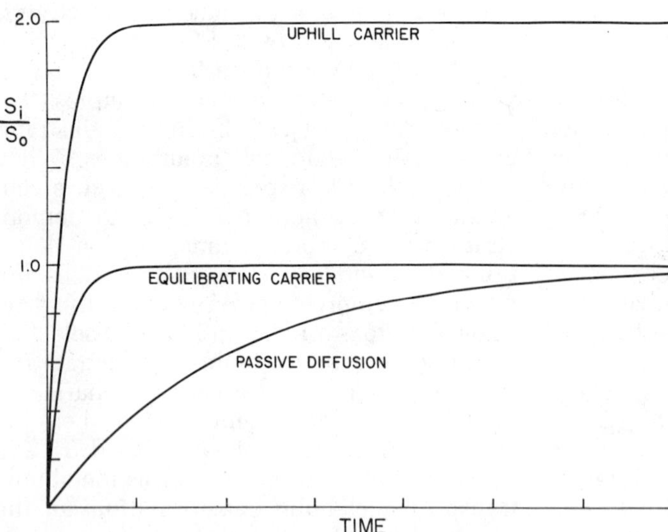

Figure 2–1. Simulated time course of uptake of drug into cells by passive diffusion, an equilibrating carrier, or an uphill carrier system. In this example the drug is neither bound to the cell surface nor to intracellular constituents, and the drug is not metabolized. S_i is the concentration of drug in the intracellular water, and S_o is the extracellular drug concentration. The latter is constant over the interval of uptake. The ordinate indicates the ratio of intracellular to extracellular drug concentrations. An equilibrating carrier increases the *rate* at which the system comes to equilibrium in comparison with passive diffusion. However, since both passive diffusion and an equilibrating carrier operate independent of cellular energy metabolism, both achieve a steady-state at "equilibrium" where, by definition, the electrochemical-potential for intracellular and extracellular drug is the same. Because the drug in this example does not carry a charge, S_i/S_o at equilibrium is 1. In the uphill carrier system simulated here, the initial rate of drug uptake is increased in comparison with the equilibrating system, and the steady-state intracellular level achieved is twofold greater than the equilibrium level. There is a transmembrane gradient that must be sustained by the coupling of cellular energy processes to the carrier system. In this example, energy is coupled to the influx mechanism to produce a twofold increase in the affinity of carrier for its substrate at the outer cell membrane.

ment at time zero and the extracellular drug concentration remains constant over the uptake interval. There is an asymptotic rise to a steady-state with the achievement of an intracellular drug concentration exactly equal to the extracellular drug level.

It is useful to visualize the molecular events that occur during this process of equilibration. The cell is exposed to a constant concentration of extracellular drug. Since the extracellular drug level is constant, the rate at which drug penetrates the cell to gain entry into the intracellular compartment is constant over the uptake interval. Initially, as drug appears within the intracellular compartment, there is, essentially, a one-way movement of drug into the cell; there are so few drug molecules within the intracellular water as compared with the extracellular compartment that the chance of drug contacting the inner cell membrane interface to leave the cell is trivial compared with the chance of drug contacting the outer cell membrane interface to enter the cell. During this period the rate of drug uptake is constant; the relationship between the drug level in the cell and time is linear and reflects solely the rate of drug entry into the cell (influx).

This phase of uptake, the unidirectional flux into the cell, is critical because it represents uptake that is determined by transport through the cell membrane alone, uninfluenced by drug binding or metabolism within the cell. When the investigator wishes to study characteristics of drug *transport* across the cell membrane, this influx phase must be distinguished from subsequent intracellular events.[4] Later, as more drug accumulates within the intracellular water, drug molecules begin to leave the cell, an efflux component becomes an increasing component of the net uptake process, and this results in a decline in the net rate of appearance of drug within the cell. As the intracellular drug concentration continues to increase, exit of drug molecules from the cell increases until ultimately a steady-state is reached.

At this point the rate of drug exit from the cell is exactly equal to the rate of drug entry, and the intracellular and extracellular drug levels are constant and equal. Hence, the steady-state is a dynamic equilibrium in which drug moves back and forth across the cell membrane. If drug is either consumed by an intracellular metabolic process or bound to an intracellular site, the exit component for unchanged drug is reduced and a net flow of drug into the cell will continue. If influx is sufficiently fast, the intracellular drug level will ultimately reach equilibrium. ("Equilibrium" refers to the condition in which the concentration of an uncharged substance free in the intracellular water is *equal* to its extracellular level. This is to be distinguished from the "steady-state" in which the intracellular and extracellular levels are *constant* but not necessarily equal.) If the extracellular drug level falls, the entry component is diminished and there is a net flow of drug out of the cell.

Intrinsic to passive diffusion is that, at steady-state, the intracellular drug concentration will be no greater, nor less, than the extracellular drug level. There can be no transmembrane gradient in a diffusional system because there is no specific interaction between the drug and any membrane constituent that could translate cellular energy processes into an uphill flow either into or out of the cell. Hence, the maximal intracellular level achieved for a pharmacologic agent transported by passive diffusion is that of the extracellular compartment (see p. 22) for exceptions related to charge or pH). Diffusion is a very inefficient mechanism of transport for large, water-soluble drugs; the rate of delivery through the lipid membrane into the intracellular compartment is very slow and the interval required to reach equilibrium very long. On the other hand, lipid-soluble compounds penetrate the cell membrane very rapidly to reach equilibrium. For a very lipid-soluble compound, transport across the cell membrane may be so rapid compared with the rate of delivery of drug to the extracellular interface that there may be, functionally, no membrane barrier at all.

Another important property of a passive diffusional process is that the bidirectional fluxes do not saturate. That is, as the extracellular or intracellular drug concentrations increase, the unidirectional drug fluxes into and out of the cell, respectively, increase in proportion. Since there is no finite number of specific membrane receptor sites with which the drug must interact to achieve translocation across the cell membrane, there is no saturable process. The flux of drug into the cell and equilibrium levels achieved are always proportional to the extracellular concentration (Figs. 2–2 and 2–3). Hence, while transport by passive diffusion

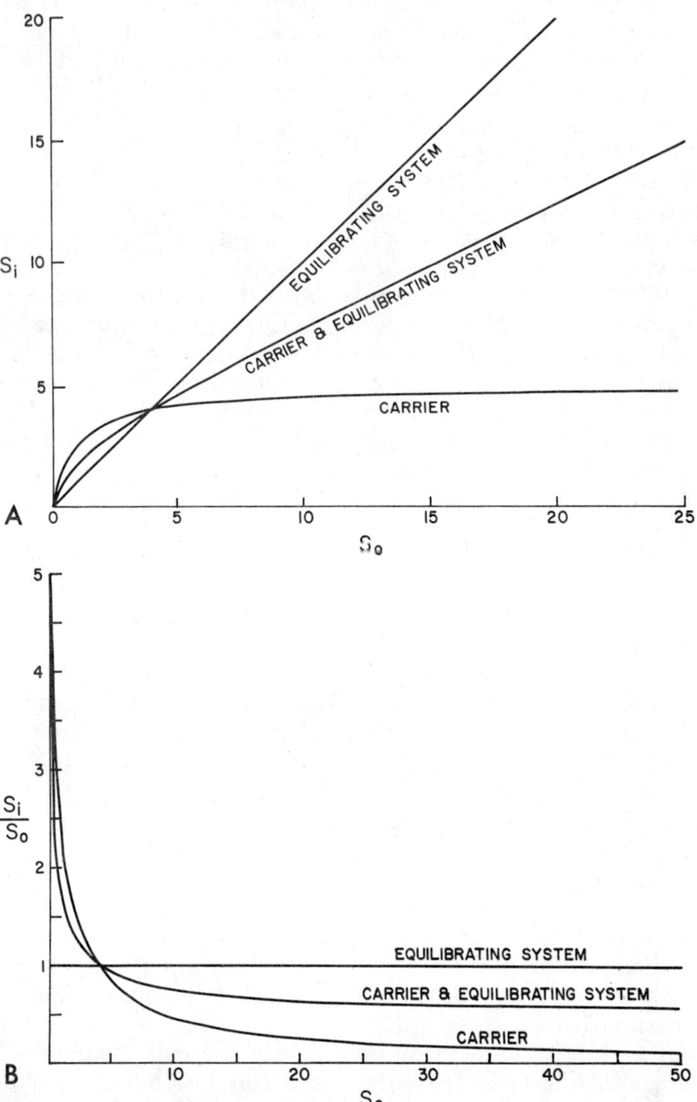

Figure 2–2. *A,* The relationship between the steady-state drug concentration in the intracellular water, S_i, and the extracellular drug concentration, S_o. For passive diffusion or an equilibrating carrier-mediated process, the steady-state intracellular drug level rises in proportion to the extracellular concentration; however, as an equilibrating carrier system saturates, the time necessary to reach the steady-state is lengthened. When transport is mediated solely by an uphill carrier system, the steady-state intracellular drug level approaches a maximum. When transport is mediated by an uphill carrier system as well as either passive diffusion or a lower-affinity equilibrating process, as the high-affinity uphill carrier system saturates, the steady-state free intracellular drug level rises as transport via the secondary route(s) increases.

B, The ratio of the steady-state intracellular to extracellular drug concentrations as the extracellular concentration is increased. For an equilibrating process — carrier-mediated or passive diffusion — this ratio is 1 (assuming the transported drug is uncharged), and independent of the extracellular concentration. For the uphill carrier system the maximal transmembrane gradient achieved is at the lowest extracellular concentration. As the extracellular concentration is increased, the carrier saturates and the gradient decreases, ultimately reverses, and approaches zero. If, however, transport is mediated by both a high-affinity carrier and also passive diffusion or a low-affinity equilibrating carrier, this produces a "leak" that permits the system ultimately to achieve a higher ratio. The greater the "leak," the closer the system comes to equilibrium when the high-affinity carrier is saturated.

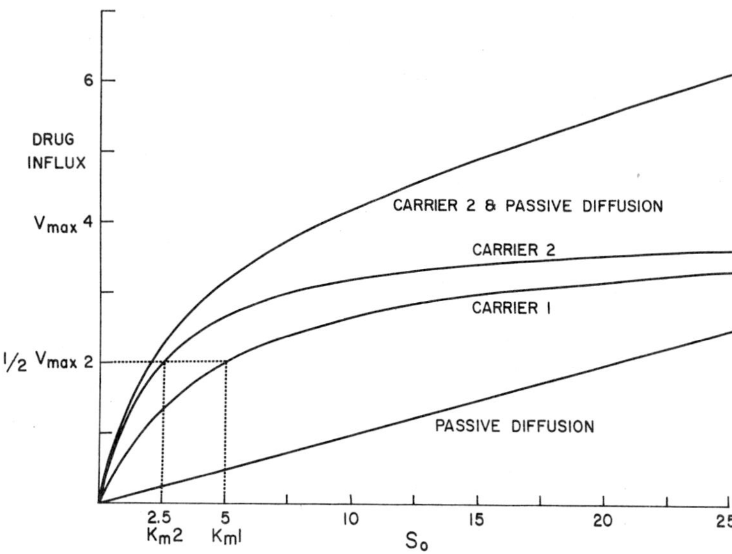

Figure 2–3. The relationship between drug influx and extracellular drug concentration, S_0, for two carrier systems. Both have the same maximal influx velocity (V_{max}). Carrier 1 has a lower affinity for the transported drug than carrier 2; the concentration at which this system reaches a velocity one-half of maximum is 5 in comparison with carrier 2, for which influx is half-saturated at a concentration of only 2.5. The figure also illustrates (lower line) the linear relationship between influx and S_0 for a passive diffusional process or a low-affinity carrier that does not saturate over the concentration range studied. Also seen is the relationship between influx and S_0 when transport is mediated by both the nonsaturating route and carrier 2. The nonsaturating process dominates influx as S_0 is increased and the carrier saturates.

(1) may limit the *rate* of drug entry into the cell, (2) may limit the *rate* of achievement of equilibrium, and (3) does not sustain transmembrane gradients, it does permit the opportunity to increase delivery of drug into the intracellular compartment as the extracellular drug concentration is raised to high levels. This may be of clinical importance, not only for the drug that penetrates the cell membrane solely by passive diffusion, but for other drugs that are transported by mediated processes as well. Hence, any substance, even if large and highly water-soluble, penetrates the cell membrane at some finite rate by passive diffusion. When a carrier-mediated process is absent, is lost, or becomes less efficient, as might occur with natural or acquired drug resistance, or when rapid intracellular drug catabolism to inactive derivative(s) requires a higher rate of drug delivery into the cell to achieve a pharmacologic effect, raising the extracellular drug concentration may allow sufficient drug accumulation by passive diffusion to result in cytotoxicity, circumventing these modes of resistance.

A variety of lipid-soluble compounds have been assumed to penetrate mammalian cell membranes by passive diffusion. Most notable are the nitrosoureas,[22] 2,4-diaminopyrimidine antifolates,[166-168] and the esterified derivatives of methotrexate.[157-159] These agents not only have the advantage of penetrating cell membranes rapidly, but also can be utilized to penetrate other body compartments, such as the central nervous system, that are less accessible to more polar cytotoxic agents. However, analysis of the transport properties of these compounds is complicated by their rapid association with the cell, precluding accurate determination of initial transport rates and reliable characterization of other transport properties. Similarly, transmembrane gradients for these compounds are difficult to interpret because of their partitioning into lipid cellular compartments. Many properties of the transport of multicyclic compounds into mammalian cells are consistent with passive diffusion. For instance, influx has not been shown to be saturable. Although the process is quite temperature-sensitive for actinomycin D, consistent with a carrier-mediated process, this was shown to be accounted for, at least in part, by the high thermal energy required to rupture hydrophilic bonds between actinomycin D and water to permit this agent to enter the lipid membrane.[41] Assessment of transmembrane gradients for actinomycin D is also complicated because of its association with a variety of sites on double-stranded DNA with different affinities for this agent.[41]

Carrier-Mediated Transport

Facilitated Diffusion or Equilibrating Carriers

As indicated above, passive diffusion represents the translocation of a pharmacologic agent across a cell membrane that, with respect to the transported substance, has the characteristics of a nonspecific physical barrier. Carrier transport mechanisms, on the other hand, are characterized by the presence of specific receptor sites within the cell membrane that facilitate the translocation of the substance into, and out of, the cell. Further, it is usually considered that the receptor site itself undergoes some physical transposition as it facilitates translocation of the transported species across the cell membrane; hence, the term "carrier."[5-8] This physical transposition, however, can be so small as to involve movements within the order of a molecule diameter.[7] Carrier processes are required to mediate transport of large, physiologically important, hydrophilic compounds that would not readily penetrate the cell membrane by passive diffusion. For some substrates at their physiologic concentrations this is the sole means of movement across the cell membrane. Carrier mechanisms permit the cell to transport substances into the intracellular compartment selectively as well as to transport catabolites out of the cell rapidly. Carrier-mediated transport maintains ionic homeostasis of the intracellular milieu critical for sustaining cell energetics, biosynthetic processes, and replication.

Within the context of this discussion, the important properties of carrier-mediated transport systems relate to saturability of bidirectional fluxes and steady-state characteristics. There is a finite number of carriers within the cell membrane with a specific affinity for the substrate to be transported. Accordingly, when the substrate concentration is sufficiently high, all the carrier sites become occupied, the system becomes saturated, and further increases in the extracellular concentration will not further increase the unidirectional flux of substrate into the cell by the carrier mechanism. "Affinity" can be related to the concentration of the substrate required to achieve a unidirectional flux one half of maximum for the carrier, (K_m). The higher the affinity, the lower the K_m, and so forth (Fig. 2–3). Hence, although a carrier system facilitates the *rate* of translocation across the cell membrane, its *capacity* is limited. At high drug concentrations, carrier-mediated flows across the cell membrane reach some maximum. At this point, influx increases, with a further increase in the extracellular drug level only if there is an additional parallel mediated transport route or a measurable passive diffusional flux.

It should also be recognized that the fact that a pharmacologic agent is transported by a carrier mechanism does not necessarily indicate that the carrier can generate a gradient for drug across the cell membrane. In thermodynamic terms, there are two kinds of carrier mechanisms. The first of these accelerates bidirectional fluxes but does not achieve gradients across the cell membrane: this is defined as an "equilibrating" carrier or "facilitated diffusion." The time course of uptake of a substance by this mechanism is illustrated in Figure 2–1. Influx and rise to the steady-state is more rapid than by passive diffusion. Within this context, equilibrating carrier flows can be distinguished from passive diffusion only by the *rate* at which the steady-state is achieved; the steady-state level is the same for both systems. However, when the extracellular concentration is high and the entry mechanism is saturated, an increased interval will be required to achieve a steady-state for the carrier system; once at steady-state again, the intracellular and extracellular levels will always be the same. The second type of carrier mechanism not only accelerates the movement of its substrates into and out of the cell, but generates gradients for the transported species as well; this "uphill" carrier system requires the expenditure of energy by the cell to sustain the gradients achieved. This type of carrier is described in the next section.

Uphill Carriers

Uphill carriers, also described as "active" transport systems, not only enhance transmembrane fluxes but also generate gradients for the transported substance across the cell membrane. A carrier system can pump a substance uphill into the cell so that the intracellular concentration is greater than the extracellular concentration (Fig. 2–1), as observed for many substrates required for biosynthetic reactions within the cell. Alternatively, active transport systems can pump out of a cell. For instance, the sodium pump maintains intracellular sodium at a level less than that of the extracellular compartment.[9] It is possible that multiple energy-dependent processes can influence transport of a drug through one or more transport carriers to achieve uphill flows into or out of the cell. For instance, methotrexate is pumped uphill into many mammalian cells, but there is evidence for a second mechanism that pumps drug out of the cell as well. When the former pump predominates (as when the exit pump is blocked by metabolic poisons), high levels of free methotrexate accumulate within the intracellular compartment. When the latter predominates (as in the presence of glucose), only low levels of free methotrexate are present within the cell.[10-14]

If a transport system generates a gradient for its substance across the cell membrane, cellular energy must be expended to account for this "work" — an energy source in the cell must "run down" to produce a transport-mediated uphill flow. There are a variety of ways in which transport systems can be "energized."[15] The hydrolysis of ATP could be "coupled" or transferred directly to a transport carrier system. For instance, intracellular phosphorylation of a carrier protein could create an asymmetry in the affinity of carrier for its substrate such that the extracellular substrate associates with carrier at the outer cell membrane interface to gain entry into the cell at a faster rate than the rate of association of intracellular substrate with carrier at the inner cell membrane as it exits from the cell. A net influx results, with the creation of a transmembrane concentration gradient.

Carrier systems may also be energized by coupling the potential energy from the gradient for one substance, maintained by an independent energized carrier, to the flow of a second substance by a second carrier mechanism. For instance, sodium is asymmetrically distributed across cell membranes by an outward sodium pump. If sodium can interact with the transport carrier for another substance at the inner and outer cell membrane interfaces to enhance the affinity of the carrier for its substrate, the asymmetry in the sodium concentration across the cell membrane (extracellular > intracellular) will produce an asymmetry in the affinities of carrier for substrate across the cell membrane. This, in turn, will generate an uphill flow of that substrate into the cell.[15-17] An analogy would be a hydraulic coupling in which an electrically driven system pumps water uphill to a high tank from where it flows downhill to drive one or more different turbines that pump one or more other fluids uphill. The advantage of this kind of coupling is that one power source (the sodium pump or the electric water pump) can drive a variety of other systems. Influx by this mechanism should be reduced as the extracellular sodium concentration is reduced, and agents that reduce the transmembrane gradient for sodium should reduce the gradient for the cotransported substrate. Transport of some antineoplastic agents is sodium-dependent. For instance, phenylalanine mustard utilizes amino acid transport systems that are, in part, sodium-dependent.[18-22] Likewise, there is evidence that organic anion gradients may be linked to the methotrexate-tetrahydrofolate cofactor carrier to drive these folates uphill into cells.[10, 23-25]

Of particular interest are the steady-state kinetics for uphill carrier systems. Just as carrier influx is saturable and reaches a maximum, so does the steady-state level achieved. As indicated in Figure 2–2A, if transport is mediated solely by an asymmetric carrier, then as the extracellular level increases, the steady-state intracellular level approaches a maximum. This process has been observed for methotrexate.[14] Hence, the maximal gradient is achieved at extracellular drug concentrations that are low with respect to the influx K_m. As the extracellular concentration increases and the carrier approaches saturation, the gradient decreases. If the concentration is sufficiently high, the gradient actually reverses and approaches zero (Fig. 2–2B). The latter is unusual, however, because as the extracellular level increases, a low-affinity carrier or passive diffusion emerges and permits the intracellular level to approach equilibrium (Fig. 2–2B).

Multiple Transport Routes Across Cell Membranes

The preceding discussion described a variety of mechanisms by which substances penetrate cell membranes — passive diffusion, and equilibrating and uphill carrier processes. Most substances, in fact, are transported by more than one process. For instance, as indicated above, irrespective of how lipophobic or large a drug, when its carrier mechanism is saturated but the extracellular concentration is sufficiently high, a finite amount of drug will continue to penetrate the cell membrane by passive diffusion. Whether or not this is pharmacologically important will depend on the intracellular level achieved in comparison with the amount required to produce a pharmacologic effect. There are various transport routes for amino acids.[26, 27] Some result in uphill transport, some are sodium-dependent, and some are not. Phenylalanine mustard utilizes several amino acid transport processes, and components of the influx of this agent can be inhibited by amino acid substrates for each of the specific transport routes.[10, 20, 22] Multiple equilibrating transport components have been suggested for cytotoxic nucleosides, but their characterization is complicated by the difficulty in obtaining accurate quantitation of unidirectional fluxes.[28, 29] At low extracellular levels, methotrexate transport is largely mediated by a high-affinity carrier system.[14] At high extracellular concentrations, the rate of transport exceeds the capacity of the high-affinity system and may represent passive diffusion and/or a second, lower-affinity process.[11, 30] However, initial rate determinations are difficult to obtain at high concentrations because of the rapid build-up of free methotrexate and the rapid decline in the net uptake rate. Evidence for two transport routes for methotrexate was obtained in resistant cells with a marked reduction in influx by the high-affinity carrier.[31]

The possibility of multiple transport routes for cytotoxic agents must be considered in clinical applications and experimental designs for the study of drug transport and action, for a variety of reasons:

1. The characteristics and rates of drug transport across the cell membrane will be influenced by the extracellular drug concentration achieved. For instance, at low extracellular drug levels when drug transport might be mediated largely by a high-affinity carrier system, the characteristics of transport may have very little relevance to the characteristics of transport at higher drug concentrations when a second, low-affinity transport route or passive diffusion might be dominant. Hence, if *in vitro* studies are to be relevant to *in vivo* drug-cell interactions, drug levels chosen for study must be comparable to those achieved *in vivo*.

2. Transport heterogeneity is an important consideration in the approach to therapy when drug resistance is transport-related. For instance, impaired transport by a high-affinity carrier could be circumvented when an increase in drug dose results in a sufficiently high extracellular level to produce drug transport by another mechanism.[31]

3. Transport heterogeneity may play an important role in selectivity. There may be differences in the expression of multiple transport routes in tumor versus susceptible host tissues that may be a basis for the selective effects of drugs.

4. The characterization of multiple transport routes may provide information that will permit drug modification to optimize transport by a route peculiar to tumor cells. For instance, there is evidence that murine bone marrow cells may lack the system L amino acid carrier, one of the several transport components for phenylalanine mustard present in L1210 leukemia cells. The suggestion was made that structural modification of the mustard to optimize transport by the L system carrier might selectively enhance transport into tumor cells.[32]

Role of Molecular Charge, Membrane Potential, and pH in Drug Transport

The above discussion considered membrane transport of drugs and, in particular, the gradients achieved across the cell membrane in terms of drug concentration and chemical gradients alone. Although this is appropriate for uncharged agents, many drugs are ionized at physiologic pH and carry a net charge. Charge is an important determinant of rates of drug flow across the cell membrane as well as of net and steady-state intracellular drug concentrations achieved. All mammalian cells sustain a negative electrical potential as compared with the extracellular compartment. This charge influences the permeation of charged species.[33] For instance, consider a pharmacologic agent that penetrates the cell membrane by passive diffusion but carries a negative charge. As this negatively charged species approaches the negatively charged cell, electrostatic forces will repel it, tending to slow entry. As the species leaves the cell, electrostatic repulsion will tend to accelerate exit. The steady-state achieved by this drug within the intracellular compartment will reflect a balance between the electrical force tending to drive the drug out and the diffusional force (the concentration gradient) tending to equalize the drug concentrations across the cell membrane. Hence, this system comes to equilibrium when the electrochemical-potential (a term that considers both electrical and diffusive forces) for the drug inside and outside the cell is the same. In this setting, equilibrium occurs when the *concentration* of drug inside the cell is *less than* its concentration outside the cell. There is a concentration gradient but no electrochemical-potential difference; the concentration gradient can be predicted by the Nernst equation* on the basis of the membrane potential and the valence of the drug.[14, 15, 33] The system is not energy-dependent. Hence chemical, but not electrochemical-potential, gradients can be achieved by passive electrical factors.

This can have important pharmacologic ramifications. For instance, methotrexate is a bivalent anion at physiologic pH. Figure 2–4 illustrates the expected ratio of intracellular to extracellular concentration of a bivalent anion at *equilibrium* as a function of the cell membrane potential. As the membrane potential rises, the ratio of intracellular to extracellular drug at equilibrium falls. At 15 to 20 millivolts, a membrane potential common for many mammalian tumor cells, the ratio is 0.2 to 0.3. At a membrane potential of 35 millivolts reported for isolated hepatocytes[34] and a level considerably lower than that observed in muscle, the predicted ratio is 0.05. Hence, passive electrical forces can have a profound effect on the concentration that methotrexate achieves within the intracellular water. Because the methotrexate transport system is capable of generating uphill flows of drug into the cell, intracellular levels are usually higher than those predicted solely from electrical considerations.[14] However, when extracellular methotrexate concentrations are increased, especially when the carrier system is saturated, transport is probably mediated to a large extent by passive diffusion or some other equilibrating process. In this situation, electrical factors will play a major role in determining the concentration gradient, and free intracellular methotrexate levels achieved will be far below those of the extracellular

*The Nernst equation provides a method of predicting the expected ratio of extracellular to intracellular concentration of a charged molecule at equilibrium across a membrane at a given electrical-potential difference:

$$\text{membrane potential} = \frac{RT}{zF} \ln \frac{S_o}{S_i}$$

R is the gas constant, T is the temperature, z is the valency of the molecule, and F is Faraday's constant. When z is unity and the temperature is 18° C the formula becomes $58 \log \frac{S_o}{S_i}$. For a bivalent anion the formula is $29 \log \frac{S_o}{S_i}$. S_o and S_i refer to the concentration of the transport substrate in the extracellular and intracellular water, respectively.

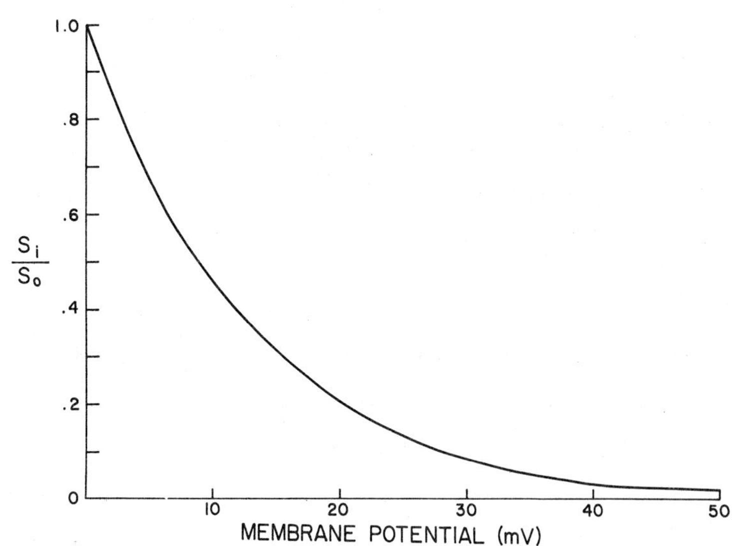

Figure 2–4. The effect of membrane potential on the chemical gradient for a bivalent anion transported by passive diffusion or an equilibrating process. The ratio of the steady-state intracellular drug concentration, S_i, to its extracellular level, S_o, is plotted as a function of a rising membrane potential. As the membrane potential increases, S_i/S_o decreases dramatically. When the charged species is transported by an uphill process, these passive electrical forces continue to retard the chemical level achieved within the cell, and the net chemical gradient will be the sum of passive electrical forces tending to decrease the intracellular drug level and the energy-requiring process tending to pump the drug into the cell.

compartment.[35] These considerations may provide a rationale, in part, for the generation of high extracellular methotrexate levels in clinical protocols in order to achieve an intracellular drug level sufficient to produce a pharmacologic effect (see pp. 26, 27).

These considerations are also of considerable experimental relevance. It is apparent that if an investigator seeks to explore the mechanism of transport of a pharmacologic agent, the demonstration of a transmembrane *concentration* gradient is not sufficient evidence for active transport. If the species is charged at physiologic pH, electrical factors must be considered, and the possibility that the electrochemical-potential difference across the cell membrane is zero must be excluded before active transport can be implicated.

Other physical gradients across the cell membrane can result in passive chemical gradients for drugs also. When the ionized species of weak acids or bases are not transported, the nonionized species can be asymmetrically distributed across the cell membrane depending on the extent of the transmembrane pH gradient.[36] For instance, marked pH-dependent changes in net accumulation of daunomycin and doxorubicin (Adriamycin) have been explained on this basis.[37]

MEMBRANE TRANSPORT OF ANTINEOPLASTIC AGENTS AS A DETERMINANT OF DRUG-TARGET INTERACTIONS WITHIN THE CELL

Membrane transport of a pharmacologic agent is often perceived solely as the penetration of drug across the cell membrane — a one-way movement of the drug into the cell that permits the subsequent association of drug with its intracellular target site. When viewed from this perspective, membrane transport is a limiting factor in cytotoxicity because it limits the *rate* at which the drug can interact with its intracellular target. This is, however, a simplistic and often misleading perception of the role of membrane transport in drug action.[15] Although the membrane transport system does, in fact, determine the rate at which the drug penetrates the cell membrane, it also influences the rate of accumulation of free drug (drug unassociated with its target site or other binding sites, and drug that does not represent a metabolite) within the intracellular water, and the final concentration of free drug achieved within the intracellular water. All, or some, of these elements may play critical roles in drug action.[15] The membrane transport system may also influence the net rate at which free drug leaves the cell as the plasma concentration falls. However, when the decline in the drug level in blood is very slow in comparison with the rate of membrane transport, the net rate of decline of free drug from the cell is determined by the characteristics of the pharmacokinetics in plasma and not by the cellular transport system (see pp. 26, 27). Likewise, the rate at which the drug penetrates the cell membrane to reach equilibrium within the intracellular water may be so rapid that, operationally, the cell membrane does not exist; as rapidly as the drug reaches the tumor cell, it is transported into the intracellular compartment, reaching a concentration at equilibrium with that of the extracellular compartment. In the latter case, the limiting factor in delivery of drug to the intracellular target is not the cell membrane but the rate of blood flow or diffusion of drug in the tumor interstitium; the factor that determines the free intracellular drug level is the extracellular drug concentration. The latter is described as a "flow-limited" system in contrast to a "membrane-limited" system in which drug transport is slow relative to the rate of drug delivery to the tumor cell.[38] The following discussion considers how the membrane transport system may influence drug action based on the nature of the interaction between the drug and its target site within the cell.

Role of Membrane Transport When There is Irreversible Interaction or High-Affinity Binding Between Drug and Target

When transport into the cell is slow relative to the rate at which drug interacts irreversibly with, or binds tightly to, its target, transport becomes a rate-limiting event. This is illustrated in Figure 2–5A. It can be seen that the rate of accumulation of drug within the cell is constant prior to saturation of the target site. During this interval, the rate of uptake is determined by the rate of drug penetration into the cell. Also, net drug uptake is equal to its unidirectional flux into the cell. As each drug molecule enters the

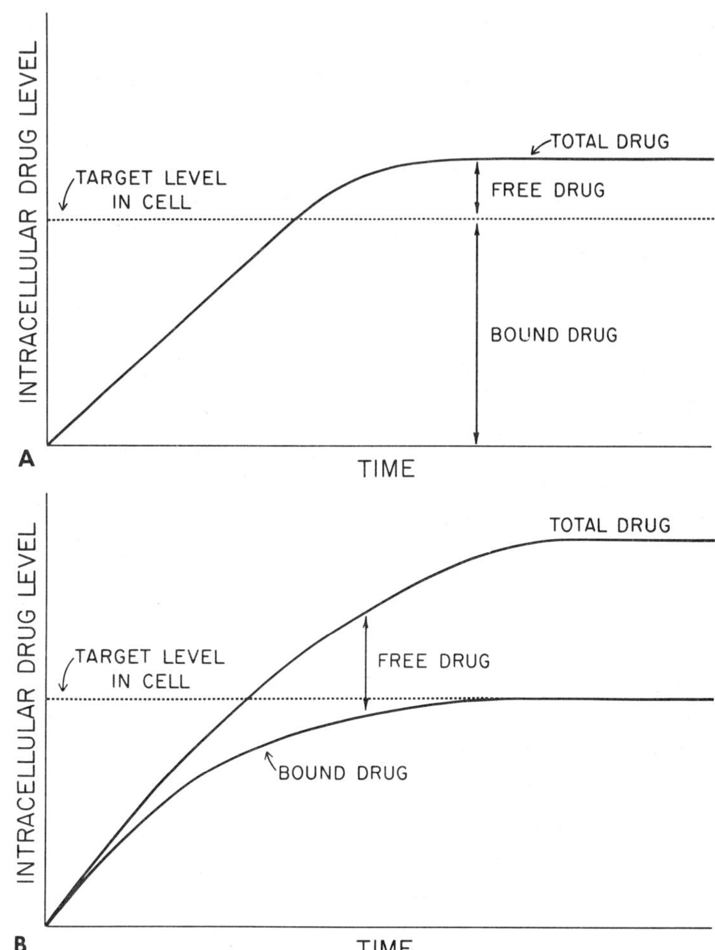

Figure 2–5. *A,* The time course of uptake of total and free drug and drug irreversibly bound or chemically associated with an intracellular target when transport is *rate*-limiting to the interaction between drug and its intracellular target. The rate of drug uptake is constant until all target sites are associated with drug, following which free drug accumulates within the cell and a steady-state for free drug is achieved. In this example the extracellular drug concentration is constant over the interval of observation.

B, The time course of appearance of drug in cells when the drug is a reversible inhibitor of the intracellular target and influx is faster than the rate of association of the drug with the target. Free drug accumulates early in the uptake process, since net interaction with the target is much slower than the rate of drug entry into the cell. A higher level of free drug is required to achieve complete inactivation of the target than with the irreversible inhibitor.

cell, it associates with a target molecule until all target sites are inactivated. It is only at this point that free drug appears within the intracellular compartment, some of which then leaves the cell. As this exit component increases, net uptake falls until a steady-state is reached (see also Fig. 2–1). A critical consideration here is the amount of drug that must be associated with the target site to achieve cytotoxicity. For instance, if an enzymic target mediates some rate-limiting step in an important biosynthetic reaction such as the synthesis of thymidylate from deoxyuridylate by thymidylate synthetase, then, as the enzyme is inhibited, the biosynthetic step will be proportionately reduced and a pharmacologic effect will be achieved immediately.[39] If, on the other hand, an enzymic target is not rate-limiting but is present in great excess with only a small fraction required to meet cellular demands for its product, a high degree of enzyme saturation by inhibitor will be required before a pharmacologic effect is perceived.[39] When transport is rate-limiting to the drug-target interaction, association with the target site sufficient to achieve cytotoxicity will be determined by the rate of drug entry into the cell, and this in turn will be determined by the extracellular concentration, the kinetics of the transport mechanism, and the interval over which the cell is exposed to drug. If an enzymic target is present in excess so that it is not limiting to a subsequent biochemical reaction, and if the exposure time is brief, the transport process slow, or the extracellular concentration low, inhibition of a sufficient number of the target sites may not be achieved and the drug will be pharmacologically inert. If the drug forms a covalent bond with its target or binds with high affinity to the target, but the *rate* of this reaction is slow, free intracellular drug must be achieved and sustained until the target is inactivated. This condition is described on pp. 26–29.

It is unclear to what extent influx limits the rate of interaction between irreversible inhibitors and their targets. Although it might be expected that alkylating agents fall into this category, there is insufficient quantitation of rates of transport relative to rates of alkylation, and the extent of alkylation required to achieve cytotoxicity, to support such a relationship. In fact, analysis of data on phenylalanine mustard[20] and nitrogen mustard[40] suggests that transport into the cell is more rapid than the rate of alkylation. Often it is very difficult to clarify whether the unidirectional drug flux into the cell is a rate-limiting event. Transport and equilibration of the drug may be so rapid compared with the rate of intracellular binding or the rate of metabolism to active derivatives that are retained within the cell, and the amount bound or metabolized so great in comparison with the free drug level within the cell, that transport may be ignored completely in the experimental design chosen for study.[4, 41, 42] The relationship between transport and binding of heterocyclic compounds also has not been established, and the extent of drug binding and the specific sites that must be bound to achieve cytotoxicity are not clear.[41]

Drugs may interact with multiple targets with different binding kinetics to achieve a pharmacologic effect. Actinomycin D interacts with a variety of base pairs as it intercalates with DNA, but the critical target, if one exists, has not been identified.[43] Alternatively, a pharmacologic effect may be based on association with a single target, but the interaction may be characterized by apparent heterogeneous kinetics. For instance, in the case of methotrexate (see below), the bulk of the drug-target interaction conforms to a model in which transport into the cell is rate-limiting relative to very tight binding to the target enzyme dihydrofolate reductase. However, because the enzyme is not rate-limiting and the substrate dihydrofolate increases within the cell as methotrexate associates with the enzyme, the interaction between methotrexate and the small fraction of dihydrofolate reductase that is necessary to sustain tetrahydrofolate synthesis has the characteristics of a very rapidly reversible competitive inhibitor.

Role of Membrane Transport When There Is Reversible Interaction Between Drug and Target

Intrinsic to reversible inhibition is the need for free drug to achieve a pharmacologic effect; the rate of drug association with target must be fast relative to the rate of dissociation from target to achieve the necessary degree of saturation of the target. Further, for enzyme inhibitors, the level of free drug required to achieve a pharmacologic effect will depend on the concentration of its competitive substrate(s) and their relative affinities for the target enzyme. Here the critical interaction between drug and the cell determined by the transport system is the rate at which free drug accumulates, the level of free drug achieved, and the duration over which free drug is sustained. The time course of cellular uptake and association of a reversible inhibitor with its intracellular target is illustrated in Figure 2–5B. Free drug accumulates prior to saturation of the target early in the uptake process. The target becomes saturated only after substantial levels of free drug accumulate within the cell. The free drug level, of course, will depend on the extracellular drug level, the specific properties of the membrane transport system, and the rate of metabolic transformations in the cell. For an uphill carrier system, energy coupling to the carrier that either enhances drug influx or retards efflux will increase the free intracellular drug level. Although drug influx may be high in a drug-sensitive tumor, this *per se* may not be the critical element. Rather, the critical factor may be the free drug level generated based on this influx.

Role of Membrane Transport With Agents That Interact With Their Cellular Targets as Both "Reversible" and "Irreversible" Inhibitors — Special Case of Methotrexate

The kinetics of drug-target interactions are usually derived from studies in cell-free systems. However, this may not necessarily be relevant to what occurs within the intracellular compartment. Cell-free analyses employ static systems with fixed initial substrate, inhibitor, and enzyme levels that may not be comparable to the relative concentrations of these constituents within the cell.

Further, the cell exists in a dynamic state in which drug-induced metabolic perturbations, in turn, can alter the drug-target interaction within the environment encapsulated by the cell membrane. For these reasons, what may appear as an irreversible inhibitor in a cell-free system may, in fact, behave as a very rapidly reversible inhibitor in the intact cell. From the foregoing discussion it can be seen that the role of membrane transport in determining drug action under these two conditions can be drastically different. Perhaps the best understood example of this phenomenon is the pharmacologic action of methotrexate. It was recognized more than two decades ago that membrane transport of methotrexate is a critical determinant of cytotoxicity, but the specific role of membrane transport has been clearly elucidated only recently. Ironically, the experimental approaches that were employed to characterize membrane transport of this agent led, at the same time, to a better understanding of the kinetics of the interaction between the drug and its target enzyme, dihydrofolate reductase, within the cell.

Shortly after methotrexate was synthesized, its high affinity for the enzyme dihydrofolate reductase was identified as a basis for its pharmacologic action. Because of the very low inhibitor constant (see Chapter 10) it was initially considered that the drug-target interaction was essentially irreversible.[62-64] Likewise, it was recognized early that the rate of transport of drug into the cell correlated well with tumor cell sensitivity and that transport was rate-limiting to binding of drug to the bulk of the enzyme within the cell.[13, 14, 65, 66] This led to the concept that the drug-target interaction in the cell was "stoichiometric"; i.e., as each drug molecule enters the cell it associates with one enzyme molecule until all enzyme is inhibited.[63] It is only after all enzyme binding sites are saturated that free drug accumulates within the cell. Membrane transport was viewed as determining cytotoxicity based solely on the rate of drug flux into the cell. According to this view, drug resistance could be related, in part, to a low rate of drug transport into the cell and/or a high enzyme level. The lower the drug influx and the higher the concentration of enzyme, the longer it would take to "inactivate" the enzyme. Although free drug was recognized as a requirement of inhibition of new enzyme as it might be synthesized, beyond this the free intracellular methotrexate component was not considered important.

A number of observations, however, seriously called into question this paradigm:

1. It became apparent that differences in tumor cell sensitivities to methotrexate could not be related solely to differences in the interval required to "saturate" dihydrofolate reductase,[15] since the times required to "saturate" the enzyme might differ by an order of minutes while the total time of exposure to the drug in excess of the binding capacity was in the order of hours.[15]

2. It became increasingly evident from *in vitro*[67-72] and *in vivo*[73-75] studies, as well as computer simulations,[39] that methotrexate inhibition of thymidylate synthesis, and ultimately tetrahydrofolate synthesis, within the cell is rapidly reversible. When cells are loaded to levels of intracellular methotrexate that abolish these biosynthetic pathways, following which extracellular methotrexate declines *in vivo*[72-75, 77] or is removed from the extracellular compartment *in vitro*,[67-72] the biosynthetic pathways rapidly resume as the free intracellular methotrexate level falls. The reversal of this pharmacologic effect *in vitro* can be observed within minutes after removal of extracellular drug.[67] A critical element in this paradoxically rapid reversibility of methotrexate action emerged when it was demonstrated that methotrexate markedly increases the intracellular dihydrofolate substrate level,[69] and that it is this perturbation that alters the interaction between methotrexate and dihydrofolate reductase, resulting in functionally reversible inhibition of this enzyme within the cell.[39, 69, 76, 78] The interaction among the enzyme, methotrexate, and dihydrofolate will be described in detail at this point because it is essential to an understanding of the role that membrane transport plays in methotrexate cytotoxicity and selectivity.

Dihydrofolate reductase is present in at least a 25- to 30-fold excess of the amount required to sustain tetrahydrofolate stores even in S-phase cells.[39, 69, 78] The high level of dihydrofolate reductase activity in comparison with the low rate of oxidation of tetrahydrofolate to dihydrofolate during the formation of thymidylate from deoxyuridylate results in a very low cell dihydrofolate level, orders of magnitude below its K_m for this enzyme. When a cell is exposed to methotrexate, the agent enters the cell slowly in comparison with the rate of binding; transport is essentially rate-limiting to its association with the target enzyme,[13, 14] and for each drug molecule that enters the cell essentially one molecule of enzyme is inactivated. As enzyme is inactivated, however, the reduction of dihydrofolate is transiently decreased, the dihydrofolate substrate level rises, and the rate of its reduction by residual free enzyme increases. This sustains a normal rate of tetrahydrofolate synthesis as the major portion of enzyme becomes associated with drug. Ultimately, however, the cell dihydrofolate level approaches its K_m, so that residual enzyme no longer sustains a normal rate of tetrahydrofolate synthesis and the tetrahydrofolate cofactor pools fall.

Another consequence of the high dihydrofolate level is that the substrate can effectively compete with methotrexate for the critical few remaining dihydrofolate reductase sites that sustain tetrahydrofolate synthesis.[39, 78] Hence, the interaction between methotrexate and the target enzyme shifts from one that is "irreversible" to one that is "competitive" with dihydrofolate. Conversely, when cells are loaded with sufficient free methotrexate to suppress tetrahydrofolate synthesis, dihydrofolate is at its maximum. When the extracellular drug level is reduced, free methotrexate leaves the cell rapidly, and dihydrofolate (presumably retained within the cell as a polyglutamate) replaces methotrexate on the few critical enzyme sites necessary to sustain tetrahydrofolate synthesis. When tetrahydrofolate synthesis resumes, dihydrofolate is rapidly consumed, and the dihydrofolate level in the cell falls by orders of magnitude to its usual low concentrations. Dihydrofolate is no longer present in a sufficiently high concentration to compete with methotrexate for enzyme, and residual drug remains tightly bound to 95 to 98 per cent of dihydrofolate reductase — a portion virtually indistinguishable, experimentally, from the total enzyme level in the cell.[39, 69, 71, 76, 78] In fact, displacement of radiolabeled methotrexate from dihydrofolate reductase by dihydrofolate has been demonstrated in a cell-free system.[78]

Figure 2–6 is a network thermodynamic simulation of this phenomenon in the intact cell, which illustrates that the "displacement" of methotrexate from 2 per cent of the enzyme by dihydrofolate is correlated with the falling free drug level, the declining dihydrofolate level, and the rising rate of thymidylate synthesis within the cell.

There is now considerable evidence from murine tumor systems that implicates membrane transport as an important element in cytotoxicity and selectivity of antifolates. Murine tumor sensitivity to drug correlates

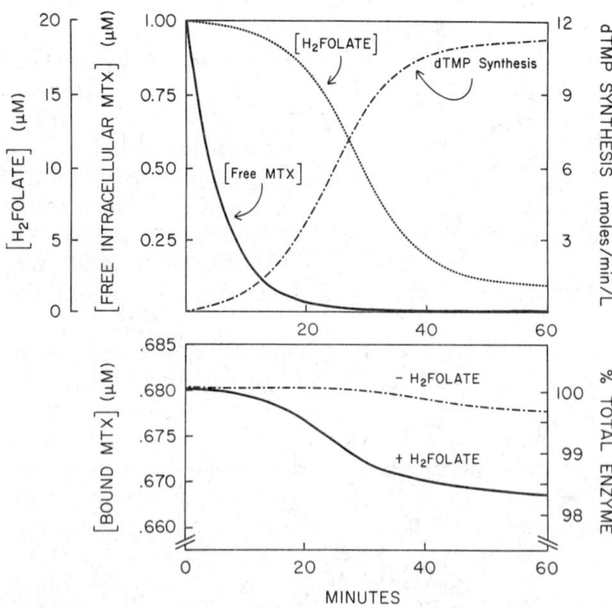

Figure 2–6. A network thermodynamic simulation of a theoretical cell that is preloaded with sufficient free methotrexate (MTX) to abolish thymidylate (dTMP) synthesis, then transferred to a methotrexate-free medium. Methotrexate rapidly leaves the cells; dihydrofolate (H_2folate) is retained as a polyglutamate. When the dihydrofolate:free methotrexate ratio is favorable, dihydrofolate displaces free methotrexate from dihydrofolate reductase (*lower panel*) binding sites. As dihydrofolate is consumed and tetrahydrofolate (H_4folate) and thymidylate (dTMP) synthesis return toward normal, the ratio of intracellular dihydrofolate to methotrexate is so low that dihydrofolate no longer competes with methotrexate for dihydrofolate reductase. The bound methotrexate level then becomes essentially constant. In this simulation, approximately 1.5 per cent of total dihydrofolate reductase is sufficient to sustain thymidylate synthesis. (Reproduced with permission from White JC: Reversal of methotrexate binding to dihydrofolate reductase by dihydrofolate. Studies with pure enzyme and computer modeling using network thermodynamics. J. Biol. Chem. 254:10889–10895, 1979.)

well with high drug influx, high free intracellular drug levels *in vitro*, and a low net rate of decline of free drug after pulse administration *in vivo*.[79, 80] The greater toxicity of methotrexate to tumor cells > murine gastrointestinal epithelial cells > murine bone marrow cells after pulse administration *in vivo* correlates with a rapid decline of free drug from bone marrow, a less rapid decline from gastrointestinal cells (the tissue with limiting host toxicity in the mouse), and the slowest loss from tumor cells with the highest degree of sensitivity to the drug.[74, 80, 81] It has been shown clearly in these systems that, as intracellular drug falls to some critical point *in vivo*, thymidylate synthesis resumes.[57, 74, 82] A slow rate of decline of the cell drug level and a slow rate of resumption of thymidylate synthesis correlates well with tumor cell sensitivity to this agent. Drug influx correlates well with cytotoxicity,[66] because it is the critical determinant of the free intracellular drug level.[15] For murine systems, at least, the parameter of influx that correlates most clearly with free drug levels and cytotoxicity is the affinity of the carrier for the drug as it transports drug into the cell.[80] At drug concentrations below carrier saturation, cells that have a lower K_m for drug influx (and therefore a higher affinity for the carrier) will have higher free intracellular drug levels and greater cytotoxicity. Further, differences in cytotoxicity among a variety of antifolates can also be related, at least in part, to their relative affinities for the tumor cell influx mechanism,[83, 84] and differences in selectivity of antifolates can be related to their relative transport in tumor versus gastrointestinal epithelial cells.[83]

The significance of the *in vivo* studies described above must be considered, however, within the context of the increasing recognition that polyglutamate derivatives of methotrexate rapidly accumulate in cells *in vivo* (see below, p. 31). These derivatives can be detected by the use of ^{3}H methotrexate,[85-87] but are not distinguished from the parent compound by assays employed in the uptake studies described above.[72, 74, 79-84] Hence, cell "drug" levels in these studies reflect not only methotrexate but also the polyglutamate derivatives, and correlations between intracellular "drug" levels and methotrexate cytotoxicity in various murine tumor cells and normal tissues may largely reflect changes in the pools of methotrexate polyglutamate derivatives rather than free parent compound. Further, when differences in the apparent half-time ($t\frac{1}{2}$) for *net* loss of cell "drug" among different tumors *in vivo* (the order of hours) is compared to the $t\frac{1}{2}$ for the unidirectional flux of methotrexate from cells (the order of minutes) and the $t\frac{1}{2}$ for the decline of the extracellular methotrexate level (the order of hours as intracellular "drug" levels approach the point at which thymidylate synthesis resumes), it becomes apparent that differences in membrane transport of methotrexate cannot account for changes in the *net* rate of decline of intracellular "drug." Membrane transport of methotrexate is so rapid in comparison with the rate of change of the extracellular methotrexate concentration that the free intracellular and extracellular methotrexate levels are always near steady-state under these conditions, and the rate of decline of free intracellular methotrexate will be controlled solely by the plasma pharmacokinetics of the drug rather than the membrane transport system.[119, 171] Accordingly, it seems likely that differences in the rate of decline of cell "drug" in tumors with different sensitivities to methotrexate are due, at least in part, to differences in the net rate of decline of methotrexate polyglutamate derivatives. The role of membrane transport may be related, in part, to the control of the free intracellular methotrexate level that is the substrate for the folylpolyglutamate synthetase. Higher free intracellular methotrexate levels will be associated with a more rapid rate of synthesis of these active methotrexate polyglutamate derivatives. Assuming that these metabolites exit the cell more slowly than methotrexate, the higher their level within the cell, the longer will be the suppression of tetrahydrofolate synthesis after administration of the drug (see below).

Inhibitors That Undergo Metabolic Transformations Within Cell Before Interaction With Their Targets

Many cytotoxic agents undergo one or more metabolic transformations within the cell before interaction with their target sites. As described in detail elsewhere in this book, nucleosides undergo phosphorylation, while bases such as 5-fluorouracil must add both a ribose or deoxyribose plus phosphate before ultimately interacting with an enzymic target site or incorporation into a macromolecule that, in turn, results in a cytotoxic or cytostatic effect. Although these metabolic conversions can be viewed as "activation" of the drug to its ultimate inhibitor structure, the metabolic step also effects a structural change that results in the retention of the metabolite within the cell based on a marked decline in the ability of the phosphorylated derivative to exit from the cell in comparison with the parent agent. The cell membrane is poorly permeable to highly charged phosphorylated compounds. Phosphorylation might be viewed, teleologically, as a mechanism that permits important biologic compounds to be retained at high concentrations within the cell in proximity to the enzymes for which they are substrates. To the extent to which these phosphorylated derivatives of cytotoxic nucleosides and bases are not hydrolyzed and do not slowly leave the cell, they represent a pool of inhibitor that has the potential for sustaining drug effects over long intervals as the extracellular drug level falls. Opposing the phosphorylating reaction, however, are intracellular catabolic processes that convert the agent to inactive forms (i.e., the deamination of cytosine arabinoside, ara-C) that may rapidly leave the cell.

Contrary to earlier perceptions,[88] most cytotoxic base and nucleoside analogues and their physiologic counterparts are transported into the cell more rapidly than they are metabolized,[28, 42, 89-94] particularly at the initial high extracellular levels achieved in most chemotherapeutic regimens. This is illustrated in Figure 2–7, which shows the rapid uptake of ^{3}H-FdUrd and its conversion to ^{3}H-FUra and ^{3}H-FdUMP in Ehrlich ascites tumor cells. Transport is very rapid! The nucleoside achieves near-equilibrium within 15 seconds; over the next 85 seconds the bulk of the ^{3}H that accumulates within the cell represents the phosphorylated derivative ^{3}H-FdUMP. Hydrolysis to FUra is also rapid, as seen by the early build-up of the base within the cell. FUra accumulates rapidly within the extracellular compartment *(not shown)*, so that in a short time (less than 30 minutes) extracellular FdUrd is almost completely converted to FUra. Because the rate of FdUrd transport into the cell and FdUMP synthesis is so rapid in this tumor line in comparison with the level of thymidylate synthetase, neither process can be important determinants of the rate at which this enzyme is initially inactivated *in vivo* when extracellular drug levels are high. However, the initial FdUMP level achieved and the net rate of decline of FdUMP appear to be important determinants, though not the sole factors, that govern the rate of recovery of thymidylate synthetase activity and cytotoxicity as the FUra level falls after administration of the base.[95, 96] Likewise, retention of ara-CTP has been shown to correlate with cytotoxicity in some tumor lines.[97] Since the net level of phosphorylated derivatives in the cell is determined by the relative rates of synthesis and hydrolysis and because blood levels of these agents decline very rapidly, transport could become an important factor in determining the intracellular level of phosphorylated derivatives as the extracel-

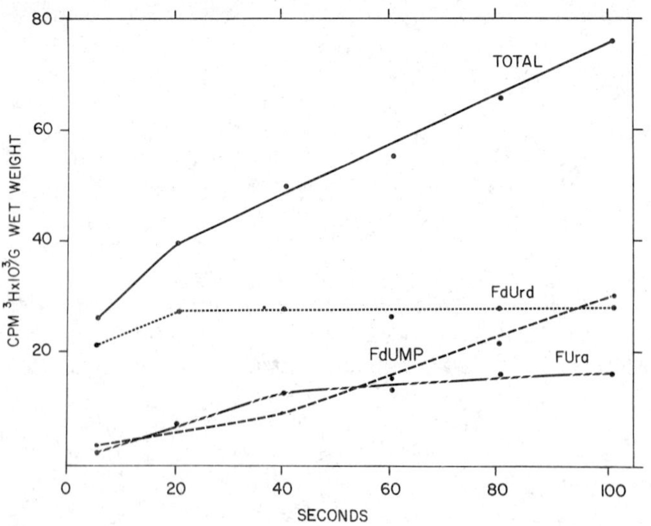

Figure 2–7. Time course of accumulation of fluorodeoxyuridine (FdUrd), fluorodeoxyuridine monophosphate (FdUMP), and fluorouracil (FUra) in the Ehrlich ascites tumor after exposure of cells to ^{3}H-FdUMP. Within 20 seconds FdUrd is at steady-state within the cell. FUra accumulates as well, but, beyond 20 seconds, continued accumulation of ^{3}H within the cell can be accounted for almost entirely by the accumulation of FdUMP. Hence, uptake beyond 20 seconds reflects the rate of phosphorylation of FdUrd to FdUMP and not transport of FdUrd across the cell membrane. (Reproduced with permission from Bowen D et al.: Distinguishing between membrane transport and intracellular metabolism of fluorodeoxyuridine in Ehrlich ascites tumor cells by application of kinetic and high performance liquid chromatographic techniques. J. Biol. Chem. 254:5333–5339, 1979.)

lular drug level falls. As drug influx falls toward the rate of phosphorylation, intracellular free drug cannot be sustained near equilibrium, the free drug level falls, and the rate of metabolism within the cell decreases and ultimately becomes rate-limiting to this process. The more rapid the rate of drug transport into the cell at any given extracellular level, the longer the free intracellular drug level can be sustained at or near equilibrium as the extracellular level declines.

As consider briefly above (p. 26) and in Chapter 10, another metabolic transformation of an antineoplastic agent that has come under increasing scrutiny is the addition of glutamyl moieties to methotrexate to form methotrexate polyglutamates.[85-87, 98-102, 173-176] In this case a biologically active antimetabolite is converted to a derivative that retains the same or a greater ability to interact with the target enzyme dihydrofolate reductase.[103] The formation of these methotrexate derivatives may play an important role in cytotoxicity, selectivity, and apparent methotrexate *cellular* pharmacokinetics *in vivo*. As indicated above (p. 26), methotrexate behaves pharmacologically as a rapidly reversible inhibitor of dihydrofolate reductase, in part because the monoglutamate rapidly leaves the cell as the extracellular level falls. However, the substrate for this enzyme, dihydrofolate, remains within the intracellular compartment, presumably because it is present as a polyglutamate derivative to which the cell membrane has a low level of permeability. If the polyglutamate derivatives of methotrexate that are synthesized within the tumor cell exit from the cell at a much lower rate than the monoglutamate, then as the extracellular methotrexate level falls, the duration over which active free 4-amino antifolates will remain within the cell will be prolonged, increasing the duration of inhibition of the target enzyme.

This metabolic conversion presents the possibility of a number of new elements in drug action. The tumor cell that synthesizes methotrexate polyglutamates most rapidly would be subject to the most prolonged inhibition of enzyme activity; differences in the rates of methotrexate polyglutamate synthesis, cellular catabolism, and rates of efflux of these polyglutamate derivatives between tumor cells and susceptible host tissues may be important determinants of selectivity. Indeed, the accumulation of methotrexate polyglutamates within the cell is associated with a sustained inhibition of thymidylate synthesis and enhanced cytotoxicity.[104, 105] This is probably related to the retention of methotrexate polyglutamate derivatives, but further verification of this relationship is required. Polyglutamate derivatives of methotrexate have been reported to exit rapidly from L1210 leukemia cells,[87, 106] and methotrexate polyglutamates appear in the medium of isolated hepatocytes incubated with the agent.[101] On the other hand, these derivatives accumulate in excess of the dihydrofolate reductase binding capacity in the Ehrlich ascites tumor and are retained within the cell for many hours.[173-174] Likewise, higher polyglutamate forms of methotrexate are retained in human breast cancer cells *in vitro*.[172] A comprehensive analysis of accumulation and exit of the different polyglutamate derivatives of methotrexate will be required, however, to better delineate the transport and pharmacologic role of these metabolites. Further, if some polyglutamate derivatives have a higher affinity for dihydrofolate reductase than methotrexate, this could also be an important element in cytotoxicity and selectivity that will require study. Finally, differences in the rates of formation of polyglutamate derivatives and their cellular efflux among different 4-amino antifolates may be a factor in differences in therapeutic efficacies among these agents. This is an area of antifolate pharmacology that will necessitate considerable additional study to clarify its potential role in drug action.

ROLE OF MEMBRANE TRANSPORT IN CELLULAR RESISTANCE TO ANTINEOPLASTIC AGENTS

Resistance to cytotoxic agents associated with alterations in membrane transport has been firmly established for 4-amino antifolates where transport-related cellular uptake can be clearly distinguished from accumulation of metabolites or binding to dihydrofolate reductase.[31, 65, 66, 75, 107-109] As indicated earlier, it is clear that the drug levels achieved and sustained within tumor cells can be related to pharmacologic activity and cytotoxicity over a broad cell-sensitivity range. Differences in *free* drug levels achieved in tumor cells are largely based on differences in the affinity of the transport carrier for a drug as it mediates entry into the cell.[80] The free drug level, in turn, determines in part the rate and extent of synthesis of methotrexate polyglutamates. In some cases, membrane transport can be so markedly impaired, either owing to deletion of the high-affinity transport carrier or to a marked reduction in affinity for the antifolate,[31, 65] that intracellular drug accumulated may be less than the enzyme binding capacity after brief intervals of exposure to low extracellular levels of this agent.

Cellular resistance to polycyclic compounds such as actinomycin D, daunorubicin, doxorubicin, colchicine, and vinca alkaloids has been associated with decreased net cellular uptake. This has been attributed to impaired transport.[49-51, 110-118, 120, 121] Evidence supporting a transport defect is derived from the following observations:

1. There is a high incidence of cross-resistance among these compounds as well as among vinca alkaloids, puromycin, and other agents.[49-51, 110-118, 120, 121] Because of the diversity of drug structures and actions, cross-resistance appeared to be best explained on the basis of a generalized change in membrane structure that would nonspecifically affect permeation of species transported by passive diffusion. In fact, changes in the lipid composition of resistant tumor cell membranes have been detected that might be expected to cause gross changes in membrane permeability.[50, 122-124]

2. Agents that affect membrane lipid properties and increase membrane permeability, such as amphotericin B and polysorbate 80 (Tween 80), increase the cytotoxicity of these heterocyclic agents in resistant cells.[59-61]

3. Differences in drug metabolism or drug binding to macromolecules in cell-free systems or the intact cell do not appear to explain the differences in cellular uptake.[49, 51, 116, 125] Of particular interest is the suggestion that decreased net accumulation of these agents may be related to the augmentation, or appearance, of an energy-dependent efflux mechanism. Hence, net uptake of daunorubicin is enhanced by metabolic poisons and decreased by glucose substrate in daunorubicin-resistant cells that are cross-resistant to vincristine, vinblastine, and doxorubicin.[49] Likewise, depressed levels of both vincristine and daunorubicin in resistant tumor cells could be increased to those of sensitive cells by inhibitors of anaerobic and aerobic energy metabolism, and markedly reduced by glucose.[49, 51, 125] An energy-dependent process that limits accumulation of daunorubicin and doxorubicin and possibly other polycyclic compounds also appears to play a role in net cellular uptake in sensitive cells, in that inhibitors of energy metabolism increase uptake of these agents in sensitive cells also.[49, 50]

Although it is clear that inhibition of energy metabolism in resistant cells can increase net accumulation of many of these agents, the mechanism by which this occurs has not been firmly established. First, there is no conclusive evidence for a carrier transport mechanism for these compounds. This is due, in part, to experimental difficulties in influx measurements that permit the discrimination of transport across the cell membrane from accumulation of drug bound to intracellular sites.[4] When initial rates were approximated, the data suggested a passive diffusional transport process.[41, 58] The possibility that an exit pump would be linked solely to a unidirectional carrier-mediated flux out of the cell, without any evidence for an inward carrier system, seems unlikely. Further, the net level of these heterocyclic compounds in the cell is influenced by pH,[37] so that alterations in transmembrane pH gradients associated with resistance and changes in energy metabolism might be related, in part, to passive factors (see p. 22). Decreased "retention" of actinomycin D[114, 126] or daunorubicin[127] has been associated with increased resistance to these agents. Although the *rate* of decline of the intracellular drug level as the extracellular levels falls *in vivo* may be influenced by membrane transport, interpretation of these studies with heterocyclic compounds is complicated by the presence of multiple binding sites within the cell.[41] Hence, differences in binding to these sites may be the basis for differences in drug retention and consequent drug sensitivity. Studies on drug binding in cell-free systems have not shown differences between sensitive and resistant tumors,[49, 51, 116, 125] but may not be relevant to binding within the intact cell.

A role for membrane transport in cellular resistance to alkylating agents has also been suggested.[21, 22, 128-131] Resistance has been related to a reduced affinity and transport maximum of the choline carrier for nitrogen mustard in L5178Y lymphoblasts.[131] Likewise, reduced uptake of melphalan has been associated with resistance in L1210 leukemia cells.[21] Of particular interest in the latter study[21] was the observation that transport in resistant and sensitive cells became comparable when one of the transport routes for melphalan in sensitive cells was blocked by a specific inhibitor of the leucine-preferring amino acid transport system, suggesting that impaired transport was related to a defect in only one of several transport routes for melphalan in these cells.

The role of drug transport in resistance to cytotoxic purine and pyrimidine nucleosides is difficult to evaluate because of the experimental difficulties that have confused interpretation of data on radiotracer uptake after exposure of cells to the radiolabeled drug. Figure 2–8A, line 1 simulates the time course of uptake of radiolabel after exposure of cells to a radiolabeled drug such as a purine or pyrimidine base or nucleoside, which is metabolized to a phosphorylated derivative. There is a rapid initial uptake phase, following which net uptake of radiolabel falls to a constant slower rate. The initial linear phase reflects membrane transport; the late linear phase represents the accumulation of phosphorylated metabolites that are retained within the cell. Line 2 simulates the time course of uptake of radiolabeled nucleoside in a cell line that is resistant owing to the loss of a kinase. The initial rate is unchanged; the late phase is eliminated. The uptake process achieves a steady-state in which intracellular drug is at equilibrium with extracellular drug.

Unfortunately, the experimental approach can often be too insensitive to detect and discriminate these two uptake phases; the phase of uptake that represents membrane transport can be overlooked completely. For instance, line 1 of Figure 2–8B illustrates the uptake of the same radiolabeled agent into the sensitive cells with the same transport and metabolic rates, but over a fivefold longer interval than in Figure 2–8A. The rapid uptake phase is not detected because the abscissa and ordinate scales are too insensitive over this interval to discriminate free drug from the total cellular radiolabel. Uptake of radiolabel appears linear and the uptake slope extrapolates through the ordinate at a point indistinguishable from the point of origin. However, this linear uptake phase does not represent the initial rate of transport; rather, it represents the rate of metabolism. In a resistant line in which the kinase is deleted, the initial uptake phase is not detectable at this scale, and "uptake" becomes almost imperceptible, leading to the erroneous conclusion that resistance is due to a permeability defect if cell kinase activity is not specifically evaluated. Hence, deletion or marked reduction in the activity of a kinase or a phosphoribosyltransferase with impaired phosphorylation of a cytotoxic nucleoside or base, respectively, will markedly retard "uptake" of the radiolabeled drug-metabolite without a primary change in transport. However, if the rate of transport in sensitive cells is not sufficiently faster than phosphorylation, the free intracellular drug level will be below equilibrium. Hence, in this situation, deletion of a kinase in a resistant strain will reduce the level of phosphorylated derivatives, but the net free drug level will increase and approach equilibrium. Resistance associated with increased deaminase or phosphorylase activity would also decrease accumulation of the active metabolite. In this case, however, the free intracellular drug level falls as its rate of catabolism is increased without any change in membrane transport.

Finally, the role of drug transport in resistance must be evaluated at drug concentrations relevant to those that characterize the clinical setting. For instance, at high drug levels, a low-affinity (high K_m) transport system[92] may transport drug into the cell much more rapidly than the drug is utilized by high-affinity (low K_m) phosphorylation system,[92] such that a reduction in transport would have little effect on the rate of phosphorylation. On the other hand, nucleoside (ara-C) and base (5-fluorouracil) blood levels fall rapidly with bolus administration or are sustained at relatively low levels during drug infusion, so that the most important phase of the drug-cell exposure might occur when the rate of transport limits the rate of phosphorylation. Hence, when transport is not clearly distinguished from metabolism of a drug, primary changes in transport might not affect intracellular drug accumulation and might not alter drug metabolism at high extracellular levels, but would limit drug availability for metabolism at lower, more relevant concentrations.

Although primary and specific alterations in membrane transport of antineoplastic agents can result in cellular resistance, other primary biochemical alterations that produce resistance may create a condition in

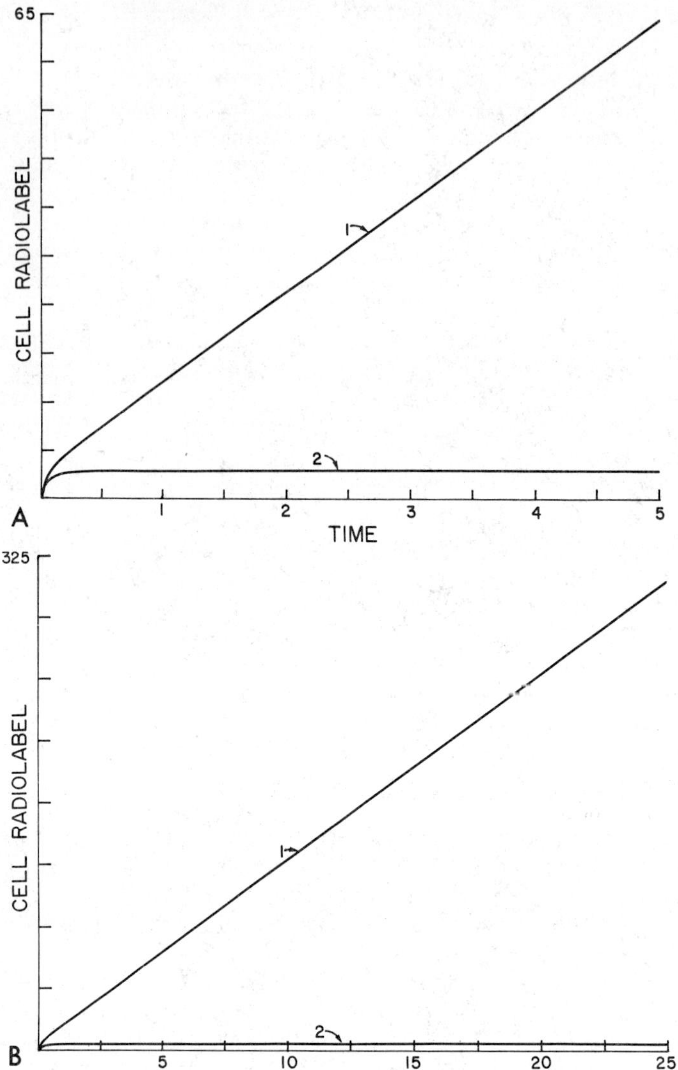

Figure 2–8. *A,* Time course of uptake of radiolabel within cells after exposure of cells to a constant concentration of a radiolabeled drug that is transported very rapidly acorss the cell membrane, followed by a slower rate of phosphorylation to a derivative that does not penetrate the cell membrane (*line 1*). There is an initial rapid appearance of drug within the cell, following which the net uptake velocity falls to a slower but constant rate. The initial linear phase reflects membrane transport; the late linear phase represents the rate of phosphorylation within the cell. Line 2 illustrates a hypothetical resistant line that loses the ability to phosphorylate the drug. The initial rate is unchanged since membrane transport is unchanged; the later linear portion that reflects phosphorylation is eliminated.

B, Data from the same tumor line, but determined over a fivefold longer interval, and plotted with one fifth the sensitivity. Initial rates of uptake that reflect membrane transport are essentially undetectable. The time course of appearance of radiolabel within the sensitive cell (*line 1*) is linear and, experimentally, the ordinate intercept cannot be distinguished from the point of origin. Hence, the assumption is made that this linear phase reflects membrane transport whereas, in fact, it represents not the *initial* linear phase but the *second* linear phase — phosphorylation. "Uptake" in the resistant line that does not phosphorylate the agent (*line 2*) is markedly reduced. giving rise to the erroneous conclusion that this represents impaired transport.

which an unchanged transport system secondarily becomes limiting to the delivery of drug into the cell. When this occurs, resistance may be circumvented if membrane transport can be enhanced, even though impaired membrane transport is not the primary basis for the resistance. For instance, transport of ara-C at high extracellular levels is usually far more rapid than its metabolism to phosphorylated derivatives or its deamination to ara-U in tumor lines in which this has been studied.[91, 92] When enhanced deaminase activity is a basis for resistance to ara-C,[132] this primary enzymatic alteration can only decrease cytotoxicity when it becomes so rapid that drug transport becomes limiting, the free cell ara-C level declines, and the rate of ara-CTP synthesis falls. Since the K_m for the transport systems is high, this is a change that could be circumvented by an increase in the flux of drug into the cell either by an agent that accelerates this process or by an increase in the extracellular drug level, provided these alterations had a selectively greater effect on tumors than normal host cells. Similarly, the effects of agents that enhance the rate of metabolism of a cytotoxic agent to its active metabolites would depend on the relative rates of metabolism versus transport in the specific tumor in which such a manipulation were proposed. For instance, enhancement of ara-CTP synthesis by a variety of agents[91, 133, 134] would depend on the availability of ara-C as substrate, and thus requires a sufficiently high rate of transport to accommodate a higher rate of ara-C phosphorylation. Thymidine enhancement of ara-CTP formation[133-135] also requires that thymidine not perturb ara-C transport as it enters the cell. However, the nucleoside transport systems are relatively unsaturated[91, 92] at the low concentrations of thymidine needed to augment ara-CTP formation and should not appreciably perturb ara-C transport.

Low levels of resistance to methotrexate based on changes in the level of dihydrofolate reductase or the affinity of methotrexate for this enzyme can be circumvented in some cases by increasing the free drug level within the cell. For instance, as the dihydrofolate reductase level in the cell increases, the inhibitory effect of any given intracellular methotrexate level on thymidylate synthesis is reduced,[119] and a greater degree of saturation of enzyme must be achieved by increasing the free intracellular drug level. When this change in resistant cells becomes very great, membrane transport of drug may not provide the levels of intracellular drug required to achieve a pharmacologic effect.

Biochemical changes that make drug transport limiting to drug action, and can be circumvented by enhanced drug transport, may not only involve specific alterations in target enzymes or in drug metabolizing enzyme, but may be related to less specific changes such as alterations in the rate of cell proliferation or the rate of thymidylate synthesis. For instance, resistance to methotrexate has been associated, in part, with decreased thymidylate synthetase activity, and thus decreased need for reduction of dihydrofolate.[119] Similarly, a fluoropyrimidine-induced reduction in the rate of thymidylate synthesis and the rate of dihydrofolate generation decreases the therapeutic efficacy of subsequent added methotrexate.[136] To achieve inhibition of this lower basal rate of enzyme activity requires higher free intracellular methotrexate levels.[39, 137]

APPROACHES TO ENHANCEMENT OF DRUG TRANSPORT

A variety of factors may produce drug resistance. Some specifically relate to impaired drug transport; others relate to alterations in drug catabolism, cell metabolism, or increases in the cell target level that could be minimized if cell transport was enhanced. When influx of the drug limits the rate at which the drug inactivates its target, drug resistance associated with decreased transport or an increased level of the target could be minimized by an increase in the extracellular drug level and duration of exposure to the drug, although this might produce intolerable host toxicity. Similarly, membrane active agents such as polysorbate 80[41, 58, 59] or amphotericin B[60, 61] enhance drug influx, but the applicability of this approach to the treatment of human neoplasms has not been established. When the critical element in drug action relates to the level of free drug that accumulates within the cell and the duration over which this is sustained, a variety of factors may be modulated that may influence these parameters.

The multiple determinants of the free drug level in uphill transport system offer a number of opportunities to modulate this intracellular component. First, the free drug level achieved will be related to the extracellular drug concentration. The higher the latter, the higher the former. However, as indicated above and in Figure 2–2, uphill carriers, unlike equilibrating carriers, only generate some maximal free drug level as the extracellular level is increased. Both the steady-state drug level as well as influx are saturable. Hence, the gradient for free drug falls and can actually reverse as the system becomes saturated. The maximal free intracellular drug level achieved by an uphill carrier system can be increased only if energy coupling to the system is increased, or transport by a low-affinity system or passive diffusion becomes a prominent component of the total fluxes across the cell membrane as the extracellular drug concentration is increased to high levels. Uphill transport of methotrexate into cells appears to be limited by an energy-dependent process that limits the accumulation of free intracellular drug and is inhibited by a variety of metabolic poisons.[10-13] Vinca alkaloids appear to block this process, slowing the rate of drug efflux to increase the free intracellular methotrexate level.[35, 44-47] This vinca-induced augmentation of net methotrexate transport augments methotrexate inhibition of thymidylate synthesis.[47] These agents synergize in mouse systems; this may be based, in part, on this interaction.[46] On the other hand, the provision of energy substrate augments this exit process to reduce the free intracellular methotrexate level.[11, 12] As in the case of methotrexate, net levels of vincristine, daunorubicin, or colchicine are reduced by energy substrate and enhanced by metabolic inhibitors.[48-51] This is especially prominent in resistant cells with depressed net drug accumulation. Uphill transport of melphalan in tumor cells is, in part, sodium-dependent.[18-22] The more active the sodium potassium ATPase, the greater the free drug level that should be achieved in the tumor cell.

Excluding passive gradients for drugs based on pH, molecular charge, and possibly other factors (see below), only uphill carrier systems can achieve sustained intracellular drug levels in excess of the extracellular concentration. The equilibrating carrier or passive diffusion only determines the *rate* at which the intracellular drug level reaches equilibrium or declines as the extracellular level falls. If the bidirectional drug flows are very slow, sufficient free drug may not accumulate to achieve a pharmacologic effect over the interval of exposure to the drug. There are, however, approaches for accelerating carrier flows that might be applied to equilibrating mechanisms. For instance, association of positively charged lipid membrane vesicles (liposomes) with cells can stimulate the *bidirectional* flows of *unencapsulated* methotrexate across the tumor cell membrane, accelerating the rate at which the steady-state is achieved without any change in the intracellular drug level at a steady-state.[52] This appears to be based on a liposome-induced augmentation of the rate of translocation of the transport carrier within the cell membrane. This may be relevant to the recent demonstration of enhanced release of methotrexate from liposomes at the site of tumors, implanted in extremities, induced by local heating of the tumor by microwave and manipulation of the phase-transition properties of the lipid membrane vesicle.[53] In this therapeutic approach the *rate* of transport of methotrexate into cells is a critical element in determining the *rate* at which drug is captured by the tumor cells as it is released from liposomes. Thus, the greater the capture of free drug by the tumor in the "first pass," the less free drug that escapes from the tumor to produce toxicity to host tissues. Hence, the composition of the liposome can influence not only the rate of methotrexate *release* but, to the extent to which the liposome or liposomal lipid can leave the vasculature and associate with the tumor cell membrane, the rate of drug entry and *capture* by the tumor cell. Similarly, alterations in the lipid diet of tumor-bearing mice causes changes in tumor plasma membrane lipid composition and fluidity, and lead to alterations in influx of methotrexate.[54] Insulin, which induces an increase in plasma membrane fluidity, causes a decrease in the influx K_m (an increase in carrier affinity) for methotrexate.[137a]

Equilibrating transport mechanisms can be made to transiently generate gradients. For instance, addition to the extracellular compartment of a physiologic substrate, that shares the same equilibrating carrier as a pharmacologic agent, when cells are at equilibrium with that agent, will result in a transient net uphill flow of the agent *out* of the cell — a "countertransport." Likewise, loading cells with such a substrate could induce a transient uphill flow of drug into the cell.[5, 15, 42] A more sustained uphill transport of adenine into the cell by its equilibrating carrier can be induced by the simultaneous exposure of cells to adenosine.[55] This is based on the following sequence of events. After adenosine is transported into the cell by its nucleoside carrier it is metabolized to inosine, then to hypoxanthine. The latter competes with adenine for exit by their common *base* carrier; the transmembrane concentration gradient for hypoxanthine resulting from its production within the cell produces an asymmetric inhibition of the interaction between adenine and the carrier, resulting in an uphill or asymmetric flow of adenine into the cell.[55] It can readily be seen how the addition of naturally occurring nucleosides along with a cytotoxic base might generate a transmembrane gradient for the agent or how a cytotoxic nucleoside might alter intracellular base levels by such a mechanism.

"Countertransport"-like interactions can also be observed for uphill carriers. Of particular interest is the interaction between methotrexate and leucovorin in "rescue."[56] When the ratio of extracellular leucovorin to methotrexate is high, leucovorin results in a net flow of free methotrexate out of the cell.[10, 14, 56] This perturbation may have important pharmacologic significance in that, with the loss of sufficient free methotrexate from the cell, endogenous cellular tetrahydrofolate synthesis can resume.

Transport fluxes by passive diffusional systems can also be stimulated. For instance, as indicated above, the detergent polysorbate 80 appears to accelerate the flow of actinomycin D across cell membranes.[41, 58, 59] Likewise, enhanced cytotoxicity of heterocyclic agents by amphotericin B has been attributed to accelerated membrane transport.[60, 61] Transmembrane concentration gradients could conceivably be enhanced for charged drugs transported by passive diffusion and equilibrating carriers if appropriate changes in transmembrane electrical-potential differences or pH gradients could be effected.

ROLE OF MEMBRANE TRANSPORT IN "RESCUE" OR "PROTECTION"

The pharmacologic effects of cytotoxic agents may be blocked by either the concurrent or subsequent administration of their naturally occurring counterparts, the synthesis of which is inhibited by the agent, or by other substances. This has been studied in detail for the antifolates. Concurrent administration of leucovorin and methotrexate ("protection") decreases the cytotoxicity of methotrexate; administration of methotrexate followed by leucovorin enhances chemotherapeutic efficacy in experimental systems.[138-149] "Rescue" from the cytotoxic effects of methotrexate is also achieved in clinical regimens by leucovorin,[150-152] although the therapeutic advantage of this approach has not been established. Leucovorin provides a source of tetrahydrofolate cofactor substrate to circumvent the antifolate block[153] and thus, in theory, should reverse methotrexate toxicity noncompetitively. However, under many conditions in which methotrexate and leucovorin are present in the extracellular compartment simultaneously, there are competitive interactions at the level of the common membrane carrier for these compounds that can influence not only the delivery of leucovorin substrate into the cell but also the free intracellular methotrexate level. When leucovorin produces a sufficient reduction in the free intracellular methotrexate level, endogenous cellular tetrahydrofolate synthesis resumes. In fact, some aspects of the competitive nature of leucovorin "rescue" *in vitro*[142, 143, 146] can be explained, at least in part, on the basis of an interaction at the level of a common transport carrier.[10, 56] This is unlike the noncompetitive reversal of methotrexate cytotoxicity by thymidine and purines, which cannot be accounted for on the basis of an interaction between methotrexate and these agents at a common site.[146] It is clear that the addition of tetrahydrofolate cofactors to the extracellular compartment can reverse the inhibitory effect of methotrexate on thymidylate synthesis by inhibition of methotrexate transport with a reduction in the free intracellular methotrexate level. Hence, the unnatural diastereoisomer of 5-methyltetrahydrofolate, which cannot be utilized as substrate to circumvent the methotrexate-induced block in tetrahydrofolate synthesis, inhibits methotrexate influx, decreases the free intracellular methotrexate level, and reverses methotrexate inhibition of thymidylate synthesis.[154, 155]

There is additional evidence that "rescue" cannot be accounted for on the basis of delivery of tetrahydrofolate substrate alone. For instance, the effects of triazinate[156] or the di-*n*-butyl ester of methotrexate[157-159] are only partially reversed by high levels of leucovorin. Since it is likely that these agents are transported largely by passive diffusion, their transport should not be perturbed by leucovorin, and leucovorin transport should be unperturbed by their extracellular presence. This suggests that delivery of leucovorin into the cell alone is not sufficient for "rescue." However, these agents may affect other tetrahydrofolate cofactor-dependent reactions. Finally, high levels of leucovorin do not protect cells from high levels of methotrexate in tumor cells resistant to methotrexate owing to a marked decrease in carrier-mediated transport.[144] While transport rates of both methotrexate and reduced folates are decreased in this tumor line[144] it would be expected, again, that at high leucovorin levels sufficient cofactor would enter the cell by diffusion or a secondary, lower-affinity route[31] to circumvent the block if this were the only element in "rescue." Another potential explanation for the competitive element in "rescue" is the extent to which leucovorin is metabolized to dihydrofolate with competition between methotrexate and dihydrofolate for dihydrofolate reductase.[160]

At this point it is clear that transport interactions occur in "rescue" protocols with methotrexate. However, it is not possible to distinguish between "rescue" (1) due to delivery of tetrahydrofolate substrate, (2) due to generation of dihydrofolate, or (3) due to perturbations of the free intracellular methotrexate level. Further, the effect of the build-up of cellular methotrexate polyglutamate pools in "rescue" protocols is uncertain. Knowledge of transport interactions between methotrexate and leucovorin, however, can be clinically useful since, when appropriate levels of leucovorin relative to methotrexate are present in the extracellular compartment, it should be possible to achieve resumption of endogenous tetrahydrofolate synthesis within the cell if free intracellular methotrexate is eliminated and appreciable levels of methotrexate polyglutamates are not present. This, as well as the build-up of high levels of dihydrofolate polyglutamate, which displace methotrexate from dihydrofolate reductase sites, may be the basis, in part, for the necessity to achieve high extracellular levels of leucovorin to circumvent methotrexate toxicity when excretion of the drug is delayed in high-dose regimens. Hence, clinically, "rescue" is a competitive phenomenon and the blood level of methotrexate will determine the dose of leucovorin required to effect "rescue."[161] The reader is referred to Chapter 10 for a discussion of the clinical use of "rescue" regimens.

The basis for selectivity with high-dose methotrexate-leucovorin "rescue" also is not clear. "Rescue" may be related to differences in the abilities of tumor versus normal susceptible host tissues to utilize leucovorin delivered into the cell. Selective toxicity may relate to the extent to which polyglutamate derivatives of methotrexate are synthesized and retained within the cells. Alternatively, selectivity may be based on differences in methotrexate and leucovorin transport into tumor versus susceptible host tissues. For instance, if the high-affinity methotrexate-tetrahydrofolate cofactor is deleted or undergoes a marked diminution in its affinity for methotrexate and leucovorin in the tumor, a long period of exposure to high levels of methotrexate will be required for drug to reach equilibrium within the tumor cell and to achieve cessation of tetrahydrofolate synthesis. However, as the drug blood level falls, drug exit from the tumor cell may also be reduced, so that drug may persist longer in these cells relative to susceptible host tissues in which transport into and out of the cell may be more rapid. Similarly, as low-dose leucovorin "rescue" is initiated, transport into the tumor cell will be slow while transport into the susceptible host tissues will be more rapid to achieve selective delivery of leucovorin to the latter. Likewise, when the transport occurs largely by passive diffusion, extracellular leucovorin, particularly at low concentrations, would not alter the intracellular methotrexate level to permit resumption of endogenous tetrahydrofolate synthesis. This formulation is supported by the observation that, as expected, leucovorin "rescues" and/or "protects" methotrexate-sensitive tumor cells (in which transport is rapid). However, this occurs to a much lesser extent, or not at all, in drug-resistant cells in which transport of methotrexate and tetrahydrofolate cofactors via their common transport carrier is impaired.[144, 147, 148] Unfortunately, there is little clinical evidence that high-dose methotrexate regimens with leucovorin "rescue" successfully overcome drug resistance.

A similar formulation for selective toxicity and "rescue" could be proposed based on differences in diffusional factors in a tumor mass versus susceptible host tissues. Poor vascularity of the tumor mass increases the distance between the capillary and tumor cells, and may decrease the rate of diffusion of the drug, increasing the time that it takes to reach an extracellular drug concentration in the tumor cell microenvironment comparable with that in the blood. Accordingly, either a higher blood level must be achieved or a lower level sustained over a longer interval to ensure drug equilibrium in the tumor interstitium and accumulation of a critical level of free drug within the tumor cell. However, once sufficient free drug is present within the tumor cell and interstitium, this will persist longer, as the diffusional barrier results in a slower decline in the cell and interstitial drug levels as the extracellular drug concentration falls. On the other hand, in the normal susceptible host tissue, drug should rapidly reach capillary-interstitial equilibrium after drug administration and decline rapidly as the extracellular drug level falls. With "rescue" or "protection," the agent appears much more rapidly in the microenvironment of the well-perfused, normal, susceptible host tissue than in the microenvironment of the tumor cell, providing earlier and more effective "rescue" or "protection" of the former tissue.

There are other examples of "protection" from the effects of antineoplastic agents by the addition of naturally occurring counterparts that compete for a common transport mechanism, or by the addition of other pharmacologic agents that are transport inhibitors. For instance, choline reverses nitrogen mustard cytotoxicity.[162] The concentrations required are high, but the level of intracellular nitrogen mustard sufficient to produce cytotoxicity may be so small that a very marked block of transport is necessary to achieve "protection." Phenylalanine mustard cytotoxicity to murine tumor cells and murine granulocyte colony-forming units *in vitro* can be prevented by the presence of amino acids that block transport of this agent.[32, 163, 164] The diminution of cytotoxicity by "protecting" amino acids can be correlated with the degree of inhibition of drug entry into the cell and the final level of drug accumulated. Finally, various nucleoside transport inhibitors, such as nitrobenzylthioinosine, related compounds, and dipyridamole, "protect" cells against the effects of cytotoxic nucleosides,[165] and there is now evidence that regimens with this agent and cytotoxic nucleosides can provide selective "protection" for host tissue to increase survival of tumor-bearing mice.[177] It is obvious that the pharmacologic effects of any antineoplastic agent that shares a common membrane transport carrier with a naturally occurring substrate can be blocked when the ratio of the competing substrate to the cytotoxic agent is sufficiently high.

MODIFICATION OF DRUG STRUCTURE TO ENHANCE MEMBRANE TRANSPORT

When membrane transport is an important limiting factor in the efficacy of a class of antineoplastic agents, alterations in drug structure to enhance transport should be considered. When the transport system is of an equilibrating type, the modification of structure can only achieve more rapid equilibration of the system. When an equilibrating transport system limits the rate of drug metabolism to active form(s) within the cell, increasing transport by structural modification can increase the level of free drug in the cell toward equilibrium, permitting an accelerated rate of activation. When drug transport is uphill, modification of the drug may permit the generation of enhanced gradients in tumor cells and may increase selectivity in that there may not be a comparable increase in uphill transport in the susceptible host tissues. This has been an area of considerable interest with antifolates because of the role of membrane transport as a factor in cytotoxicity and resistance. New methotrexate analogues have been identified with enhanced transport into tumor cells and increased chemotherapeutic efficacy.[83] As indicated above, a variety of factors limit the accumulation of free methotrexate in tumor cells, in particular the anionic nature of the methotrexate molecule. Hence, alterations in structure that decrease or eliminate the molecular charge and increase lipophilicity have been attempted, not only to augment drug uptake into the tumor but also to augment transport across other compartmental barriers such as the blood-brain barrier. Esterified derivatives of methotrexate have been synthesized[157-159] that produce inhibition of thymidylate synthesis comparable with that of methotrexate in methotrexate-sensitive tumor cells.[159] Since the esters have a lower affinity than methotrexate for dihydrofolate reductase,[158] this action comparable with that of methotrexate may be due to a higher level of accumulation of esterified drug within the intracellular compartment. Of interest is the observation that the di-*n*-butyl ester of methotrexate is a more potent inhibitor of thymidylate synthesis than methotrexate in cells resistant to methotrexate owing to impaired transport.[159] Further evaluation of these compounds will require analysis of their membrane transport properties. Ultimately, their utility *in vivo* may be limited by plasma esterase activity and their rapid 7-hydroxylation.[157]

Another approach has been the synthesis of other 2,4-diamino compounds lacking the benzoylglutamate moiety, such as DDMP.[166]

Although the latter is a less effective inhibitor of dihydrofolate reductase than is methotrexate, DDMP achieves considerably higher intracellular levels than methotrexate[167] and is effective against murine tumors *in vivo* with and without leucovorin "rescue."[168] Although net uptake of DDMP is decreased in cells resistant to methotrexate owing to reduced carrier-mediated methotrexate transport,[145] the cytotoxicity to these cells *in vitro* is somewhat greater than that of methotrexate.[147]

Finally, poly(L-lysine) conjugation of methotrexate is another approach reported to enhance drug uptake into resistant cells, possibly by a pinocytotic mechanism.[169] Similarly, methotrexate covalently linked to proteins retains the same therapeutic efficacy as free methotrexate *in vivo*.[170] Although the data suggest that the complex enters cells by pinocytosis, the determinants of methotrexate action in this drug complex and the possible advantages of such an approach in contrast to that of free methotrexate requires further clarification.

References

1. Stein WD: *In* The Movement of Molecules across Cell Membranes. Academic Press, New York, 1967, pp. 1–35, 65–125.
2. Tsien RW: Ion permeation through membrane channels. *In* Stevens DF (ed.): Membrane Transport Processes, Vol. 3. Raven Press, New York, 1979.
3. Chapman D: Recent physical studies of phospholipids and natural membranes. *In* Chapman D, and Wallach DFH (eds.): Biological Membranes: Physical Fact and Function. Academic Press, New York, 1968.
4. Goldman ID, Bowen D, and Gewirtz DA: Some considerations in the experimental approach to distinguishing between membrane transport and intracellular disposition of antineoplastic agents with specific references to fluorodeoxyuridine, actinomycin D, and methotrexate. Cancer Treat. Rep., in press.
5. Wilbrandt W, and Rosenberg T: The concept of carrier transport and its corollaries in pharmacology. *In* Koelle GB (ed.): Pharmacologic Review. Williams & Wilkins Co., Baltimore, 1961, pp. 109–183.
6. Hladsky SB: *In* Bonner F, and Kleinseller A (eds.): Current Topics in Membranes and Transport, Vol. 12. Academic Press, New York, 1979, pp. 53–164.
7. Patlak CS: Contributions to the theory of active transport: II. The gate type non-carrier mechanism and generalizations concerning tracer flow, efficiency, and measurement of energy expenditure. Bull. Math. Biophys. 19:209–235, 1957.
8. LeFevre PG: The present state of the carrier hypothesis. *In* Bonner F, and Kleinzeller A (eds.): Current Topics in Membranes and Transport, Vol. 7. Academic Press, New York, 1975, pp. 109–215.
9. Dean RB: Theories of electrolyte equilibrium in muscle. Biol. Sym. 3:331–348, 1941.
10. Goldman ID: The characteristics of the membrane transport of amethopterin and the naturally occurring folates. Ann. N.Y. Acad. Sci. 186:400–422, 1971.
11. Goldman ID: Transport energetics of the folic acid analogue, methotrexate, in L1210 leukemia cells. Enhanced accumulation by metabolic inhibitors. J. Biol. Chem. 244:3779–3785, 1969.
12. Fry DW, White JC, and Goldman ID: Effects of 2,4-dinitrophenol and other metabolic inhibitors on the bidirectional carrier fluxes, net transport, and intracellular binding of methotrexate in Ehrlich ascites tumor cells. Cancer Res. 40:3669–3673, 1980.
13. Hakala MT: On the role of drug penetration in amethopterin resistance of sarcoma-180 cells *in vitro*. Biochim. Biophys. Acta 102:198–209, 1965.
14. Goldman ID, Lichtenstein NS, and Oliverio VT: Carrier-mediated transport of the folic acid analogue, methotrexate, in L1210 leukemia cells. J. Biol. Chem. 243:5007–5017, 1968.
15. Goldman ID: Uptake of drugs and resistance. *In* Mihich E (ed.): Drug Resistance and Selectivity: Biochemical and Cellular Basis, Vol. 1. Academic Press, New York, 1973, pp. 299–358.
16. Schafer JA, and Barfuss DW: Mechanisms of transmembrane transport in isolated cells and their experimental study. Pharmacol. Ther. 10:223–260, 1980.
17. Heinz E: Sodium Linked Transport of Organic Solutes. Springer-Verlag, New York, 1972.
18. Vistica DT: Cytotoxicity as an indicator for transport mechanism. Evidence that melphalan is transported by two leucine-preferring carrier systems in the L1210 murine leukemia cell. Biochim. Biophys. Acta 550:300–317, 1979.
19. Goldenberg GJ, Lam HYP, and Begleiter A: Active carrier-mediated transport of melphalan by two separate amino acid transport systems in LPC-1 plasmacytoma cells *in vitro*. J. Biol. Chem. 254:1057–1064, 1979.
20. Begleiter A, Lam HYP, Grover J, et al.: Evidence for active transport of melphalan by two amino carriers in L5178Y lymphoblasts *in vitro*. Cancer Res. 39:353–359, 1979.
21. Redwood WR, and Colvin M: Transport of melphalan by sensitive and resistant L1210 cells. Cancer Res. 40:1144–1149, 1980.
22. Goldenberg GJ, and Begleiter A: Membrane transport of alkylating agents. Pharmacol. Ther. 8:237–274, 1980.
23. Goldman ID: Membrane transport of antifolates as a critical determinant of drug cytotoxicity. *In* Proceedings of the Ninth Rochester International Conference on Environmental Toxicity — Membrane Transport. Plenum Publishing Corp., New York, 1977, pp. 85–113.
24. Jennette JC, and Goldman ID: Inhibition of the membrane transport of folates by anions retained in uremia. J. Lab. Clin. Med. 86:834–843, 1975.
25. Bobzien WF III, and Goldman ID: The mechanism of folate transport in rabbit reticulocytes. J. Clin. Invest. 51:1688–1696, 1972.
26. Christensen HN: Recognition sites for material transport and information transfer. *In* Bonner F, and Kleinzeller A (eds.): Current Topics in Membranes and Transport, Vol. 6. Academic Press, New York, 1975, pp. 227–258.
27. Christensen HN: Amino acid transport systems in animal cells: interactions and energization. J. Supramol. Struct. 6:205–213, 1977.
28. Heichal O, Bibi O, Katz J, et al.: Nucleoside transport in mammalian cell membranes. III. Kinetic and chemical modification studies of cytosine-arabinoside and uridine transport in hamster cells in culture. J. Membrane Biol. 39:133–157, 1978.
29. Kessel D: Transport of a nonphosphorylated nucleoside, 5′-deoxyadenosine, by murine leukemia L1210 cells. J. Biol. Chem. 253:400–403, 1978.
30. Warren RD, Nichols AP, and Bender RA: Membrane transport of methotrexate in human lymphoblastoid cells. Cancer Res. 38:668–671, 1978.
31. Hill BT, Bailey BD, White JC, et al.: Characteristics of transport of 4-amino antifolates and folate compounds by two lines of L5178Y lymphoblasts, one with impaired transport of methotrexate. Cancer Res. 39:2440–2446, 1979.
32. Vistica DT: Cytotoxicity as an indicator for transport

mechanism: evidence that murine bone marrow progenitor cells lack a high-affinity leucine carrier which transports melphalan in murine L1210 leukemia cells. Blood 56:427–429, 1980.

33. Arndt RA, and Roper LD: Simple membrane electrodiffusion theory. *In* Physical Biological Sciences Misc., Blacksburg, VA, 1972.
34. Baur H, Kasperak S, and Pfaff E: Criteria of variability of isolated liver cells. Hoppe-Seyler's Z. Physiol. Chem. 356:827–838, 1975.
35. Goldman ID, Gupta V, White JC, et al.: Exchangeable intracellular methotrexate levels in the presence and absence of vincristine at extracellular drug concentrations relevant to those achieved in high-dose methotrexate-folinic acid "rescue" protocols. Cancer Res. 36:276–279, 1976.
36. Jollow DJ, and Brodie BB: Mechanisms of drug absorption and of drug solution. Pharmacology, 8:21–32, 1972.
37. Skovsgaard T: Transport and binding of daunorubicin, adriamycin, and rubidazone in Ehrlich ascites tumor cells. Biochem. Pharmacol. 26:215–222, 1977.
38. Lutz RJ, Dedrick RL, and Zaharko DS: Physiological pharmacokinetics: an *in vivo* approach to membrane transport. Pharmacol. Ther. 11:559–592, 1980.
39. Jackson RC, and Harrap KR: Studies with a mathematical model of folate metabolism. Arch. Biochem. Biophys. 158:827–841, 1973.
40. Kessel D, Myers M, and Wodinsky I: Accumulation of two alkylating agents, nitrogen mustard and busulfan, by murine leukaemia cells *in vitro*. Biochem. Pharmacol. 18:1229–1234, 1969.
41. Bowen D, and Goldman ID: The relationship among transport, intracellular binding, and inhibition of RNA synthesis by actinomycin D in Ehrlich ascites tumor cells *in vitro*. Cancer Res. 35:3054–3060, 1975.
42. Bowen D, Diasio RB, and Goldman ID: Distinguishing between membrane transport and intracellular metabolism of fluorodeoxyuridine in Ehrlich ascites tumor cells by application of kinetic and high performance liquid chromatographic techniques. J. Biol. Chem. 254:5333–5339, 1979.
43. Müller W, and Crothers DM: Studies of the binding of actinomycin and related compounds to DNA. J. Mol. Biol. 35:251–290, 1968.
44. Zager RF, Frisby SA, and Oliverio VT: The effects of antibiotics and cancer chemotherapeutic agents on the cellular transport and antitumor activity of methotrexate in L1210 murine leukemia. Cancer Res. 33:1670–1676, 1973.
45. Fyfe MJ, and Goldman ID: Characteristics of the vincristine-induced augmentation of methotrexate uptake in Ehrlich ascites tumor cells. J. Biol. Chem. 248:5067–5073, 1973.
46. Chello PL, Sirotnak FM, and Dorick DM: Different effects of vincristine on methotrexate uptake of L1210 cells and mouse intestinal epithelia *in vitro* and *in vivo*. Cancer Res. 39:2106–2112, 1979.
47. Goldman ID, and Fyfe MJ: The mechanisms of action of methotrexate. II. Augmentation by vincristine of inhibition of deoxyribonucleic acid synthesis by methotrexate in Ehrlich ascites tumor cells. Mol. Pharmacol. 10:275–282, 1974.
48. Skovsgaard T: Carrier-mediated transport of daunorubicin, adriamycin, and rubidazone in Ehrlich ascites tumor cells. Biochem. Pharmacol. 27:1221–1227, 1978.
49. Skovsgaard T: Mechanism of cross-resistance between vincristine and daunorubicin in Ehrlich ascites tumor cells. Cancer Res. 38:4722–4727, 1978.
50. Ling V: Drug resistance and membrane alteration in mutants of mammalian cells. Can. J. Genet. Cytol. 17:503–515, 1975.
51. Dano K: Active outward transport of daunomycin in resistant Ehrlich ascites tumor cells. Biochim. Biophys. Acta 323:466–483, 1973.
52. Fry, DW, White JC, and Goldman ID: Alterations of the carrier-mediated transport of an anionic solute, methotrexate, by charged liposomes in Ehrlich ascites tumor cells. J. Membrane Biol. 50:123–140, 1979.
53. Weinstein JN, Magin RL, Yatvin MB, et al.: Liposomes and local hyperthermia: selective delivery of methotrexate to heated tumors. Science 204:188–191, 1979.
54. Burns CP, Luttenegger DG, Dudley DT, et al: Effect of modification of plasma membrane fatty acid composition of fluidity and methotrexate transport in L1210 murine leukemia cells. Cancer Res. 39:1726–1732, 1979.
55. Cybulski RL, Fry DW, and Goldman ID: Adenosine stimulation of uphill adenine transport in L1210 leukemia cells. Evidence for a novel countertransport mechanism. J. Biol. Chem. 256:4455–4459, 1981.
56. Goldman ID: Membrane transport of methotrexate (NSC-740) and other folate compounds: relevance to rescue protocols. Cancer Chemother. Rep. 6:63–72, 1975.
57. Sirotnak FM, and Donsbach RC: Biochemical and pharmacokinetic effects of leucovorin after high-dose methotrexate in a murine leukemia model. Cancer Res. 36:4679–4686, 1976.
58. Polet H: Role of the cell membrane in the uptake of ^{3}H-actinomycin D by mammalian cells *in vitro*. J. Pharmacol. Exp. Ther. 192:270–279, 1975.
59. Riehm H, and Biedler JL: Potentiation of drug effect by Tween 80 in Chinese hamster cells resistant to actinomycin D and daunomycin. Cancer Res. 32:1195–1200, 1972.
60. Medoff J, Medoff G, Goldstein MN, et al.: Amphotericin B-induced sensitivity to actinomycin D in drug-resistant HeLa cells. Cancer Res. 35:2548–2552, 1975.
61. Valeriote F, Medoff G, and Dieckman J: Potentiation of anticancer agent cytotoxicity against sensitive and resistant AKR leukemia by amphotericin B. Cancer Res. 39:2041–2045, 1979.
62. Peters JM, and Greenberg DM: Studies on folic acid reduction. Biochim. Biophys. Acta 32:273–274, 1959.
63. Werkheiser WC: Specific binding of 4-amino folic acid analogues by folic acid reductase. J. Biol. Chem. 236:888–893, 1961.
64. Werkheiser WC: Limitations on the therapeutic effectiveness of the folic acid antagonists. Cancer Res. 25:1608–1613, 1965.
65. Fischer GA: Defective transport of amethopterin (methotrexate) as a mechanism of resistance to the antimetabolite in L5178Y leukemia cells. Biochem. Pharmacol. 11:1233–1234, 1962.
66. Kessel D, Hall TC, and Roberts DW: Uptake as a determinant of methotrexate response in mouse leukemia. Science 150:752–754, 1965.
67. Goldman ID: The mechanism of action of methotrexate. I. Interaction with a low-affinity intracellular site required for maximum inhibition of deoxyribonucleic acid synthesis in L-cell mouse fibroblasts. Mol. Pharmacol. 10:257–274, 1974.
68. White JC, Loftfield S, and Goldman ID: The mechanism of action of methotrexate. III. Requirements of free intracellular methotrexate for maximal suppression of [^{14}C] formate incorporation into nucleic acids and protein. Mol. Pharmacol. 11:287–297, 1975.
69. White JC, and Goldman ID: The mechanism of action of methotrexate. IV. Free intracellular methotrexate required to suppress dihydrofolate reduction to tetrahydrofolate by Ehrlich ascites tumor cells *in vitro*. Mol. Pharmacol. 12:711–719, 1976.
70. Goldman ID: Analysis of the cytotoxic determinants for methotrexate (NSC-740): a role for "free" intracellular drug. Cancer Chemother. Rep. 6:51–61, 1975.
71. Goldman ID: Effects of methotrexate on cellular metabolism: some critical elements in the drug-cell interaction. Cancer Treat. Rep. 61:549–558, 1977.
72. Sirotnak FN, and Donsbach RC: The intracellular concentration dependence of antifolate inhibition of DNA synthesis in L1210 leukemia cells. Cancer Res. 34:3332–3340, 1974.
73. Chabner BA, and Young RC: Threshold methotrexate concentration for *in vivo* inhibition of DNA synthesis in normal and tumorous target tissues. J. Clin. Invest. 52:1804–1811, 1973.
74. Sirotnak FM, and Donsbach RC: Differential cell perme-

ability and the basis for selective activity of methotrexate during therapy of the L1210 leukemia. Cancer Res. 33:1290–1294, 1973.

75. Sirotnak FM: Correlates of folate analog transport, pharmacokinetics and selective antitumor action. Pharmacol. Ther. 8:71–103, 1980.
76. Jackson RC, Niethammer D, and Hart LI: Reactivation of dihydrofolate reductase inhibited by methotrexate or aminopterin. Arch. Biochem. Biophys. 182:646–656, 1977.
77. Zaharko DS, Fung WP, and Yang KH: Relative biochemical aspects of low and high doses of methotrexate in mice. Cancer Res. 37:1602–1607, 1977.
78. White JC: Reversal of methotrexate binding to dihydrofolate reductase by dihydrofolate. Studies with pure enzyme and computer modeling using network thermodynamics. J. Biol. Chem. 254:10889–10895, 1979.
79. Sirotnak FM, and Donsbach RC: Further evidence for a basis of selective activity and relative responsiveness during antifolate therapy of murine tumors. Cancer Res. 35:1737–1744, 1975.
80. Sirotnak FM, and Donsbach RC: Kinetic correlates of methotrexate transport and therapeutic responsiveness in murine tumors. Cancer Res. 36:1151–1158, 1976.
81. Sirotnak FM, and Moccio DM: Pharmacokinetic basis for differences in methotrexate sensitivity of normal proliferative tissues in the mouse. Cancer Res. 40:1230–1234, 1980.
82. Sirotnak FM, and Donsbach RC: Tissue pharmacokinetics, inhibition of DNA synthesis, and tumor cell kill after high-dose methotrexate in murine tumor models. Cancer Res. 36:4672–4678, 1976.
83. Chello PL, Sirotnak FM, Dorick DM, et al.: Therapeutic relevance of differences in the structural specificity of the transport system for folate analogs in L1210 tumor cells and in isolated murine intestinal epithelial cells. Cancer Res. 37:4297–4303, 1977.
84. Sirotnak FM, and Donsbach RC: A basis for the difference in toxicity of methotrexate, aminopterin and methasquin in mice. Biochem. Pharmacol. 24:156–158, 1975.
85. Baugh CM, Krumdieck CL, and Nair MG: Polygammaglutamyl metabolites of methotrexate. Biochem. Biophys. Res. Commun. 52:27–34, 1973.
86. Whitehead VM, Perrault MM, and Stelcner S: Tissue-specific synthesis of methotrexate polyglutamates in the rat. Cancer Res. 35:2985–2990, 1975.
87. Poser RG, Sirotnak FM, and Chello PL: Extracellular recovery of methotrexate-polyglutamates following efflux from L1210 leukaemia cells. Biochem. Pharmacol. 29:2701–2704, 1980.
88. Plagemann PGW, and Richey DP: Transport of nucleosides, nucleic acid bases, choline and glucose by animal cells in culture. Biochim. Biophys. Acta 344:263–305, 1974.
89. Wohlhueter RM, Marz R, Graff JC, et al.: The application of rapid kinetic techniques to the transport of thymidine and 3-0-methyl-glucose into mammalian cells in suspension culture. Cell. Physiol. 89:605–612, 1976.
90. Rozengurt E, Stein WD, and Wigglesworth NM: Uptake of nucleosides in density-inhibited cultures of 3T3 cells. Nature 267:442–444, 1977.
91. Plagemann PGW, Marz R, and Wohlhueter RM: Transport and metabolism of deoxycytidine and 1-β-D-arabinofuranosylcytosine into cultured Novikoff rat hepatoma cells, relationship to phosphorylation, and regulation of triphosphate synthesis. Cancer Res. 38:978–989, 1978.
92. Koren R, Shohami E, and Yeroushalmi S: A kinetic analysis of the uptake of cytosine-β-D-arabinoside by rat-B77 cells. Differentiation between transport and phosphorylation. Eur. J. Biochem. 95:333–339, 1979.
93. Marz R, Wohlhueter RM, and Plagemann PGW: Purine and pyrimidine transport and phosphoribosylation and their interaction in overall uptake by cultured mammalian cells. J. Biol. Chem. 254:2329–2338, 1979.
94. Wohlhueter RM, McIvor RS, and Plagemann PGW: Facilitated transport of uracil and 5-fluorouracil, and permeation of orotic acid into cultured mammalian cells. J. Cell. Physiol. 104:309–319, 1980.
95. Rustum YM, Danhauser L, and Wang G: Selectivity of action of 5-FU: biochemical basis. Bull. Cancer 66:43–47, 1979.
96. Mandel HG, Klubes P, and Fernandes DJ: Studies of the antitumor action of 5-fluorouracil (FU). Bull. Cancer 66:49–54, 1979.
97. Rustum YM: Metabolism and intracellular retention of 1-β-D-arabinofuranosylcytosine as predictors of response of animal tumors. Cancer Res. 38:543–549, 1978.
98. Shin YS, Buehring KU, and Stokstad ELR: The metabolism of methotrexate in *Lactobacillus casei* and rat liver and the influence of methotrexate on metabolism of folic acid. J. Biol. Chem. 249:5772–5777, 1974.
99. Rosenblatt DS, Whitehead VM, Dupont MM, et al.: Synthesis of methotrexate polyglutamates in cultured human cells. Mol. Pharmacol. 14:210–214, 1978.
100. Galivan J: Transport and metabolism of methotrexate in normal and resistant cultured rat hepatoma cells. Cancer Res. 39:735–743, 1979.
101. Gewirtz DA, White JC, Randolph JK, et al.: Formation of methotrexate polyglutamates in rat hepatocytes. Cancer Res. 39:2914–2918, 1979.
102. Whitehead VM: Synthesis of methotrexate polyglutamates in L1210 murine leukemia cells. Cancer Res. 37:408–412, 1977.
103. Jacobs SA, Adamson RH, Chabner BA, et al.: Stoichiometric inhibition of mammalian dihydrofolate reductase by the γ-glutamyl metabolite of methotrexate, 4-amino-4-deoxy-N^{10}-methylpteroylglutamyl-γ-glutamate. Biochem. Biophys. Res. Commun. 63:692–698, 1975.
104. Rosenblatt DS, Whitehead VM, Vera N, et al.: Prolonged inhibition of DNA synthesis associated with the accumulation of methotrexate polyglutamates by cultured human cells. Mol. Pharmacol. 14:1143–1147, 1978.
105. Galivan J: Evidence for the cytotoxic activity of polyglutamate derivatives of methotrexate. Mol. Pharmacol. 17:105–110, 1980.
106. Sirotnak FM, Chello PL, Piper JR, et al.: Growth inhibitory, transport and biochemical properties of the γ-glutamyl and γ-aspartyl peptides of methotrexate in L1210 leukemia cells *in vitro*. Biochem. Pharmacol. 27:1821–1825, 1978.
107. Sirotnak FM, Kurita S, and Hutchison DJ: On the nature of a transport alteration resistance to amethopterin in the L1210 leukemia. Cancer Res. 28:75–80, 1968.
108. Niethammer D, and Jackson RC: Changes of molecular properties associated with the development of resistance against methotrexate in human lymphoblastoid cells. Eur. J. Cancer 11:845–854, 1975.
109. Jackson RC, Niethammer D, and Huennekens FM: Enzymic and transport mechanisms of amethopterin resistance in L1210 mouse leukaemia cells. Cancer Biochem. Biophys. 1:151–155, 1975.
110. Goldstein MN, Hamm K, and Amrod E: Incorporation of tritiated actinomycin D into drug-sensitive and drug-resistant HeLa cells. Science 151:1555–1556, 1966.
111. Biedler JL, and Riehm H: Cellular resistance to actinomycin D in Chinese hamster cells *in vitro*: cross-resistance, radioautographic, and cytogenetic studies. Cancer Res. 30:1174–1184, 1970.
112. Riehm H, and Biedler JL: Cellular resistance to daunomycin in Chinese hamster cells. Cancer Res. 31:409–412, 1971.
113. Cremisi C, Sonenshein GE, and Tournier P: Studies on the mechanism of actinomycin D resistance of an SV 40-transformed hamster cell line. Exp. Cell Res. 89:89–94, 1974.
114. Inaba M, and Johnson RK: Decreased retention of actinomycin D as the basis for cross-resistance in anthracycline-resistant sublines of P388 leukemia. Cancer Res. 37:4629–4634, 1977.
115. Peterson RHF, O'Neil JA, and Biedler JL: Some biochemi-

cal properties of Chinese hamster cells sensitive and resistant to actinomycin D. J. Cell Biol. 63:773–779, 1974.

116. Inaba M, and Johnson RK: Uptake and retention of adriamycin and daunorubicin by sensitive and anthracycline-resistant sublines of P388 leukaemia. Biochem. Pharmacol. 27:2123–2130, 1978.

117. Dano K: Development of resistance to daunomycin (NSC-82151) in Ehrlich ascites tumor. Cancer Chemother. Rep. 55:133–141, 1971.

118. Dano K: Development of resistance to adriamycin (NSC-123127) in Ehrlich ascites tumor *in vivo*. Cancer Chemother. Rep. 56:321–326, 1972.

119. White JC, and Goldman ID: Methotrexate resistance in an L1210 cell line resulting from increased dihydrofolate reductase, decreased thymidylate synthetase activity, and normal membrane transport. J. Biol. Chem. 256:5722–5727, 1981.

120. Dano K: Cross-resistance between vinca alkaloids and anthracyclines in Ehrlich ascites tumor *in vivo*. Cancer Chemother. Rep. 56:701–708, 1972.

121. Biedler JL, Riehm H, Peterson RHF, et al.: Membrane-mediated drug resistance and phenotypic reversion to normal growth behavior of Chinese hamster cells. J. Natl. Cancer Inst. 55:671–680, 1975.

122. Bosmann NB: Mechanism of cellular drug resistance. Nature 233:566–569, 1971.

123. Peterson RHF, and Biedler JL: Plasma membrane proteins and glycoproteins from Chinese hamster cells sensitive and resistant to actinomycin D. J. Supramol. Struct. 9:289–298, 1978.

124. Juliano R, Ling V, and Graves J: Drug-resistant mutants of Chinese hamster ovary cells possess an altered cell surface carbohydrate component. J. Supramol. Struct. 4:521–526, 1976.

125. Skovsgaard T: Mechanisms of resistance to daunorubicin in Ehrlich ascites tumor cells. Cancer Res. 38:1785–1791, 1978.

126. Kessel D, and Wodinsky I: Uptake *in vivo* and *in vitro* of actinomycin D by mouse leukaemias as factors in survival. Biochem. Pharmacol. 17:161–164, 1968.

127. Kessel D, Botterill V, and Wodinsky I: Uptake and retention of daunomycin by mouse leukemia cells as factors in drug response. Cancer Res. 28:938–941, 1968.

128. Rutman RJ, Chun EHL, and Lewis FS: Permeability difference as a source of resistance to alkylating agents in Ehrlich tumor cells. Biochem. Biophys. Res. Commun. 32:650–657, 1968.

129. Wolpert MK, and Ruddon RW: A study on the mechanism of resistance to nitrogen mustard (HN2) in Ehrlich ascites tumor cells: comparison of uptake of HN2-^{14}C into sensitive and resistant cells. Cancer Res. 29:873–879, 1969.

130. Goldenberg GJ, Lyons RM, Lepp JA, et al.: Sensitivity to nitrogen mustard as a function of transport activity and proliferative rate in L5178Y lymphoblasts. Cancer Res. 31:1616–1619, 1971.

131. Goldenberg GJ, Vanstone GL, Israels LG, et al.: Evidence for a transport carrier of nitrogen mustard in nitrogen mustard-sensitive and -resistant L5178Y lymphoblasts. Cancer Res. 30:2285–2291, 1970.

132. Stewart CD, and Burke PJ: Cytidine deaminase and the development of resistance to arabinosyl cytosine. Nature [New Biol.] 233:109–110, 1971.

133. Jackson RC: The regulation of thymidylate biosynthesis in Novikoff hepatoma cells and the effects of amethopterin, 5-fluorodeoxyuridine, and 3-deazauridine. J. Biol. Chem. 253:7440–7446, 1978.

134. Harris AW, Reynolds EC, and Finch LR: Effect of thymidine on the sensitivity of cultured mouse tumor cells to 1-β-D-arabinofuranosylcytosine. Cancer Res. 39:538–541, 1979.

135. Danhauser LL, and Rustum YM: Effect of thymidine on the toxicity, antitumor activity, and metabolism of 1-β-D-arabinofuranosylcytosine in rats bearing a chemically induced colon carcinoma. Cancer Res. 40:1274–1280, 1980.

136. Bertino JR, Sawicki WL, Lindquist CA, et al.: Schedule-dependent antitumor effects of methotrexate and 5-fluorouracil. Cancer Res. 37:327–328, 1977.

137. Bowen D, White JC, and Goldman ID: A basis for fluoropyrimidine-induced antagonism to methotrexate in Ehrlich ascites tumor cells *in vitro*. Cancer Res. 38:219–222, 1978.

137a. Schilsky RL, Bailey BD, and Chabner BA: Characteristics of membrane transport of methotrexate by cultured human breast cancer cells. Biochem. Pharmacol. 30:1537–1542, 1981.

138. Goldin A, Mantel N, Venditti JM, et al.: An analysis of dose-response for animals treated with aminopterin and citrovorum factor. J. Natl. Cancer Inst. 13:1463–1471, 1953.

139. Goldin A, Mantel N, Greenhouse SW, et al.: Effect of delayed administration of citrovorum factor on the antileukemia effectiveness of aminopterin in mice. Cancer Res. 14:43–48, 1954.

140. Goldin A, Venditti JM, Humphreys SR, et al.: Studies on the management of mouse leukemia (L1210) with antagonists of folic acid. Cancer Res. 15:724–747, 1955.

141. Goldin A, Venditti JM, Kline I, et al.: Eradication of leukaemic cells (L1210) by methotrexate and methotrexate plus citrovorum factor. Nature 212:1548–1550, 1966.

142. Borsa J, and Whitmore GF: Studies relating to the mode of action of methotrexate. II. Studies on sites of action in L-cells *in vitro*. Mol. Pharmacol. 5:303–317, 1969.

143. Borsa J, and Whitmore GF: Studies relating to the mode of action of methotrexate. III. Inhibition of thymidylate synthetase in tissue culture cells and in cell-free systems. Mol. Pharmacol. 5:318–332, 1969.

144. Goldie JH, Harrison SI, Price LA, et al.: Impaired responsiveness to folinic acid protection in methotrexate-resistant L5178Y cells. Eur. J. Cancer 11:627–632, 1975.

145. Hill BT, Price LA, and Goldie JH: Methotrexate resistance and uptake of DDMP by L5178Y cells. Selective protection with folinic acid. Eur. J. Cancer 11:545–554, 1975.

146. Pinedo HM, Zaharko DS, Bull JM, et al.: The reversal of methotrexate cytotoxicity to the mouse bone marrow cells by leucovorin and nucleosides. Cancer Res. 36:4418–4424, 1976.

147. Hill BT, Price LA, Harrison SI, et al.: The difference between "selective folinic acid protection" and "folinic acid rescue" in L5178Y cells culture. Eur. J. Cancer 13:861–871, 1977.

148. Groff JP, and Blakley RL: Rescue of human lymphoid cells from the effects of methotrexate *in vitro*. Cancer Res. 38:3847–3853, 1978.

149. Sirotnak FM, Moccio DM, and Dorick DM: Optimization of high-dose methotrexate with leucovorin rescue therapy in the L1210 leukemia and sarcoma 180 murine tumor models. Cancer Res. 38:345–353, 1978.

150. Capizzi RL, DeConti RC, Marsh JC, et al.: Methrotrexate therapy of head and neck cancer: improvement in therapeutic index by the use of leucovorin "rescue." Cancer Res. 30:1782–1788, 1970.

151. Pratt CB, Roberts DW, Shanks EC, et al.: Clinical trials and pharmacokinetics of intermittent high-dose methotrexate-"leucovorin rescue" for children with malignant tumors. Cancer Res. 34:3326–3331, 1974.

152. Levitt M, Mosher MB, DeConti RC, et al.: Improved therapeutic index of methotrexate with "leucovorin rescue." Cancer Res. 33:1729–1734, 1973.

153. Werkheiser WC: The biochemical, cellular, and pharmacologic action and effects of the folic acid antagonists. Cancer Res. 23:1277–1285, 1963.

154. White JC, Bailey BD, and Goldman ID: Lack of stereospecificity at carbon 6 of methyltetrahydrofolate transport in Ehrlich ascites tumor cells. J. Biol. Chem. 253:242–245, 1978.

155. White JC, and Goldman ID: Lack of stereospecificity at carbon 6 of methyltetrahydrofolate transport: possible relevance to rescue regimens with methotrexate and leucovorin. *In* Kisliuk RL, and Brown GM (eds.): Chemistry and Biology of Pteridines. Elsevier North Holland, New York, 1979.

156. Skeel RT, Sawicki WL, Cashmore AR, et al.: The basis for the disparate sensitivity of L1210 leukemia and Walker 256 carcinoma to a new triazine folate antagonist. Cancer Res. 33:2972–2976, 1973.
157. Johns DG, Farquhar D, Wolpert MK, et al.: Dialkyl esters of methotrexate and 3′,5′-dichloromethotrexate: synthesis and interaction with aldehyde oxidase and dihydrofolate reductase. Drug Metab. Dispos. 1:580–589, 1973.
158. Johns DG, Farquhar D, Chabner BA, et al.: Effect of carboxyl group esterification of methotrexate on its properties as an inhibitor of dihydrofolate reductase and a substrate for aldehyde oxidase. Biochem. Soc. Trans. 2:602–604, 1974.
159. Curt GA, Tobias JS, Kramer RA, et al.: Inhibition of nucleic acid synthesis by the di-*n*-butyl ester of methotrexate. Biochem. Pharmacol. 25:1943–1946, 1976.
160. Moran RG, Mulkins M, and Heidelberger C: Role of thymidylate synthetase activity in development of methotrexate cytotoxicity. Proc. Natl. Acad. Sci. USA 76:5924–5928, 1979.
161. Bertino JR: "Rescue" techniques in cancer chemotherapy: use of leucovorin and other rescue agents after methotrexate treatment. Semin. Oncol. 4:203–216, 1977.
162. Goldenberg GJ, and Sinha BK: Protection of L5178Y lymphoblasts by choline and ethanolamine against cytocidal effect of nitrogen mustard *in vitro*. Cancer Res. 33:1253–1257, 1973.
163. Vistica DT, Rabon A, and Rabinovitz M: Amino acid conferred protection against melphalan: comparison of amino acids which reduce melphalan toxicity to murine bone marrow precursor cells (CFU-C) and murine L1210 leukemia cells. Res. Commun. Chem. Pathol. Pharmacol. 23:171–183, 1979.
164. Vistica DT, Toal JN, and Rabinovitz M: Amino acid conferred protection against melphalan: interference with leucine protection of melphalan cytotoxicity by the basic amino acids in cultured murine L1210 leukemia cells. Mol. Pharmacol. 14:1136–1142, 1978.
165. Paterson ARP, Kolassa N, and Cass CE: Transport of nucleoside drugs in animal cells. Pharmacol. Ther. 12:515–536, 1981.
166. Clarke DA, Buckley SM, Sternberg SS, et al.: Effects of 2,4-diaminopyrimidines on mouse sarcoma 180. Cancer Res. 12:255, 1952.
167. Hill BT, Price LA, Harrison SI, et al.: Studies on the transport and distribution of diaminopyrimidines in L5178Y lymphoblasts in cell culture. Biochem. Pharmacol. 24:535–538, 1975.
168. Sirotnak FM, Dorick DM, and Moccio DM: Experimental chemotherapy with 5-arylpyrimidine antifolates: preliminary studies of toxicity and responsiveness of sarcoma 180 to DDMP (NSC-19494) and DDMP with citrovorum factor (NSC-3590). Cancer Treat. Rep. 60:547–553, 1976.
169. Ryser HJP, and Shen WC: Conjugation of methotrexate to poly(L-lysine) increases drug transport and overcomes drug resistance in cultured cells. Proc. Natl. Acad. Sci. USA 75:3867–3870, 1978.
170. Chu BCF, and Whitley JM: The interaction of carrier-bound methotrexate with L1210 cells. Mol. Pharmacol. 17:382–387, 1980.
171. White JC, and Mikulecky DC: Application of network thermodynamics to the computer modeling of the pharmacology of anticancer agents: a network model for methotrexate action as a comprehensive example. *In* Goldman ID (ed.): Pharmacology and Therapeutics. The International Encyclopedia of Pharmacology and Therapeutics. Pergamon Press, New York, in press.
172. Schilsky RL, Bailey BD, and Chabner BA: Methotrexate polyglutamate synthesis by cultured human breast cancer cells. Proc. Natl. Acad. Sci. USA 77:2919–2922, 1980.
173. Fry DW, Yalowich JC, Hess ML, et al.: Intracellular synthesis and disposition of polygammaglutamyl derivatives of the folic acid analog, methotrexate, in Ehrlich ascites tumor cells *in vitro*. Fed. Proc. 40:1748, 1981.
174. Yalowich JC, Fry DW, and Goldman ID: Rapid accumulation of methotrexate polyglutamates in Ehrlich ascites tumor cells *in vitro*: a marked augmentation by vincristine. Proc. Am. Assoc. Cancer Res. 22:207, 1981.
175. Gewirtz DA, Randolph JK, and Goldman ID: Potent bile salt and organic anion inhibition of methotrexate uptake and accumulation in the freshly isolated rat hepatocyte. Cancer Res. 40:1852–1857, 1980.
176. Witte A, Whitehead VM, Rosenblatt DS, et al.: Synthesis of methotrexate polyglutamates by bone marrow cells from patients with leukemia and lymphoma. Dev. Pharmacol. Ther. 1:40–46, 1980.
177. Lynch TP, Paran JH, and Paterson ARP: Therapy of mouse leukemia L1210 with combinations of nebularine and nitrobenzylthioinosine 5′-monophosphate. Cancer Res. 41:560–565, 1981.

CELL KINETICS

3

Stanley E. Shackney
Paul S. Ritch

INTRODUCTION

The field of cell kinetics is concerned with quantitative aspects of the growth behavior of normal and malignant cell populations. Cell proliferative characteristics play an important role in determining whether exposure to cytotoxic drugs will result in a lethal outcome. Cytotoxic drugs also produce transient changes in the proliferative behavior of normal and malignant cells, changes that may affect the outcome of subsequent therapy. Because of the interrelationships between cell proliferative behavior and the effects of drugs on cell survival, the pharmacologist often finds himself dealing with issues that generally fall within the purview of the field of cell kinetics when he wishes to use pharmacologic principles in the treatment of cancer.

Example 1. Johnson et al.[1] have reported that growing 3T6 mouse fibroblast cells exposed to methotrexate were subject to time-dependent and dose-dependent lethality. More than 95 per cent of such cells were killed following exposure to MTX at a concentration of 1×10^{-6}M for 24 hours. In contrast, resting 3T6 cells showed no loss of cloning efficiency even after exposure to MTX at concentrations of 1×10^{-3}M for as long as seven days. This resistance was shown not to be due to a defect in drug transport since MTX was taken up by both growing and resting cells. Furthermore, intracellular dihydrofolate reductase activity was abolished in both growing and resting cells at similar extracellular MTX concentrations. To explain their findings, the authors claimed that resting 3T6 cells do not traverse the cell cycle and therefore should be resistant to thymidine starvation induced by methotrexate. They noted that, in other published studies, starving or stationary phase cells *were* killed by MTX, and suggested that starving cells traverse the cell cycle slowly, while their 3T6 cells were in a truly quiescent "G_0" state.

Here is a concrete example of the importance of cell proliferative state in determining the ultimate effects of exposure to a cytotoxic drug. Proliferating 3T6 cells were sensitive to MTX at drug concentrations and drug exposure durations that can be achieved readily *in vivo*, whereas the same 3T6 cells in a "resting" state were highly resistant to very high MTX concentrations and exceedingly long drug exposure times.

In reviewing the broad clinical chemotherapy experience of the past two decades, the one generalization that cuts across histologic lines and treatment modalities is that human tumor growth rate is a major determinant of therapeutic responsiveness and curability.[2]

It is relatively easy to estimate the clinical growth rate of a human tumor by making serial measurements of tumor size and calculating the tumor doubling time.[3] The population *doubling time* is simply the time required for population mass (or cell number) to double in size. The minimal detectable body burden of tumor in man is generally of the order of 1×10^9 cells (approximately 1 gm of tissue) or more; i.e., when the tumor cell population has already undergone about 30 doublings. Generally, a lethal body tumor burden is reached when tumor cell mass approaches or exceeds 1 kg or 1×10^{12} cells (40 doublings). Tumors undergo progressive growth retardation with increasing size. In many tumors, particularly in the slowly growing ones, this process of growth retardation is already far advanced by the time they are large enough to be detected clinically.

Human solid tumors can be divided con-

TABLE 3–1. Human Tumor Doubling Times

Mean Tumor Doubling Time		
<30 DAYS	30–70 DAYS	>70 DAYS
Burkitt's lymphoma	Hodgkin's disease	Small cell carcinoma, lung
Testicular cancer	Osteogenic sarcoma	Squamous cell carcinoma
Ewing's sarcoma	Fibrosarcoma	Adenocarcinoma, lung
Non-Hodgkin's lymphoma (predominantly large cell types)		Adenocarcinoma, colon
		Adenocarcinoma, breast (advanced)
Choriocarcinoma (subclinical)		
Wilms' tumor (subclinical)		
Adenocarcinoma, breast (subclinical)		

veniently into three groups by doubling time (Table 3–1). Ewing's sarcoma, testicular carcinoma, and the non-Hodgkin's lymphomas (primarily the large cell lymphomas) have mean doubling times that are shorter than 30 days. Hodgkin's disease, osteogenic sarcoma, and fibrosarcoma have intermediate growth rates, with mean doubling times ranging from 30 to 70 days. Lung carcinomas and adenocarcinomas of the colon and breast have mean doubling times that exceed 70 days.

Clinical experience has shown that the more rapidly growing tumors have higher rates of complete response and that these complete responses are often quite durable. In contrast, the complete response rates of slowly growing tumors are generally low (except for small cell carcinoma of the lung); when complete responses do occur, they are rarely durable, and patients usually die of their disease, despite an initial response to treatment.

One may hope that a better understanding of the basic processes that underlie these empirical observations will lead to improvements in cancer treatment. This chapter explains the basic principles that govern the proliferative behavior and drug response behavior of normal and malignant cell populations, and considers the applications of these principles to clinical cancer therapy.

BASIC PRINCIPLES OF CELL KINETICS

The Cell Cycle

The Chronologic Age of Proliferating Cells. Each proliferating cell goes through a sequential process of growth and division. Since this process repeats itself with each successive generation of cells, it has come to be known as the *cell cycle* (Fig. 3–1). The cyclic nature of cell proliferation can best be appreciated by comparing Figure 3–1 with the face of a clock. The hour of day increases progressively until the stroke of twelve, at which point the hour is reset instantaneously to zero and the clock cycle begins again. Similarly, a cell increases in chronologic age as it progresses through its physiologic growth cycle until it reaches mitosis, at which point the ages of both daughter cells are set to zero and their age cycles begin again. Obviously, the clock-face representation of the cell cycle is an apt one when both daughter cells take the same length of time to complete the cycle and when the duration of the cell cycle does not vary from

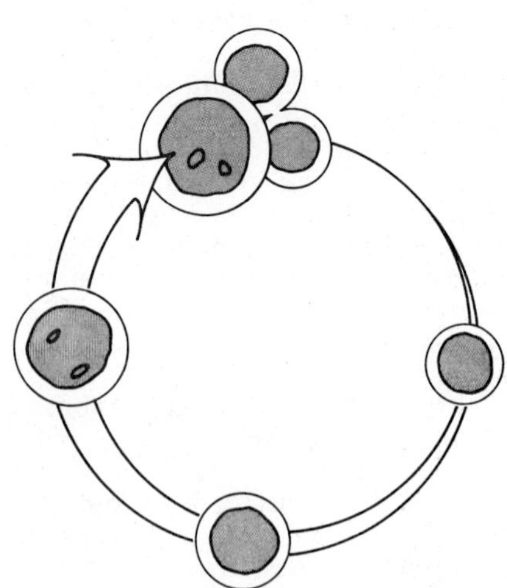

Figure 3–1. The proliferative cell cycle.

one cell generation to the next. Although this is a highly oversimplified assumption, we shall use it initially for the sake of clarity, and replace it later on.

The Physiologic Age of Proliferating Cells. Since it is rarely possible to make sequential observations on individual living cells *in situ*, it is difficult to measure the chronologic age of individual cells or the duration of the cell cycle directly. However, there are other, more easily measured cell properties that also must change cyclically with cell proliferation. For example, in cell populations that maintain stable overall morphologic characteristics through successive cell generations, individual cell volumes and nuclear volumes must, on the average, double between divisions and halve at the time of cell division. Other biochemical constituents of cells, which are maintained at constant levels overall through successive cell divisions (e.g., overall protein content/cell or the cellular levels of individual constitutive enzymes), must also double in amount between cell divisions and halve at mitosis.

In principle, then, it should be possible to identify the relative position of cells in the cell cycle by making static measurements of one or more of their cyclically varying properties. In practice, certain cell constituents are better suited for cell cycle analysis than others. A cyclically varying constituent should lend itself to rapid and accurate measurement in individual cells and should be chemically and biologically stable. A cell constituent that doubles exactly between divisions and is distributed exactly equally to both daughter cells with cell division is preferable to one that exhibits considerable variability from one postmitotic cell to the next and which doubles *on the average* between divisions. It is not surprising, then, that cell kineticists focused their attention on the process of DNA synthesis from the beginning, since cell DNA content meets many of the requirements of an ideal parameter of cell age within the cycle.

Early cytologic studies of cell division had emphasized the sequence of morphologic changes associated with the mitotic process itself. Before 1950 it was assumed that the interval between mitoses, or interphase, was an inactive stage of the cell cycle. It was thought that the new chromosomal DNA that appeared during mitosis was synthesized early in mitosis or very shortly before its onset. However, in the early 1950s, several lines of evidence converged to establish that DNA synthesis occurred much earlier in the cell cycle.

Walker and Yates,[4] using microspectrophotometric methods, showed that the DNA content of individual cells increased progressively during interphase. Walker[5] showed that cellular DNA content does not increase at a uniform rate as cells progress through the cell cycle. Rather, the curve of cellular DNA content, as a function of time elapsed since last mitosis, exhibits a sigmoidal shape (Fig. 3–2*A*). This was inferred from frequency histograms of cell DNA content measurements obtained in asynchronously growing cell populations (Fig. 3–2*C*). In simple terms, at any given moment, cells are found throughout the cell cycle during unperturbed growth (Fig. 3–2*B*). The high frequency of 2N cells in the DNA histogram (Fig. 3–2*C*) reflects the presence of cells distributed throughout a relatively long period in the cell cycle during which there is no appreciable change in cellular DNA content from the 2N or diploid value (Fig. 3–2*A*). Similarly, the high frequency of 4N cells in the DNA histogram reflects a significant fraction of cells in the premitotic segment of the cell cycle, during which DNA content also does not change appreciably. The cells with intermediate DNA contents in the DNA histogram are cells in the process of DNA synthesis at the time the cell sample is obtained. The fact that cell DNA content increases in sigmoidal rather than linear fashion indicates that the rate of DNA synthesis is higher in midcycle than in the pre- and postmitotic periods.

Early Radioautographic Studies. At about the same time that Walker and Yates published their early studies of cell DNA content, Howard and Pelc[6] used radioautography to demonstrate that DNA synthesis took place during interphase. By this technique, cells are exposed to a radioactive precursor that is incorporated into a marker macromolecule such as DNA. These cells are then fixed on glass slides and coated with a photographic emulsion. After a period of incubation in the dark, the slides are processed as photographic negatives. Cells labeled with radioactive material are identified by the black silver grains in the overlying photographic emulsion.

Howard and Pelc[6] studied DNA synthesis in growing bean root tips that were exposed continuously to ^{32}Phosphate. They observed that 20 per cent of the interphase cells were

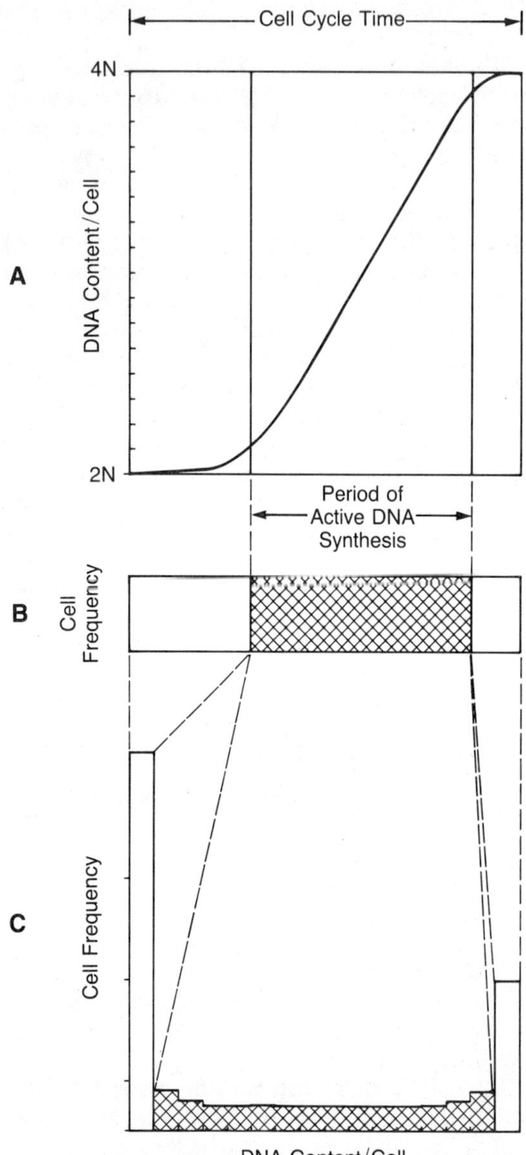

Figure 3–2. The relations among cell DNA content as a function of position in the cell cycle (*A*), the frequency distribution of cells throughout the cell cycle (*B*), and the observed DNA histogram (*C*).

labeled within two hours of initial exposure, and concluded that the duration of the period of active DNA synthesis must be about 20 per cent of the total cell cycle time. They concluded further that this period of active DNA synthesis, which they called "S phase," does not immediately precede mitosis, since labeled mitotic cells did not appear in appreciable numbers until ten hours after exposure to ^{32}P.

Howard and Pelc proposed a model that subdivided interphase into discrete subphases, as shown in Figure 3–3. This model included an early gap (G_1) between mitosis and the onset of S phase, in addition to the gap (G_2) between S phase and the succeeding mitosis. This was necessary because the duration of S, G_2, and M (T_S, T_{G_2} and T_M, respectively) added up to something less than T_C, the total duration of the cell cycle (estimated independently).

Tritiated Thymidine Pulse Labeling. Tritiated thymidine (^{3}H-TdR) was introduced as a radiotracer for DNA synthesis in the late 1950s and offered several important advantages over ^{32}P in radioautographic studies. ^{3}H-TdR is rapidly converted to thymidylate (dTMP), then dTTP, and is incorporated exclusively into DNA following brief exposure. Since the weak tritium β particle travels only short distances (1–2 microns) in tissue, ^{3}H-TdR provided improved spatial localization of DNA synthesis over ^{32}P in radioautographs. Since ^{3}H-TdR administered in tracer amounts is metabolized rapidly — the plasma half-life of a pulse dose is about two minutes in man[7] — it became practical to carry out studies utilizing *pulse* doses of ^{3}H-TdR *in vivo*.

The Thymidine Pulse Labeling Index (LI). This represents the fraction of cells that incorporate radioactivity into their nuclei following pulse exposure to ^{3}H-TdR. Assuming that cells are distributed uniformly throughout the cell cycle (an oversimplifi-

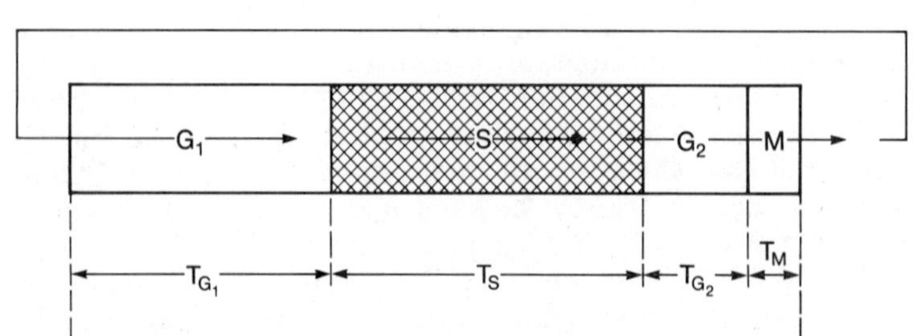

Figure 3–3. The discrete phase model of the cell cycle.

cation, but adequate for our purposes), the fraction of cells in S should be equal to the fraction of the cell cycle time devoted to DNA synthesis, as in the initial studies of Howard and Pelc. That is:

$$\text{Observed LI} = N_S/N_{total} = T_S/T_C \qquad \text{[eq. 1]}$$

where N_S = number of cells in S, N_{total} = total number of cells, T_S is the duration of S phase, and T_C is the duration of the cell cycle. The validity of this relationship depends on several additional assumptions, namely:

1. that all the cells included in N_{total} are actively progressing through the cell cycle;
2. that the variation in T_S and T_C is small; or
3. if the variation in T_C is large, that the ratio T_S/T_C remains constant over a broad range of T_C's.

In retrospect, these were reasonable working assumptions for the rapidly proliferating tissues, such as mouse intestinal epithelium, that were studied initially. Again, we shall treat these assumptions as valid for the present, recognizing that more realistic ones will be needed to replace them in later discussions.

In rapidly proliferating, relatively homogeneous experimental cell systems, pulse LIs of 0.4 to 0.7 can be observed. In most human tumors the LI is less than 0.2 and is commonly less than 0.1 (Table 3–2). It is uncommon for the LI to exceed 0.3 in human tumors. There is a considerable degree of variability within tumor types and a great deal of overlap in the range of LIs among tumor types in man. Despite this variability, it has been observed that tumors with short doubling times tend to have higher LIs than tumors with long doubling times.[8] Thus, one would expect a correlation between tumor LI and responsivness to therapy. Although this is true in a general sense, single LI values obtained in individual patients are of limited usefulness for prognostic purposes.

The Percent Labeled Mitosis Curve. A major concern of cell kineticists during most of the 1960s was the measurement of the durations of the cell cycle and its component phases in mammalian cell populations.

Even under the best of circumstances, all that the LI can provide is the ratio, T_S/T_C. The method of *percent labeled mitoses (PLM,* or alternatively *FLM,* for *fraction of labeled mitoses)* was developed in 1959 by Quastler

TABLE 3–2. Labeling Indices in Human Tumors

Cell Type	*Site*	*Mean or Median LI*	*No. of Patients*	*Ref.*
Adenocarcinoma	Pooled data	0.02	45	8
	Breast	0.02	170	9
		0.02	92	10
	Colon	0.03	134	9
	Lung	0.05	18	11
Squamous cell carcinoma	Pooled data	0.08	7	8
	Head and neck	0.11	3	12
		0.05	12	13
	Lung	0.08	38	11
	Cervix	0.05	2	12
		0.19	13	14
Small cell carcinoma	Lung	0.15	12	15
		0.24	5	16
		0.11	14	11
Sarcoma	Pooled data	0.05	28	8
	Brain tumors	0.03	14	17
Melanoma		0.03	8	18
		0.03	25	16
Multiple myeloma		0.02	13	19
Lymphoma, pooled data		0.09	20	20
Burkitt's lymphoma		0.29	13	8

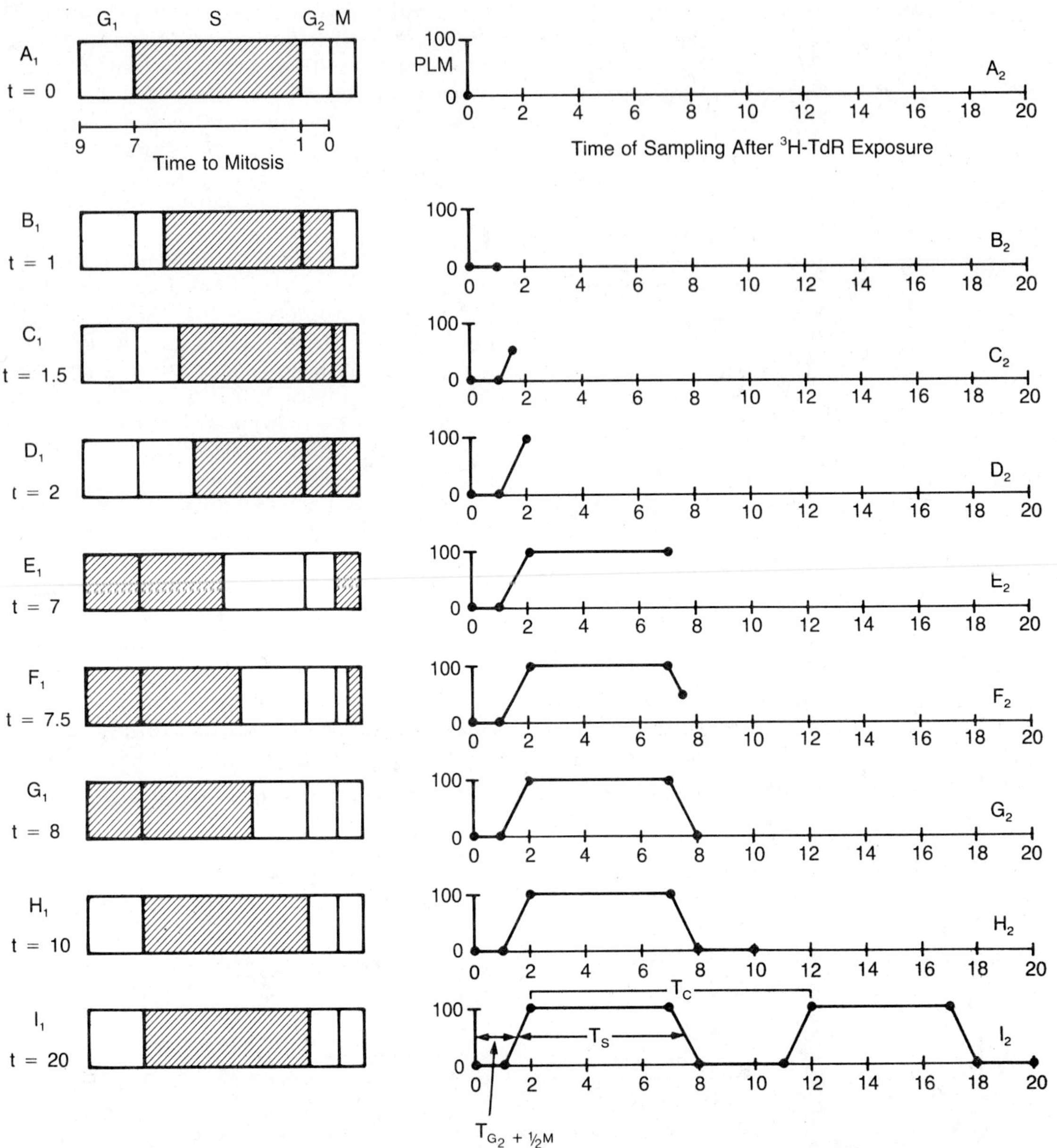

Figure 3–4. A schematic representation of the basis for PLM curve analysis.

and Sherman[21] for estimating the durations of the component phases of the cell cycle.

The PLM curve method is explained in the following example:

Example 2. Let us consider a hypothetical cell population in which T_{G_1} is 2 hours, T_S is 6 hours, T_{G_2} is 1 hour, and T_M is 1 hour, as shown in Figure 3–4A_1. Their sum, T_C, is 10 hours. Let us now consider cell position in the cell cycle on a scale of time required to reach the *next* mitosis instead of time elapsed since the last mitosis. Following a pulse of ^{3}H-TdR, only cells in the S phase will incorporate labeled tritium, but it will take at least 1 hour (the duration of T_{G_2}) for any of these labeled cells to move into mitosis. If mitotic cells are examined within 1 hour of pulse ^{3}H-TdR exposure (Fig. 3–4B_1), none will be labeled (Fig. 3–4B_2). From 1 to 7 hours after ^{3}H-TdR exposure, labeled cells will enter mitosis (Fig. 3–4C_1 to G_1), and can be detected and quantitated by radioautography (Fig. 3–4C_2 to G_2). At the time of ^{3}H-TdR pulse exposure, the G_1 cells were not synthesizing DNA; thus, 7 to 9 hours later they will enter the mitotic pool as unlabeled cells (Fig. 3–4G_1,G_2). Ten hours after pulse exposure, all the cells will have cycled through mitosis, and the daughter cells will be in the same relative positions that were occupied by their parents at the time of original pulse ^{3}H-TdR exposure (Fig. 3–4H_1). During the next 10 hours after pulse, the PLM curve of the daughter cells should recapitulate that of their parents (Fig. 3–4I_1,I_2).

In principle, T_{G_2} + ½M can be estimated from the delay in the upstroke of the first wave of labeled mitosis, and T_S from the width of the labeled mitotic wave (Fig. 3–4I_2). Since the interval between successive labeled mitotic waves is that of the cell cycle itself, T_C can also be estimated from the PLM curve. T_{G_1} can be calculated from the simple relation that the sum of the durations of the individual phases is equal to the total cell cycle time. That is:

$$T_{G_1} + T_S + T_{G_2} + M = T_C \qquad \text{[eq. 2]}$$

Of course, this analysis assumes that the cell cycle and its subphases are of uniform duration. Experience has shown that few cell populations exhibit PLM curves similar to those of the ideal curve shown in Figure 3–4. These have included such very rapidly proliferating cell populations as embryonic mouse tissues,[22] rat intestinal epithelium,[23] and log phase mouse tumor cells in tissue culture.[24] In reality it is exceedingly rare for the trough between the first and second wave to fall to zero, and the greater the degree of kinetic heterogeneity, the broader and lower the second wave of the PLM curve. In most human tumors the second labeled mitotic wave is low, broad, and often difficult to identify at all.

Nonetheless, in the early 1960s, T_C and the phase durations were thought to be tightly clustered about their respective mean values. The method shown in Figure 3–4I_2, or closely related variants,[25] was used to analyze a wide variety of PLM curves, despite the deviations of these curves from the ideal. Later in the 1960s, computer-based automated curve-fitting methods were developed for PLM curve analysis.[26, 27] These methods assumed the existence of independent distributions of the cell cycle phase durations. These phase-duration distributions were fitted to the PLM curve data by numerical methods, and the putative distribution of T_C's could then be calculated.

Other methods have been developed for estimating T_C. We might note, for example, that the ^{3}H-TdR label acquired during pulse exposure is divided approximately equally between both daughter cells at mitosis. Hence, the mean radioautographic grain count of labeled cells should fall by half with each successive round of cell division, and T_C can be estimated from the time required for the mean grain count to halve.[22]

The reader should be aware that each of the various radioautographic methods used for estimating T_C and the durations of the cycle phases is associated with its own technical pitfalls. However, a comprehensive and detailed treatment of radioautographic methodology is beyond the scope of this chapter.

Overall, the PLM technique provides more information regarding population proliferative characteristics than any other single method, but it alone is insufficient to characterize population proliferative characteristics completely, as described later in this chapter.

The Growth Fraction. It was recognized from the beginning that all cells in a population were not identical with respect to their proliferative behavior. According to early conceptual formulations, cells were classified as either dividing or nondividing. As we have seen, dividing cells were treated as having a uniform cell cycle time and uniform cycle phase durations. The nondividing cells were considered to be indistinguishable morphologically from dividing cells, but they did not incorporate ^{3}H-TdR or contribute to the mitotic cell pool. In the early 1960s, Mendelsohn[28] proposed that the fraction of dividing cells, or the *growth fraction*, could be estimated from the discrepancy between the LI that would be expected for the population if all cells were dividing and the LI that is actually observed.

Example 3. Again, let us assume that T_C is 10 hours and T_S is 6 hours. Half of the cells are nonproliferating cells (Fig. 3–5A_1). Since the duration of S phase represents 60 per cent of the total cell cycle time, an LI of 0.6 would be expected if all cells were dividing. Since the nonproliferating cells contribute to the denominator but not to the numerator of the observed LI, the observed LI is only 0.3. It is easy to verify that:

$$\text{Growth fraction} = \frac{\text{observed LI}}{\text{expected LI}} \qquad \text{[eq. 3]}$$

When PLM curve data are available, one can obtain T_S and T_C separately (Fig. 3–5A_2), and

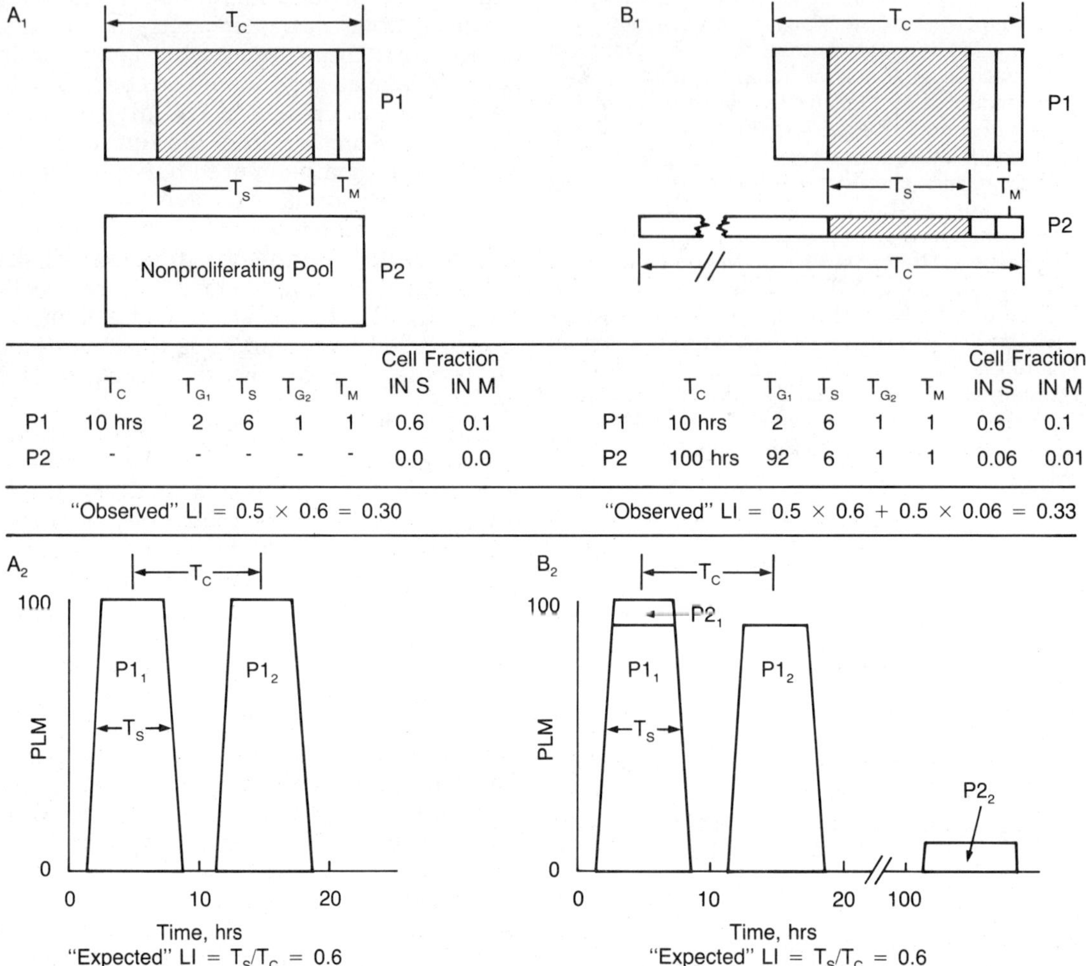

	T_C	T_{G_1}	T_S	T_{G_2}	T_M	Cell Fraction IN S	Cell Fraction IN M
P1	10 hrs	2	6	1	1	0.6	0.1
P2	-	-	-	-	-	0.0	0.0

"Observed" LI = 0.5 × 0.6 = 0.30

	T_C	T_{G_1}	T_S	T_{G_2}	T_M	Cell Fraction IN S	Cell Fraction IN M
P1	10 hrs	2	6	1	1	0.6	0.1
P2	100 hrs	92	6	1	1	0.06	0.01

"Observed" LI = 0.5 × 0.6 + 0.5 × 0.06 = 0.33

Figure 3–5. The effects of the presence of a nonproliferating pool on kinetic measurements (*A₁* and *A₂*); for comparison, the effects of a slowly proliferating population are also shown (*B₁* and *B₂*).

calculate the LI that would be expected for the dividing cells from the ratio T_S/T_C (equation 1). Given the observed LI for the entire population, one can then calculate the growth fraction using equation [3].

The Nondividing Cell Compartment and the G_0 State. The nondividing cell compartment was thought to contain cells of two basic types: end-stage cells that would never divide again and nondividing cells that retain the potential for proliferation.[29] Quastler suggested that these potentially proliferative cells produced new cells either at a low rate or only upon stimulation. He proposed the term G_0 for this potentially reversible nondividing state.

The distinction between a truly nonproliferative G_0 state and a very long G_1 phase was to occupy the attention of cell kineticists for years to come, and remains a controversial issue to this day. This distinction is difficult to make on conceptual as well as experimental grounds. A cell that "left" the cell cycle from G_1, resided in the G_0 state, and then "returned" to the cell cycle at a later time would be indistinguishable from a cell that never left the cell cycle at all, but remained in the G_1 phase for a long period.

Quastler's original definition of G_0 was deliberately vague in distinguishing between slowly dividing and truly nondividing cells. His purpose was to distinguish these slowly dividing or potentially proliferative nondividing cells from rapidly proliferating cells on the one hand, and end-stage nondividing cells on the other.

The exclusion of G_0 cells from the growth fraction was based on the premise that the cell cycle time of rapidly proliferating cells was uniform, or nearly so. As Mendelsohn stated in 1963[30]:

> There is a distinction between a model based entirely on cell cycle time and one including growth fraction as well. In the first case one could include the effects of nonproliferating cells by assuming a monotonic skewed distribution of cell cycle times extending far out to the right, perhaps reaching to infinity. By introducing growth fraction, two distributions of cell cycle time are implied. One is at infinity, and the other has a finite mean with a limited spread to each side. In the absence of the appropriate data on the distributions of cell cycle times, the choice between these approaches is arbitrary, but the use of growth fraction is more amenable to analysis and perhaps easier to comprehend.

In early experimental studies, the average cell cycle times in many mouse tissues were often found to be in the range of 8 to 12 hours; cells with cycle times exceeding 24 to 36 hours were often considered either to be slowly proliferating or in G_0 for all practical purposes. Later studies in human tumors indicated mean or median cell cycle times of 2 to 3 days,[31] with considerable variability in cell cycle time, both within and among tumors. More recent computer modeling studies have suggested that the range of cell cycle times is such that one might find some cells dividing every 24 hours and others dividing every 40 days in the same tumor cell population.[32] This degree of kinetic heterogeneity was not anticipated in early studies and it should prompt us to re-examine early basic concepts in the light of this new information.

The Identification of Slowly Proliferating Cells in the Presence of Rapidly Proliferating Cells. Let us consider the illustrative example shown in Figure $5B_1$ and B_2:

Example 4. The population is composed of two subpopulations represented with equal frequency, one with a 10-hour cell cycle time and the other with a cycle time of 100 hours. Assigned cycle phase durations are shown in the illustration. The overall "observed" labeling index for the population is 0.33. In this example, 10 per cent of the rapidly growing cells and 1 per cent of the slowly growing cells are in mitosis at any given time. Thus, although rapidly growing cells and slowly growing cells are equally represented in the *interphase* cell pool, in the *mitotic* cell pool the slowly proliferating cells are outnumbered by 10 to 1. Hence, the second labeled mitotic wave of the PLM curve appears 10 hours after the first and achieves a height exceeding 90 per cent labeled mitoses (Fig. 3–$5B_2$). Given an S-phase duration of 6 hours and a cell cycle time of 10 hours (obtained from the PLM curve directly), one can calculate an "expected" labeling index of 0.6. This is almost twice the "observed" value. If half the population were composed of truly nonproliferating cells rather than slowly proliferating cells (Fig. 3–$5A_1$), there would be a comparable discrepancy between the observed labeling index and that expected from the PLM curve.

This example illustrates two important points. First, the PLM curve is always dominated by the most rapidly proliferating cells in the population; this results in a false impression of cell cycle time uniformity. Second, since only a small fraction of slowly proliferating cells are detected by ^{3}H-TdR labeling, they contribute little to cell kinetic measurements and are virtually indistinguishable from truly nonproliferating cells both in theory and in practice.

In the foregoing example we considered a mixture of two populations with cell cycle times that differed by a factor of 10. In this instance the distinction between slowly proliferating cells and G_0 cells would be of little practical consequence.

However, cells with intermediate cell cycle times are also subject to the biases inherent in the PLM curves method. Such cells are also underrepresented in the PLM curve, but in varying degrees. When large numbers of cells with intermediate cell cycle times are present, the resultant PLM curves have very different properties from those obtained in kinetically homogeneous cell populations.

Example 5. Let us consider a population that contains 10 cell cycle time classes ranging from 10 hours to 100 hours, as shown in Figure 3–6A. In this example, cell cycle time classes are represented equally in interphase, but the most rapidly proliferating cells are better represented in the mitotic cell pool (Fig. 3–6B). The resultant PLM curve is shown in Figure 3–6C, together with the relative contributions of each cycle time class. For simplicity, only the contribution of the 10-hour cycle time class is identified explicitly *(shaded areas)*. It is readily apparent that the second mitotic wave is low and broad; it is not sharply peaked as in the example in Figures 3–4 and 3–5.

A

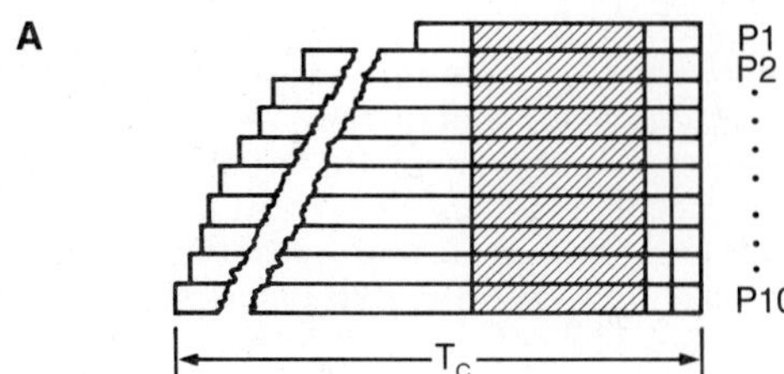

B

	T_C	T_{G_1}	T_S	T_{G_2}	T_M	Interphase Cell Frequency	Mitotic Cell Frequency
P1	10	2	6	1	1	0.1	0.342
P2	20	12	6	1	1	0.1	0.171
P3	30	22	6	1	1	0.1	0.113
P4	40	32	6	1	1	0.1	0.086
P5	50	42	6	1	1	0.1	0.069
⋮	⋮	⋮	⋮	⋮	⋮	⋮	⋮
P10	100	92	6	1	1	0.1	0.034

C

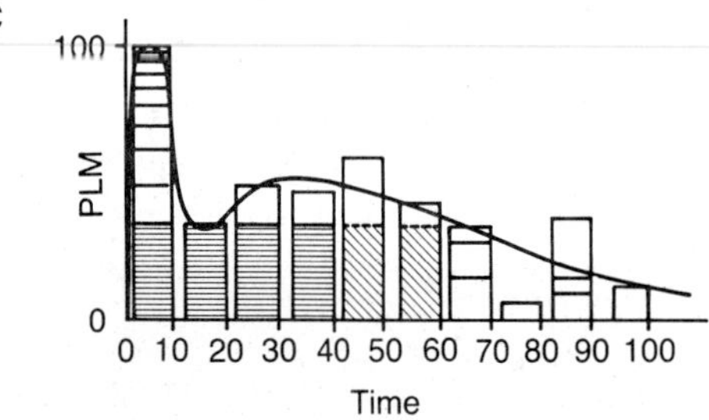

Figure 3–6. The effects of cell cycle time heterogeneity on the PLM curve.

While all the cycle time classes contribute to this low, broad second wave, it consists mostly of the repeated divisions of the most rapidly proliferating cells. The *height* of the second wave depends largely on the *relative abundance* of rapidly proliferating cells. Since the amount of label per cell is diluted with successive cell divisions, the *breadth* of the second wave depends largely on the number of divisions that can be detected radioautographically before cells become too lightly labeled to be detected as such. This, in turn, depends on such factors as initial interphase cell labeling intensity and the grain count detection threshold. For example, if the interphase cell mean grain count of the rapidly proliferating cells is 16 grains/cell initially, and the detection threshold is 2 grains/cell, three successive divisions of labeled rapidly proliferating cells will be detected. If the initial mean grain count of the most rapidly proliferating cells is 64 grains/cell, the second wave of the PLM curve will include five successive divisions of labeled rapidly proliferating cells (*dashed bars*, Fig. 3–6C).

The foregoing example is still highly oversimplified for purposes of exposition. For example, transitions among cycle time classes during the course of the observation period are not considered; however, more extensive and more rigorous computer modeling studies have supported the essential elements of PLM curve analysis described above.[32]

The simulated PLM curve in Figure 3–6 conforms with observations in kinetically heterogeneous populations. Many experimental tumors and virtually all human tumors lack sharply peaked second waves, yet there is progressive mitotic label dilution that results in light labeling in the middle and late portions of the second PLM wave. This may account for well-recognized discrepancies between human PLM curve data and theoretical PLM curves derived from conventional models,[31] since conventional models for PLM curve analysis make no provision for label dilution.

If the PLM curve is relatively insensitive to the presence of the more slowly proliferating cells, how *can* the cell cycle time distribution be studied? It is apparent from Figure 3–6 that changes in mitotic grain counts over time strongly reflect the kinetic behavior of the most rapidly proliferating cells in the

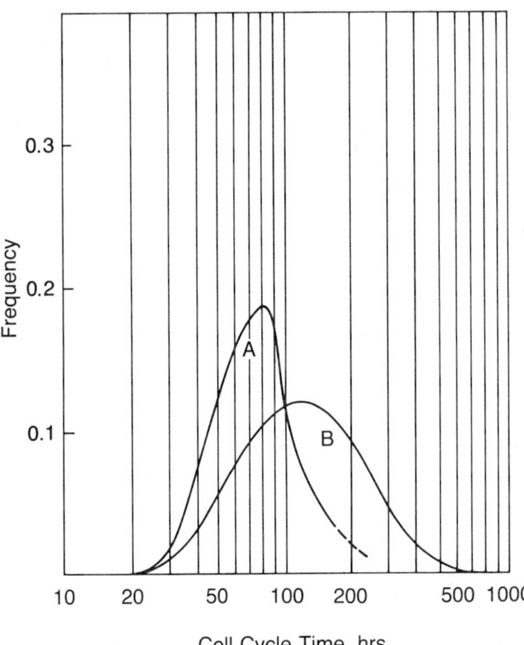

Figure 3–7. A comparison of calculated cell cycle time distributions in human malignant melanoma, obtained by two different methods of kinetic analysis.

population. On the other hand, since interphase cells are not subject to the biases inherent in mitotic cell studies, changes in *interphase* cell grain counts would reflect the kinetic behavior of the overall cell population. A comparison of differences in the behavior of the mitotic grain count distribution over time and the behavior of the interphase cell grain count distribution over time can be used to reconstruct the overall cell cycle time distribution, using computer simulation techniques. The details of this approach are described elsewhere.[32] To date, two human malignancies — adult acute leukemia and human melanoma — have been analyzed extensively using this approach.

The cell cycle time distribution in adult acute leukemia ranges from 16 to approximately 600 hours. In Figure 3–7 the cell cycle time distribution in human melanoma that was obtained in these studies *(curve B)* is compared with that obtained by conventional PLM curve analysis *(curve A)*. It should be noted that the abscissa is plotted on a log scale and that the simulated cell cycle time distribution ranges from 24 to over 960 hours (40 days). Many of the cells with cycle times in the range of 120 to 960 hours would be excluded from the growth fraction by conventional methods of kinetic analysis.[33]

After all is said and done, why not simply consider these excluded slowly proliferating cells to be G_0 cells, as shown in Figure 3–8A? Conceptually, it would be simpler to think of growth retardation in terms of a reduction in the growth fraction and entry into the G_0 compartment rather than in terms of a shift in the cell cycle time distribution to longer values (Fig. 3–8B). By the same token, it would be simpler to think of cell recruitment as a discrete transition from the G_0 compartment to the proliferating cell compartment than as a shift in the cell cycle time distribution from longer to shorter values (Fig. 3–8C).

Indeed, for most qualitative purposes, the growth fraction-G_0 two compartment model may be quite serviceable. However, the two-compartment model is not suited for quanti-

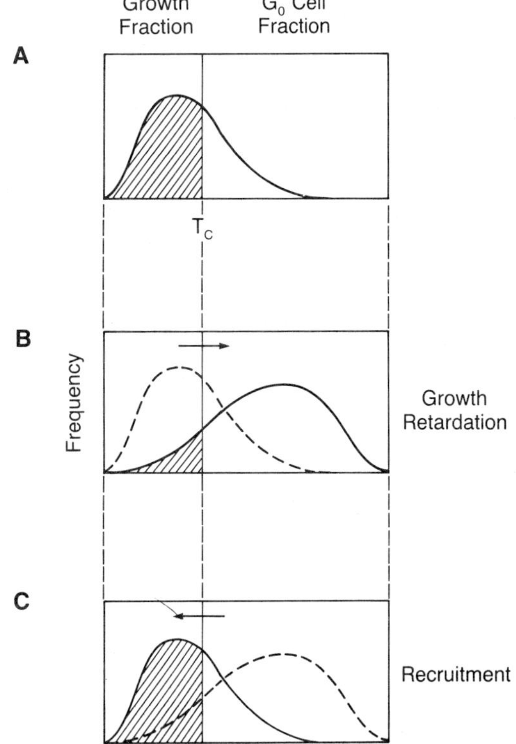

Figure 3–8. *A,* The relationships among the growth fraction, the nonproliferating pool, and the cell cycle time distribution. *B,* The conceptual equivalence of entry into G_0 and a shift of the cell cycle time distribution to longer values. *C,* The conceptual equivalence of recruitment from G_0 into rapid cycle and a shift of the cell cycle time distribution to shorter values.

tative applications. In populations that contain large numbers of slowly proliferating cells, when the more slowly proliferating cells are systematically excluded from the cell cycle time distribution, the calculated mean (or median) cell cycle time is spuriously low and the range of cell cycle times is spuriously narrow (see Fig. 3–7, for example). Published estimates of average cell cycle times in human tumors based on conventional methods of analysis are generally in the range of two to three days.[31, 34] The upper limit of the range has been estimated to be about five to seven days.[34] In retrospect, the apparent kinetic homogeneity of human tumors may well be due to the fact that conventional methods of PLM curve analysis "see" only a narrow region of the cell cycle time distribution containing the rapidly proliferating cells.

This apparent kinetic homogeneity within and among most human tumors has tended to discourage the collection of additional kinetic data in man, yet it is among the more slowly proliferating cells that the greatest kinetic differences among tumors are likely to be found. In those human tumors for which sufficient data are available, computer modeling studies that utilize both mitotic and interphase cell data have demonstrated distinctly different patterns of DNA synthesis among the slowly proliferating cell fractions of different tumor types.[35] It remains to be determined whether these distinctive patterns are subject to therapeutic exploitation. However, the distinctive kinetic features of the more slowly proliferating cells raise interesting possibilities. Cells with intermediate cell cycle times (say, three to 12 days) might be of particular interest as potential targets for treatment optimization with currently available drugs, especially in tumors that are responsive to therapy but are not often curable (e.g., small cell carcinoma of the lung or small cleaved cell lymphomas).

The Distinction Between Proliferating Cells and End-Stage Cells

Cell Death and Cell Differentiation. Cell death is often a protracted process that occurs in stages (Fig. 3–9); advanced stages can be appreciated morphologically, whereas the detection of early stages may require more elaborate functional studies. From the standpoint of cell kinetics, cell viability is defined strictly in terms of cell reproductive integrity. To a cell kineticist, a cell is viable if it retains the unrestricted capacity to divide and produce other cells like itself. A cell becomes nonviable when it loses the capacity for continued proliferation. Cells that are nonviable in the kinetic sense may continue to occupy space and carry on many normal metabolic processes. However, such cells are doomed to undergo physical destruction sooner or later.

Mature granulocytes, mature erythrocytes, and neurons are examples of cells that cannot divide to produce other cells like themselves. Most mature granulocytes are lost within 24 hours. Most mature erythrocytes are lost within four months. Although some

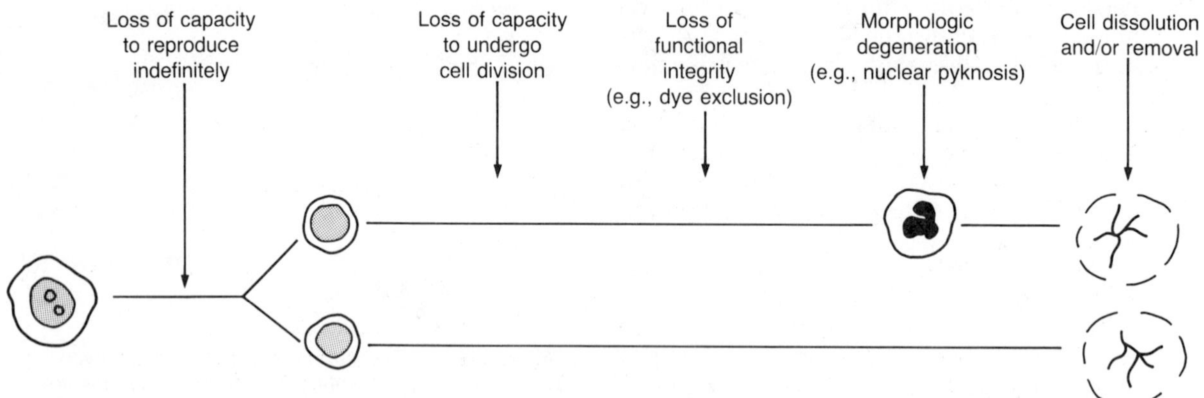

Figure 3–9. Schematic representation of cell death as a multistage process, beginning with subtle functional changes associated with loss of the capacity to reproduce indefinitely and terminating with physical cell dissolution or removal. Nonviable cells may or may not exhibit morphologic evidence of cell death prior to their dissolution and/or removal.

neuronal cell loss occurs throughout adult life, most neurons survive through advanced host age. Despite the broad range of clearance times exhibited by these cell types, they share in common certain fundamental properties of cells that are nonviable in the kinetic sense. Such cells are unable to contribute to normal tissue growth or to tissue repopulation after a cytotoxic insult, and they cannot be used to establish cell lines in tissue culture.

The kinetic definition of cell viability is especially useful in defining the goals and assessing the effectiveness of cancer treatment. This is discussed in greater detail later in this chapter.

In normal tissues, the loss of cell viability is often associated with cell differentiation. However, the term differentiation does not necessarily imply loss of cell viability in the kinetic sense. Thus, the small lymphocyte is often described as "mature" or "differentiated," but it is not an end-stage cell.

In normal tissues, nonviable cells often perform highly specialized functions that are vital to host survival (e.g., mature granulocytes, erythrocytes, and neurons). However, the performance of specialized functions is not restricted to end-stage differentiated cells, nor does it necessarily imply normal proliferative behavior. Thus, the induction of specialized normal functions in cytogenetically abnormal malignant cells may be of little practical therapeutic benefit in and of itself unless it is achieved by inducing *end-stage* differentiation in most, if not all, tumor cells.

The Residual Proliferative Capacity of Nonviable Cells. Early studies on the effects of radiation on mammalian cells in the mid-1950s showed that lethally damaged cells can undergo one or more preterminal rounds of cell division before dying.[36]

With the recognition of agonal proliferative behavior of nonviable cells, it became considerably more difficult to draw a clear distinction between viable and nonviable cells. It was perceived that both classes of cells could synthesize DNA and divide. Differences in behavior or morphology might not become apparent until one or more cell generations after the lethal insult (Fig. 3–9). For example, this type of delayed death appears to occur after cells incorporate 6-thiopurine analogues into DNA (see Chapter 9). Thus, in principle, the fundamental difference between viable and nonviable cells was conceived to be that viable cells were capable of cell division indefinitely, whereas nonviable cells were restricted to a finite number of cell divisions.

This distinction was concordant with concepts of stem cell biology promulgated in the late 1950s and early 1960s (see below).

The Stem Cell. The earliest ideas regarding stem cells were derived from classical histology and embryology. A primitive progenitor cell, or stem cell, was placed at the head of a given histologic series and was thought to progress through a linear sequence of gradual morphologic changes that terminated in differentiated cells characteristic of that series.

The concept of linear maturation sequences had two serious weaknesses. First, since the construction of such sequences was based on the premise that cytomorphologic changes were gradual and progressive, no provision was made for the cyclic and discontinuous changes associated with cell progression through the cell cycle and cell division. Second, the linear sequence model did not *really* shed light on the nature of the first cell in the series, since the origin of the earliest recognizable cell in any given series was still left unresolved.

The realization that stem cells must undergo cyclic growth and cell division came in the late 1950s. Osgood[37] was the first to recognize that stem cells were defined by two properties, namely, the capacity for perpetual self-maintenance through cell division, and the ability to produce differentiated cells. These concepts were later extended and applied to hematopoietic cell proliferation and differentiation by Lajtha[38], Patt,[39] and others.[40, 41] In these hematopoietic models, cell differentiation was viewed as a discrete and irreversible transition from a state characterized by the capacity to proliferate without limit to a state characterized by a limited number of cell divisions. Conceptually, then, the classic linear sequence of cell differentiation was replaced by a separate, perpetually self-renewing stem cell pool and a simple branching sequence that originated at the point of transition from stem cell to differentiated cell.

Stem Cell Assays. Obviously, one cannot show that a given cell is a stem cell by demonstrating its capacity to proliferate indefinitely. However, one can identify stem cells operationally by showing that they are capable of undergoing some arbitrarily large, but finite, number of divisions. For example, Skipper and co-workers[42] showed that a single L1210 leukemia cell injected into a mouse could proliferate to produce a lethal body burden of tumor cells (approximately 1×10^9 cells, or 30 cell divisions). The capacity to undergo 30 successive cell divisions is convincing evidence that the cell that was injected originally was a stem cell. In these studies, the progeny of the original leukemia cell were not counted directly; rather, the death of the host was used as an end point. This is an example of a stem cell *bioassay*.

In contrast, in *clonogenic* stem cell assays, cells are transplanted from their native milieu to a specialized growth environment that permits each stem cell to produce a separate multicellular clone. Each clone (and therefore each original stem cell) is identified and counted. In 1961 Till and McCullough showed that if donor mouse bone marrow cells are injected into heavily irradiated recipient mice, some of these cells lodge in the spleen and produce discrete macroscopic colonies.[43] Such colonies have been estimated to contain approximately 1×10^6 cells after 10 days of growth, indicating that the original colony-forming cell, and its progeny, had undergone at least 20 divisions. Spleen colony-forming cells (CFU-S) are considered pluripotent hematopoietic stem cells, since the colonies derived from them contain myeloid and erythroid elements as well as megakaryocytes.

Various *in vitro* clonogenic assays have been developed also for other hematopoietic cells. Different assays select for different colony-forming subclasses. CFU-C are cells that produce myeloid or macrophage colonies in soft agar in the presence of specific growth-promoting factors. Erythroid colonies of two types can be produced by BFU-E and CFU-E, respectively, under appropriately selected growth conditions.[44]

In vitro cloning assays have also been developed for a variety of experimental tumors. More recently, conditions have been established for *in vitro* colony assays of human tumor cells.[45, 46]

We cannot consider all these assays in detail here. However, it should be appreciated that not all clonogenic cells are stem cells, and not all stem cells are clonogenic. In the *in vitro* clonogenic assays, cell clones are much smaller than in the spleen colony assay, often consisting of fewer than 64 cells (less than six demonstrated clonogenic cell divisions). In the CFU-E assay system, cell clusters consisting of as few as eight cells are counted as colonies.[44] The demonstrated capacity to undergo only three divisions would hardly qualify the CFU-E as a stem cell.

Conversely, not all stem cells produce colonies in the clonogenic cell assays. For example, the overall yield of CFU-S in mouse bone marrow cell suspensions is of the order of one to three CFU-S per 10,000 nucleated marrow cells. The true frequency of stem cells is much higher than this, since (1) only 4 to 17 per cent of injected CFU-S will lodge in the spleen,[47, 48] and (2) the spleen colony assay selects for a specific class of stem cells and excludes all others (e.g., the CFU-C and BFU-E present in the original marrow cell suspension). An additional theoretical consideration is that there may be a class of stem cells that functions quite well *in situ*, but which would not survive transplantation to a new environment. Since such stem cells would not be detected in any of the clonogenic assays, it may never be possible to estimate true tissue stem cell content *in vivo*.

Clonogenic cell yield (colonies observed/-*nucleated* cells plated or injected) should not be confused with stem cell cloning efficiency (colonies observed/*stem* cells plated or injected). The clonogenic cell yield can be determined directly. Stem cell cloning efficiency is not subject to experimental evaluation except under the special circumstance when the clonogenic cell yield approaches 100 per cent.

One can obtain an estimate of *relative* assay efficiency for tumor stem cells by comparing the yield obtained by the clonogenic technique with that obtained by bioassay. For example, the clonogenic stem cell yield in L1210 leukemia *in vivo* is about 2 per cent,[49] whereas the yield by bioassay is greater by an order of magnitude.[42] Studies in experimental tumor systems have suggested that the efficiency of stem cell bioassays is highly sensitive to the growth conditions under which the assay is performed. For example, in mouse B16 melanoma, the admixture of radiation-killed cells with the tumor at the time of inoculation increases stem cell yield by 1000-fold[50] to between 50 and 100 per cent. This so-called Revesz effect has been seen in other experimental tumors.[51, 52] The addition of growth-promoting factors has improved tumor stem cell yields in the clonogenic assays for human tumors also.[45, 46, 53]

Overall, it would seem reasonable to treat a low clonogenic tumor stem cell yield as an underestimate of tumor stem cell frequency *in situ*, since stem cell assay efficiency is likely to be much less than 100 per cent.

The fact that stem cell assay efficiency is indeterminate has far-reaching clinical implications. For example, the relevance of data obtained by flow cytometry or from ^{3}H-TdR incorporation studies has been questioned by some[34] on the grounds that it is only the tumor stem cells that are important from a therapeutic standpoint, and the stem cells may have different kinetic properties from the overall cell population. Now, human tumor stem cell yields are in the range 0.1 to 1 per cent. If, for example, the observed yield is 1 per cent, and assay efficiency is 100 per cent, the true frequency of tumor stem cells is one stem cell per 100 cells in the tumor. If the observed yield is 1 per cent, and assay efficiency is 5 per cent, 20 per cent of the tumor cells that one might observe under a microscope would be stem cells. If the observed stem cell yield is 1 per cent and assay efficiency is also 1 per cent, nearly all the cells of the tumor are stem cells, and flow cytometry studies and ^{3}H-TdR incorporation studies would be of unquestioned validity.

From a practical standpoint, the clinical approach to the stem cell problem is quite straightforward. If the objective of treatment planning is to achieve cures, then not even one stem cell must be left behind. Since it is likely that true tumor stem cell content is much higher than the observed yield of 0.1 to 1 per cent in clonogenic assays, it would be safer to consider *all* cells as potential stem cells until it was proved otherwise. Thus, the kinetic behavior of all cells and the details of their kinetic responses to drugs are of direct interest and are relevant to the development of drug treatment strategies.

Another major drawback of clonogenic stem cell assays is that they provide little information regarding the kinetic heterogeneity of the cells being studied, unless they are combined with other techniques.

Example 6. In early studies, few mouse CFU-S cells were found to be susceptible to hydroxyurea or to toxic doses of ^{3}H-TdR. This was interpreted to mean that few CFU-S cells were in S, i.e., that they were "out of cycle" or that their cell cycle time was very long.[54] Lord et al.[55] made use of an ingenious marrow coring technique to obtain cells from different regions of the marrow. They found that subendosteal CFU-S were highly susceptible to thymidine suicide, whereas CFU-S cells in the central region were not. Thus, these studies revealed the presence of a small fraction of cells with high T_S/T_C ratios among a much larger fraction of cells with low T_S/T_C ratios.

Unfortunately, the coring technique used in the studies of Lord et al. does not lend itself for use in other cell systems, and especially not in human tumors.

The Population Growth Curve and Growth Retardation

Biologic populations do not grow at a constant rate. Limitations of space, limitations on the delivery of oxygen and nutrients, limitations relating to the removal of waste products, and various other factors lead to a progressive decrease in overall population growth rate as population size increases. Over the years, various equations have been suggested to describe population growth curves that feature lower growth rates in late stages of growth.[56-59] The Gompertz function[57] is commonly used to describe the attenuation in growth rate of malignant tumors.

It may be possible to fit many different equations of different types to a given set of biologic data, so that no single equation should be considered an inviolate "law of growth." Furthermore, none of these equations provides an explanation for the underlying causes of growth retardation (e.g., nutrient deprivation versus waste product accumulation) or the kinetic processes that are responsible for producing the observed changes in the slope of the growth curve.

In the kinetic studies reviewed by Lala,[60] growth retardation with increased population size could be accounted for in kinetic terms by one or a combination of the following: lengthening of cell cycle time, a decrease in the growth fraction, and increased cell loss. As noted earlier (Fig. 3–8 and associated discussion), the first two factors are equivalent operationally, so that we really must focus only on the relation between two processes: a decrease in proliferative rate due to a shift in the cell cycle time distribution to longer values, and an increase in the rate of cell death and/or cell loss.

The very existence of a distribution of cell cycle times raises several important questions. How are the relative numbers of slowly proliferating cells maintained, much less increased, during population growth in the continued presence of a more rapidly proliferating cell component? That is, why don't the most rapidly proliferating cells overgrow all the others? This mathematical paradox has two possible biologic explanations. Either there is preferential loss of rapidly proliferating cells, or many of the rapidly proliferating cells *become* slowly proliferating cells before they are lost. There is evidence to suggest that the latter (conversion from fast to slow cycle times) is the major biologic route for the removal of excess rapidly proliferating cells, whereas the former (preferential cell death of rapidly proliferating cells) is, at best, a minor cell disposal pathway.

First, the establishment of a relatively broad cell cycle time distribution occurs early in the course of population growth, long before the growth curve exhibits prominent changes in slope. For example, in sarcoma 180 grown *in vitro*, one already sees changes in the DNA content distribution that are consistent with major shifts in the cell cycle time distribution during early- and midlog phase growth.[61] By the time the growth curve shows a significant decrease in slope, the changes in the cell cycle time distribution are so extensive that they are even apparent in the less sensitive PLM curve studies.[61, 62] In L1210 leukemia *in vivo*, changes in drug responsiveness reflect shifts in the cell cycle time distribution over tumor size ranges as low as 10^3 to 10^6 cells, long before changes in the slope of the growth curve can be appreciated.[63, 64]

During fairly early stages of growth, then, there is an increase in both the relative and absolute numbers of slowly proliferating cells. That is, throughout the course of population growth, a fraction of the rapidly proliferating cells must undergo growth retardation in order to expand and later maintain the slowly proliferating fraction of the cell population. As we shall see below, in late stages of growth it is the slowly proliferating cells that preferentially undergo orderly end-stage differentiation and/or cell removal in normal tissues, and a more disorganized form of cell loss in tumors.

Growth Retardation and Cell Loss; Spatial Correlates. In many mammalian tissues the rapidly proliferating cells are generally found in close proximity to the microvascular blood supply; under steady-state growth conditions, many of these rapidly proliferating cells migrate physically to separate regions of lower proliferative rate and undergo growth retardation themselves in the process. Cell loss (cell necrosis in tumors) and/or end-stage differentiation are found in association with the regions of low proliferative rate.

This type of kinetic microarchitectural organization has been observed in epidermis,[65, 66] intestinal epithelium,[21] regenerating liver,[67] lymphoid germinal centers,[68, 69] thymus,[70, 71] adrenal gland,[72-74] bone marrow,[75, 76] and certain tumors.[77]

Thus, in many tissues, the cell cycle time distribution has a spatial representation, and the physical migration of cells from one region to another provides directly observable evidence for the sequence of cell cycle lengthening, and loss of reproductive capacity and/or cell removal.

Growth Retardation and Cell Loss; Cytomorphologic Correlates. In some tissues, notably in the reticuloendothelial system, the process of cell migration with growth retardation is associated also with distinctive changes in cell morphology. In the normal lymphoid germinal center the cells of the dark zone become smaller as they migrate into the light zone, and undergo growth retardation over the course of one or more divisions.[68, 69] In the normal bone marrow the large, rapidly proliferating myeloid cells are found in the subendosteal region of the marrow and become smaller as they migrate from the subendosteal region to the central region of the marrow, undergoing growth retardation in the process.[75]

The cytomorphologic changes accompanying growth retardation are often present even in the absence of clearly demonstrable microarchitectural organization and in the absence of clearly demonstrable physical migration of cells from one region to another. The large lymphoid cells of the normal bone marrow proliferate more rapidly than the small lymphoid cells, and the latter are derived from the former.[78-80] The transition from rapidly proliferating large cells to slowly proliferating small cells has been demonstrated in experimental and human leukemias.[81-84] Recent studies in our own

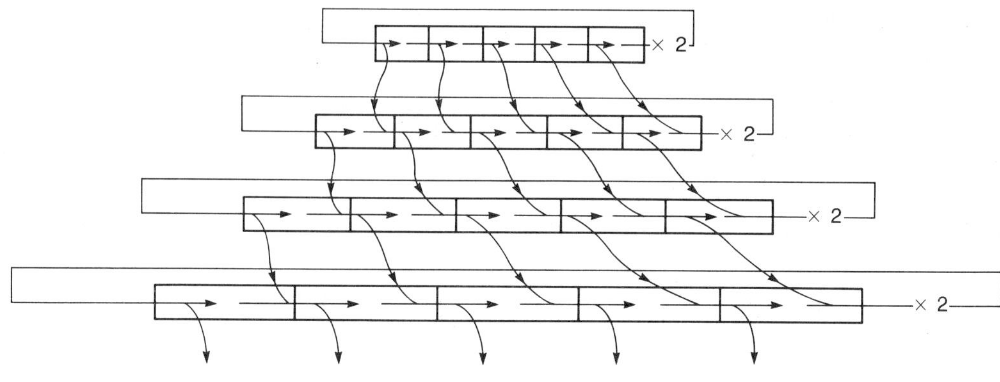

Figure 3–10. Diagrammatic representation of cell cycle pathways in a cell population with structured kinetic heterogeneity. Rapidly proliferating cells (usually found in close proximity to the arteriolar blood supply) may cycle "in place" or spiral into longer cell cycles. Similarly, cells at other levels may cycle "in place" or spiral into longer cell cycles. The net flow of cells is from shorter to longer cell cycles.

laboratory have demonstrated a correlation between G_1 cell size and proliferative rate in human lymphomas also.[85]

Structured Kinetic Heterogeneity. The foregoing observations suggest that the kinetic heterogeneity of mammalian cell populations is not random, but is highly structured. For example, in a population with random heterogeneity, cells and their progeny may either speed up or slow down at random. In a population with structured heterogeneity, there is a *net* flow of cells from short cell cycles to long cell cycles under steady-state conditions (Fig. 3–10).

Smith and Martin[86] have proposed an alternative to the classic cell cycle model in which a cell's life is divided into what they call "A" and "B" states. A cell is assumed to remain in the A state (equivalent to a variable G_1 or G_0 state) for any length of time, but with a constant probability of leaving the A state to enter the B state. The B state, encompassing at least S, G_2, and M, is envisioned as the deterministic portion of the cell cycle that is directed toward replication. Upon completion of mitosis, a cell is presumed to re-enter the A state.

The Smith and Martin model has the advantage of formally dispensing with the seemingly futile attempt to distinguish long G_1 from G_0. However, the model implies complete randomness of cell cycle time. It does not take into account the organized kinetic structure of tissues and the spatial separation of rapidly growing and slowly growing cells. It also disregards the correlations between mother and daughter cells, and between daughter cells, that are inherent in kinetically structured tissues.

THE INTERACTIONS OF CYTOTOXIC DRUGS WITH PROLIFERATING CELL POPULATIONS

An understanding of the principles of cell kinetics described in the earlier sections of this chapter is essential for an understanding of the effects of cytotoxic drugs.

In this section we will examine the interactions of drugs with proliferating cell populations on two levels. First, we will consider concepts that relate drug lethality to overall changes in the tumor cell population growth curve. In this area the concept of log kill proposed by Skipper and coworkers[42] has been of central importance. These concepts are relevant to the development of basic principles of clinical treatment strategy, dealing with such issues as the overall duration of treatment, the role of treatment intensification, the value of low-dose maintenance therapy, and the role of adjuvant therapy.

In this section we will also deal with the lethal and sublethal effects of drugs on cells in relation to cell proliferative state and proliferative rate. Cell cycle phase–specific lethality, cell cycle blockade, and cell recruitment will be considered in detail. These concepts are relevant to the optimization of therapeutic tactics, i.e., in choosing the most appropriate drugs for a given schedule and in choosing the best drug sequences and treatment intervals.

Many of the concepts dealing with the effects of cytotoxic drugs on proliferating cells were developed in the late 1960s, before the nature and extent of population kinetic heterogeneity were fully appreciated. Historically, concepts that focus on drug effects within "the" cell cycle, such as cell cycle phase–specific lethality and cell cycle blockade, have received the most attention. More recently, with the recognition that the therapist must deal with a broad spectrum of tumor cell cycles, the concept of recruitment has come to assume greater importance.

Lethal Drug Effects

The Concept of Log Kill. The log kill concept was developed by Skipper and colleagues[42] to account for their observations in mouse L1210 leukemia that multiple courses of treatment with cytotoxic drugs could be curative although individual courses of treatment were not.

The essential element of the log kill concept is the notion that, quite apart from any other forms of drug resistance that might be present, cells can survive a course of treatment purely by chance, even though they are essentially *no different* in their susceptibility from the cells that *were* killed. The same surviving cells might be killed by a dose of the same drug in a subsequent course of treatment. To appreciate this better, we might consider a simplified model borrowed from the field of radiation biology.

Example 7. Let us assume that a given dose of radiation produces a given average number of randomly distributed "active events" per unit area within the radiation field and that the number of "active events" greatly exceeds the initial number of cells in the field. Let us assume further in this example that any cell within the field has a 50 per cent chance of being "hit" by an "active event" and killed. When there are 20 cells within the field, 10 cells are killed by a given radiation dose (Fig. 3–11A). The 10 cells that survive are intrinsically no different in their susceptibility to radiation from the cells that were killed. A second dose of radiation will be just as effective as the first and is likely to kill another 50 per cent of the population (Fig. 3–11B).

It is clear from this example that a treatment regimen that reduces a population of 20 cells by 75 per cent overall is hardly curative, considering that even one surviving viable cell can regenerate the entire population. If the cell fraction killed per treatment were higher, say 0.9, then approximately two cells, on the average, would survive the first dose, and the probability of at least one viable cell surviving a second dose would be low. When the cell popula-

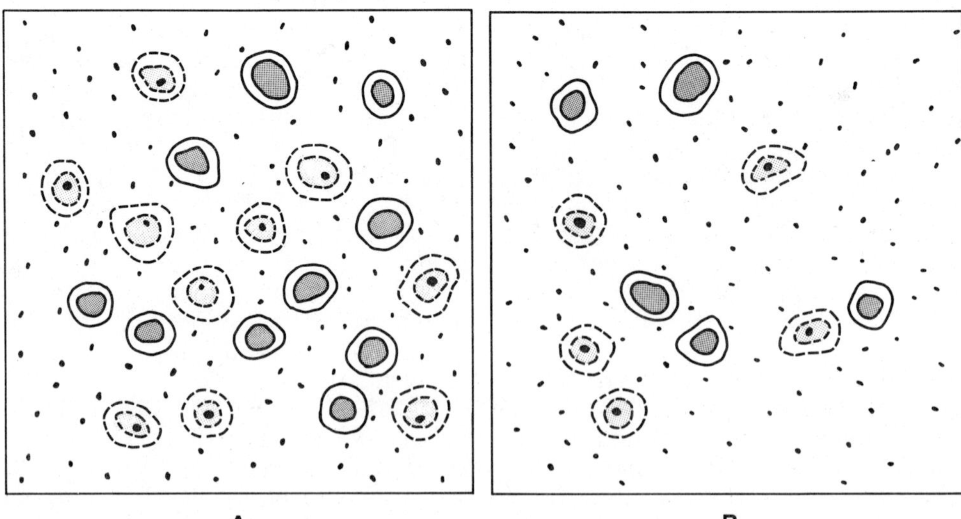

Figure 3–11. Schematic illustration of cell survival due to chance following radiation. Small dots represent "active" radiation "events" randomly distributed throughout the radiation field. Cells shown with broken lines represent lethally damaged cells.

TABLE 3–3. The Relationship of Fractional Cell Kill To Log Kill

Cell Fraction Killed	*Surviving Cell Fraction*	*Log Surviving Cell Fraction*	*Log Kill*
.9	.1	−1	1
.99	.01	−2	2
.999	.001	−3	3
.999999999	.000000001	−9	9

tion is large (e.g., 1×10^9 cells), a much greater fractional cell kill, or multiple courses of therapy, are needed to achieve cure. Large overall fractional cell kills (for example 0.99999) can be cumbersome to deal with in decimal notation. Hence, the log kill notation where

$$\text{log kill} = -\log\ (\text{surviving cell fraction}) \quad \text{[eq. 4]}$$

Sample calculations are shown in Table 3–3. Thus, for example, to eradicate a tumor containing 1×10^9 cells (~1 gm of tissue) one must achieve a log kill that exceeds 9.

One might infer from the example shown in Figure 3–11 that a given dose of drug will kill a constant fraction of the population *regardless* of population size. Originally, Skipper's group did, in fact, make this assumption in interpreting their drug response data. For simplicity, they also assumed the ideal case of simple exponential growth for L1210 leukemia, as shown schematically in Figure 3–12A.

Skipper et al. studied the schedule-dependent effects of cytosine arabinoside in mouse L1210 leukemia.[63] This drug preferentially kills cells that are actively engaged in DNA synthesis (see below). Using host survival time as a bioassay for estimating the number of cells surviving treatment, these authors showed that by increasing the frequency of doses and thereby prolonging exposure to cytosine arabinoside progressively for up to 24 hours, increasingly larger

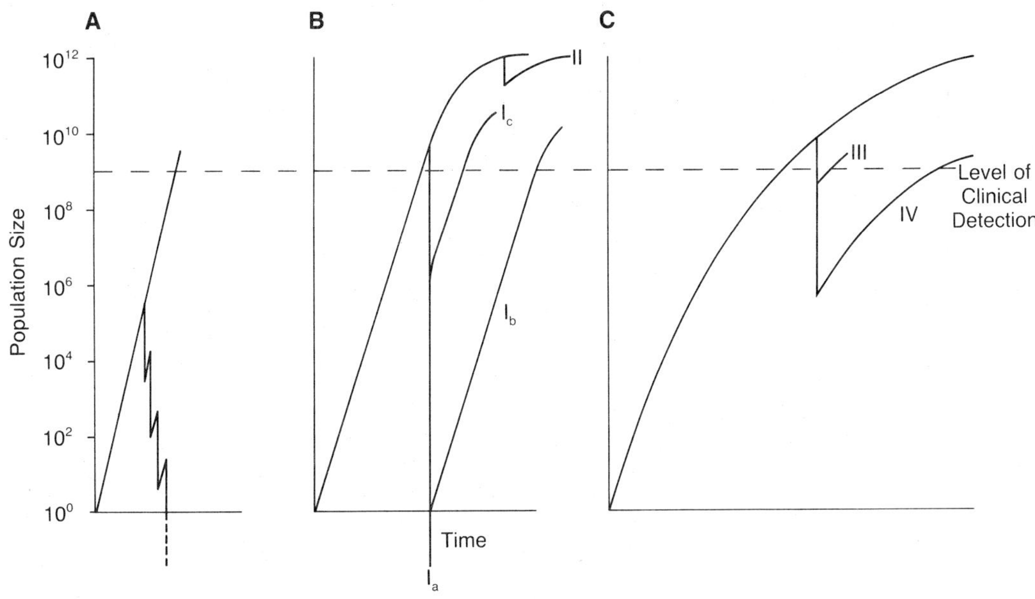

Figure 3–12. Schematic illustration of the interrelationships among tumor growth rate, log kill, and cure or relapse. *A,* Simple exponential growth is assumed. Log kill is assumed to be independent of population size and population growth rate. Repeated courses of treatment produce a progressive reduction in tumor size until cure is achieved. *B,* Schematic representation of a rapidly growing human tumor. Growth retardation occurs in late stages of growth. Log kill is assumed to be dependent on population growth rate. Large log kills in early clinical stages of disease may be curative (*curve I_a*) or nearly curative (*curve I_b*). Intermediate log kills lead to early relapse (*curve I_c*). Low growth rates in advanced disease are associated with small log kills (*curve II*). *C,* Schematic representation of a slowly growing human tumor. Growth retardation occurs in subclinical stages of growth. Small log kills in clinical stages of growth are followed by early relapses (*curve III*). A long period of disease-free survival may not imply a large log kill (*compare curve IV with curve I_b*).

cell kills were produced. Skipper and his group assumed that this was due to continual entry of cells into the vulnerable S phase during the period of drug exposure.

Skipper showed that a single 24-hour course of cytosine arabinoside (eight drug injections q3h) would not cure mice inoculated with 1×10^5 leukemic cells, but that three to four courses given at four-day intervals *were* curative.[63] These observations could be explained by the log kill concept (see Fig. 3–12A) if all the viable tumor cells had gone through the vulnerable S phase during the course of each 24-hour treatment. This was a reasonable premise, assuming that:

1. the cell cycle time of L1210 leukemia cells was 12 hours with little variability (from PLM curve data);
2. the growth fraction was 1;
3. cells exposed to drug in nonsensitive phases of the cell cycle proceeded without impediment into S phase; and
4. the kinetic behavior of cells that were exposed to drug in S phase and survived treatment in early courses was no different from that of cells that had never been exposed to drug.

In retrospect, virtually all the various assumptions regarding population growth and drug response that formed the basis for interpreting these studies have proved to be so highly oversimplified that they could not be applied to clinical cancer treatment in their original form. The broad cell cycle time distributions of human tumors and the ubiquitous phenomenon of growth retardation with increasing population size have been considered in previous sections. Detailed computer modeling studies of Skipper's own L1210 leukemia data have demonstrated the importance of growth retardation even in this rapidly proliferating cell system, and have indicated that log kill varies with population growth rate.[64] In late stages of growth there is a progressive decrease in log kill that accompanies a progressive decrease in growth rate.

In spite of the oversimplification of early assumptions associated with the log kill concept, it did represent a major advance in the effort to quantitate the post-treatment residual body burden of tumor in experimental systems. More recent refinements of this concept have made it possible to estimate the post-treatment residual body burden of tumor in man and to assess the efficacy of clinical treatment regimens.[2]

Clinical applications of the log kill concept are based on the following principles:

Despite variability from patient to patient, human tumors are distinctive and predictable in their overall growth behavior. This principle was first proposed by Collins and co-workers[87] and formed the basis for the "period of risk" method that they introduced. Collins hypothesized that the growth pattern of a given tumor from the time of its inception from a single malignant cell to the time of clinical diagnosis would be characteristic and reproducible in each patient. If a single viable tumor were left after therapy, the time of tumor growth to clinical recurrence should be comparable to the time of growth from inception of the original tumor to initial clinical diagnosis. This, then, is the period of risk. If the tumor did not recur within the period of risk, one could infer that the last tumor cell had been eradicated and that the patient would continue to remain free of disease.

Although Collins and colleagues assumed the case of simple exponential growth (Fig. 3–12A), much as Skipper and his group did later, the principle that tumors exhibit characteristic growth rates in individual patients or groups of patients could also apply to growth curves that exhibit late growth retardation. Of course, since all tumors eventually become slowly growing tumors, we must define more carefully what we mean by slowly growing and rapidly growing tumors.

Slowly growing human tumors undergo much of their growth retardation during the subclinical stage of growth; they are likely to exhibit low growth rates (long doubling times) throughout the clinically observable range of growth (Fig. 3–12C). Although rapidly growing human tumors also undergo growth retardation, this occurs late in the course of growth; the property that defines rapidly growing human tumors is that high subclinical growth rates are maintained during early stages of clinically observable tumor growth (Fig. 3–12B).

Another important principle is that the responsiveness of human tumors to therapy is dependent on tumor growth rate (see Table 3–1 and associated discussion). Large log kills are achievable in rapidly growing tumors in early stages of clinical growth, and with adequate treatment such tumors are often curable (*curve* I_a, Fig. 3–12B). Slowly growing tumors respond less well to therapy. Complete responses tend to be shallow, in that the residual subclinical body tumor burden is still substantial; relatively small log kills lead to relapses on therapy, or within months of cessation of therapy (*curve III*, Fig. 3–12C). A long, disease-free remission following treatment of a slowly growing tumor does not have the same implications as a prolonged, disease-free remission following treatment of a rapidly growing tumor (compare log kill achieved in *curve* I_b, Fig. 3–12B, with that of *curve IV*, Fig. 3–12C).

The concept of the period of risk can provide a quantitative measure of the efficacy of cancer treatment in biologic terms. Early tumor recurrences after termination of therapy, in patients with slowly growing tumors who achieve complete clinical responses to treamment, would suggest that log kills were small and that the subclinical body tumor burden was still substantial when therapy was stopped. That is, it is likely that the therapy given was ineffective to begin with (see *curves III* and *IV*, Fig. 3–12C). On the other hand, late tumor recurrences in patients with rapidly growing tumors would suggest that significant reductions in body tumor burden were achieved. That is, late recurrences would suggest that therapy *was* effective but that too few treatment courses may have been given to eradicate the tumor completely (see *curve* I_b, Fig. 3–12B). Of course, the definition of early and late relapses would depend to a large extent on the period of risk for the tumor under consideration. In Burkitt's lymphoma, for example, relapses occurring within six weeks of termination of therapy might be considered early relapses, whereas those occurring after six weeks would have to be considered late relapses. In the large cell non-Hodgkin's lymphomas, relapses occurring as late as six to nine months after termination of therapy might still be considered early relapses, whereas in Hodgkin's disease the dividing line might be between one and two years.

From a practical standpoint, in patients with late tumor recurrences, more prolonged retreatment with the initially effective regimen should be given serious consideration. In contrast, patients with early tumor recurrences might be expected to respond poorly to the initial regimen, and a change in treatment would be appropriate. This strategy is supported by the good responses to retreatment in patients with late tumor recurrences in Hodgkin's disease[88] and large cell non-Hodgkin's lymphoma.[89] As might be expected, early recurrences in MOPP-treated patients with Hodgkin's disease do not respond well to retreatment with MOPP.[88]

One aspect of the period of risk concept is the notion that true tumor cure requires the eradication of the last viable tumor cell. This is essentially an all-or-none phenomenon. It follows that intermittent or low-level maintenance therapy has no rational justification in the primary treatment of responsive tumors. If a small body burden of residual tumor is presumed to be present following treatment induction and consolidation, prudence dictates prolongation of the period of intensive consolidative therapy. If, on the other hand, the last tumor cell is presumed to have been eradicated, no further therapy is warranted.

Phase-Specific Drug Lethality. The concept of cell cycle phase–specific lethality of cytotoxic drug was developed by Bruce and colleagues,[90] based on their studies of dose-response relationships using a modification of the spleen colony assay for clonogenic murine AKR lymphoma cells. They administered various drugs in multidose schedules (usually q4h over a 24-hour period) and found that survival curves could be classified broadly either as exponentially decreasing or as plateau-type curves. Drugs that exhibited exponential dose-response curves were considered noncycle stage–specific; drugs exhibiting plateau-type dose-survival curves were interpreted as having cell cycle phase–specific properties. That is, the plateau in survival despite increasing dosage was attributed to the invulnerability of cells that had not passed through the drug-sensitive phase during the period of drug availability, and thus would not be killed by the drug even at very high drug concentrations. Alkylating agents and ionizing radiation clearly produced exponential dose-response curves.[90] The vinca alkaloids, methotrexate, and cytosine arabinoside clearly produced plateau-type curves.[90, 91] Phase-specific lethality was explained on the basis of mitotic arrest in the case of the vinca alkaloids (Chapter 11) and on the basis of inhibition of DNA synthesis in the case of methotrexate and cytosine arabinoside (Chapters 10 and 18).

It should be emphasized that cell cycle phase–specific drug lethality was not demonstrated directly in the studies of Bruce and colleagues, but was inferred from cell survival patterns following multidose drug treatment schedules. The development of

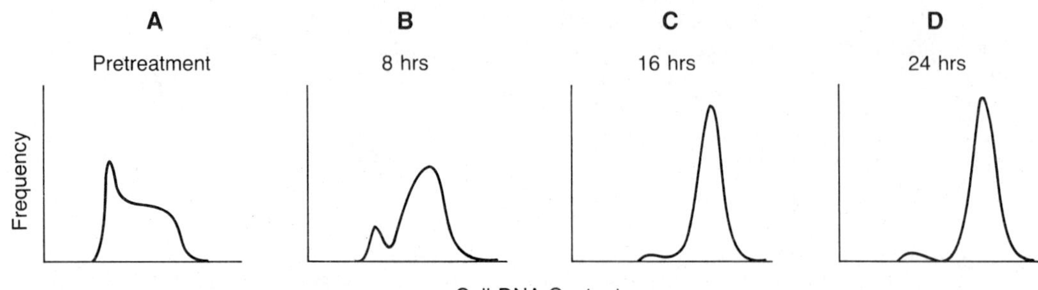

Figure 3–13. The effects of doxorubicin (Adriamycin) on the DNA histogram in sarcoma 180 *in vitro*. Cells progress from the G_1 and early S region (*A* and *B*) and accumulate in the G_2M region of the histogram (*C* and *D*).

techniques for cell synchronization *in vitro*[92] enabled more direct studies of the the cycle phase–specific drug lethality. Cell killing following brief exposure to hydroxyurea[93, 94] or cytosine arabinoside[94, 95] was greatest when these drugs were administered when cells were passing through S phase. This evidence, taken together with the known inhibitory effects of hydroxyurea and cytosine arabinoside on DNA synthesis, made a strong case for the preferential lethality of these two agents for S-phase cells.

There are pitfalls in the interpretation of data relating to phase–specific lethality that could lead to the misuse of this principle in the design of optimized drug treatment regimens.

When the effects of cytotoxic drugs involve multiple intracellular biochemical sites of action, drug lethality may not be linked exclusively to cell cycle phase–dependent processes. For example, cytosine arabinoside inhibits DNA polymerase[96, 97] and is also incorporated into both DNA and RNA.[97-99] It is not entirely clear which of these mechanisms is responsible for drug lethality, or whether the same mechanism(s) would apply under different conditions of drug exposure. Methotrexate inhibits DNA synthesis, but also affects purine synthetic pathways that could affect RNA and protein synthesis as well. The binding of vincristine to tubulin could account for metaphase arrest during and after drug exposure. However, the relative resistance of synchronized premitotic and mitotic cells to the lethal effects of vincristine in comparison with cells in late S phase[93, 100] suggests that tubulin binding may not be its only pharmacologic action.

Many of the commonly used antineoplastic drugs produce a common and distinctive sequence of kinetic changes in the DNA histogram following drug exposure, namely, an accumulation of cells in the G_2 region of the histogram over the course of time. This pattern has been observed following doxorubicin (Adriamycin) and daunomycin,[101-104] nitrosoureas,[105] streptozotocin and chlorozotocin,[106] bleomycin,[107] and various alkylating agents.[108] A representative DNA histogram sequence following exposure to doxorubicin is shown in Figure 3–13. This general pattern has been interpreted as indicating cell cycle arrest in G_2. However, it seems unlikely that there is any direct connection between the mechanism of drug lethality and the accumulation of cells in the G_2 region of the DNA histogram. Most of these agents exhibit exponential or quasi-exponential pulse dose survival curves in experimental systems,[104, 106, 109, 110] with log kills in the range of 1 to 3 following brief exposure to high drug concentrations, suggesting the absence of cell cycle phase–specific lethality of any kind.

Rather than focus on the fact that these drugs produce an accumulation of cells in the G_2 region of the DNA histogram, we might direct our attention to the fact that these drugs do not prevent G_1 cells from traversing the S region. That is, they do not prevent cells from synthesizing their full complement of DNA. The failure of these drugs to prevent the initiation and completion of DNA synthesis points to the primacy of a lethal mechanism of drug action that involves some other metabolic process in the cell that is critical for cell division.

Nonlethal Drug Effects

Cell Cycle Blockade. In the early studies of Skipper et al.[63] and Bruce et al.,[90] it was assumed that there was no impediment to the flow of cells through nonsensitive phases of the cell cycle following pulse drug exposure or during continuous exposure to phase-specific agents. In subsequent work, Bruce et al. found that survival curves during continued drug exposure *did* exhibit decreased cell killing with time, most notably in the case of methotrexate, but also in the case of vinblastine and cytosine arabinoside.[91] These later studies were interpreted as possibly indicating cell cycle blockade, i.e., interference with the progression of cells into the drug-sensitive phase of the cell cycle.

Many of the early studies of hydroxyurea were carried out in tissue culture, where the effects of the drug on both cell survival and cell cycle traverse could be examined directly. Sinclair[111] and others[112, 113] showed that synchronized G_1 cells were prevented from incorporating ^{3}H-TdR in the presence of a drug, but proceeded through S phase after the drug was removed. The same was also shown to be true of cytosine arabinoside.[113] Synchronized G_1 cells that were exposed to cytosine arabinoside for prolonged periods showed no decrease in cell survival in the presence of the drug.[94] In asynchronous populations exposed to hydroxyurea, the rapid inhibition of DNA synthesis was followered several hours later by an overshoot in ^{3}H-TdR incorporation and/or the LI.[114-116] Cytosine arabinoside produced similar effects.[117] These findings suggested a block at the G_1/S boundary in the presence of these drugs, with subsequent release and progression of a synchronized cohort of cells through S phase after drug removal (Fig. 3–14).

Although the concept of cell cycle blockade with cell synchronization does provide a plausible explanation for the post-treatment increase in LI and cell labeling intensity that is often observed in experimental cell systems, the recruitment of slowly proliferating cells into rapid cycle could also account for these observations (see below). Additional data would be required in order to distinguish between these two processes. The features that distinguish cell cycle blockade and cell synchronization from cell recruitment are listed in Table 3–4.

If cell cycle blockade is the underlying mechanism responsible for cell synchronization, the degree of cell synchronization should depend on the duration of the drug-induced block, as shown in Figure 3–14. For example, if there is a block at the G_1/S boundary, all G_1 cells less than one hour away from the G_1/S boundary would be blocked and synchronized after a drug exposure period of one hour; cells earlier in G_1 that are four hours away from the G_1/S boundary at the time the block was imposed would be neither blocked nor synchronized unless the block were maintained for longer than four hours. If it cannot be shown experimentally that the degree of synchronization increases with increasing drug exposure duration, the synchronization that *is* observed may be due to a kinetic mechanism other than cell cycle blockade. By the same token, the inclusion of an unexpectedly large fraction of the cell population in the synchronized wave after only brief drug exposure would also favor an underlying mechanism other than cell cycle blockade.

Dethlefsen et al.[118] reviewed the literature prior to 1977 and were unable to find convincing evidence for increased cell synchronization with prolongation of exposure to either hydroxyurea or cytosine arabinoside. In more recent studies by the authors of this chapter,[119] the degree of synchronization of sarcoma 180 cells as determined by flow cytometry was no greater after 12 hours to exposure to hydroxyurea than after one hour of drug exposure.

Radioautographic and flow cytometry data obtained in sarcoma 180 cells grown *in vitro* following brief exposure to hydroxyurea[119] are shown in Figure 3–15. ^{3}H-TdR incorporation (as evidenced by the cell fractions with high grain counts) falls rapidly after a two-hour exposure to drug, reflecting a rapid reduction in the rate of DNA synthesis (Fig. 3–15A). ^{3}H-TdR incorporation resumes within several hours, peaking eight to ten hours after initial drug exposure. The DNA histogram shows a cohort of partially synchronized cells starting to traverse the S region within two hours of drug removal (Fig. 3–15B_2) and passing through mid-S phase at about eight to ten hours (Fig. 3–15B_4 and B_5).

One might wish to explain these data simply on the basis of drug-induced cell cycle blockade with cell synchronization. However, the cell cycle time distribution in these cells ranges from eight to 18 hours or longer, with a median of approximately 12 hours.[62] It seems unlikely that a period of drug-induced cell cycle blockade of only

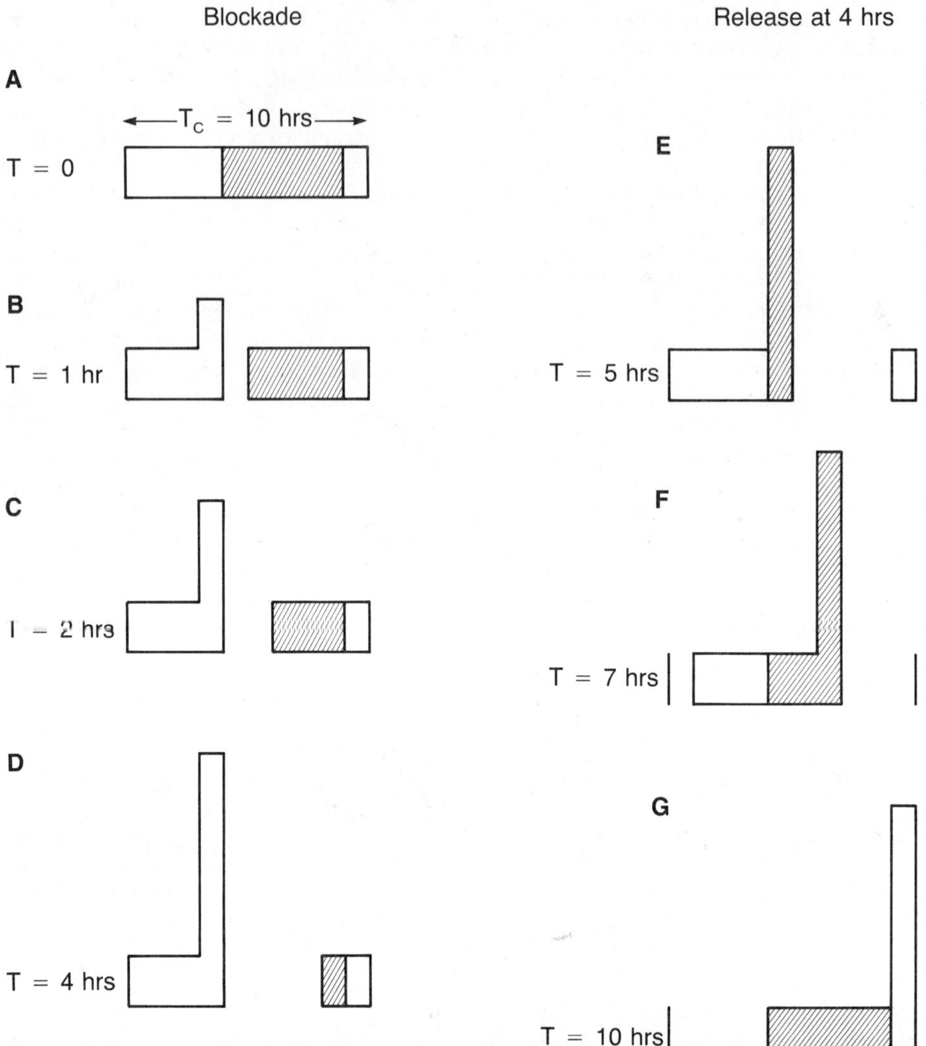

Figure 3–14. Schematic representation of cell cycle blockade with cell synchronization at the G_1/S interface (*A–D*), followed by movement of the synchronized cell cohort through the cell cycle after release from the block (*E–G*).

two hours' duration could account for the early appearance of so prominent a wave of synchronized cells.

The theoretical basis for preferential blockade and synchronization of rapidly proliferating cells (Table 3–4) is shown schematically in Figure 3–16. In a kinetically heterogeneous cell population the rapidly proliferating cells should be more extensively affected by a block of given duration than are the slowly proliferating cells. Significant involvement of slowly proliferating cells in the post-treatment increase in LI would favor recruitment over cell cycle blockade with synchronization as the underlying kinetic process (see below).

TABLE 3–4. The Distinguishing Features of Cell Cycle Blockade with Synchronization

1. Greater synchronization with prolongation of block duration
2. Preferential blockade and synchronization of rapidly proliferating cells
3. Rapid appearance of synchronized cell cohort (hours) after block removal
4. Rapid desynchronization (within a time period equivalent to 2 to 3 rapid cell cycles)

If cell cycle blockade is to be followed by the progression of a synchronized wave of cells beyond the blockade point, the effects of the block should be reversed promptly and completely upon drug removal. A gradual increase in LI following drug removal

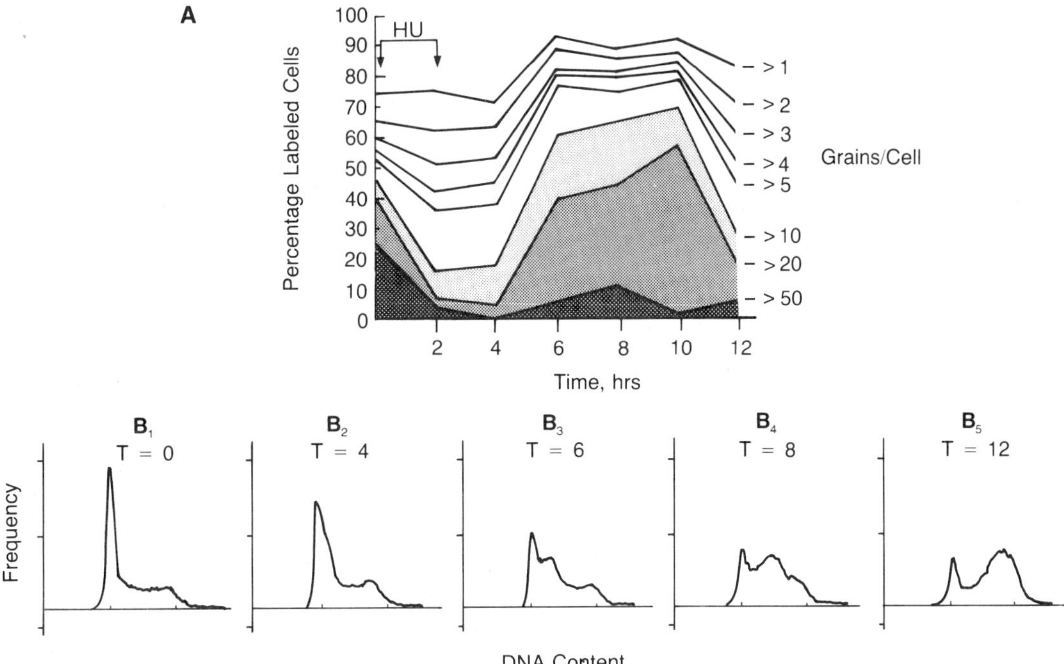

Figure 3–15. *A,* Changes in the LI obtained at several different grain count thresholds as a function of time after brief exposure of sarcoma 180 cells to hydroxyurea *in vitro.* There is a rapid fall in the fractions of heavily labeled cells at 2–4 hours, followed by an increase in the heavily labeled cell fractions at 6–10 hours. B_1–B_5, Sequential changes in the DNA histogram following exposure of sarcoma 180 cells to hydroxyurea *in vitro.*

would suggest the presence of lingering drug effects. A delayed increase in LI (e.g., by several days) would favor a kinetic process other than cell cycle blockade with synchronization.

The desynchronization of synchronized cells is generally quite rapid; it is usually apparent within a period equivalent to one rapid cycle time and is far advanced over a period equivalent to two rapid cycle times. Thus, a post-treatment increase in LI that is sustained for longer than the equivalent of two to three rapid cell cycles is likely to be due to the recruitment of slowly proliferating cells into rapid cycle rather than to cell cycle blockade with synchronization.

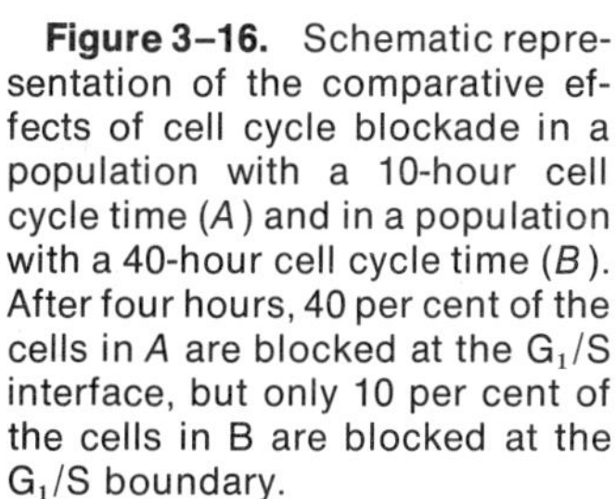

Figure 3–16. Schematic representation of the comparative effects of cell cycle blockade in a population with a 10-hour cell cycle time (*A*) and in a population with a 40-hour cell cycle time (*B*). After four hours, 40 per cent of the cells in *A* are blocked at the G_1/S interface, but only 10 per cent of the cells in B are blocked at the G_1/S boundary.

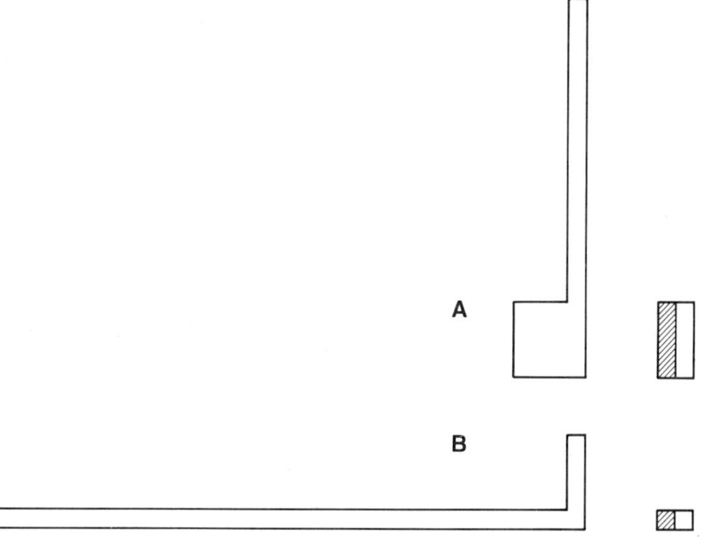

The schema shown in Figure 3–13 is based on the assumptions that (1) drug-induced blockade is restricted to a single point; i.e., there is no inhibition of cell cycle progression proximal to the block; and (2) blocked cells are brought to a complete halt rather than being slowed in their progress through the cell cycle. If either of these conditions is not met, cell cycle blockade may not be accompanied by cell synchronization. Although the question of single-point blockade versus blockade at multiple points is far from settled, it is clear that hydroxyurea and cytosine arabinoside can retard but not completely block the progression of cells into and through early S phase. Tobey and Crissman showed that synchronized G_1 cells exposed to hydroxyurea or cytosine arabinoside[113] for prolonged periods incorporated ^{3}H-TdR after a delay of several hours, but that the grain counts of the labeled cells were low. Using flow cytometry, Yataganas et al. demonstrated a broadening of the G_1 peak in asynchronous populations exposed to cytosine arabinoside[120] or hydroxyurea[121] for prolonged periods. They interpreted these findings as indicating that cells crossed the G_1/S boundary but that there was greater inhibition of cell progression through S phase, especially at higher drug concentrations.

Under conditions of prolonged exposure to drugs that directly inhibit DNA synthesis but do not abolish it completely, the very concept of a discrete G_1/S boundary tends to break down. In this setting, postmitotic cells that undertake DNA synthesis at very low rates may remain indistinguishable from nonsynthesizing postmitotic cells for a long time with respect to cell DNA content, and their incorporation of ^{3}H-TdR may be too low to be detected under ordinary radioautographic processing conditions. Since the rate of DNA synthesis is a major determinant of S-phase–specific drug lethality,[122] cells in early S phase that are synthesizing DNA slowly may also be relatively resistant to prolonged exposure to S-phase–specific drugs.

Regardless of whether cell cycle blockade produces cell synchronization, it *is* a major effect of treatment with cytotoxic drugs. Cell cycle blockade and a variety of related terms, including *inhibition* of cell cycle progression, cell cycle progression *delay* or division delay (a prolonged reduction in the mitotic index), *arrest* within a phase or at a phase boundary, and *inhibition* or interference with specific cell cycle–dependent reactions, like DNA synthesis, all describe one common kinetic process: affected cells undergo a provisional lengthening of cell cycle time. This is true regardless of whether the block is complete or incomplete (provided, of course, that the block is reversible upon drug removal). Obviously, when there is a drug-induced shift in the cell cycle time distribution to longer values, the pretreatment mean (or median) and range of the distribution cannot be relied on to determine optimal intervals between pulse doses of drug or the optimal duration of treatment by prolonged drug infusion.

Cell Recruitment. Cell recruitment may be defined as the mobilization of slowly proliferating or nonproliferating cells to more rapid proliferation. Conceptually, this may be viewed either as a discrete transition from G_0 to the cycling state or as a shift in the cell cycle time distribution from longer to shorter values (see Fig. 3–8C). Recruitment is commonly achieved by "uncrowding" the population, i.e., by reducing overall population size, but recruitment can also be effected by chemical means in the absence of extensive cell loss, as with the addition of fresh serum-containing medium *in vitro*.[123-125]

The magnitude and time course of the recruitment response depend on a variety of factors, such as the nature, intensity, and duration of the recruitment stimulus; the degree of kinetic heterogeneity in the population; and intrinsic cell properties that govern the rates at which slowly proliferating cells can be mobilized to proliferate more rapidly.

When relatively large numbers of slowly proliferating G_1 cells are telescoped rapidly into short cell cycles, they may traverse these short cell cycles in a synchronized wave (Fig. 3–17A_1 to A_3). Depending on the intensity and duration of the original recruitment stimulus, these cells and their progeny may continue to cycle rapidly, or they may return to longer cell cycles within one or two cell generations.

Detailed computer modeling studies have indicated that the wave of synchronized cells revealed by the data shown in Figure 3–15 consists of two components. The early component is attributable to the rapid recruitment of slowly proliferating G_1 cells. Cells recovering from drug-induced growth retardation (i.e., G_1 blockade and inhibition of DNA synthesis) contribute to the partially

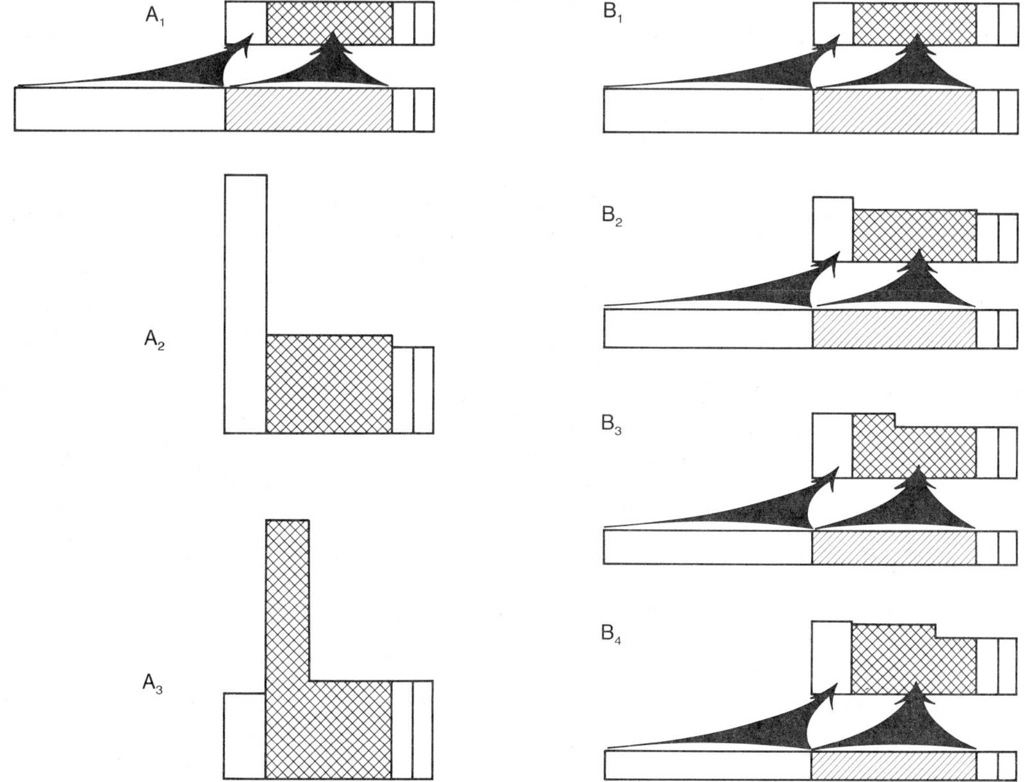

Figure 3–17. The relation between recruitment and cell synchronization (*shaded regions represent S phase*). With rapid cell recruitment (A_1), slowly cycling G_1 cells are telescoped into a short G_1 period in short cycles, producing a synchronized wave of cells (A_2), which is propagated through the cell cycle (A_3). When cell recruitment is gradual (B_1–B_4), recruitment does not produce a synchronized wave. However, there is a sustained increase in LI and MI that is due to higher T_S/T_C and T_M/T_C ratios.

synchronized wave at later times. Overall, the wave of partially synchronized cells could not be accounted for in quantitative terms in these studies without invoking the recruitment of slowly proliferating cells following drug exposure. Computer modeling studies of the kinetic response to hydroxyurea in mouse duodenum[118] and the EMT6 mouse tumor[126] have also led to the conclusion that cell recruitment is a major component of the kinetic recovery sequence following drug exposure.

Serial radioautographic studies have provided more concrete demonstrations of recruitment following exposure to hydroxyurea in small bowel mucosa[127] and bone marrow.[128] In both tissues there is a clear spatial localization of slowly proliferating and rapidly proliferating cells, and in both tissues a rapid increase in the proliferative rate of the slowly cycling cells is observed following drug exposure.

When the recruitment of slowly proliferating cells proceeds gradually, the transition from longer to shorter cell cycles may *not* be accompanied by significant synchronization within a particular phase of the cell cycle (see Fig. 3–17B_1 to B_4). Nonetheless, gradual recruitment can still produce an increase in the LI (due solely to a decrease in average T_C relative to average T_S (see [eq. 1]). Similarly, the mitotic index (MI), where

$$MI = \frac{N_{mitosis}}{N_{total}} = \frac{T_M}{T_C} \qquad [eq. 5]$$

may also increase during the gradual recruitment of slowly proliferating cells, owing solely to a decrease in average T_C relative to T_M. Thus, increases in LI and MI may be associated with either synchronization or recruitment, or both. When increases in LI and MI are sustained for longer than the equivalent of two to three rapid cell cycles, they are likely to be due primarily to the recruitment of slowly proliferating cells into rapid cycle rather than to cell synchronization, especially when they are also accompanied by sustained increases in radioautographic labeling intensity.

Although cell recruitment and recovery from cell cycle blockade often overlap in time in experimental cell systems, the time courses of these processes may differ considerably in man. Changes in LI in acute human leukemia following treatment with cytosine arabinoside are summarized in Table 3–5. In most of these studies, drug-induced changes in LI were monitored over the first 24 to 72 hours after drug administration. A decrease in LI was commonly observed within two to eight hours of drug administration. Post-treatment increases in LI were most commonly observed at 24 to 48 hours. Increases above pretreatment values were of modest proportions in most instances, with the maximal LI rarely exceeding 0.3. In several studies, 20 to 30 per cent of patients showed no post-treatment increases in LI above pretreatment values. From these observations one would expect marginal improvements in tumor response from treatment regimens that employ drugs directed specifically against the fraction of cells synchronized in S phase.

Bleomycin has been proposed for cell cycle blockade in G_2 with synchronization upon release.[136] The LI in two patients with human melanoma showed only a modest increase 48 to 72 hours after termination of a four-day bleomycin infusion;[136] the maximal LI observed in this study was 0.32. Here, too, therapy directed specifically against cells synchronized in S phase would be of marginal value.

Most clinical studies of drug-induced kinetic changes have tended to focus on the potential role of cell synchronization in the early post-treatment period, but evidence has been accumulating that significant post-treatment changes in LI extend through the second and third weeks following drug treatment. The nadir in the LI of leukemic myeloblasts following daunomycin treatment was found to extend over a period ranging from one to four days after drug exposure.[137] Presumably, recovery to pretreatment levels occurred in these patients at later times. Increases in LI have been observed in human leukemic marrow eight days after daunomycin and cytosine arabinoside were given together.[138] In the marrow of a neuroblastoma patient treated with a combination of vincristine, cyclophosphamide, and doxorubicin, the nadir in LI was not observed until day 4, and a progressive rise in LI and cell labeling intensity was under way on day 9 when the study was terminated.[139] Peak labeling indices in normal human marrow are observed during the second and third week after cyclophosphamide administration.[140]

The time course of such changes in LI is so protracted that they cannot be accounted for by cell cycle blockade with synchronization and must be attributed to recruitment of slowly proliferating cells into rapid cycle. Treatment strategies based on recruitment need not depend on drug effects that are

TABLE 3–5. The Effects of Cytosine Arabinoside on the LI In Human Leukemia

Dose	Tissue/Tumor	No. of Pts.	LI Range Pre Rx	LI Range Post Rx	Times of Max. LI Post Rx	Ref.
2–2.5 μg/kg single dose	AML, myeloblasts	6	0.07–0.18	0.10–0.2	12–36 hrs	129
4.3–6.1 μg/kg single dose	CML, myeloblasts	3	0.12–0.18	0.21–0.34	15 hrs	130
	Promyeloblasts and myeloblasts		0.19–0.23	0.26–0.30	15 hrs	
100 mg/m² single dose	AML	21	0.06–0.18	0.02–0.32	24–48 hrs	131, 132
5 mg/kg single dose	ALL	7	0.02–0.16	0.02–0.40	24–48 hrs	133
5 mg/kg single dose	AML	18	0.02–0.15	0.05–0.22	18–36 hrs	133, 134
5 mg/kg single dose	AML	13	0.09–0.14	0.05–0.23	24 hrs	135
100 mg/m²	AML	3	0.02–0.06	0.06–0.13	48–96 hrs	130
100 mg/m² 48-hr infusion	AML	4	0.03–0.19	0.10–0.14	48–120 hrs	130

restricted to cells in a particular phase of the cell cycle, but can take advantage of the greater overall sensitivity of rapidly proliferating cells to a wide variety of chemotherapeutic agents. We might note that a number of commonly used empirical clinical regimens (e.g., MOPP, CMF) include drug treatment on days 1 and 8 of each treatment cycle. The utility of this treatment schedule may be due in part to the increased susceptibility of cells recruited into rapid cycle during this interval. Clearly, additional studies are required to define the magnitude and time course of cell recruitment in human tumors *in situ*, and their relation to optimal clinical drug scheduling.

CLINICAL APPLICATIONS OF CELL KINETICS: AN OVERVIEW

Although a great deal has been learned over the past 30 years about tumor growth behavior and the perturbation effects of drugs, the principles of cell kinetics have yet to be applied successfully in the design of clinical cancer treatment regimens.

Historically, cell kinetics began as a basic experimental discipline and not as an applied clinical science. The main thrust of early studies was to break down complex problems into simpler components that could be isolated and studied separately under well-controlled conditions. Often, experimental investigators deliberately chose to work with cell systems that exhibited relatively little kinetic heterogeneity and highly reproducible patterns of growth behavior (e.g., mouse intestinal epithelium, mouse L1210 leukemia, and HeLa cells or CHO cells in tissue culture) in order to obtain clear answers to basic questions. Early analytical methods, and particularly the classic approach to PLM curve analysis, fostered a false sense of cell cycle time uniformity by virtue of their bias in favor of rapidly proliferating cells. This was reinforced further by early conceptual formulations (e.g., the growth fraction and G_0 concepts) that effectively excluded slowly proliferating cells from the cell cycle time distribution and lumped them together with nonproliferating cells in a separate category.

In retrospect, these early methodologic approaches and conceptual formulations were not well suited for clinical applications. Nowhere is this reflected more clearly than in early treatment strategies that focused on such concepts as cell cycle blockade with cell synchronization and S-phase–specific therapy. Such strategies might be appropriate for homogeneous, rapidly growing cell populations with large fractions of cells in S phase, but they are inappropriate for populations with the extensive kinetic heterogeneity found in human tumors. With this in mind, it is not surprising that attempts to optimize treatment with S-phase–specific drugs during the early (24–48-hour) post-treatment period have not produced dramatic improvements in tumor response.

In recent years, attention has begun to shift to the process of cell recruitment and its potential exploitation by means of drug schedule manipulation. At present, clinical data on the magnitude and time course of the recruitment response in man are scant. The data that are available, mostly in normal and leukemic bone marrow, suggest that peak recruitment responses occur in the second and third weeks after initial drug therapy. The studies of Burke et al.[138] in acute adult human leukemia indicate that log kills of considerable magnitude can be achieved with single courses of treatment containing an 8- to 14-day interval between drugs.

There is much yet to be learned about the details of the recruitment response in normal and malignant tissues in man, particularly in the common solid tumors. As a practical matter, such data are difficult to obtain. Few patients have tumors that are accessible for multiple serial biopsies. Patients must be willing to undergo the discomfort of serial biopsies, knowing full well that the results of such studies may be of no direct and immediate benefit to them. Ultimately, advances in this area can come about only through the perception by both patient and physician that orderly progress in clinical cancer treatment depends on the availability of detailed information on the effects of anticancer drugs in man. This area of scientific study is likely to be of common concern to pharmacologists and cell kineticists for some time to come.

References

1. Johnson LF, Fuhrman CL, and Abelson HT: Resistance of resting 3T6 mouse fibroblasts to methotrexate cytotoxicity. Cancer Res. 38:2408–2412, 1978.
2. Shackney SE, McCormack GW, and Cuchural GJ Jr: Growth rate patterns of solid tumors and their relation to

responsiveness to therapy: an analytical review. Ann. Intern. Med. 89:107–121, 1978.

3. Schwartz M: A biomathematical approach to clinical tumor growth. Cancer 14:1272–1294, 1961.
4. Walker PMB, and Yates HB: Nuclear components of dividing cells. Proc. R. Soc. Lond. B 140:274–299, 1952.
5. Walker PMB: The mitotic index and interphase processes. J. Exp. Biol. 31:8–15, 1954.
6. Howard A, and Pelc SR: Synthesis of desoxyribonucleic acid in normal and irradiated cells and its relation to chromosome breakage. Heredity (Suppl.) 6:261–273, 1953.
7. Rubini JR, Cronkite EP, Bond VP, et al.: The metabolism and fate of tritiated thymidine in man. J. Clin. Invest. 39:909–918, 1960.
8. Malaise EP, Chavaudra N, and Tubiana M: The relationship between growth rate, labelling index and histological type of human solid tumours. Eur. J. Cancer 9:305–312, 1973.
9. Wolberg WH, and Ansfield FJ: The relation of thymidine labeling index in human tumors *in vitro* to the effectiveness of 5-fluorouracil chemotherapy. Cancer Res. 31:448–450, 1971.
10. Meyer JS, and Bauer WC: Tritiated thymidine labeling index of benign and malignant human breast epithelium. J. Surg. Oncol. 8:165–181, 1976.
11. Hainau B, Dombernowsky P, Hansen HH, et al.: Cell proliferation and histologic classification of bronchogenic carcinoma. J. Natl. Cancer Inst. 59:1113–1118, 1977.
12. Coons H, Norman A, and Nahum AM: *In vitro* measurements of human tumor growth. Cancer 19:1200–1204, 1966.
13. Fabrikant JI: The kinetics of cellular proliferation in normal and malignant tissues: a review of methodology and the analysis of cell population kinetics in human tissues. Am. J. Roentgenol. 111:700–711, 1971.
14. Yanagita T, Herman GG, and Gusberg SB: Autoradiographic studies in cervical cancer before and after a test dose of irradiation. Am. J. Obstet. Gynecol. 95:1051–1058, 1966.
15. Muggia FM, Krezoski SK, and Hansen HH: Cell kinetic studies in patients with small cell carcinoma of the lung. Cancer 34:1683–1690, 1974.
16. Livingston RB, Ambus U, George SL, et al.: *In vitro* determination of thymidine-^{3}H labeling index in human solid tumors. Cancer Res. 34:1376–1380, 1974.
17. Kury G, and Carter HW: Autoradiographic study of human nervous system tumors. Arch. Pathol. 80:38–42, 1965.
18. Steel GG: Cell loss as a factor in the growth rate of human tumours. Eur. J. Cancer 3:381–387, 1967.
19. Drewinko B, Brown BW, Humphrey R, et al.: Effect of chemotherapy on the labeling index of myeloma cells. Cancer 34:526–531, 1974.
20. Cooper EH, Peckham MJ, Millard RE, et al.: Cell proliferation in human malignant lymphomas. Analysis of labelling index and DNA content in cell populations obtained by biopsy. Eur. J. Cancer 4:287–296, 1968.
21. Quastler H, and Sherman FG: Cell population kinetics in the intestinal epithelium of the mouse. Exp. Cell Res. 17:420–438, 1959.
22. Wimber DE: Methods for studying cell proliferation with emphasis on DNA labels. *In* Lamerton LF, and Fry RJM (eds.): Cell Proliferation. Blackwell Scientific Publications, Oxford, 1963, pp. 1–17.
23. Cairnie AB, Lamerton LF, and Steel GG: Cell proliferation studies in the intestinal epithelium of the rat. Exp. Cell Res. 39:528–538, 1965.
24. Lala PK, and Patt HM: Cytokinetic analysis of tumor growth. Proc. Natl. Acad. Sci. USA 56:1735–1742, 1966.
25. Painter RB, and Drew RM: Studies on deoxyribonucleic acid metabolism in human cancer cell cultures (HeLa). 1. The temporal relationships of deoxyribonucleic acid synthesis to mitosis and turnover time. Lab. Invest. 8:278–285, 1959.
26. Takahashi M, Hogg GD, and Mendelsohn ML: The automatic analysis of FLM curves. Cell Tissue Kinet. 4:505–518, 1971.
27. Steel GG and Hanes S: The technique of labelled mitoses: analysis by automatic curve-fitting. Cell Tissue Kinet. 4:93–105, 1971.
28. Mendelsohn ML: Autoradiographic analysis of cell proliferation in spontaneous breast cancer of C3H mouse. III. The growth fraction. J. Natl. Cancer Inst. 28:1015–1029, 1962.
29. Quastler H: The analysis of cell population kinetics. *In* Lamerton LF, and Fry RJM (eds.): Cell Proliferation. Blackwell Scientific Publications, Oxford, 1963, pp. 18–34.
30. Mendelsohn ML: Cell proliferation and tumour growth. *In* Lamerton LF, and Fry RJM (eds.): Cell Proliferation. Blackwell Scientific Publications, Oxford, 1963, pp. 190–210.
31. Steel GG: Growth Kinetics of Tumours. Clarendon Press, Oxford, 1977, pp. 194–216.
32. Shackney SE: A cytokinetic model for heterogeneous mammalian cell populations. III. Tritiated thymidine studies. Correlations among multiple kinetic parameters in human tumours. J. Theor. Biol. 65:421–464, 1977.
33. Shirakawa S, Luce JK, Tannock I, et al.: Cell proliferation in human melanoma. J. Clin. Invest. 49:1188–1199, 1970.
34. Tannock I: Cell kinetics and chemotherapy: a critical review. Cancer Treat. Rep. 62:1117–1133, 1978.
35. Shackney SE: The role of radioautographic studies in clinical investigative oncology and chemotherapy. Cancer Treat. Rep. 60:1873–1886, 1976.
36. Puck TT, and Marcus PI: Action of x-rays on mammalian cells. J. Exp. Med. 103:653–666, 1956.
37. Osgood EE: A unifying concept of the etiology of the leukemias, lymphomas, and cancers. J. Natl. Cancer Inst. 18:155–166, 1957.
38. Lajtha LG, Oliver R, and Gurney CW: Kinetic model of a bone marrow stem-cell population. Br. J. Haematol. 8:442–460, 1962.
39. Patt HM, and Maloney MA: A model of granulocyte kinetics. Ann. N.Y. Acad. Sci. 113:515–522, 1964.
40. Boggs DR, Athens JW, Cartwright GE, et al.: Leukokinetic studies. IX. Experimental evaluation of a model of granulopoiesis. J. Clin. Invest. 44:643–656, 1965.
41. Cronkite EP, and Vincent PC: Granulocytopoiesis. *In* Stohlman F Jr (ed.): Hemopoietic Cellular Proliferation. Grune & Stratton, New York, 1970, p. 211–228.
42. Skipper HE, Schabel FM Jr, and Wilcox WS: Experimental evaluation of potential anticancer agents. XIII. On the criteria and kinetics associated with "curability" of experimental leukemia. Cancer Chemother. Rep. 35:1–111, 1964.
43. Till JE, and McCulloch EA: A direct measurement of the radiation sensitivity of normal mouse bone marrow. Radiat. Res. 14:213–222, 1961.
44. Iscove NN, Sieber F, and Winterhalter KH: Erythroid colony formation in cultures in mouse and human bone marrow: analysis of the requirement for erythropoietin by gel filtration and affinity chromatography on agarose-concanavalin A. J. Cell Physiol. 83:309–320, 1974.
45. Hamburger AW, and Salmon SE: Primary bioassay of human tumor stem cells. Science 197:461–463, 1977.
46. Hamburger A, and Salmon SE: Primary bioassay of human myeloma stem cells. J. Clin. Invest. 60:846–854, 1977.
47. Siminovitch L, McCulloch EA, and Till JE: The distribution of colony-forming cells among spleen colonies. J. Cell Comp. Physiol. 62:327–336, 1963.
48. Matioli G, Vogel H, and Niewisch H: The dilution factor of intravenously injected hemopoietic stem cells. J. Cell Physiol. 72:229–234, 1968.
49. Wodinsky I, Swiniarski J, and Kensler CJ: Spleen colony studies of leukemia L1210. I. Growth kinetics of lymphocytic L1210 cells *in vivo* as determined by spleen colony assay. Cancer Chemother. Rep. 51:415–421, 1967.
50. Steel GG: Growth Kinetics of Tumours. Clarendon Press, Oxford, 1977, p. 241.
51. Hewitt HB, Blake E, and Porter EH: The effect of lethally irradiated cells on the transplantability of murine tumours. Br. J. Cancer 28:123–135, 1973.
52. Peters LJ, and Hewitt HB: The influence of fibrin formation

on the transplantability of murine tumour cells: implications for the mechanism of the Revesz effect. Brit. J. Cancer 29:279–291, 1974.

53. Carney DN, Gadar AF, Bunn PA, et al.: *In vitro* cloning of small cell carcinoma of the lung in small cell lung cancer. *In* Greco FA, Oldham RK, and Bunn PA, Jr (eds.): Small Cell Cancer. Grune & Stratton, New York, 1980, pp. 79–94.
54. Becker AJ, McCulloch EA, Siminovitch L, et al.: The effect of differing demands for blood cell production on DNA synthesis by hemopoietic colony-forming cells of mice. Blood 26:296–308, 1965.
55. Lord BI, Testa NG, and Hendry JH: The relative spatial distributions of CFU-S and CFU-C in the normal mouse femur. Blood 46:65–72, 1975.
56. Mayneord WV: On a law of growth of Jensen's rat sarcoma. Am. J. Cancer 16:841–846, 1932.
57. Laird AK: The dynamics of tumour growth. Br. J. Cancer 18:490–502, 1964.
58. Summers WC: Dynamics of tumor growth: a mathematical model. Growth 30:333–338, 1966.
59. Burton AC: Rate of growth of solid tumors as a problem of diffusion. Growth 30:157–176, 1966.
60. Lala PK: Studies on tumor cell population kinetics. *In* Busch H (ed.): Methods in Cancer Research, Vol. VI. Academic Press, New York, 1971, pp. 3–95.
61. Shackney SE, and Ford SS: Correlations between the DNA content distribution and tritiated thymidine studies in relation to population size in sarcoma 180 *in vitro*. Cancer Res. 34:1401–1407, 1974.
62. Shackney SE, Ford SS, and Wittig AB: The effects of counting threshold and emulsion exposure duration on the percent-labeled mitosis curve and their implications for cell cycle analysis. Cancer Res. 33:2726–2731, 1973.
63. Skipper HE, Schabel FM Jr, and Wilcox WS: Experimental evaluation of potential anticancer agents. XXI. Scheduling of arabinosylcytosine to take advantage of its S-phase specificity against leukemia cells. Cancer Chemother. Rep. 51:125–165, 1967.
64. Shackney SE: A computer model for tumor growth and chemotherapy, and its application to L1210 leukemia treated with cytosine arabinoside. Cancer Chemother. Rep. 54:399–429, 1970.
65. Leblond CP, Greulich RC, and Periera JPM: Relationship of cell formation and cell migration in the renewal of stratified squamous epithelia. *In* Montagna W, and Billingham RE (eds.): Advances in Biology of Skin. V. Wound Healing. Pergamon Press, Oxford, 1964, pp. 39–67.
66. Iversen OH, Bjerknes R, and Devik F: Kinetics of cell renewal, cell migration and cell loss in the hairless mouse dorsal epidermis. Cell Tissue Kinet. 1:351–367, 1968.
67. Grisham JW: A morphologic study of deoxyribonucleic acid synthesis and cell proliferation in regenerating rat liver; autoradiography with thymidine-H^3. Cancer Res. 22:842–849, 1962.
68. Hanna MG Jr: An autoradiographic study of the germinal center in the spleen white pulp during early intervals of the immune response. Lab. Invest. 13:95–104, 1964.
69. Ishii Y, Mori M, and Onoe T: Studies on the germinal center. IV. Autoradiographic study of lymph node germinal centers in relation to zonal differentiation. J. Reticuloendothel. Soc. 11:383–393, 1972.
70. Borum K: Pattern of cell production and cell migration in mouse thymus studied by autoradiography. Scand. J. Haematol. 5:339–352, 1968.
71. Borum K: Cell kinetics in mouse thymus studied by simultaneous use of ^{3}H-thymidine and colchicine. Cell Tissue Kinet. 6:545–552, 1973.
72. Diderholm H, and Hellman B: The cell migration in the adrenal cortex of rats studied with tritiated thymidine. Acta Physiol. Scand. 50:197–202, 1960.
73. Ford JK, and Young RW: Cell proliferation and displacement in the adrenal cortex of young rats injected with tritiated thymidine. Anat. Rec. 146:125–137, 1963.
74. Wright NA: Cell proliferation in the prepubertal male rat adrenal cortex: an autoradiographic study. J. Endocrinol. 49:599–609, 1971.
75. Shackney SE, Ford SS, and Wittig AB: Kinetic-microarchitectural correlations in the bone marrow of the mouse. Cell Tissue Kinet. 8:505–516, 1975.
76. Shackney SE, Bunn PA Jr, and Ford SS: The effects of colcemid on mouse bone marrow. Cell Tissue Kinet. 9:363–369, 1976.
77. Tannock IF: The relation between cell proliferation and the vascular system in a transplanted mouse mammary tumour. Br. J. Cancer 22:258–273, 1968.
78. Miller SC, and Osmond DG: The proliferation of lymphoid cells in guinea-pig bone marrow. Cell Tissue Kinet. 6:259–269, 1973.
79. Osmond DG, and Everett NB: Radioautographic studies of bone marrow lymphocytes *in vivo* and in diffusion chamber cultures. Blood 23:1–17, 1964.
80. Yoshida Y, and Osmond DG: Identity and proliferation of small lymphocyte precursors in cultures of lymphocyte-rich fractions of guinea pig bone marrow. Blood 37:73–86, 1971.
81. Metcalf D, and Wiadrowski M: Autoradiographic analysis of lymphocyte proliferation in the thymus and in thymic lymphoma tissue. Cancer Res. 26:483–491, 1966.
82. Omine M, Sarna GP, and Perry S: Composition of leukaemic cell populations in AKR leukaemia and effects of chemotherapy. Eur. J. Cancer 9:557–565, 1973.
83. Clarkson BD, Sakai Y, Kimura T, et al.: Studies of cellular proliferation in human leukemia. II. Variability in rates of growth and cellular differentiation in acute myelomonoblastic leukemia and effects of treatment. *In* The Proliferation and Spread of Neoplastic Cells. Williams & Wilkins Co., Baltimore, 1968, pp. 295–330.
84. Gavosto F, Pileri A, Gabutti V, et al.: Non-self-maintaining kinetics of proliferating blasts in human acute leukaemia. Nature (Lond.) 216:188–189, 1967.
85. Shackney SE, Skramstad KS, Cunningham RE, et al.: Dual parameter flow cytometry studies in human lymphomas J. Clin. Invest. 66:1281–1294, 1980.
86. Smith JA, and Martin L: Do cells cycle? Proc. Natl. Acad. Sci. USA 70:1263–1267, 1973.
87. Collins VP, Loeffler RK, and Tivey H: Observations on growth rates of human tumors. Am. J. Roentgenol. 76:988–1000, 1956.
88. Fisher RI, DeVita VT, Hubbard SP, et al.: Prolonged disease-free survival in Hodgkin's disease with MOPP reinduction after first relapse. Ann. Intern. Med. 90:761–763, 1979.
89. Sweet DL, Golomb HM, Ultmann JE, et al.: Cyclophosphamide, vincristine, methotrexate, with leucovorin rescue, and cytarabine (COMLA) combination sequential chemotherapy for advanced diffuse histiocytic lymphoma. Ann. Intern. Med. 92:785–790, 1980.
90. Bruce WR, Meeker BE, and Valeriote FA: Comparison of the sensitivity of normal hematopoietic and transplanted lymphoma colony-forming cells to chemotherapeutic agents administered *in vivo*. J. Natl. Cancer Inst. 37:233–245, 1966.
91. Bruce WR, Meeker BE, Powers WE, et al.: Comparison of the dose- and time-survival curves for normal hematopoietic and lymphoma colony-forming cells exposed to vinblastine, vincristine, arabinosylcytosine, and amethopterin. J. Natl. Cancer Inst. 42:1015–1025, 1969.
92. Terasima T, and Tolmach LJ: Growth and nucleic acid synthesis in synchronously dividing populations of HeLa cells. Exp. Cell Res. 30:344–362, 1963.
93. Mauro F, and Madoc-Jones H: Age responses of cultured mammalian cells to cytotoxic drugs. Cancer Res. 30:1397–1408, 1970.
94. Bhuyan BK, Fraser TJ, Gray LG, et al.: Cell-kill kinetics of several S-phase–specific drugs. Cancer Res. 33:888–894, 1973.
95. Bhuyan BK, Scheidt LG, and Fraser TJ: Cell cycle phase specificity of antitumor agents. Cancer Res. 32:398–407, 1972.
96. Furth JJ, and Cohen SS: Inhibition of mammalian DNA polymerase by the 5′-triphosphate of 1-B-D-arabinofuranosylcytosine and the 5′-triphosphate of 9-B-D-arabinofuranosyladenine. Cancer Res. 28:2061–2067, 1968.
97. Graham FL, and Whitmore GF: Studies in mouse L-cells on the incorporation of 1-B-D-arabinofuranosylcytosine

into DNA and on inhibition of DNA polymerase by 1-B-D-arabinofuranosylcytosine 5′-triphosphate. Cancer Res. 30:2636–2644, 1970.

98. Chu MY, and Fischer GA: The incorporation of ^{3}H-cytosine arabinoside and its effect on murine leukaemic cells (L5178Y). Biochem. Pharmacol. 17:753–767, 1968.

99. Grant S, Lehman C, and Cadman E: Enhancement of 1-B-D-arabinofuranosylcytosine accumulation within L1210 cells and increased cytotoxicity following thymidine exposure. Cancer Res. 40:1525–1531, 1980.

100. Wibe E: Age-dependent cell inactivation by vincristine alone or in combination with 1-propargyl-5-chloropyrimidin-2-one. Cancer Res. 40:2069–2073, 1980.

101. Linden WA, Baisch H, Canstein LV, et al.: Impulse cytophotometric studies on the effects of daunomycin on synchronized L-cells. Eur. J. Cancer 10:647–651, 1974.

102. Krishan A, and Frie E III: Effect of Adriamycin on the cell cycle traverse and kinetics of cultured human lymphoblasts. Cancer Res. 36:143–150, 1976.

103. Barlogie B, Drewinko B, Johnston DA, and Freireich EJ: The effect of Adriamycin on the cell cycle traverse of a human lymphoid cell line. Cancer Res. 36:1975–1979, 1976.

104. Tobey RA, Crissman HA, and Oka MS: Arrested and cycling CHO cells as a kinetic model: studies with Adriamycin. Cancer Treat. Rep. 60:1829–1837, 1976.

105. Tobey RA, and Crissman HA: Comparative effects of three nitrosourea derivatives on mammalian cell cycle progression. Cancer Res. 35:160–170, 1975.

106. Tobey RA, Oka MS, and Crissman HA: Differential effects of two chemotherapeutic agents, streptozotocin and chlorozotocin, on the mammalian cell cycle. Eur. J. Cancer 11:433–441, 1975.

107. Barlogie B, Drewinko B, Schumann J, et al.: Pulse cytophotometric analysis of cell cycle perturbation with bleomycin *in vitro*. Cancer Res. 36:1182–1187, 1976.

108. Barlogie B, and Drewinko B: Cell cycle–related induction of cell progression delay. *In* Drewinko B, and Humphrey RM (eds.): Growth Kinetics and Biochemical Regulation of Normal and Malignant Cells. Williams & Wilkins Co. Baltimore, 1977, pp. 315–327.

109. Barranco SC, Novak JF, and Humphrey RM: Response of mammalian cells following treatment with bleomycin and 1,3-bis(2-chloroethyl)-1-nitrosourea during plateau phase. Cancer Res. 33:691–694, 1973.

110. Barranco SC, Novak JK, and Humphrey RM: Studies on recovery from chemically induced damage in mammalian cells. Cancer Res. 35:1194–1204, 1975.

111. Sinclair WK: Hydroxyurea: differential lethal effects on cultured mammalian cells during the cell cycle. Science 150:1729–1731, 1965.

112. Pfeiffer SE, and Tolmach LJ: Inhibition of DNA synthesis in HeLa cells by hydroxyurea. Cancer Res. 27:124–129, 1967.

113. Tobey RA, and Crissman HA: Use of flow microfluorometry in detailed analysis of effects of chemical agents on cell cycle progression. Cancer Res. 32:2726–2732, 1972.

114. Rajewsky MF: Synchronization *in vivo*: kinetics of a malignant cell system following temporary inhibition of DNA synthesis with hydroxyurea. Exp. Cell Res. 60:269–276, 1970.

115. Dethlefsen LA, and Riley RM: Hydroxyurea effects in the C3H mouse. I. Duodenal crypt cell kinetics. Cell Tissue Kinet. 6:3–16, 1973.

116. Malkinson FD, Griem ML, and Marianovic R: Effects of hydroxyurea and radiation on hair matrix cells. Cell Tissue Kinet. 6:395–405, 1973.

117. Gibson MHL, and Bertalanffy FD: *In vivo* synchrony of solid B16 melanoma by cytosine arabinoside, an inhibitor of DNA synthesis. J. Natl. Cancer Inst. 49:1007–1018, 1972.

118. Dethlefsen LA, Ohlsen JD, and Roti Roti JL: Cell synchronization *in vivo*: fact or fancy? *In* Drewinko B, and Humphrey RM (eds.): Growth Kinetics and Biochemical Regulation of Normal and Malignant Cells. Williams & Wilkins Co., Baltimore, 1977, pp. 491–507.

119. Ford SS, and Shackney SE: Lethal and sublethal effects of hydroxyurea in relation to drug concentration and duration of drug exposure in sarcoma 180 *in vitro*. Cancer Res. 37:2628–2637, 1977.

120. Yataganas X, Strife A, Perez A, et al.: Microfluorimetric evaluation of cell kill kinetics with 1-B-D-arabinofuranosylcytosine. Cancer Res. 34:2795–2806, 1974.

121. Yataganas X, Strife A, Perez A, et al.: Cell kill kinetics with hydroxyurea. Med. Pediatr. Oncol. 2:39–54, 1976.

122. Shackney SE, Erickson BW, and Lengel CE: Schedule optimization of cytosine arabinoside and hydroxyurea in sarcoma 180 *in vitro*. Proc. Am. Assoc. Cancer Res. 19:225, 1978.

123. Todaro GJ, Lazar GK, and Green H: The initiation of cell division in a contact-inhibited mammalian cell line. J. Cell Physiol. 66:325–334, 1965.

124. Wiebel F, and Baserga R: Early alterations in amino acid pools and protein synthesis of diploid fibroblasts stimulated to synthesize DNA by addition of serum. J. Cell Physiol. 74:191–202, 1969.

125. Temin HM: Stimulation by serum of multiplication of stationary chicken cells. J. Cell Physiol. 78:161–170, 1971.

126. Demeestere M, Rockwell S, Valleron A-J, et al.: Cell proliferation in EMT6 tumours treated with single doses of x-rays or hydroxyurea. II. Computer simulations. Cell Tissue Kinet. 13:309–317, 1980.

127. Al-Dewachi HS, Wright NA, et al.: The effect of a single injection of hydroxyurea on cell population kinetics in the small bowel mucosa of the rat. Cell Tissue Kinet. 10:203–213, 1977.

128. Newburger A, Ritch P, Occhipinti S, et al.: Regional kinetic effects of hydroxyurea in normal mouse bone marrow. Cell Tissue Kinet. 12:679–680, 1979.

129. Ernst P, Faille A, and Killmann SA: Perturbation of cell cycle of human leukaemic myeloblasts *in vivo* by cytosine arabinoside. Scand. J. Haematol. 10:209–218, 1973.

130. Baccarani M, Santucci AM, Tura S, et al.: Arabinosyl cytosine in chronic myeloid leukaemia: evidence for high cytokinetic sensitivity of myeloblasts. Scand. J. Haematol. 16:335–352, 1976.

131. Vogler WR, Cooper LE, and Groth DP: Correlation of cytosine arabinoside-induced increment in growth fraction of leukemic blast cells with clinical response. Cancer 33:603–610, 1974.

132. Vogler WR, Kremer WB, Knospe WH, et al.: Synchronization with phase-specific agents in leukemia and correlation with clinical response to chemotherapy. Cancer Treatment Rep. 60:1845–1859, 1976.

133. Lampkin BG, Nagao T, and Mauer AM: Synchronization and recruitment in acute leukemia. J. Clin. Invest. 50:2204–2214, 1971.

134. Lampkin BC, McWilliams NB, Mauer AM, et al.: Manipulation of the mitotic cycle in the treatment of acute myelogenous leukaemia. Br. J. Haematol. 32:29–40, 1976.

135. Wantzin GL: Effect of cytosine arabinoside on nuclear labelling of leukaemic myeloblasts with tritiated thymidine triphosphate. Leuk. Res. 3:7–13, 1979.

136. Barranco SC, Luce JK, Romsdahl MM, et al.: Bleomycin as a possible synchronizing agent for human tumor cells *in vivo*. Cancer Res. 33:882–887, 1973.

137. Wantzin GL, and Killmann S-A: Nuclear labelling of leukaemic blast cells with tritiated thymidine triphosphate after daunomycin. Eur. J. Cancer 13:647–655, 1977.

138. Burke PJ, Karp JE, Braine HG, et al.: Timed sequential therapy of human leukemia based upon the response of leukemic cells to humoral growth factors. Cancer Res. 37:2138–2146, 1977.

139. Shackney SE, Bunn PA, Ford SS, et al.: A study of drug-induced kinetic perturbations in the marrow of a patient with neuroblastoma. Cancer 45:882–892, 1980.

140. Burke PJ, Diggs CH, and Owens AH Jr: Factors in human serum affecting the proliferation of normal and leukemic cells. Cancer Res. 33:800–806, 1973.

PHARMACOKINETICS OF ANTICANCER DRUGS 4

Jerry M. Collins
Robert L. Dedrick

INTRODUCTION

Pharmacokinetics has become a principal component of clinical pharmacology. In particular, pharmacokinetic studies of anticancer drugs have been increasing in frequency in the past decade and are now almost routine in Phase I/II clinical trials. Since these studies are very demanding in terms of professional manpower and analytical resources, it is reasonable to expect a return commensurate with this investment. This chapter describes the two major branches of pharmacokinetics, empirical (classical or curve-fit) and physiologic, including major concepts and formulas. Before becoming involved in the details of this discipline, we need to step back and evaluate the possible benefits of pharmacokinetic studies, both at the population level ("average" patient) and at the level of the individual patient.

First, a clear distinction needs to be made between the effects of a drug (dynamics) and its concentration-time history (kinetics). The role of pharmacodynamics is to define therapeutic goals, which are then attained by using kinetics to formulate an administration strategy to achieve these goals. For infectious diseases, the goal is prolonged maintenance of plasma concentration above a minimal inhibitory concentration (MIC) or minimal bactericidal concentration (MBC), but below levels toxic to the host. In anticancer chemotherapy, while the general goal of killing tumor cells is clearly defined, we are severely limited in most cases by an inability to select concentration-time parameters that separate antitumor effect from normal tissue toxicity. Current guidelines for selecting drug dose are summarized by the empirical strategy of escalating the dose to the maximal tolerated toxicity and hoping that this schedule will achieve adequate tumor kill. Much remains to be learned about differences between normal and tumor tissues that can be exploited therapeutically. Thus, although pharmacokinetics is a tool that can be used to evaluate the feasibility of a strategy based on pharmacodynamics, it is not a replacement for a knowledge of exploitable differences between host and tumor.

Benefits for the Average Patient: Scheduling and Dosage

For the average patient, pharmacokinetics can help answer the fundamental questions in delivery of drugs: (1) what route of administration?, (2) how often (schedule)?, and (3) how much (dose)? These questions are answered on the basis of empirical observation (what works best in an experimental or clinical setting) and on the basis of biochemical, cell kinetic, and pharmacokinetic considerations. Table 4–1 lists some of the important considerations in the design of drug regimens. It is clear that many of these factors are related to the absorption, distribution, metabolism, and elimination of drug, i.e., to the pharmacokinetic characteristics of the agent.

The choice of drug administration *route* is primarily based on pharmacokinetic assessment of bioavailability (the ability of drug to reach its target site in an active form) and the

TABLE 4–1. Pharmacokinetic Considerations in Drug Scheduling in Man

Route of Administration
1. Oral—especially useful for lipid-soluble drugs or drugs taken up by specific transport mechanisms. Drugs may be unstable in gastric acid, hydrolyzed by intestinal enzymes, or eliminated by hepatic first-pass metabolism.
2. Intramuscular—not used for drugs that cause tissue necrosis or in patients at risk of bleeding.
3. Intravenous—most secure route, but possible only for drugs of sufficient aqueous solubility.
4. Local administration — effective for control of local tumor. Best for organs with low blood flow and drugs with high body clearance.

Schedule of Administration
1. Duration of individual dose
   a. Bolus achieves high peak, but rapid fall-off.
   b. Prolonged infusion provides set duration of exposure at set concentration.
2. Frequency of dose repetition—depends on patient tolerance, tumor kinetics.

Dose—For a Specific Schedule, Determined by Phase I Study
1. May be set to provide a pharmacokinetic objective: a specific drug concentration for a specific time interval.
2. Must be adjusted for dysfunction of organ crucial to drug elimination.

ability to formulate an acceptable dose preparation for oral, intravenous, or intramuscular use. Bioavailability for oral preparations is judged by measurement of plasma drug concentrations, by measurement of nonabsorbed compound in the stool, and by therapeutic efficacy. Absorption through the lipid bilayer cell membrane of the intestinal mucosa is determined by molecular size, lipid solubility, and the presence of specific transport systems such as the folate transport mechanism for antifolates. Absorption is also affected by drug stability in gastric acid and breakdown by intestinal enzymes such as cytidine deaminase (which hydrolyzes cytosine arabinoside). The physiologic state of the intestinal tract may be adversely affected by disease or by previous drug therapy. Vomiting induced by chemotherapeutic drugs may lead to a loss of a major portion of an oral dose. Thus, highly emetic agents such as *cis*-DDP cannot be used in combination with orally administered drugs. In addition to intestinal absorption, hepatic metabolism or uptake and biliary excretion may prevent orally administered drug from reaching the systemic circulation in an active form.

The intravenous route, although it necessitates a venipuncture, is the preferred route for water-soluble compounds since complete absorption is guaranteed if the intravenous infusion is performed correctly. The primary disadvantage is the greater danger of acute toxicities owing to the presentation of high peak drug levels to target organs. Particularly for neurotoxic or cardiotoxic compounds, rapid intravenous infusion may present unacceptable dangers.

On occasion, tumor may grow in a body compartment, such as the central nervous system or peritoneal cavity, which is not penetrated rapidly by systemically administered drug. The rate of penetration of these compartments is influenced by the same factors that determine intestinal absorption (size, lipid solubility, specific transport processes). Direct intrathecal, intraperitoneal, or topical administration may be advantageous in these cases, but the relative advantage as compared with that of systemic therapy will be determined by pharmacokinetic factors such as relative rates of clearance from the central and peripheral compartment. These considerations are dealt with in detail later in this chapter.

In addition to route, the *schedule* of drug administration is highly dependent on pharmacokinetic considerations and requires a choice of the duration of administration (bolus versus prolonged infusion), frequency of repetition of dose, and the sequencing of multiple drugs, or drugs and other modalities such as radiation. Bolus dosing provides maximal drug peak levels in plasma, but a rapid decline thereafter as drug is eliminated from the plasma compartment by metabolism or excretion. This form of dosing is optimal for drugs that are non-cell cycle–phase-dependent and therefore do not have to be present during a specific phase of the cell cycle. Examples are the nitrosoureas, alkylating agents, procarbazine, and other drugs that chemically interact with DNA. For agents that act preferentially in specific phases of the cell cycle, such as S-phase–specific drugs (cytosine arabinoside or methotrexate), prolonged intravenous infusion has advantages, particularly if the drug has a short plasma half-life. Prolonged infusions have the additional advantage of providing a specific and constant plasma concentration of drug, a desirable feature if one has information regarding the sensitivity of the tumor, as provided by the human tumor stem cell assay.

The specific sequence of administering

multiple drugs in combination therapy regimens is usually determined by knowledge of the biochemical and cell kinetic effects of the individual agents, as reviewed in Chapter 1, and by their possible synergistic interactions. Pharmacokinetic considerations are less important in this phase of schedule development, although drug interactions that lead to altered elimination of one member of a combination are possible. Few such interactions are known for anticancer drugs, the best example being thymidine inhibition of 5-fluorouracil metabolism.[1] Drug interactions that produce therapeutic synergism are outlined in Table 1–5, and are reviewed in detail in the appropriate drug-related chapters. Many of these interactions depend on the appropriate timing and sequencing of drugs.

The frequency of repetition for cycles of drug administration is usually determined by patient tolerance and must allow time for recovery of normal tissues. Cell kinetic considerations may also dictate the frequency with which treatment must be repeated. For example, virtually continuous marrow ablative treatment is used for the more rapidly growing acute leukemias and lymphomas, whereas more indolent tumors such as the nodular lymphomas and chronic leukemias are treated on intermittent schedules.

The final consideration in drug administration is the choice of *dose*. Dose is usually determined by an empirical Phase I trial using a set schedule, with stepwise evaluation of toxicity at progressively higher doses. Information derived from group studies does not allow for interindividual variability, a subject that will be central to our later discussion of drug level monitoring in cancer treatment (Chapter 5). However, if one knows the pharmacokinetics of a given agent, specifically its route of elimination, adjustments in dose can be made for altered renal or hepatic function to accommodate abnormalities in individual patients. Examples of such adjustments are provided in individual drug chapters. In general, these adjustments are only crude approximations and poor substitutes for adjustments based on drug level measurement.

Dose may also be determined by setting pharmacologic objectives, such as a target drug concentration in a specific body compartment such as plasma, cerebrospinal fluid, or ascites. This type of regimen planning requires pharmacokinetic planning and verification by drug level monitoring and has been used in only a few clinical oncologic settings, such as intrathecal chemotherapy with methotrexate[2] and intraperitoneal therapy with methotrexate and 5-fluorouracil.[3,4] Additional information on the relationship of drug concentration to tumor cell kill, as provided by stem cell assay *in vitro*, may provide a basis for more precise pharmacokinetic adjustment of dosage.

Benefits for the Individual Patient

For the individual, pharmacokinetics offers the possibility of tailoring the drug delivery to the particular patient's needs. Measurements of plasma drug levels might reveal unusually low levels of drug in a nonresponding patient or excessive levels in an unusually toxic patient, as demonstrated by Bleyer in his studies of intrathecal methotrexate.[2] Simple adjustment of dosage or schedule would lead to more appropriate plasma levels. Precedent for this manipulation is found in the use of cytosine arabinoside by bolus administration,[5] in which investigators found that responding patients had a longer half-time than nonresponders, presumably allowing drug concentrations to be maintained in an effective range for a longer time, as is achieved on constant infusion schedules. If an excessively toxic dose is given, "rescue" strategies such as hemodialysis or antidotes may sometimes be employed. An example of this approach is the methotrexate study of Stoller et al.,[6] in which the leucovorin rescue strategy is tailored to plasma drug concentrations measured 48 hours after drug administration. Adjustment of dose in the presence of renal or hepatic disease has also been proposed. depending on the route of elimination for a given drug. The rationale and implementation of drug monitoring in cancer treatment are discussed in depth in Chapter 5.

Pharmacokinetics and the Future of Chemotherapy

The fundamental obstacle to greater success in application of pharmacokinetics to anticancer therapy is our limited knowledge of pharmacodynamics. We need the perspective of other medical specialties to evaluate our dilemma. In both infectious diseases and cardiology, pharmacokinetics has made a larger impact in the treatment of patients than in oncology. However, the therapeutic goal, or pharmacokinetic prescription, is very straightforward: to maintain a reasonably constant, effective plasma level of drug until the invading organism is overcome (infectious diseases) or to control blood pressure or enhance cardiac contractility for as long as required (cardiology). In cancer chemotherapy a constant, effective plasma level usually results in unacceptable patient toxicity. We need strategies based on intermittent dosing, to allow recovery of normal tissue from drug-induced toxicity.

Furthermore, treatment of infectious diseases can be guided by *in vitro* incubation of a patient's serum with drugs proposed for treatment to determine cytotoxic or inhibitory levels. For patients infected with "resistant" organisms that require very large concentrations for therapeutic effect with a particular drug, standard treatment with that drug will result in therapeutic "failure." Relative resistance might be overcome by use of doses higher than usual. Similarly, not all patients respond to antiarrhythmic drugs, regardless of dose or plasma level. The lack of response to anticancer chemotherapy in some patients is analogous to these situations.

The intensive effort to establish *in vitro* biochemical and clonogenic screening tests offers the potential for more efficacious use of pharmacokinetics, primarily for reasons of efficiency. In these tests, an individual patient's tumor cells (and possibly normal tissue) are exposed to potential drugs and then evaluated for cytotoxic or biochemical effects. In the test situation, drug concentration and exposure duration required for cell kill can be defined and these conditions can be used to select specific drugs and schedules of administration. In acute myelogenous leukemia, efforts have focused on the ability of cells *in vitro* to form the active triphosphate nucleotide from ara-C, ara-CTP, the formation of which appears to correlate with *in vivo* responses.[7] For fluorinated pyrimidines, activation to a variety of nucleotides *in vitro* is being related to therapeutic effect.[8, 9] Clonogenic assays have been developed,[10] particularly for tumors offering ready access, such as ascites cells from ovarian cancer. An alternative to these *in vitro* tests is the measurement of tumor tissue parameters, such as rates of DNA synthesis or other intracellular biochemical process following treatment.[11] Serial studies might determine the optimal timing for the next treatment, although they might be prohibitively invasive.

Those patients whose tumors are potentially sensitive to a given drug become candidates for extensive pharmacokinetic workup, both to tailor the treatment to the individual and to unravel effective delivery patterns for the average patient. If a given treatment yields 15 per cent complete responders, 25 per cent partial responders, and 60 per cent nonresponders, a large fraction of the nonresponders presumably could be prescreened and placed on alternative therapy. Without a prescreen, aggressive treatment forces many patients to maximal toxicity with little improvement in overall success, especially in diseases such as colorectal cancer, with only a 20 per cent response rate.[6] Those patients whose tumors are inherently insensitive to a given drug can be spared this fruitless toxicity.

PHARMACOKINETIC MODELING

Drug concentration measurements are the heart of any pharmacokinetic study. No model or application of a model is better than the data on which it is built. Many anticancer drugs are difficult to measure because of inherent instability, either spontaneously degrading or being degraded by enzymes in blood or tissues. Although the study of many anticancer drugs has been facilitated by the use of radiolabeled drugs, separation methods are required since the majority are extensively metabolized. Recent advances in separation methodology, such as high-pressure liquid chromatography, combined with improved sensitivity from radiolabeled drugs and mass spectrometric detectors and the development of competitive protein binding assays, have provided an improved basis for drug concentration measurement.

A pharmacokinetic model is a mathematical model, i.e., an equation or set of equations that can be used to describe the concentration versus time history of a drug. By convention, pharmacokinetic models are often presented in terms of box diagrams. Each box is called a compartment and corresponds to a region in the body with specific kinetic properties. The compartments may or may not represent real, identifiable anatomic regions. For some purposes a model is merely a summary of the data, and the data itself may answer questions without the need for a model construction. Simple concentration-time measurements of drug levels in plasma may be used to determine the basis of a population's therapeutic or toxic response, as in the case of high-dose methotrexate.[3] These measurements may be used directly to adjust an individual patient's dose when levels outside the target range are encountered. When models are not available this strategy is the only one available other than a titration based on apparent response or toxicity. This type of dosage adjustment becomes particularly difficult for those drugs with nonlinear kinetics or for situations in which a change in the drug delivery pattern must be made. A model can improve the adjustment process by identifying the range of nonlinearity and suggesting adjustment ratios, so that excessive escalations in concentration, $C \times t$, or time above an inhibitory concentration are avoided while the number of adjustments is minimized to avoid overcautious creeping up toward a target level.

Even for those models that are empirically constructed from concentration-time data, a model may provide insight that is not obvious from examination of the raw data. For data that exhibit great variation, a model may suggest which variables (e.g., binding or elimination) are likely sources of this variation and may lead to adjustments of drug delivery based on clinical laboratory tests, such as glomerular filtration rate or plasma protein analysis. For cases in which routine drug level measurement is not feasible, a high-risk population might be identified for selective monitoring. For drugs that exhibit multicompartmental behavior, a model may be able to predict concentrations in a compartment not accessible to sampling, such as a site of toxicity. Such extrapolations must be undertaken with great caution, but the study by Schentag et al.[12] on gentamicin nephrotoxicity provides an example of the possible benefits. Use of a two-compartment analysis of plasma data following the initial gentamicin dose made it possible to predict the patients likely to accumulate toxic drug levels in kidney tissue, despite the fact that plasma levels observed in the course of repeated dosing were not different for toxic and nontoxic patients.

Perhaps the ultimate use of a model would be in a case in which no data at all were available, e.g., when drug concentrations were too low to measure or no reliable assay method existed. This type of predictive modeling requires tremendous confidence in the modeling process. Such confidence might be gained from interspecies comparison and the success of *a priori* physiologic models, discussed below. These models are constructed largely from animal studies with the same drug. Perhaps most important, the modeling process forces us to make judgments about a drug's kinetic behavior, and this process clarifies the importance of what is unknown and the uncertainty of what is "known."

Models for drug distribution have existed for some time, but the widespread availability of computers has contributed to the growth of interest in modeling over the last 20 years. Models can be so complex that a computer is required for their study, but useful models frequently can be constructed and applied without sophisticated mathematics or any computer. "Modern" pharmacokinetic models evolved from similar models used to describe the behavior of diving gases, and intravenous and inhalation anesthetics were the first areas to capitalize on the power of models to help elucidate puzzling phenomena such as accumulation kinetics, multiphase decay, and redistribution behavior. Anticancer drugs have become prime modeling targets, because the therapeutic index for each of these drugs is so low that the modeling effort is thought to be worthwhile.

Like any other tool, the primary rule in model selection is that the model chosen should be the simplest description consistent with known details, yet general enough to serve its intended purpose. Many models have been published, with the principal delineation among them based either on whether they are derived from an empirical analysis of concentration-time data or on a physiologic description of the body, which includes chemical and physical data for a particular drug. Both types of models are compartmental, i.e., boundaries are drawn around kinetically homogeneous regions connected by transport processes. Although both types have been used extensively for anticancer drugs, it is unfortunate that there is little overlap between the users of each type. Pharmacokinetic models of both types have usually been developed to deal only with pure compounds such as the parent drug. Modifications to deal with metabolites substantially increase the complexity of the models and must be justified by the importance of these metabolites for either therapy or toxicity.

Mass Balance Concepts

Once the structure for the model (whether physiologic or empirical) has been established, the next step is formulation of mass balances, i.e., equations to describe the transfer processes between the compartments and reaction or excretory processes within the compartments. A mass balance for a compartment is simply an overall accounting of the rate processes that influence the amount of drug in the compartment:

$$\text{Net change} = \text{input(s)} - \text{output(s)} - \text{reaction(s)} \quad \text{[eq. 1]}$$

$$\begin{bmatrix}\text{rate of change of}\\ \text{drug in compartment}\end{bmatrix} = \begin{bmatrix}\text{rate of absorption}\\ \text{or injection}\end{bmatrix} + \begin{bmatrix}\text{rate of inflow}\\ \text{with blood}\end{bmatrix} + \begin{bmatrix}\text{rate of}\\ \text{diffusion in}\end{bmatrix} - \begin{bmatrix}\text{rate of outflow}\\ \text{with blood}\end{bmatrix} - \begin{bmatrix}\text{rate of}\\ \text{diffusion out}\end{bmatrix} - \begin{bmatrix}\text{rate of}\\ \text{conversion by}\\ \text{reaction}\end{bmatrix} - \begin{bmatrix}\text{rate of}\\ \text{excretion}\end{bmatrix} \quad \text{[eq. 2]}$$

The mass balances constitute a set of differential equations that form the basis of the model. Details of the various rate processes may be well understood (e.g., in terms of active or passive transport), or empirically observed, or inferred to account for conservation of mass. A complete mass balance considers all species: free (un-ionized), free (ionized), and bound forms. Since such equations can be quite complex structurally, and since only total drug concentration is normally measured, the balances are usually expressed in terms of total drug. If the free concentration is desired, it may be calculated from binding relationships.

A fundamental property of the mass balance is that the units for both the left and right side of the equation are identical: mass/time. Mass may be expressed in units such as mg, mmoles, and so on.

After the differential mass balances have been formulated and initial conditions specified, these equations are integrated to yield mass as a function of time. In some cases, analytical solutions are possible, as illustrated in the Empirical Modeling section below. For those cases without an analytical solution, numerical integration procedures are used.

A frequently useful conceptual approach invokes the steady-state, i.e., a situation in which there is constant input of drug balanced by constant removal by the elimination processes. Practically, this is achieved by a constant intravenous infusion. The major advantage of this approach is that the set of differential equations simplifies to a set of algebraic equations, which are far easier to use. For example, the differential mass balance for a generalized multicompartment model with input to and elimination from the body only in the central compartment is:

$$V_c \frac{dC_p}{dt} = G - Cl\, C_p + \sum_i \left[K_{ic}\,(C_i/R_i - C_p)\right] \quad \text{[eq. 3]}$$

V_c is the volume and C_p is the concentration (usually measured in the plasma) in the central compartment, G is the drug input function, Cl is total body clearance, and K_{ic} is the exchange rate between the i-th compartment and the central compartment. At steady-state, G is a constant (G_0), $dC_p/dt = 0$, and the net exchanges between compartments are zero. Concentration in any compartment, C_i, can be expressed in terms of a partition coefficient, R_i, between that compartment and the central compartment:

$$C_i = R_i C_p \quad \text{[eq. 4]}$$

The central compartment concentration at steady-state, C_{SS}, is found from the mass balance:

$$G_o = Cl\, C_{SS} \quad \text{[eq. 5]}$$

or

$$C_{SS} = G_0/Cl \quad \text{[eq. 6]}$$

For linear pharmacokinetic models all transfer and elimination processes are first-order, i.e., proportional to drug concentration. Inputs are arbitrary. The most commonly used are short bolus injection, constant infusion, and exponentially declining absorption. The steady-state concentration during constant infusion represents the time-averaged concentration for intermittent administration.

Empirical (Curve-Fit) Modeling

Empirical modeling remains the workhorse of clinical pharmacokinetics. Owing to its widespread applications (mostly in areas outside anticancer chemotherapy), there are several textbooks[13,14] that describe these models and compile a myriad of formulas associated with this approach. The interested reader can consult these texts for details; we will limit our approach to conceptual features of empirical modeling.

One-Compartment Model

The one-compartment model, in which the whole body is assumed to be kinetically homogeneous, is the most commonly used clinical model. There are two situations in which the one-compartment model is applicable:

1. Drugs that are injected intravenously and do not escape from plasma. This behavior is exhibited by very large molecules, such as the enzyme carboxypeptidase,[15] and by drugs that are tightly bound to plasma proteins, such as diagnostic contrast dyes.
2. Drugs that have slow elimination phases compared to the time scale for distribution to body tissues. Although any drug departs from a single compartment behavior if samples are taken early and/or late enough, one phase may dominate to the extent that the one-compartment model is a useful approximation. Additionally, the concepts learned in the analysis of one-compartment kinetics can be transferable to more complex models. The linear one-compartment model will be analyzed for several drug delivery patterns and then extended to nonlinear problems.

Figure 4–1 is a representation of the kind of concentration-time curve that is observed after bolus administration of a drug that behaves according to a one-compartment model. Our approach for the analysis of this type of curve is to begin with the mass balance and to compare the mathematical features of the model with figures that display the commonly observed characteristics of the model.

The mass balance for the *linear* one-compartment model is simplified from [eq. 3] by the removal of intercompartment transfer terms, so that the rate of change in drug mass equals the drug infusion rate minus the drug elimination rate:*

$$V_d \frac{dC_p}{dt} = G - k_{el}V_dC_p \qquad \text{[eq. 7]}$$

For this model, input is defined by the function G (units: mass/time), which may represent intermittent or continuous drug delivery. All excretory and reaction terms are considered as parallel elimination pathways, with the overall elimination rate constant, k_{el}(time^{-1}), representing the sum of these individual processes:

$$k_{el} = \sum_i k_i = k_{renal} + k_{bile} + k_{enzymatic} + \cdots \qquad \text{[eq. 8]}$$

Measured concentration (usually plasma), C_p, has units of mass/volume. The apparent volume of distribution, V_d, is simply the mass in the compartment divided by concentration in the compartment. As presented in [eq. 7], V_d is assumed to be constant for the time scale of interest. In [eq. 7], the product of the elimination rate constant and the volume of distribution is identical to total body clearance, Cl, as presented in [eq. 3].

When drug input is by bolus injection, the input is assumed to be instantly mixed throughout the compartment volume, providing the initial condition for the differential equation: C_0 = dose/V_d, and G = 0. Integration of the differential model, [eq. 7], yields:

$$\ln C_p(t) = \ln C_0 - k_{el}t \qquad \text{[eq. 9]}$$

or

$$C_p(t) = C_0 \exp(-k_{el}t) \qquad \text{[eq. 10]}$$

---

*Some readers may be more familiar with model equations that have been rearranged to express concentration changes rather than mass changes. So long as the mass balance is written first, any desired rearrangements may then be made. For example, [eq. 7] can be rewritten in terms of concentration changes by dividing both sides by V_d:

$$\frac{dC_p}{dt} = \frac{G}{V_d} - K_{el}C_p$$

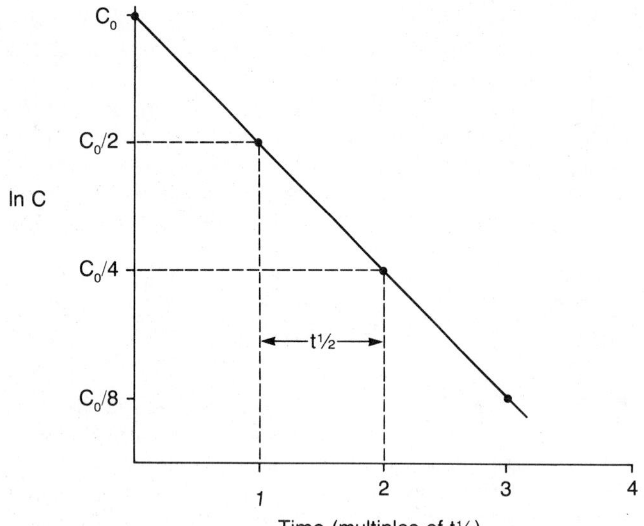

Figure 4–1. Concentration-time profile observed after bolus input to one-compartment model.

which is a straight line on semilogarithmic paper (Fig. 4–1), with a slope of $-k_{el}$. The notation "exp(x)" is equivalent to "e^x." Some form of [eq. 10] can be found in all textbooks on pharmacokinetics, and could be easily memorized and applied without use of the mass balance concept. The major advantage of the mass balance approach is flexibility, since once the derivation is understood, the equation can be readily modified. For example, the volume of distribution may not be constant, the drug delivery schedule may be novel, or other changes in assumptions may present the kineticist with a previously undescribed solution.

One of the more popular features of the one-compartment model is the "half-time," t½, which is the time required for the concentration (at any point on the concentration-time curve) to achieve one half its value (Fig. 4–1). This formula may be repetitively applied, so that in two half-times 25 per cent of drug is present, and so forth. This half-time is inversely related to the elimination rate constant. From [eq. 9], when $t = t½$ and $C(t½) = C_0/2$:

$$\ln(C_0/2) = \ln C_0 - k_{el} t½ \quad \text{[eq. 11]}$$

$$t½ = (\ln 2)/k_{el} = 0.693/k_{el} \quad \text{[eq. 12]}$$

Constant infusion of drug may be preferred to bolus injection. Although it requires more support services, this route provides constant levels of drug, especially in cases in which the drug half-time is short. The same mass balance [eq. 7] applies, except that $G = G_0$ (constant). When therapy is initiated, $C_p = 0$, and the integration yields:

$$C_p(t) = C_{ss}\,(1 - \exp(-k_{el}t)) \quad \text{[eq. 13]}$$

$$C_{ss} = G_0/(k_{el}V_d) \quad \text{[eq. 14]}$$

Substitution of Cl for $k_{el}V_d$ in [eq. 14] yields the same result as [eq. 6].

As shown in Figure 4–2, there is a rapid increase in drug concentration that levels off toward a plateau concentration, C_{ss}, which is then maintained for the duration of the infusion. Regardless of when the infusion is terminated, first-order decay of drug concentration is observed with the same rate constant, k_{el}, exhibited after bolus administration. The time to achieve plateau level depends on k_{el} only, and is independent of the infusion rate. The time required to reach one half the plateau level, t½, is identical to the time required for concentration decrease of 50 per cent after bolus injection. Also, 75 per cent of the plateau level is reached in two half-times, and so forth. For practical purposes, the plateau level is said to be reached in three to five half-times.

Many combinations of drug injection schedules might be utilized. For all *linear* kinetic models, each injection can be analyzed independently and the analyses combined to yield the resultant concentration-time profile. For example, if it is desirable to achieve the steady-state concentration rapidly, a "loading dose" may be given as a bolus at the same time the infusion is started. Total

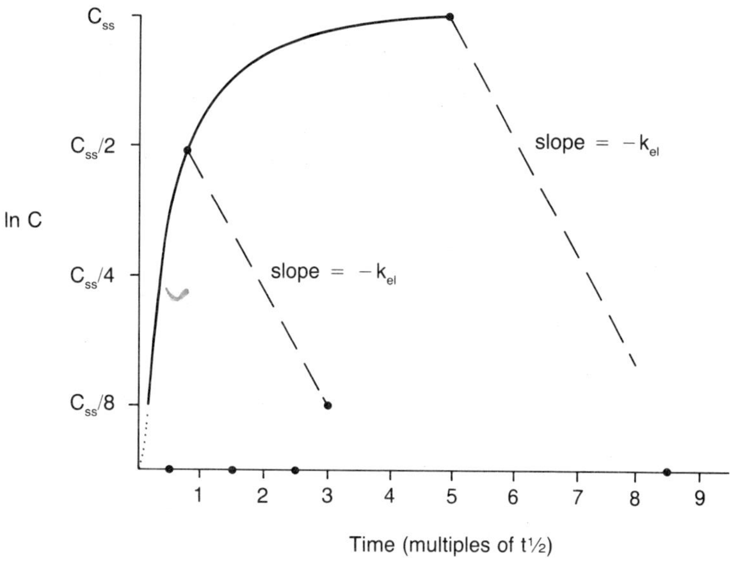

Figure 4–2. Constant infusion input to one-compartment model. Slope observed after cessation of input is independent of infusion length.

concentration at any time is the sum of the bolus and infusion contributions:

$$\text{total } C_p(t) = \text{bolus } C_p(t) + \text{infusion } C_p(t) \qquad \text{[eq. 15]}$$

The bolus dose is usually selected to achieve an initial concentration $C_0 = C_{ss}$ by administering a dose calcuated as follows: dose = $V_d C_{ss}$. In this way the time lag to plateau is eliminated:

$$C_p(t) = C_{ss}\exp(-k_{el}t) + C_{ss}(1 - \exp(-k_{el}t)) = C_{ss} \qquad \text{[eq. 16]}$$

As an alternative to continuous drug insion, periodic bolus injections may be given to maintain reasonably constant levels. As with the infusion, there is an approach to steady values (peaks and valleys), or the steady-state can be reached immediately with proper choice of loading dose. The most popular schedule is illustrated in Figure 4–3, where the peak concentration is designed to be twice the valley concentration. The design requires dosing once each half-time. An initial dose of twice the successive (maintenance) doses abolishes the time lag. The effect of changing the dose interval, τ, is illustrated as a ratio of peak and valley concentrations:

$$\frac{C_{max}}{C_{min}} = 2^{(\tau/t_{1/2})} \qquad \text{[eq. 17]}$$

As the dosing frequency increases or as τ gets smaller, the ratio of C_{max}/C_{min} approaches 1, and the concentration-time curve looks more like a constant infusion.

Oral, subcutaneous, intramuscular, and intraperitoneal routes of administration are not as commonly used for anticancer drugs as the intravenous modes, but deserve some mention. All these routes are usually thought to give an exponentially decreasing rate of drug delivery after initial dosing. This process is referred to as "first-order absorption," and the mass balance is:

$$V_d \frac{dC_p}{dt} = k_a F X_0 \exp(-k_a t) - k_{el} V_d C_p \qquad \text{[eq. 18]}$$

X_0 is the dose given, k_a is the first-order absorption rate constant (time^{-1}), and F is the fractional bioavailability. For subcutaneous or intramuscular administration, F is usually 1. For oral and intraperitoneal routes, absorption may be erratic and/or subject to first-pass elimination by the liver before reaching the systemic circulation. This differential model may be integrated subject to an initial condition of zero concentration:

$$C_p(t) = \frac{k_a F X_0/V_d}{k_a - k_{el}}(\exp(-k_{el}t) - \exp(-k_a t)) \qquad \text{[eq. 19]}$$

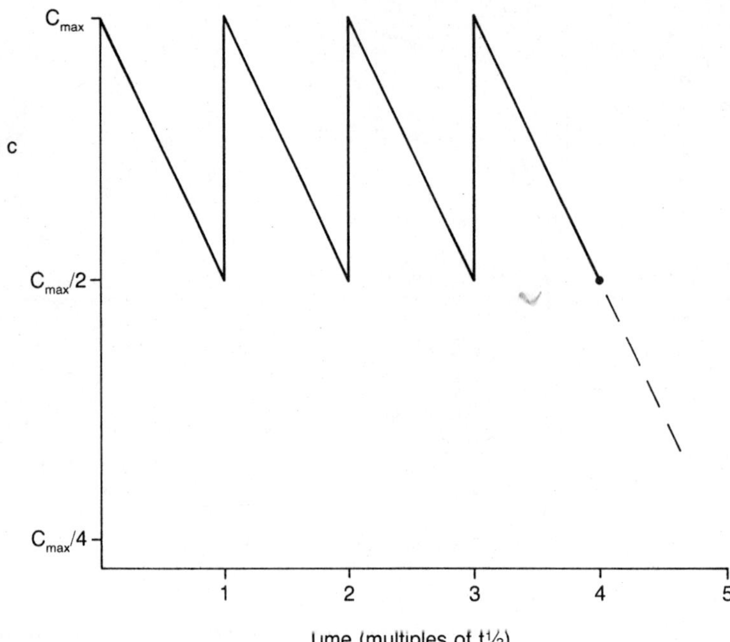

Figure 4–3. Concentration-time profile for intermittent bolus input to one-compartment model. Doses at t = 1, 2, and 3 are one half as large as dose at t = 0.

As shown in Figure 4–4, the concentration rises to a peak value and then declines. It is useful to know what this peak concentration is and when it occurs. The time of maximal concentration, t_{max}, is found when $dC_p/dt = 0$, which is:

$$t_{max} = \frac{\ln(k_a/k_{el})}{k_a - k_{el}} \quad \text{[eq. 20]}$$

The maximal concentration, C_{max}, is found by substituting t_{max} for t in [eq. 19]:

$$C_{max} = C(t_{max}) = \frac{FX_0}{V_d} \exp(-k_{el} t_{max}) \quad \text{[eq. 21]}$$

Usually the absorption rate is faster than the elimination rate, so that absorption is essentially complete while elimination continues to proceed, and this "postabsorptive" phase exhibits behavior similar to postbolus:

$$C_p(t) = \frac{k_a FX_0/V_d}{k_a - k_{el}} \exp(-k_{el} t) \quad \text{[eq. 22]}$$

Nonlinear One-Compartment Model

The linear models are quite useful for studying concentrations in certain ranges and also for concept formation. We would expect, however, that anticancer drugs that

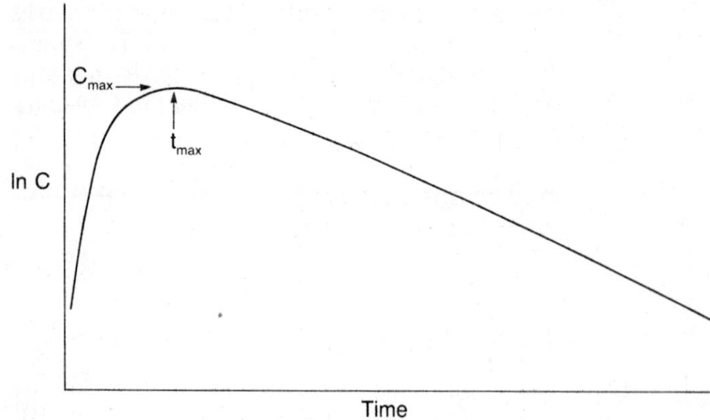

Figure 4–4. Concentration-time profile for first-order input to one-compartment model.

are given to maximally tolerated doses might exhibit deviations from linear behavior. Following bolus administration, deviations due to nonlinearities are expressed as convex curves on semilogarithmic plots, while multicompartment (but still linear) deviations are expressed as concave curvature.

There are three types of nonlinearities that may be encountered, all of which are saturation effects that may be approximated by linear models below saturation levels:

1. *Excretion.* For example, there may exist limited capacity for tubular secretion in kidneys or biliary secretion. From recent clinical studies[16] it can be inferred that methotrexate (MTX), which is now given over a wide range of doses, exhibits saturation of its elimination. This finding is consistent with earlier reports that demonstrated inhibition of MTX elimination by probenecid in animals[17] and humans.[18]

2. *Metabolism.* Michaelis-Menten enzyme kinetics have been demonstrated for ara-C and 5-fluorouracil in clinically relevant concentration ranges. This means that the rate of drug removal (amount/time) is independent of drug concentration above a threshold that saturates the degradative enzyme.

3. *Protein binding.* In plasma or tissue sites, a fixed number of binding sites can be expected to result in saturation effects. Unlike the first two mechanisms, this nonlinearity may lead to increased elimination rates (% dose/time) at high concentrations by making more drug available to elimination mechanisms in free form.

We will concentrate our analysis on the first two mechanisms, which are mathematically similar. The mass balance for nonlinear elimination from a one-compartment model is a straightforward modification of the elimination term in [eq. 7]:

$$V_d \frac{dC_p}{dt} = G - \frac{v_{max} C_p}{K_M + C_p} \quad \text{[eq. 23]}$$

The maximal capacity of the body to eliminate drug (mass/time) is v_{max}, and K_M is the concentration (mass/volume) at which the mass rate of elimination is half-maximal.

For bolus administration ($G = 0$), this differential model ([eq. 23] plus the initial condition $C_0 = \text{dose}/V_d$) cannot be integrated and solved *explicitly* for C_P as a function of time. Implicit analytical solutions or numerically integrated solutions are available and can be used to generate simulations such as Figure 4–5, which illustrate the convex curvature characteristic of Michaelis-Menten processes. In Figure 4–5, the effect of increasing dose is seen for the illustrative parameters $K_M = 5$ mg/l, $V_d = 40$ l, and $v_{max} = 25$ mg/hour. At concentrations below the K_M, the model behavior becomes nearly first-order. Above the K_M, increasingly longer times are required to decrease concentration by a factor of 2. "Half-time" is now dependent on concentration and is a less useful concept than for linear models. If the therapeutic or toxic effect of a drug depends on either $C \times t$ or time above some inhibitory concentration, disproportionate increases in effect are produced by dose increases.

When a drug with nonlinear kinetics is administered by continuous infusion ($G = G_0$), the mass balance at steady-state is given by [eq. 23] with $dC_p/dt = 0$:

$$G_0 = \frac{v_{max} C_{ss}}{K_M + C_{ss}} \quad \text{[eq. 24]}$$

which is readily solved for the plateau concentration:

$$C_{ss} = \frac{G_0 K_M}{v_{max} - G_0} \quad \text{[eq. 25]}$$

The form of the denominator suggests rapid increases in C_{ss} as the infusion rate G_0 approaches the maximal capacity of the body to remove drug.

Two-Compartment Linear Model

Although the one-compartment model has provided an important introduction to kinetic analysis, most drugs require two compartments for satisfactory analysis.[19] The two-compartment model has become the most widely published research model. Figure 4–6 illustrates a typical plasma concentration-time curve resulting from bolus drug input to a two-compartment model, also referred to as a biphasic model (two phases seen on semilogarithmic plot) or biexponential model (the mathematical description is a summation of two exponential terms). The two major reasons for adopting a two-compartment model are:

1. inappropriate doses will be given if based upon a one-compartment analysis, and
2. the drug target (receptor) may be located

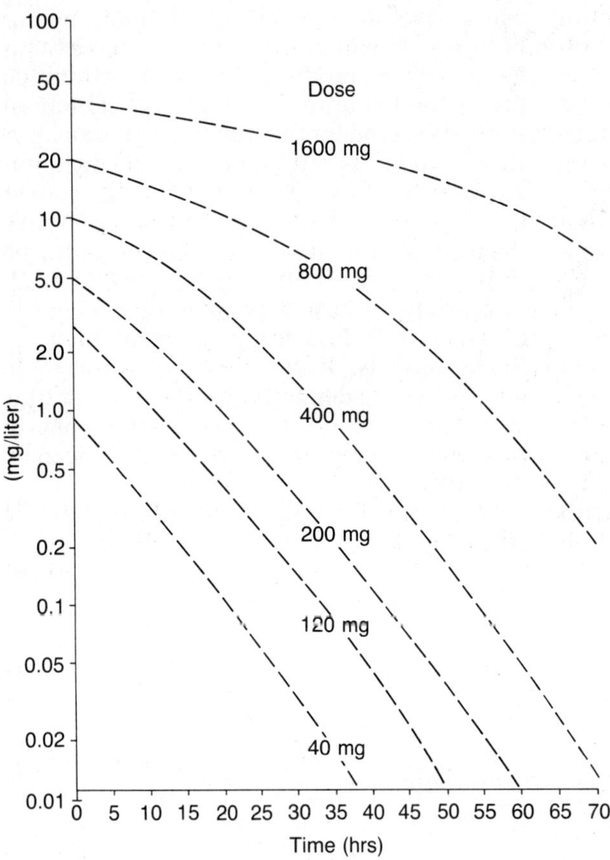

Figure 4–5. Dose-dependency in one-compartment model with Michaelis-Menten elimination after bolus input. K_M = 5 mg/liter; v_{max} = 25 mg/hr; v_d = 40 liters.

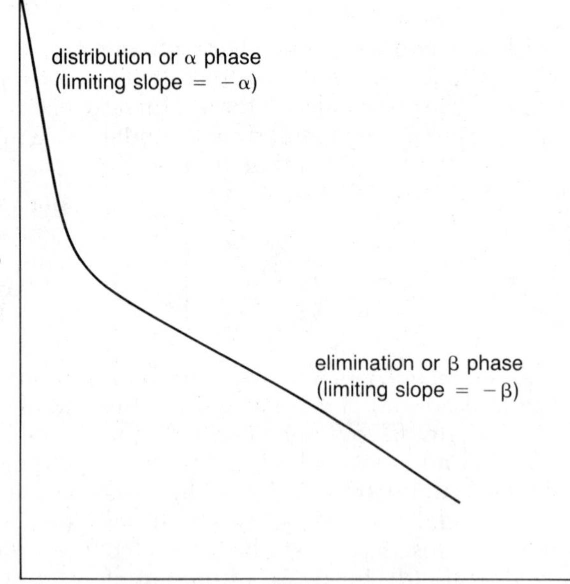

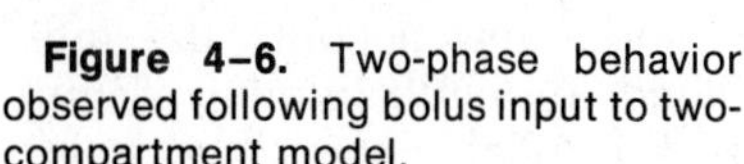
Figure 4–6. Two-phase behavior observed following bolus input to two-compartment model.

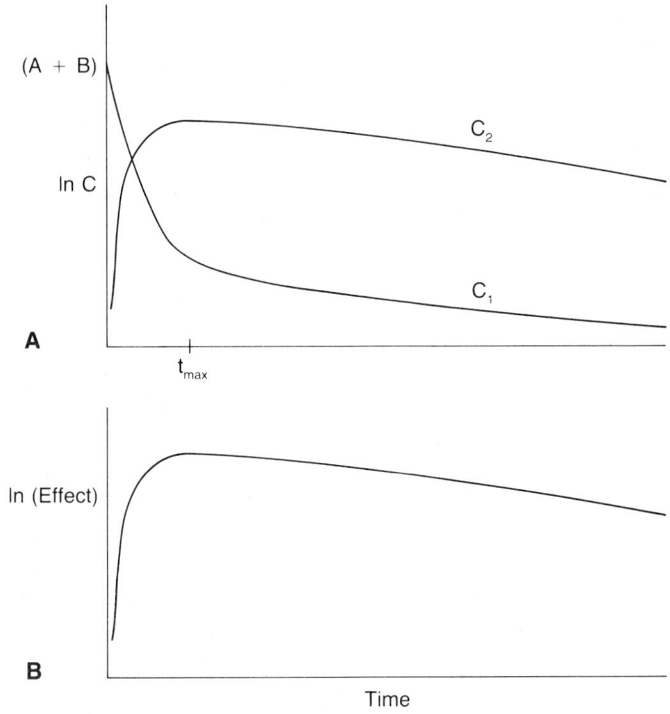

(A + B)

ln C

C_2

C_1

A

t_{max}

ln (Effect)

B

Time

Figure 4–7. *A,* Concentration-time history for compartments C_1 and C_2 of two-compartment model, following bolus injection. *B,* Pharmacodynamic effect observed after the bolus, plotted on the same time scale. (Adapted from Reuning et al.: Role of pharmacokinetics in drug dosage adjustment. I. Pharmacologic effect, kinetics, and apparent volume of distribution of digoxin. J. Clin. Pharmacol. 13:127–141, 1973.)

outside the compartment that is accessible to sampling, normally the plasma.

Since the correlation of effect and concentration is not well understood for most drugs in anticancer chemotherapy, we will borrow an example from the cardiovascular literature. Figure 4–7 shows that digoxin effect does not correlate well with initial plasma levels, but seems to follow the concentration in the second compartment (adopted from the study of Reuning et al.[20]). The previously cited gentamicin nephrotoxicity example is also relevant. Of course, such extrapolations of unmeasured concentrations must be done cautiously. The site(s) of action is (are) *never* the same as the second compartment, which is a mathematical concept. The site of action usually is also small in volume relative to the total volume of drug distribution, so that it has little effect on observable pharmacokinetics. Classical curve-fit models can be combined with a physiologic description of the site of action to produce a "hybrid" model, as discussed below.

In general, input and elimination can occur in either compartment, but the most common situation is illustated in Figure 4–8: input and elimination located only in compartment 1, which includes plasma and is also called the "central" compartment. The second compartment is often referred to as the "peripheral" compartment. Conceptually, the biphasic behavior arises from the process of distribution, in which transfer of drug from compartment 1 to 2 dominates, and elimination, during which the two compartments have "equilibrated," and elimination of drug dominates.

The mass balances for the two compartments include terms for transfer between the compartments, as well as input and output terms in compartment 1:

$$\frac{dX_1}{dt} = V_1 \frac{dC_1}{dt} = -k_{12}V_1C_1 + k_{21}V_2C_2 - k_{el}V_1C_1 + G \quad \text{[eq. 26]}$$

$$\frac{dX_2}{dt} = V_2 \frac{dC_2}{dt} = k_{12}V_1C_1 - k_{21}V_2C_2 \quad \text{[eq. 27]}$$

X_1 and X_2 are the amounts (mass) of drug in compartments 1 and 2, k_{12} is the rate constant ($time^{-1}$) for drug transfer from compartment 1 to compartment 2, and k_{21} is the corresponding rate constant for transfer from compartment 2 to compartment 1.

For a bolus injection ($G = 0, C_1(0) = dose/V_1$

and $C_2(0) = 0$), the differential mass balances can be integrated:

$$C_1(t) = A \exp(-\alpha t) + B \exp(-\beta t) \quad \text{[eq. 28]}$$

$$C_2(t) = H (\exp(-\beta t) - \exp(-\alpha t)) \quad \text{[eq. 29]}$$

A, B, H, α, and β are algebraic functions of the rate constants, volumes, and dose:

$$A = \frac{\text{dose}}{V_1}\left(\frac{\alpha - k_{21}}{\alpha - \beta}\right) \quad \text{[eq. 30]}$$

$$B = \frac{\text{dose}}{V_1}\left(\frac{k_{21} - \beta}{\alpha - \beta}\right) \quad \text{[eq. 31]}$$

$$H = \frac{\text{dose}}{V_2}\left(\frac{k_{12}}{\alpha - \beta}\right) \quad \text{[eq. 32]}$$

$$\alpha, \beta = \tfrac{1}{2}\left[(k_{12} + k_{21} + k_{el}) \pm \sqrt{(k_{12} + k_{21} + k_{el})^2 - 4k_{12}k_{el}}\right] \quad \text{[eq. 33]}$$

Figure 4–7A demonstrates the concentration-time profiles generated from these functions. Only $C_1(t)$ is usually measurable. The zero-time concentration for C_1 is A + B, B is the zero-time intercept for C_1 extrapolated from the elimination phase, α is the initial disappearance rate, and β is the terminal disappearance rate. $C_2(t)$ reaches a peak value at $t = t_{max}$:

$$t_{max} = \frac{\ln(\alpha/\beta)}{\alpha - \beta} \quad \text{[eq. 34]}$$

The half-time for C_1 is continuously increasing and is bounded by the terminal slope (elimination phase). After the distribution phase is essentially complete, curves for C_1 and C_2 are nearly parallel, and the system becomes a pseudo–one-compartment model.

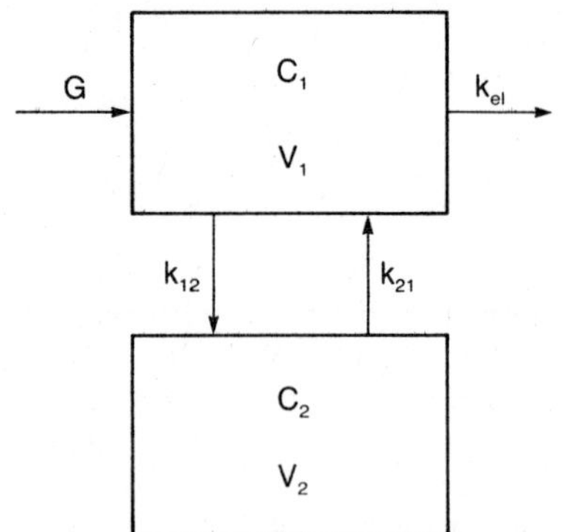

Figure 4–8. Two-compartment model, box diagram.

When a drug is given by constant infusion, there is an accumulation of drug until steady-state is reached, and the plateau concentration is the same as for the one-compartment model:

$$C_{ss} = G_0/Cl \quad \text{[eq. 35]}$$

However, the behavior after the infusion has stopped is no longer independent of the infusion time. Figure 4–9 illustrates post-delivery behavior for a bolus dose and an infusion that has reached steady-state. The α-phase is clearly seen postbolus, but is barely perceptible postinfusion.

As with one-compartment linear analysis, each injection in a multidose regimen behaves independently of other doses. However, rapid achievement of a plateau is not possible with a single loading dose. A complex time-dependent infusion schedule would be required. As shown in Figure 4–10, if the plateau value is immediately achieved with a loading dose, the concentration subsequently decreases before rising again toward the plateau. In order to ensure that the concentration remains at or above the plateau, higher initial levels must be tolerated.

Three or More Compartments

In reality, there is a continuous spectrum of blood:tissue exchange rates in the body. Any separation of tissues into various boxes is somewhat arbitrary. The complexity (number of compartments) of the model is dictated by the application for the model. It is difficult to justify more than two or at most three compartments on statistical grounds; therefore, a pharmacologic or physiologic rationale is needed. Any compartment large enough to influence the drug's distribution must be included. Additionally, a compartment that may not be important in terms of overall distribution may be required if it functions as a target organ.

Physiologic Pharmacokinetic Models

In the most general form, physiologic pharmacokinetic models are overly complex and require too large a data base for routine clinical use. However, they provide a basis

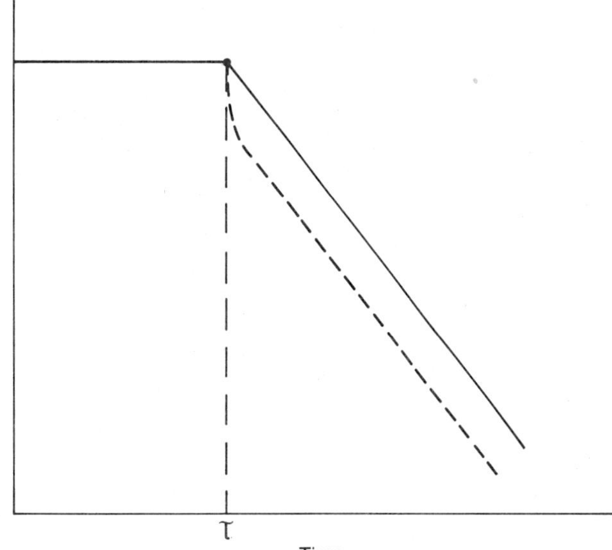

Figure 4–9. Postdelivery kinetics: bolus vs. infusion that has reached steady-state (two-compartment model). (-------) bolus at t = τ; (——) infusion stopped at t = τ.

for understanding a drug's kinetic behavior that can be incorporated into simpler models, either physiologic or hybrid, incorporating both empirical observations and physiologic information. Physiologic modeling goes beyond the usual goals of empirical pharmacokinetic modeling to allow for incorporation of data into the model that has been obtained in other species or *in vitro*.

Examples of physiologic pharmacokinetic models of anticancer drugs are given in Table 4–2. Verification of model predictions in man is generally limited to a comparison of predicted and actual plasma concentration; extensive tissue analysis is possible and often undertaken in other mammalian species.

Figure 4–10. Approach to steady-state: infusion plus one of two loading dose strategies (two-compartment model).

Five categories of data are essential in the construction of a physiologic pharmacokinetic model:

1. *Blood flow and tissue volume.* These values are obtained from standard references (e.g., textbooks or handbooks), and are ordinarily constant for all models, i.e., drug-independent. A particularly useful compilation has been made by Mapleson,[21] shown in Table 4–3.

2. *Drug binding to plasma proteins and tissues.* These data can be estimated from *in vitro* studies or from experiments in other species.

3. *Drug metabolism.* These data are usually obtained *in vivo*; however, there is some

TABLE 4–2. Physiologic Pharmacokinetic Models for Anticancer Drugs

Drug	*Ref.*	*Species*
Actinomycin D	32	Dog
Doxorubicin (Adriamycin)	33, 34	Rabbit, human
Cyclocytidine	35	Human
Cytosine arabinoside	22, 23	Mouse, dog, monkey, human
Mercaptopurine	36	Human
Methotrexate	26, 27	Mouse, rat, dog, monkey, human
Cis-Platinum	37	Dog

TABLE 4–3. Volumes and Blood Supply for a Standard Human*†

Tissue	*Volume, liters*	*Blood Flow, ml/min*
Adrenals	0.08	100
Kidneys	1.07	1240
Thyroid	0.07	80
Gray matter	1.12	600
Heart	0.45	240
Small glands and organs	0.16	80
Liver plus portal system	4.90	1580
White matter	0.85	160
Red marrow	2.10	120
Muscle	30.00	600
Skin, nutritive	3.00	60
Nonfat subcutaneous	4.80	70
Fatty marrow	2.20	60
Fat	10.00	200
Arterial blood plus lung parenchyma	2.00	–
Totals	62.80	5190
NOT INCLUDED IN MODEL		
Bone cortex	6.40	0
Skin, shunt blood	0.80	1290
Full Total	70.00	6480

*Tissue volumes include equilibrium blood.
†Adapted from Mapleson.[21]

evidence that properly designed *in vitro* experiments can be employed. Several model systems have been used to study *in vitro* metabolism: subcellular (e.g., microsomes), cellular (e.g., hepatocytes), tissue homogenates, and whole organs (e.g., isolated perfused liver). In each case, a determination of the drug metabolism parameters v_{max} and K_M can be made and these values are incorporated into the model. The cytosine arabinoside model[22, 23] is an example of this approach. Nonenzymatic drug disappearance can also be studied *in vitro* and incorporated into the model.[34, 36]

4. *Excretory processes.* It is difficult to obtain this information *in vitro*. Some guidance may be obtained from experiments in other species.

5. *Transport.* The rate of drug entry into a tissue, if not blood flow–limited, depends on the permeability characteristics of capillary and cell membranes. Such processes may be active (and saturable) or passive, and require *in vivo* experiments to elucidate model parameters.

The compartments comprising a physiologic pharmacokinetic model have an anatomic basis, and the transfer processes in the model have physiologic or pharmacologic identity. A typical example is shown in Figure 4–11 for the anticancer drug cytosine arabinoside (ara-C). We will analyze several of these models in detail, but first it is interesting to examine certain features of the mass balance and to derive some useful results from simplified models.

We will first focus on a single organ (Figure 4–12: volume, V_i; concentration, C_i; blood perfusion, Q_i). For simplicity, we will assume that the drug we are studying is not bound in this organ or blood and has partition coefficients of 1 between the organ and blood and between blood cells and plasma. The rate at which drug enters the organ from the blood can be controlled by the rate it can leave capillaries and the rate at which it can move from extracellular into intracellular space. For each organ, a separate transport equation can be written for each of these two processes. However, if both processes are rapid relative to the rate at which blood supplies drug to the organ, the two processes are lumped into a single mass balance.

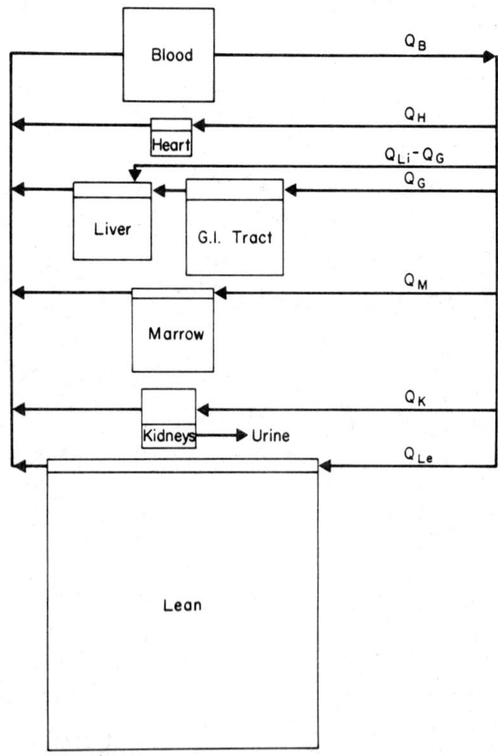

Figure 4–11. Physiologic pharmacokinetic model for ara-C.

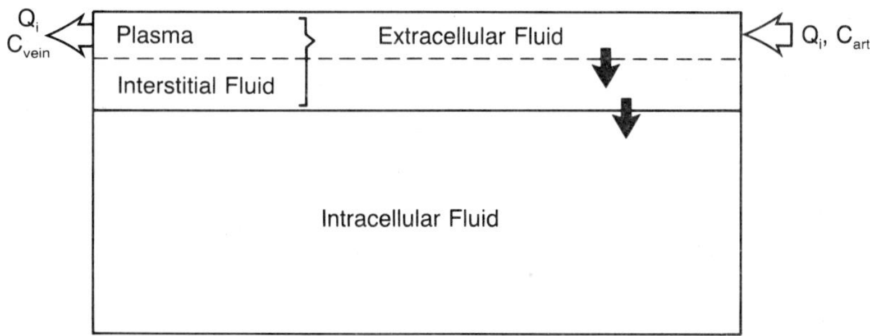

Figure 4–12. Schematic drawing of an individual compartment. (Revised from Dedrick et al.: Transport and binding of methotrexate in vivo. J. Pharm. Sci. 62:882–890, 1973.)

$$V_i \frac{dC_i}{dt} = Q_i C_{art} - Q_i C_{vein} - Cl_i C_i \quad \text{[eq. 36]}$$

C_{art} is the concentration of drug in arterial blood supplying the organ, C_{vein} is the mixed-venous blood draining the organ, and Cl_i is the intrinsic drug clearance of the organ, a measure of its maximal capacity to remove drug by all routes. Since the transcapillary and transcellular processes are rapid, the organ concentration is said to be "blood flow–limited." In this case, the organ concentration is in equilibrium with the venous blood exiting the tissue. These are identical when the partition coefficient is unity:

$$V_i \frac{dC_i}{dt} = Q_i (C_{art} - C_i) - Cl_i C_i \quad \text{[eq. 37]}$$

The concept of clearance introduced in [eq. 36] requires further exploration. For an organ that removes drug from the body, we can express a steady-state extraction, E, in terms of arterial and venous concentration:

$$E = (C_{art} - C_{vein})/C_{art} \quad \text{[eq. 38]}$$

From our usual reference point external to the organ, elimination by the organ is based on the fraction of its blood flow "cleared" by the organ:

$$Cl_e = Q_i E = Q_i (C_{art} - C_{vein})/C_{art} \quad \text{[eq. 39]}$$

We have designated this clearance with the subscript "e" to indicate a reference external to the organ. From the reference of the organ, an intrinsic clearance is defined by the steady-state mass balance ($dC_i/dt = 0$ in [eq. 36]):

$$Q_i C_{art} = Q_i C_{vein} + Cl_i C_i \quad \text{[eq. 40]}$$

$$Cl_i = Q_i (C_{art} - C_{vein})/C_i \quad \text{[eq. 41]}$$

While external clearance (Cl_e) is often the most useful operationally, intrinsic clearance (Cl_i) is required to model first-pass effects and is also the quantity derived from *in vitro* experiments such as tissue homogenate incubations. Therefore, a relationship between these terms is required. Comparison of [eq. 39] and [41] yields:

$$\frac{Cl_e}{Cl_i} = \frac{Q_i (C_{art} - C_{vein})/C_{art}}{Q_i (C_{art} - C_{vein})/C_i} = \frac{C_i}{C_{art}} \quad \text{[eq. 42]}$$

Substitution of C_i for C_{vein} in [eq. 40], flow-limitation, yields (with rearrangement):

$$\frac{C_i}{C_{art}} = \frac{Q_i}{Q_i + Cl_i} \quad \text{[eq. 43]}$$

Finally, [eq. 42] and [43] are combined to yield:

$$\frac{Cl_e}{Cl_i} = \frac{Q_i}{Q_i + Cl_i} \quad \text{[eq. 44]}$$

or

$$Cl_e = \frac{Q_i Cl_i}{Q_i + Cl_i} \quad \text{[eq. 45]}$$

This expression has two limiting cases. The maximal external clearance is the blood flow, Q_i. If intrinsic clearance is much lower than blood flow, the magnitude of external clearance approaches that of intrinsic clearance.

Simple exercises with physiologic mass balances are often adequate to describe the most important features of a drug's kinetics in the body. It is important to realize that compartments such as muscle and fat, which may have no drug receptors and usually have no role in drug elimination, profoundly influence drug concentrations (and hence, response) throughout the body by acting as reservoirs for redistribution of drugs. Therefore, the most demanding test of physiologic modeling is whole body simulation. A list of published models is presented in Table 4–2. Next, we will examine whole body physiologic models for the anticancer drugs ara-C and methotrexate (MTX) to illustrate the interplay of kinetic variables throughout the body. The ara-C model incorporates simplified mass balances coupled with large interspecies differences in elimination. The MTX mass balances are complicated by intracellular binding and membrane permeability limitations, but there is a high degree of species similarity.

Ara-C Model

Cytosine arabinoside (ara-C) is a drug with considerable usefulness in the treatment of leukemias. Its mechanism of action and other pharmacologic properties are summarized in Chapter 18. It requires intracellular conversion to the triphosphate nucleotide, ara-CTP, but much of the drug is deactivated instead by deaminating enzymes (ara-C → ara-U) in various body tissues. The distribution of these enzymes is a source of considerable variation in mammalian species. The structure for this model is presented in Figure 4–11.

The mass balances are simplified because the drug is freely transported across cell membranes, and thus flow limitation is assumed. There is no binding or partitioning of ara-C between blood and other tissues. The mass balance for the blood is:

$$V_B \frac{dC_B}{dt} = \left[\sum_i (Q_i C_i)\right] - \left[C_B \sum_i Q_i\right] - \frac{v_{max,B}\, C_B}{K_M + C_B} + G \qquad \text{[eq. 46]}$$

Because drug clearance depends on enzymatic degradation, clearance is expressed as a Michaelis-Menten process. Mass balances for the heart, gastrointestinal tract, bone marrow, and lean compartments have identical form:

$$V_i \frac{dC_i}{dt} = Q_i(C_B - C_i) - \frac{v_{max,i}\, C_i}{K_M + C_i} \qquad \text{[eq. 47]}$$

The mass balance for the kidney is similar, except for an additional elimination term for urinary removal. The liver mass balance incorporates input from both the hepatic artery and portal vein. Simulations[22,23] compared favorably with data for mouse, monkey, dog, and human parameters, despite considerable variation in elimination rates in these four species.

Data from four of the five categories required to construct a physiologic model were obtained in an *a priori* fashion, at least for some species:

1. blood flow and tissue volumes were primarily literature values;
2. binding was not present (as suspected from structure of ara-C and confirmed in a single species);
3. drug metabolism was determined entirely from *in vitro* experiments (tissue homogenates);
4. kidney clearance of ara-C and ara-U was determined from *in vivo* data; and
5. transport processes were not modeled, since there was *a priori* expectation of flow limitation.

From a pharmacokineticist's view, the ara-C model remains today as one of the most satisfying ever published. In light of this success, Morrison[24] and Lincoln[25] have extended the model by incorporating more details of cellular metabolism, namely, the formation of the active agent, ara-CTP, and its effect on tumor-bearing mice.

Methotrexate

Methotrexate (MTX) was the first anticancer drug for which a physiologic pharmacokinetic model was developed.[26] The original model (structure in Fig. 4–13) incorporated two features not required in the ara-C model, but essential to MTX distribution: strong intracellular binding and biliary secretion with possible enterohepatic circulation of drug. Flow limitation was assumed, but a nonlinear expression was used for the description of the tissue binding:

$$C_{tissue} = RC_p + \frac{aC_p}{\epsilon + C_p} \quad \text{[eq. 48]}$$

where "a" is the strong binding capacity (dihydrofolate reductase [DHFR]), ϵ is the dissociation constant of the MTX:DHFR complex, and "R" is the nonsaturable binding component. Transport from the liver into bile and from the gut lumen into gut tissue were also modeled as saturable processes. No metabolism was incorporated into the model. Kidney clearance was measured. An impressive presentation comparing simulations with experimental data required four cycles of semilogarithmic paper to illustrate all tissues simultaneously.

The assumption of flow limitation has been modified in subsequent papers[27–29] to focus on transport in particular tissues such as spontaneous canine lymphosarcoma[27] and murine[28] experimental tumors, and sensitive normal tissues in the mouse and rat.[28,29] A complete presentation of the currently used model is available.[30] Improvements in MTX assay methods[31] have demonstrated that limited metabolism does occur. This can confound pharmacokinetic calculations based on total radioactivity, particularly at long times following a single dose when a significant fraction of the radioactivity administered as MTX is no longer the parent compound.

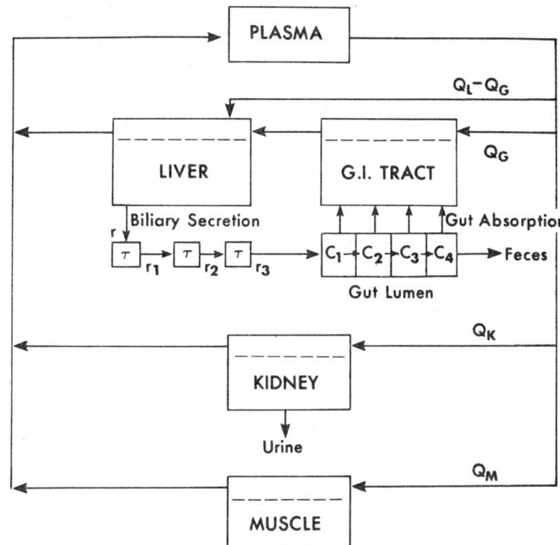

Figure 4–13. Physiologic pharmacokinetic model for MTX.

Review of Other Physiologic Models for Anticancer Drugs

Actinomycin D. This drug has been modeled for the beagle dog,[32] but not in humans. It is highly bound to tissues, although the binding was found to be rapid, reversible, and linear in the range studied. Fourteen compartments were included; only the testes compartment was found to be membrane-limited. Binding parameters and kidney and biliary clearances were determined from experimental data obtained from bile duct–cannulated dogs. No metabolism was observed in previous experiments.

Doxorubicin (Adriamycin). This drug was first modeled in the rabbit.[33] Elimination and binding parameters were derived from the data, and flow limitation was assumed for all tissues. The spleen appears to have deviated from this assumption. This model was slightly modified and scaled up for humans.[34] Human plasma data were reported to be reasonably simulated in 11 of 17 patients with normal liver function. Assay of doxorubicin is complicated by the photosensitivity of the compound, and no separation method has gained universal acceptance, which complicates model development and interpretation.

Cyclocytidine (cyclo-C). This is a prodrug for ara-C, and was modeled[35] by extension of the ara-C model[22,23] to include hydrolysis of cyclo-C to ara-C in all compartments. The only experimental data presented were plasma values from two human subjects, so that a thorough evaluation is not possible. Renal elimination of cyclo-C was obtained from the data. The hydrolysis rate constant obtained *in vitro* differed by a factor of 2 from that which provided adequate simulation *in vivo*.

Mercaptopurine (6-MP). This drug was modeled for the rat and humans by using the structure of the MTX model, but many of the binding, transport, and excretory parameters were determined by curve-fitting of the experimental data.[36] A serious methodologic problem is that total radioactivity data were used to build the model, but the paper states that a "large proportion of mercaptopurine undergoes biotransformation *in vivo*."

***cis*-Dichlorodiammineplatinum (II) (DDP).** For this drug the kinetics were modeled for the beagle dog,[37] and are dominated by nonenzymatic conversion of parent drug to other species, extensive binding to tissue, and renal elimination. Tissue binding and kidney clearance parameters were obtained from the data, but the conversion rate was obtained from *in vitro* experiments. Unlike the cyclo-C model, it did not have to be modified to provide reasonable simulations.

Hybrid Models

It is rather unfortunate that a dichotomy exists in the literature between empirical and physiologic models. Features of both can be combined in the development of "hybrid" models, of which there are two major useful types.

Having met the formidable challenge of whole body pharmacokinetic simulation, we expect that more effort will be spent by physiologic modelers on detailed models of "local" kinetics. In such problems, most of the body is considered a black box that provides an empirical concentration-time history to the tissue compartment of interest. For methotrexate, this approach has been used to study drug uptake in two tumors: spontaneous canine lymphosarcoma[27] and transplanted murine Lewis lung.[28] Plasma concentration was presented as a multi-exponential function, and drug transport into the tumor was examined as transport parameters were varied. The simplified analysis of peritoneal dialysis discussed in the next section is a similar hybrid in which local uptake is physiologically described while the rest of the body is lumped into a single compartment.

Another type of hybridization is the substitution of information derived from empirical models into a physiologic model. For example, clearance can be derived from an empirical analysis and incorporated into liver or kidney compartments. The value of the clearance and its concentration dependence may provide some clues regarding the mechanism for drug removal from the body. Since "clearance" has the same meaning and same numerical value in both types of models, this concept can serve as a bridge between the two modeling approaches.

REGIONAL ADMINISTRATION

Owing to the low therapeutic index of most anticancer drugs, several unusual routes of administration have been implemented in order to deliver drugs close to the site of the tumor and reduce the deleterious effects associated with ordinary systemic administration. Examples of these are the intra-arterial, intrathecal, and intraperitoneal routes. Pharmacokinetic analysis can help to evaluate the potential usefulness of these approaches; the functional form of the equations is quite similar.

Intra-Arterial

Intra-arterial infusion is a delivery mode unique to anticancer chemotherapy. It has been applied to a number of arteries in the body, most commonly in head and neck disease, in conjunction with limb isolation procedures, and for liver perfusion. Fenstermacher and Cowles[38] have used a physiologic pharmacokinetic model to simulate drug concentration in tumor and various body tissues as a result of a carotid artery infusion. Eckman et al.[39] have developed equations that quantitate the potential concentration advantage expected from intra-arterial infusion compared with intravenous infusion. They have also discussed the possible impact on pharmacodynamics (drug effects), with emphasis on our lack of understanding in that area.

The quantitative advantage of intra-arterial infusion is most easily expressed in terms of the area-under-the-concentration curve (AUC), although this may not be the most appropriate measure for some drugs, such as antimetabolites. As long as all transfer processes are linear, this area is independent of the particular time course of delivery. To examine the selective advantage of intra-arterial versus intravenous infusion, the key index is the ratio of drug concentration in the tumor (AUC_T) which is perfused (or the circulation exiting the tissue) to drug concentration in the systemic circulation (AUC_S) which is supplying potential sites of toxicity (such as bone marrow). The therapeutic advantage for drug delivery, R_d, can be expressed as the ratio of the index value for intra-arterial versus the index value for intravenous administration:

$$R_d = \frac{(AUC_T/AUC_S)IA}{(AUC_T/AUC_S)IV} \quad \text{[eq. 49]}$$

For a region that does not eliminate drug from the body, R_d is a function only of the local artery flow rate (Q_i) and the total body clearance (Cl_{TB}) observed after IV administration:

$$R_d = \frac{Cl_{TB}}{Q_i} + 1 \quad \text{[eq. 50]}$$

This equation suggests that the smaller the blood flow in the artery being infused, the greater the advantage for intra-arterial administration. Also, for a given artery, the advantage can be increased by selection of a drug with a high body clearance. For example, methotrexate infusion (assume Cl_{TB} = 200 ml/min) into a carotid artery (assume Q_i = 300 ml/min) yields an R_d of 1.67, while doxorubicin infusion (assume Cl_{TB} = 600 ml/min) yields an R_d of 3. Naturally, tumor sensitivity to the drug must also be considered. Since there is no elimination by the perfused tissue, the AUC in all other body tissues is unchanged (same for IA or IV). Thus, tumor exposure can be increased, while systemic exposure is not. R_d for this case, [eq. 49], is simply the ratio of AUC_T (IA)/AUC_T (IV).

For a tissue that does eliminate drug (such as the liver), there is an additional advantage. R_d is now related to the fraction of drug, E, eliminated on a single pass through the tissue:

$$R_d = \frac{Cl_{TB}}{Q(1 - E)} + 1 \quad \text{[eq. 51]}$$

For the particular case of elimination only in the perfused region (e.g., hepatic artery infusion of certain drugs),

$$R_d = \frac{1}{1 - E} \quad \text{[eq. 52]}$$

since $E = Cl_{TB}/Q_i$.

Intrathecal

Intrathecal administration has been used primarily to obtain adequate drug levels in the CSF to eradicate cancer cells that are otherwise protected from effective therapy. Assuming that the brain is a lumped compartment (at least for illustrative purposes), its mass balance is:[40]

$$V_{brain} \frac{dC_{brain}}{dt} = K(C_p - C_{brain}) - Q_{CSF} C_{CSF} + P + G \quad \text{[eq. 53]}$$

K is the blood brain barrier permeability, Q_{CSF} is the rate of CSF formation and removal from the brain, and P represents any active transport of drug into the CSF (assume negligible for this analysis). G is the input function. G is included in the brain mass balance for intrathecal administration, but is left out for intravenous input. When all transfer processes are linear, the advantage for intrathecal administration is determined only by the permeability and total body clearance:

$$R_d = \frac{Cl_{TB}}{K} + 1 \quad \text{[eq. 54]}$$

Although Q_{CSF} strongly affects the concentration in CSF regardless of administration route, its effects are equally felt by all routes. Methotrexate has been most often studied by this route.[2]

Intraperitoneal

Peritoneal dialysis is currently being evaluated[3,4,30,41] as an intraperitoneal delivery vehicle for anticancer drugs when disease is localized to the abdomen. The pharmacokinetic rationale suggests that tumor tissue may be exposed to very high local drug concentration, while systemic levels are no greater than normally encountered in intravenous therapy. For a drug that is not subject to "first-pass" elimination by the liver, the therapeutic advantage for intraperitoneal versus intravenous administration is:

$$R_d = \frac{Cl_{TB}}{PA} + 1 \quad \text{[eq. 55]}$$

assuming all transfer processes are linear.

PA is the permeability-area product for peritoneal drug administration. It is determined by multiplying the volume of intraperitoneal fluid by the slope obtained from a semilogarithmic plot of peritoneal concentration versus time. For most hydrophilic anticancer drugs, PA ranges from 5 to 20 ml/min and Cl_{TB} ranges from about 100 to several thousand ml/min. R_d of about 25 was found[41] for methotrexate, and R_d of approximately 300 was found[4] for 5-fluorouracil.

The structural similarity of [eq. 50], [54], and [55] emphasizes the conceptual similarity (Fig. 4–14) of these three modes of regional administration. Furthermore, the same concepts apply to the oral route, which is occasionally used for anticancer drugs. Presumably, higher local drug concentration in the gastrointestinal tract and portal vein can be achieved than with intravenous dosing, but incomplete and/or erratic absorption often make the oral route unacceptable. Furthermore, delivery of drug to the liver via the portal vein for "first-pass" metabolism is a disadvantage for treatment of systemic disease.

CONCLUDING REMARKS

The ultimate goal of pharmacokinetics is to assist in the optimization of therapy. Before pharmacokinetics can make substantial contributions to the treatment process, several preliminary steps are required. A substantial data base is needed, i.e., measurement of concentration-time profiles after drug administration. Another important step is the development of kinetic models, both physiologic and empirical. There is a continuing need for these steps in the progression toward our ultimate goal, but sufficient headway has been made to justify more emphasis being placed on studies designed to provide fundamental information.

One such study, as previously discussed, is the use of hybrid pharmacokinetic modeling to determine transport parameters for a particular tissue or site of interest. Another relatively unexplored area, particularly for anticancer drugs, is that of drug–drug interactions. Virtually all treatment protocols include combinations of drugs, encompassing two or more anticancer agents as well as various other drugs related to general supportive therapy of the patient. Several types of interactions between these agents may occur, resulting in alteration of clearance, volume of distribution, binding, membrane transport, and other properties of the interacting compounds. These changes might result in unexpected toxicity due to increased concentrations or in lessened effectiveness due to decreased concentrations. Well-formulated pharmacokinetic models can help distinguish between the various interactions and possibly predict which drugs are likely to have adverse interactions.

Although progress has been made in pharmacokinetic areas, the limiting step for optimization of therapy is inadequate knowledge of the relationship between drug concentration-time profiles and drug effects. Pharmacokinetics can serve as a useful tool to help elucidate these pharmacodynamic relationships by determining which profiles are feasible and by helping to design administration strategies. Also, since overall drug effect results from both kinetic and dynamic variables, studies can be designed to adjust doses individually so that kinetic differences between patients can be minimized and attention can be solely focused upon drug dynamics.

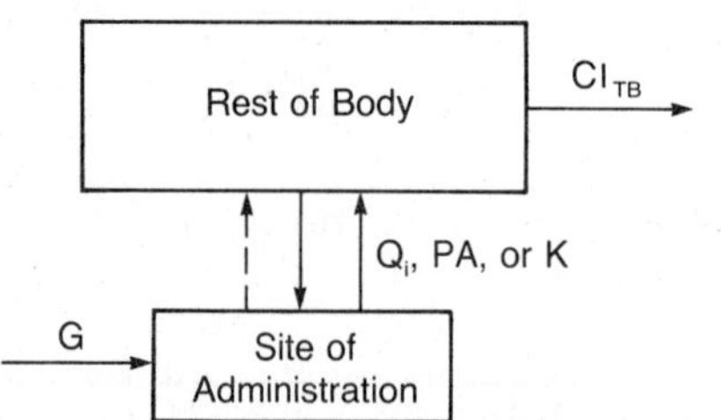

Figure 4–14. Regional drug administration. Solid arrows illustrate symmetric intercompartmental transfer, designated in text as Q_i for intra-arterial administration, PA for intraperitoneal administration, and K for intrathecal administration. Asymmetric routes of transfer such as lymph or cerebrospinal fluid flow are shown as a dotted arrow.

References

1. Woodcock TM, Martin DS, Damin LEM, et al.: Clinical trials with thymidine and fluorouracil: a phase I and clinical pharmacologic evaluation. Cancer 45:1135–1143, 1980.
2. Bleyer WA: The clinical pharmacology of intrathecal methotrexate. II. An improved dosage regimen derived from age-related pharmacokinetics. Cancer Treat. Rep. 61:1419–1425, 1977.
3. Jones RB, Myers CE, Guarino AM, et al.: High volume intraperitoneal chemotherapy for ovarian cancer: pharmacologic basis and early results. Cancer Chemother. Pharmacol. 1:161–166, 1978.
4. Speyer JL, Collins JM, Dedrick RL, et al.: Phase I and pharmacologic studies of 5-fluorouracil administered intraperitoneally. Cancer Res. 40:567–572, 1980.
5. van Prooijen R, van der Kleijn E, and Haanen C: Pharmacokinetics of cytosine arabinoside in acute myeloid leukemia. Clin. Pharmacol. Ther. 21:744–750, 1977.
6. Stoller RG, Hande KR, Jacobs SA, et al.: Use of plasma pharmacokinetics to predict and prevent methotrexate toxicity. N. Engl. J. Med. 297:630–634, 1977.
7. Chabner BA, Hande KR, and Drake JC: Ara-C metabolism: implications for drug resistance and drug interactions. Bull. Cancer (Paris) 66:89–92, 1979.

8. Ardalan B, MacDonald JS, Cooney D, et al.: Studies on mechanisms of 5-fluorouracil resistance in murine and human tumors. Bull. Cancer (Paris) 66:55–59, 1979.
9. Moran RG, and Heidelberger C: Determinants of 5-fluorouracil sensitivity in human tumurs. Bull. Cancer (Paris) 66:79–83, 1979.
10. Salmon SE, Hamburger AW, Soehnlen B, et al.: Quantitation of differential sensitivity of human-tumor stem cells to anticancer drugs. N. Engl. J. Med. 298:1321–1327, 1978.
11. Young, RC: Kinetic aids to proper chemotherapeutic scheduling: Labeled nucleoside incorporation studies *in vivo*. Cancer Treat. Rep. 60:1947–1958, 1976.
12. Schentag JJ, Jusko WJ, Vance JW, et al.: Aminoglycoside nephrotoxicity in relation to tissue accumulation. *In* Fillastre JP (ed.): Nephrotoxicity: Interaction of Drugs with Membrane Systems, Mitochondria-Lysosomes. Masson Publishing, New York, 1978, pp. 63–82.
13. Gibaldi M, and Perrier D: Pharmacokinetics. Marcel Dekker, New York, 1975.
14. Wagner JG: Fundamentals of Clinical Pharmacokinetics. Drug Intelligence Publications, Hamilton, IL, 1975.
15. Howell, SB, Blair, HE, Uren J, et al.: Haemodialysis and enzymatic cleavage of methotrexate in man. Eur. J. Cancer 14:787–792, 1978.
16. Marty JJ: Methotrexate pharmacokinetics: long and short infusions. Clin. Exp. Pharmacol. Physiol. (Suppl.) 5:29–34, 1979.
17. Bourke RS, Chheda G, Bremer A, et al.: Inhibition of renal tubular transport of methotrexate by probenecid. Cancer Res. 35:110–116, 1975.
18. Liegler DG, Henderson ES, Hahn MA, et al.: The effect of organic acids on renal clearance of methotrexate in man. Clin. Pharmacol. Ther. 10:849–857, 1969.
19. Oates J, and Wilkinson G: Principles of drug therapy. *In* Harrison's Principles of Internal Medicine. McGraw-Hill Book Co., New York, 1977, pp. 334–346.
20. Reuning RH, Sams RA, and Notari RE: Role of pharmacokinetics in drug dosage adjustment. I. Pharmacologic effect, kinetics, and apparent volume of distribution of digoxin. J. Clin. Pharmacol. 13:127–141, 1973.
21. Mapleson WW: An electric analogue for uptake and exchange of inert gases and other agents. J. Appl. Physiol. 18:197–204, 1963.
22. Dedrick RL, Forrester DD, Cannon JN, et al.: Pharmacokinetics of 1-β-D-arabinofuranosylcytosine (ara-C) deamination in several species. Biochem. Pharmacol. 22:2405–2417, 1973.
23. Dedrick RL, Forrester DD, and Ho DHW: *In vitro–in vivo* correlation of drug metabolism — deamination of 1-β-D-arabinofuranosylcytosine. Biochem. Pharmacol. 21:1–16, 1972.
24. Morrison PF, Lincoln TL, and Aroesty J: Disposition of cytosine arabinoside (NSC-63878) and its metabolites: a pharmacokinetic simulation. Cancer Chemother. Rep. 59:861–876, 1975.
25. Lincoln T, Morrison P, Aroesty J, et al.: Computer simulation of leukemia therapy: combined pharmacokinetics, intracellular enzyme kinetics, and cell kinetics of the treatment of L1210 leukemia by cytosine arabinoside. Cancer Treat. Rep. 60:1723–1739, 1976.
26. Bischoff KB, Dedrick RL, Zaharko DS, et al.: Methotrexate pharmacokinetics. J. Pharm. Sci. 60:1128–1133, 1971.
27. Lutz RJ, Dedrick RL, Straw JA, et al.: The kinetics of methotrexate distribution in spontaneous canine lymphosarcoma. J. Pharmacokinet. Biopharm. 3:77–97, 1975.
28. Yang KH, Fung WP, Lutz RJ, et al.: *In vivo* methotrexate transport in murine Lewis lung tumor. J. Pharm. Sci. 68:941–945, 1979.
29. Dedrick RL, Zaharko DS, and Lutz RJ: Transport and binding of methotrexate *in vivo*. J. Pharm. Sci. 62:882–890, 1973.
30. Dedrick RL, Myers CE, Bungay PM, et al.: Pharmacokinetic rationale for peritoneal drug administration in the treatment of ovarian cancer. Cancer Treat. Rep. 62:1–11, 1978.
31. Jacobs SA, Stoller RG, Chabner BA, et al.: Dose-dependent metabolism of methotrexate in man and rhesus monkeys. Cancer Treat. Rep. 61:651–656, 1977.
32. Lutz RJ, Galbraith WM, Dedrick RL, et al.: A model for the kinetics of distribution of actinomycin-D in the beagle dog. J. Pharmacol. Exp. Ther. 200:469–478, 1977.
33. Harris PA, and Gross JF: Preliminary pharmacokinetic model for Adriamycin (NSC-123127). Cancer Chemother. Rep. 59:819–825, 1975.
34. Chan KK, Cohen JL, Gross JF, et al.: Prediction of Adriamycin disposition in cancer patients using a physiologic, pharmacokinetic model. Cancer Treat. Rep. 62:1161–1171, 1978.
35. Himmelstein KJ, and Gross JF: Mathematical model for cyclocytidine pharmacokinetics. J. Pharm. Sci. 66:1441–1444, 1977.
36. Tterlikkis L, Ortega E, Solomon R, et al.: Pharmacokinetics of mercaptopurine. J. Pharm. Sci. 66:1454–1457, 1977.
37. LeRoy AF, Lutz RJ, Dedrick RL, et al.: Pharmacokinetic study of *cis*-dichlorodiammineplatinum (II) in the beagle dog: thermodynamic and kinetic behavior of DDP in biologic milieu. Cancer Treat. Rep. 63:59–71, 1979.
38. Fenstermacher JD, and Cowles AL: Theoretic limitations of intracarotid infusions in brain tumor chemotherapy. Cancer Treat. Rep. 61:519–526, 1977.
39. Eckman WW, Patlak CS and Fenstermacher JD: A critical evaluation of the principles governing the advantages of intra-arterial infusions. J. Pharmacokinet. Biopharm. 2:257–285, 1974.
40. Dedrick RL, Zaharko DS, Bender RA, et al.: Pharmacokinetic considerations on resistance to anticancer drugs. Cancer Chemother. Rep. 59:795–804, 1975.
41. Jones RB, Collins JM, Myers CE, et al.: High volume intraperitoneal chemotherapy with methotrexate in patients with cancer. Cancer Res. 41:55–59, 1981.

5 CLINICAL PHARMACOKINETICS AND DRUG MONITORING

Bruce A. Chabner

In Chapter 4 we examined the basic principles of pharmacokinetics and their application to the modeling of drug disposition in the experimental setting. Preclinical modeling has considerable value for the clinician in aiding the initial design of clinical trials. However, for important reasons to be discussed below, these studies are insufficient to provide a reliable basis for drug usage in man. The primary difficulty in extrapolation from preclinical to clinical settings is the variability of drug metabolism and elimination rates between species; in addition, there is well-established variability among patients in their handling of drugs, as compared with the relatively uniform handling of drugs by inbred strains of subprimate species.

Pharmacokinetic differences between man and experimental animals have been observed in the case of many anticancer drugs. For example, methotrexate (MTX) is rapidly converted to an inactive metabolite, 7-OH-MTX, in rabbits, but small quantities of this metabolite are formed in man.[1] Cytosine arabinoside (ara-C) is deaminated by cytidine deaminase. The concentration of this enzyme in various tissues varies greatly among preclinical species.[2] It is found in particularly high concentration in mouse kidney, human liver, and monkey plasma (Table 5–1). These differences make extrapolation between species an unreliable basis for treatment planning in man, and emphasize the need for clinical pharmacokinetic studies, which become the basis for the development of rational drug schedules.

Although very complete information can be obtained on blood and tissue levels of drugs in experimental animals, access to clinical samples is usually limited to the few biologic fluids that can be repetitively sampled. Thus, the extensive mathematical modeling and complex pharmacokinetics, which are feasible in experimental studies, are impossible to duplicate in patients. In general, clinical studies are confined to the sampling of blood, urine, cerebrospinal fluid, stool, bile, and third-space collections such as ascites. Occasionally, surgical biopsies performed following drug administration may provide single time-point measurements for solid tissues,[3-5] including tumor, but these latter samples rarely supply enough information to enable a kinetic profile of drug concentration to be constructed.

Not only does pharmacokinetic *variability between species* present problems for rational drug usage in man, but there also exists a marked *interindividual variability* in the handling of drugs. This variability results

TABLE 5–1. Cytidine Deaminase Activity in Tissues of Various Species

Species	Cytidine Deaminase Activity* LIVER	KIDNEY
Man	1180	210
Rhesus monkey	860	770
Rabbit	120	<50
Rat	<50	<50
Mouse	<50	800

*nmoles product per incubation. See Camiener and Smith[27] for details of assay.

both from genetic factors, such as the concentration of drug-metabolizing enzymes in the liver, and from physiologic factors arising from the effects of illness, previous drug treatment, and indeed the life history of the patient. More obvious factors are hepatic or renal dysfunction in patients receiving drugs that are eliminated by one of these routes. Any of these factors may lead to deviation from expected serum levels of drugs such as procainamide, phenytoin, digoxin, hydralazine, and many others.[6] Among the anticancer agents, variability in peak serum levels of hexamethylmelamine,[7] phenylalanine mustard,[8] 5-fluorouracil (5-FU),[9] and MTX[10] has been documented in studies of patients receiving medication by the oral route, implying variation in either gastrointestinal absorption or first-pass elimination of drug in the liver. Further variability has been demonstrated in the plasma half-life of ara-C,[11] 5-FU,[12] and MTX.[13] The importance of these findings is that they emphasize the fallacy of assuming uniform drug exposure for a patient population treated with a "standard dose" of drugs, as is the usual practice in clinical oncology. These studies further suggest that, in addition to the comprehensive type of pharmacokinetic study, there may be a role for *routine drug level monitoring* of drugs used in schedules known to provide variable drug levels.

DRUG CONCENTRATION: RELATIONSHIP TO DRUG EFFECT

Central to the role of drug monitoring is the assumption, still unproved for most antineoplastic drugs, that drug concentration in plasma bears a consistent relationship to pharmacologic effect. This thesis has been validated for many non-oncologic drugs, for which a "therapeutic range" has been defined, including the cardiac glycosides, theophylline, procainamide, and others. A therapeutic range has been more difficult to define for antineoplastic agents. Perhaps the best understood of these drugs is MTX; the serum concentrations required to inhibit DNA synthesis in gastrointestinal epithelium (5×10^{-9}M) and bone marrow (1×10^{-8}M) have been established in the mouse and partially verified in man.[14] This relationship is less well defined for tumor cells, which, on the basis of laboratory studies and clinical experience, are known to exhibit wide variation in their response to drugs. The relationship between drug levels and pharmacologic effects is poorly understood for drugs other than MTX. The primary source of information has come from tissue culture experiments, and more recently from the human tumor stem cell assay. These studies have indicated the threshold concentrations for kill of various tumor cell lines[15] (Table 5–2). This information has uncertain relevance to dose-response relationships in the clinic since nutritional, immunologic, cytokinetic, and other factors *in vivo* may alter susceptibility to drugs.

The relationship between drug concentration and cell killing involves a second dimension, the duration of exposure.[16] For example, brief exposure times lead to limited cell kill for antimetabolites such as MTX and ara-C, with progressively greater cytotoxicity as the period increases up to and beyond the cell cycle time. Thus, it is difficult to predict cytotoxicity on the basis of a single time-point drug concentration. This factor (duration of exposure) lends additional uncertainty to the effort to predict drug effect on the basis of measurement of drug levels.

MONITORING AND DOSE ADJUSTMENT

In many instances the clinical effects of a drug (e.g., myelosuppression or mucositis) or the lack thereof may serve as the basis for dose modification. For example, oncologists usually modify the dose of myelosuppressive drugs so that tolerable, but not life-threatening, depression of the white blood cell count and platelet count results. This type of dose modification is inexact because of the narrow therapeutic index (ratio of therapeutic to toxic dose) of anticancer drugs, and is fraught with danger in the case of dose escalation. Therefore, the usual increase in dosage called for by "sliding scales" is only a fraction of the protocol dose, and not enough to accommodate for major changes in pharmacokinetics. Second, because drugs with common patterns of toxicity are often used in combination, it may be impossible to use a toxicity end point in adjusting the dose of individual components of a regimen. A more rational approach would be to modify dose on the basis of pharmacokinetic measurements. However, because of the unavailability of suitable drug

TABLE 5–2. Minimal Inhibitory Concentrations for Selected Anticancer Drugs in Tissue Culture

Drug	Cell Type*	Inhibitory Concentration (μM) CD_{50}*	ID_{50}*	Duration of Exposure (hrs)	Ref.
Actinomycin D	CHO		0.002	3 days	41
	PCI		1	24 hrs	42
	EMT_6	0.01		1 hr	46
Bleomycin	T_1	10†		1 hr	40
	EMT_6	25		1 hr	46
BCNU	L1210	9		1 hr	33
	LoVo	100		1 hr	38
CCNU	L1210	9		1 hr	33
	T_1	15†		1 hr	40
MeCCNU	T_1	180†		1 hr	40
Cytosine arabinoside	L1210	1		6 hrs	31
	L1210	5		5 hrs	52
	HM-19-4	10		1 hr	51
	Mouse L cells	30		1 hr	53
Daunomycin	HeLa	0.02		21 hrs	45
Doxorubicin (Adriamycin)	CHO	1		1 hr	43
	T_1	0.2		1 hr	48
	EMT_6	0.01		1 hr	
	L1210	0.01		4 hrs	47
	HeLa	0.14		1 hr	44
5-Fluorouracil	Fibroblasts (human U cells)	1		At least 24 hours	32
	Wilms' tumor	1.5			
	HeLa	3			
Hydroxyurea	Sarcoma 180	5000		4 hrs	49
	HeLa	1000		24 hrs	50
Melphalan	L1210	0.8–1.5		0.4 hr	34
	Murine CFU-C	~0.5		0.25 hr	34
	T_1	3†		1 hr	39
Methotrexate	HCT-8	~0.1		24 hrs	28
	ZR-7	~0.04		48 hrs	29
	Mouse CFU-C	~0.01		continuous	30
	CHO	~0.2		24 hrs	36
	HeLa	~0.06		24 hrs	36
Mitomycin C	LoVo	0.075		24 hrs	37
		2.7		1 hr	37
	EMT_6	1		1 hr	46
cis-Platinum	LoVo	~20		1 hr	35
	T_1	17†		1 hr	40
6-Thioguanine	HeLa	4		21 hrs	45
Vinblastine	CEM	0.1		24 hrs	55
Vincristine	Murine leukemia	0.01		6 hrs	54
	EMT_6	1		1 hr	46
VP-16	T_1	30†			40

*Cell lines: CEM — human lymphoblastic leukemia; CHO — Chinese hamster ovary; EMT_6 — mouse mammary tumor; HeLa — human cervical carcinoma; HCT-8 — human colon carcinoma; HM-19-4 — human malignant melanoma; LoVo — human colon adenocarcinoma; PCI — human lung adenocarcinoma; T_1 — human lymphoma; ZR-7 — human breast adenocarcinoma. CD_{50} — concentration producing 50% inhibition of number of colonies in clonal assay; ID_{50} — concentration producing 50% inhibition of cell growth.

†D_0 or concentration producing 63 per cent cell kill.

assay procedures, the more desirable approach (i.e., dose modification based on drug level monitoring) is used only occasionally in cancer treatment. Again, the best example is the modification of MTX dosage in accordance with drug clearance, as calculated from a test dose.[13] In one exemplary study, drug clearance rates varied from 40 to 400 ml per hour. Adjustment of drug infusion rates to accommodate these differences in clearance yielded very close approximation of the desired plasma concentration.

An additional important use for pharmacokinetics in treatment planning is the value of drug studies for dosage modification in patients with potentially altered drug distribution, metabolism, or renal elimination. Since the therapeutic index of cancer drugs is very narrow — the margin between successful tumor therapy and serious or life-threatening toxicity is slight — the clinician is obliged to alter dosage if abnormal renal function is present in patients being treated with MTX, bleomycin, or hydroxyurea. Similarly, abnormal hepatic function signals the need for a change in doxorubicin or vinca alkaloid usage. In each case, pharmacokinetic analysis of drug disappearance from plasma could play an important role in dose adjustment. Only in the case of MTX[13] is such information available. For the remainder, crude guidelines have been based on the correlation between organ function tests (such as creatinine clearance or serum bilirubin) and the toxicity of full drug doses.

PREDICTION OF TOXICITY BY DRUG LEVEL MONITORING

Routine drug level monitoring may also be useful in predicting (and preventing) drug toxicity, but is possible only in selected clinical situations and with specific agents. The requirements for a successful monitoring program are outlined in Table 5–3. Assuming the availability of suitable assay methods, the primary obstacle to useful monitoring is the identification of an appropriate time point after drug administration for collection of the clinical sample. This time point may be chosen after comparison of the drug disappearance curve from plasma (or other body fluids) of patients showing the desired pharmacologic response (tolerable toxicity and therapeutic effect), as opposed to patients exhibiting signs of inappropriate dosage (intolerable toxicity or lack of therapeutic effect). If the curves of the two patient groups demonstrate clear segregation with respect to drug levels or plasma half-lives, as in Figure 5–1*A*,[17, 18] an appropriate time point can be chosen that will allow the clinician to detect under- or overdosage in comparison with the desired level.

TABLE 5–3. Components of Drug Level Monitoring

A. Rapid, Sensitive, and Specific Assay Procedure
1. Competitive ligand assay (radioimmunoassay or competitive protein-binding assay)
2. Enzyme-linked immunoassay

B. Defined Relationship Between Drug Concentration and Drug Effect
1. An appropriate time point for monitoring
2. A clear segregation of therapeutic or toxic properties based on drug levels

C. Clinical Decision Possible Based on Drug Level Measurement
1. Modification of dosage or schedule
2. Institution of "rescue" procedures

This monitoring point is usually chosen at a point in the plasma disappearance curve that reflects steady-state drug levels: e.g., several hours into a constant infusion regimen, or during the less steep portion of the drug disappearance curve for drugs administered as a bolus dose. A steady state is achieved during constant drug infusion only after multiple (at least three) half-lives of drug disappearance have elapsed. For drugs given orally, a steady-state concentration may not be achieved for several days, depending again on the drug half-life and the frequency of administration. After bolus intravenous administration, a monitoring point well into the elimination phase should be chosen, since early points (in the first few minutes) may reflect distribution rather than elimination (the primary determinant of under- or overdosing in intravenous therapeutics). Measurement of multiple sequential time points, while increasing the assay load, allows a more accurate calculation of drug disappearance rate,[19] but is unnecessary for most clinical monitoring purposes. Thus, for MTX, the usual monitoring point is 24 or 48 hours after drug administration, a time that is well into the second phase of drug elimination.[19] The choice of monitoring point may also be influenced by the need to institute protective or preventive measures, such as administration of an antidote, within a certain period after drug administration. Thus, in MTX regimen monitoring, drug levels are obtained within 48 hours of administration in order to allow an increase in leucovorin dosage before irreparable damage is done to bone marrow or gastrointestinal epithelium. Extensive damage is incurred if high drug concentrations are allowed to persist unopposed by leucovorin for longer than 48 hours.

The final requirement for a successful drug monitoring effort is the capacity to utilize the drug level result in a beneficial way. Based on the drug level determination, the clinical pharmacologist must be able to suggest changes in dosage or clinical care that will result in greater efficacy or decreased toxicity. The value of clinical drug level monitoring is best illustrated by its use in MTX chemotherapy.[17-19] "Preventive monitoring" is commonly used to detect *delayed* drug excretion and to predict a high risk of serious bone marrow toxicity in patients receiving high-dose MTX (greater than 1.5 gm/m²) in six- to 42-hour infusions. Drug concentration in plasma 24 or 48 hours after the beginning of the infusion can be measured by any one of several rapid and relatively specific assays — radioimmunoassay and competitive protein-binding assay — and can be compared with the drug levels in a patient population that did not develop toxicity. The results of one such study (Fig. 5–1*B*) illustrate the excellent correlation between drug concentration and the risk of toxicity. Thus, it is possible to predict which patients are at high risk of developing myelosuppression on the basis of a 48-hour timepoint measurement. In patients receiving the Jaffe regimen (50 to 250 mg/kg for six hours) (Fig. 5–1*B*), drug concentrations greater than 9×10^{-7}M are usually associated with toxicity, but these complications can be prevented in most cases by increasing the dose and duration of administration of the antidote, leucovorin. The rationale and design of high-dose MTX regimens are considered in greater detail in Chapter 10.

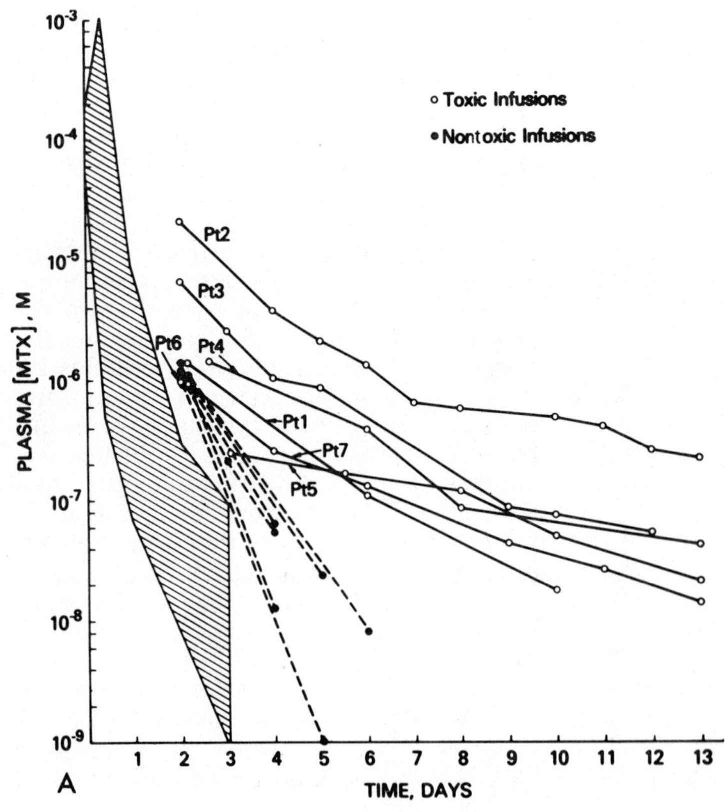

Figure 5–1. *A,* Methotrexate plasma disappearance curves in patients receiving six-hour infusions of 50 to 250 mg/kg, followed by leucovorin rescue, 15 mg/m² every six hours for seven doses. Curves for toxic patients are shown by solid lines; those for patients with elevated levels who received increased leucovorin and experienced no toxicity are depicted by dashed lines; and plasma levels of nontoxic patients are shown by the hatched area.

Illustration continued on opposite page

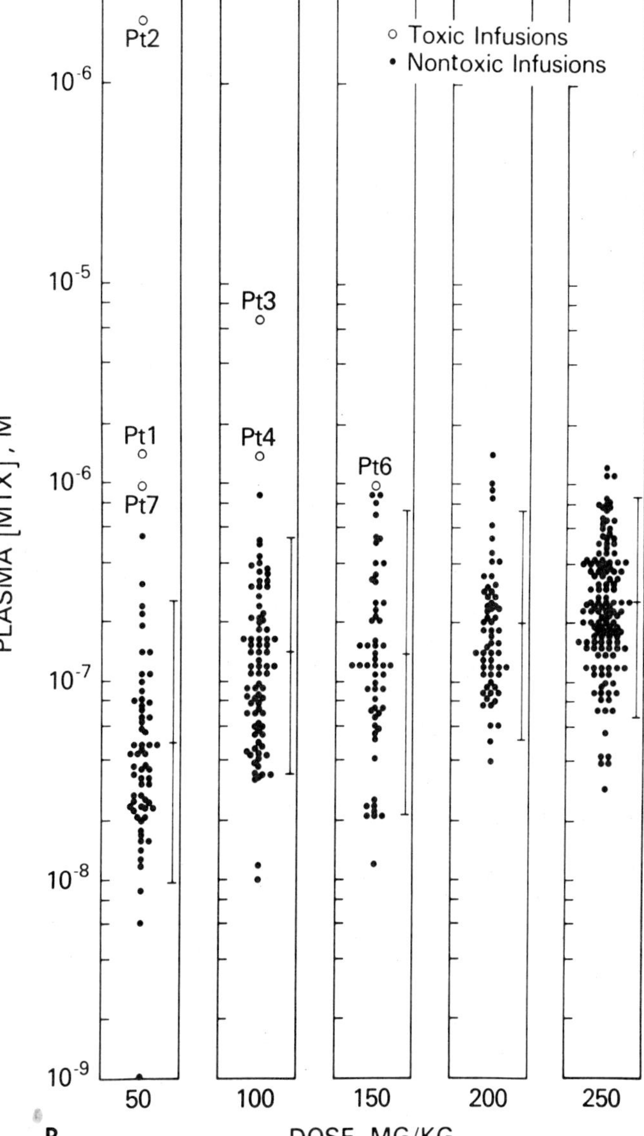

Figure 5–1 *Continued B,* Concentration of methotrexate in plasma 48 hours after MTX infusion. Levels for toxic patients (indicated by patient number) are all 9×10^{-7}M or greater, and correspond to the 48-hour point from the curves in *A.* (Reproduced with permission from Stoller et al.: Use of plasma pharmacokinetics to predict and prevent methotrexate toxicity. N. Engl. J. Med. 297:630–634, 1977.)

MONITORING OF DRUG LEVELS IN CSF

The measurement of MTX concentrations in the cerebrospinal fluid (CSF) serves as an example of the value of pharmacokinetic monitoring to allow dose adjustment, selection of route, and prediction of toxicity, particularly in the treatment of leukemic meningitis.[20-22] CSF pharmacokinetic studies have been helpful in the following respects:

1. Distinguishing drug-induced neurotoxicity from progression of leukemic meningitis.[20] The former is associated with delayed drug clearance from the CSF and with abnormally elevated CSF MTX levels.

2. Detection of underdosage of patients receiving intrathecal MTX.[22] Again, CSF drug monitoring can detect patients with low drug levels who, as a consequence, are at increased risk of developing leukemic meningitis.

3. Design of systemic high-dose infusion regimens that provide cytotoxic MTX concentrations in the CSF.[23] In an attempt to circumvent the combined use of intrathecal MTX and cranial irradiation, a combination associated with delayed neurotoxicity, many

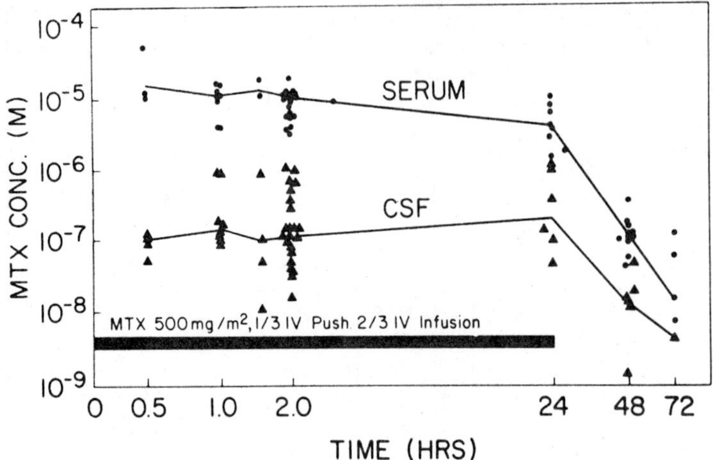

Figure 5–2. Gradient of methotrexate from plasma to cerebrospinal fluid during constant intravenous infusion. (Reproduced with permission from Freeman AI, Wang JJ, and Sinks LF: High-dose methotrexate in acute lymphocytic leukemia. Cancer Treat. Rep. 61:727–731, 1977.)

investigators are investigating the possibility of using high-dose systemic MTX. These new regimens are designed to provide cytotoxic drug levels in the CSF, and depend on CSF drug level monitoring for validation. Typically, a 1:30 gradient in drug concentration exists between CSF and plasma (Fig. 5–2). Thus, extremely high systemic drug concentrations are required to provide minimal cytotoxic CSF levels. The specific concentration needed to prevent leukemic meningeal relapse in the CSF is not known, but most investigators aim for at least 1 μM MTX in the CSF.

Routine pharmacokinetic monitoring has not played an important role in the clinical use of any other antineoplastic drug, with the possible exception of intraperitoneal 5-FU.[24] The reasons for this lack of utilization of routine monitoring are the converse of those outlined in Table 5–3: i.e., a lack of suitable assay techniques, the absence of a clear relationship between drug concentration and specific drug effects, and the lack of measures for preventing toxicity if delayed elimination is detected. Nonetheless, the potential of routine monitoring for contributing to the rational design of cancer treatment has been amply demonstrated by these MTX studies.

DRUG INTERACTIONS AND PHARMACOKINETICS

In addition to its value in allowing compensations for interindividual variations in pharmacokinetics, drug level monitoring may be helpful in clarifying the interaction of drugs used in combination. Most effective regimens employ combinations of antineoplastic drugs that may produce synergistic or, inadvertently, antagonistic actions (see Table 1–5). Although most of these interactions occur at the biochemical level of drug action, some result from pharmacokinetic effects. For example, thymidine administered prior to 5-FU blocks the reduction of the pyrimidine ring of 5-FU, greatly extending the 5-FU half-life from 10 to 90 minutes[24a] in some combination regimens. Probenicid blocks the tubular secretion of MTX and extends the plasma half-life of the antifolate.[25] These are only a few examples of the interactions that are described in detail in subsequent chapters, and which illustrate the utility of pharmacokinetic studies of drug interactions.

Microsomal activation is required for a number of anticancer drugs, including cyclophosphamide, dimethyltriazinoimidazole carboxamide, procarbazine, and hexamethylmelamine. Microsomal oxidative reactions are known to be subject to induction by substrates or broad classes of compounds such as anticoagulants, tranquilizers, and hormones. However, because of the major difficulties in measuring the active intermediates of the antineoplastic agents, there exists very little information regarding the potentially important interactions mediated by microsomal inducers.

Similarly important information may be obtained from studies of drug interactions in the competition for binding to plasma proteins. Aspirin displaces MTX from binding to albumin;[26] it has not been proved that this interaction affects MTX toxicity. Drugs that cause renal toxicity, such as *cis*-dichlorodiammineplatinum, must be used cautiously in patients who are being treated with agents requiring elimination by the kidney, such as MTX, bleomycin, or hydroxyurea. Thus, drug interactions may occur at multiple stages in the absorption, distribution, metabolism, and excretion of these compounds; pharmacokinetic analysis can provide an important insight into these effects and can prevent serious toxicity or ineffective therapy.

In summary, the discipline of pharmacokinetics is essential to the rational treatment of cancer with drugs. The range of applications of this specialty, encompassing comprehensive pharmacokinetic studies, drug level monitoring, and the analysis of drug interactions, is constantly expanding. In the clinical as well as the laboratory sphere, a thorough understanding of pharmacokinetics is indispensable to valid chemotherapy investigations, but then dividends of this analysis are only beginning to be appreciated.

References

1. Stewart DJ, Leavens M, Friedman J, et al: Penetration of N-(phosphonacetyl)-L-aspartate in human central nervous system and intracerebral tumor. Cancer Res. 40:3163–3166, 1980.
2. Chabner BA, Stoller RG, Hande KR, et al.: Methotrexate disposition in humans: case studies in ovarian cancer and following high-dose infusion. Drug Metab. Rev. 8:107–117, 1978.
3. Fraile RJ, Baker LH, Buroker TR, et al.: Pharmacokinetics of 5-fluorouracil administered orally by rapid intravenous and by slow infusion. Cancer Res. 40:2223–2228, 1980.
4. Goldman ID: A model system for the study of heteroexchange diffusion: methotrexate-folate interactions in L1210 leukemia and Ehrlich ascites tumor cells. Biochim. Biophys. Acta 233:624–634, 1971.
5. Camiener GW, and Smith CG: Studies of the enzymatic deamination of cytosine arabinoside. I. Enzyme distribution and species specificity. Biochem. Pharmacol. 14:1405, 1965.
6. Koch-Weser J: Serum concentrations of drugs as guides to pharmacotherapy. *In* Merkus FWHM (ed.): The Serum Concentration of Drugs: Clinical Relevance, Therapy, and Practice. Elsevier, Amsterdam, 1979, pp. 3–17.
7. D'Incalci M, Bolis G, Mangioni C, et al.: Variable absorption of hexamethylmelamine in man. Cancer Treat. Rep. 62:2117–2119, 1978.
8. Tattersall MHN, Jarman M, Newlands ES, et al.: Pharmacokinetics of melphalan following oral or intravenous administration in patients with malignant disease. Eur. J. Cancer 14:507–513, 1978.
9. Cohen JL, Irwin LW, Marshall OJ, et al.: Clinical pharmacology of oral and intravenous 5-fluorouracil (NSC-19893). Cancer Chemother. Rep. 58:723–731, 1974.
10. Steele WH, Stuart JFB, Lawrence JR, et al.: Enahancement of methotrexate absorption by subdivision of dose. Cancer Chemother. Pharmacol. 3:235–237, 1979.
11. van Proojien R, van der Kleijn R, and Haanen C: Pharmacokinetics of cytosine arabinoside in acute myeloid leukemia. Clin. Pharmacol. Ther. 21:744–750, 1977.
12. MacMillan WE, Wolberg WH, and Welling PG: Pharmacokinetics of fluorouracil in humans. Cancer Res. 38:3479–3482, 1978.
13. Monjanel S, Rigault JP, Cano JP, et al.: High-dose methotrexate: preliminary evaluation of a pharmacokinetic approach. Cancer Chemother. Pharmacol. 3:189–196, 1979.
14. Chabner BA, and Young RC: Threshold methotrexate concentration for *in vivo* inhibition of DNA synthesis in normal and tumorous target tissues. J. Clin. Invest. 52:1804–1811, 1973.
15. Alberts DS: Tabular summary of pharmacokinetic parameters relevant to *in vitro* drug assay. Prog. Clin. Biol. Res. 48:351–359, 1980.
16. Pinedo HM, Zaharko DS, Bull JM, et al.: The relative contribution of drug concentration and duration of exposure to mouse bone marrow toxicity during continuous methotrexate infusion. Cancer Res. 37:445–450, 1977.
17. Stoller RG, Hande KR, Jacobs SA, et al.: Use of plasma pharmacokinetics to predict and prevent methotrexate toxicity. N. Engl. J. Med. 297:630–634, 1977.
18. Nirenberg A, Mosende C, Mehte B, et al.: High-dose methotrexate with citrovorum factor rescue: predictive value of serum methotrexate concentrations and corrective measures to avert toxicity. Cancer Treat. Rep. 61:779–783, 1977.
19. Isacoff WH, Morrison PF, Aroesty J, et al.: Pharmacokinetics of high-dose methotrexate with citrovorum rescue. Cancer Treat. Rep. 61:1665–1674, 1977.
20. Bleyer WA, Drake JC, and Chabner BA: Neurotoxicity and elevated cerebrospinal fluid methotrexate concentration in meningeal leukemia. N. Engl. J. Med. 298:770–773, 1973.
21. Bleyer WA, Poplack DG, and Simon RM: "Concentration × time" methotrexate via a subcutaneous reservoir: a less toxic regimen for intraventricular chemotherapy of central nervous system neoplasms. Blood 51:835–842, 1978.
22. Bleyer WA: The clinical pharmacology of methotrexate. Cancer 41:36–51, 1978.
23. Shapiro WR, Young DG, and Mehta BM: Methotrexate distribution in cerebrospinal fluid after intravenous, ventricular, and lumbar injections. N. Engl. J. Med. 293:161–166, 1975.
24. Speyer JL, Collins JM, Dedrick RL, et al.: Phase I and pharmacological studies of intraperitoneal 5-fluorouracil. Cancer Res. 40:567–572, 1980.

24a. Woodcock TM, Martin DS, Damin LEM, et al.: Clinical trials with thymidine and fluorouracil: a phase I and clinical pharmacologic evaluation. Cancer 45:1135–1143, 1980.

25. Aherne GW, Prall E, Marks V, et al.: Prolongation and enhancement of serum methotrexate concentrations by probenecid. Br. Med. J. 1:1097–1099, 1978.
26. Liegler DG, Henderson ES, Hahn MA, et al.: The effect of organic acids on renal clearance of methotrexate in man. Clin. Pharmacol. Ther. 10:849–857, 1969.
27. Camiener GW, and Smith CG: Studies of the enzymatic deamination of cytosine arabinoside. I. Enzyme distribution and species specificity. Biochem. Pharmacol. 14:1405–1416, 1965.
28. Cadman E: Modulation of 5-fluorouracil metabolism and cytoxicity by antimetabolite pretreatment in human colorectal adenocarcinoma HCT-8. Cancer Res. 41:994–999, 1981.
29. Donehower RC, Allegra JC, Lippman ME, et al: Combined effects of methotrexate and 5-fluoropyrimidine on human breast cancer cells in serum-free culture. Eur. J. Cancer 16:655–661, 1980.
30. Pinedo HM, Zaharko DS, Bull JM, et al.: The reversal of methotrexate cytotoxicity to mouse bone marrow cells by leucovorin and nucleosides. Cancer Res. 36:4418–4424, 1976.
31. Kufe DW, Major PP, Egan EM, et al.: Correlation of cytotoxicity with incorporation of ara-C into DNA. J. Biol. Chem. 255:8997–9000, 1980.
32. Laskin JD, Evans RM, Slocum HK, et al.: Basis for natural variation in sensitivity to 5-fluorouracil in mouse and human cells in culture. Cancer Res. 39:383–390, 1979.

33. Kann HE Jr: Comparison of biochemical and biological effects of four nitrosoureas with differing carbamoylating activities. Cancer Res. 38:2363–2366, 1978.
34. Vistica DT, Rabon A, and Rabinovitz M: Amino acid conferred protection against melphalan: comparison of amino acids which reduce melphalan toxicity to murine bone marrow precursor cells (CFU-C) and murine L1210 leukemia cells. Res. Commun. Chem. Pathol. Pharmacol. 23:171–183, 1979.
35. Bergerat JP, Drewinko B, Corry P, et al.: Synergistic lethal effect of *cis*-dichlorodiammineplatinum and 1-beta-D-arabinofuranosylcytosine. Cancer Res. 41:25–30, 1981.
36. Eichholtz CH, and Trott KR: Effect of methotrexate concentration and exposure time on mammalian cell survival *in vitro*. Br. J. Cancer 41:277–284, 1980.
37. Barlogie B, and Drewinko B: Lethal and cytokinetic effects of mitomycin C on cultured human colon cancer cells. Cancer Res. 40:1973–1980, 1980.
38. Drewinko B, Barlogie B, and Freireich EJ: Response of exponentially growing, stationary-phase, and synchronized cultured human colon carcinoma cells to treatment with nitrosourea derivatives. Cancer Res. 39:2630–2636, 1979.
39. Barlogie B, and Drewinko B: Lethal and kinetic response of cultured human lymphoid cells to melphalan. Cancer Treat. Rep. 61:425–436, 1977.
40. Drewinko B, Roper P, and Barlogie B: Patterns of cell survival following treatment with antitumour agents *in vitro*. Eur. J. Cancer 15:93–99, 1979.
41. Biedler JL, and Hansjong R: Cellular resistance to actinomycin D in Chinese hamster cells *in vitro*: cross-resistance, radioautographic, and cytogenic studies. Cancer Res. 30:1174–1184, 1970.
42. Tsukeda H, Satoshi M, and Hitta K: Susceptibilities of normal and malignant human lung cells in culture to the cytocidal action of antitumor agents. Cancer Res. 38:2529–2532, 1978.
43. Barranco SC, and Novak JK: Survival responses of dividing and nondividing mammalian cells after treatment with hydroxyurea, arabinosylcytosine, or Adriamycin. Cancer Res. 34:1616–1618, 1974.
44. Kim SH, and Kim JH: Lethal effect of Adriamycin on the division cycle of HeLa cells. Cancer Res. 32:323–325, 1972.
45. Fried J, Perez AG, Doblin JM, et al.: Cytotoxic and cytokinetic effects of 1-beta-D-arabinofuranosylcytosine, daunorubicin, and 6-thioguanine on HeLa cells in culture. Cancer Res. 41:1127–1132, 1981.
46. Teicher BA, Lazo JS, and Sartorelli AC: Classification of antineoplastic agents by their selective toxicities toward oxygenated and hypoxic tumor cells. Cancer Res. 41:73–81, 1981.
47. Wilkott LJ, Dulmadge EA, and Lloyd HH: Effect of Adriamycin on the reproductive integrity of cultured leukemia L1210 and P388 cells. J. Natl. Cancer Inst. 60:1117–1120, 1978.
48. Roper PR, and Drewinko B: Comparison of *in vitro* methods to determine drug-induced cell lethality. Cancer Res. 36:2182–2188, 1976.
49. Ford SS, and Shackney SE: Lethal and sublethal effects of hydroxyurea in relation to drug concentration and duration of drug exposure in sarcoma 180 *in vitro*. Cancer Res. 37:2628–2637, 1977.
50. Kim JH, Gelbard AS, and Perez AG: Action of hydroxyurea on the nucleic acid metabolism and viability of HeLa cells. Cancer Res. 27:1301–1305, 1967.
51. Barranco SC, Ho DH, Drewinko B, et al.: Differential sensitivities of human melanoma cells grown *in vitro* to arabinosylcytosine. Cancer Res. 32:2733–2736, 1972.
52. Grant S, Lehman C, and Cadman E: Enhancement of 1-beta-D-arabinofuranosylcytosine accumulation within L1210 cells and increased cytotoxicity following thymidine exposure. Cancer Res. 40:1525–1531, 1980.
53. Graham FL, and Whitmore GF: The effects of 1-beta-D-arabinofuranosylcytosine on growth viability and DNA synthesis of mouse L-cells. Cancer Res. 30:2627–2635, 1970.
54. Jackson DV Jr, and Bender RA: Cytotoxic thresholds of vincristine in a murine and a human leukemia cell line *in vitro*. Cancer Res. 39:4346–4349, 1979.
55. Kishan A, and Frei E III: Morphological basis for the cytolytic effect of vinblastine and vincristine on cultured human leukemic lymphoblasts. Cancer Res. 35:497–501, 1975.

LATE COMPLICATIONS OF CHEMOTHERAPY: INFERTILITY AND CARCINOGENESIS

6

Richard L. Schilsky

Charles Erlichman

Cytotoxic chemotherapy has produced sustained clinical remissions and cures for many patients with Hodgkin's disease,[1] acute lymphoblastic leukemia,[2] choriocarcinoma,[3] testicular carcinoma,[4] and other malignant and nonmalignant disorders. As detailed in subsequent chapters, most of the commonly used antineoplastic drugs produce immediate toxicities in organs composed of self-renewing cell populations such as bone marrow, skin, and gastrointestinal tract epithelium. Pancytopenia, stomatitis, alopecia, and nausea and vomiting occur frequently, but generally are not prolonged or irreversible once chemotherapy is completed. Antitumor agents are associated with more delayed toxic effects, such as the cardiomyopathy of doxorubicin (Adriamycin) or the pulmonary fibrosis associated with bleomycin, which may become clinically apparent even after chemotherapy is completed. However, as patients continue to survive longer following chemotherapy, previously unrecognized toxic effects are becoming manifest. Most important among these late effects are infertility and carcinogenesis, which assume particular concern for successfully treated patients hoping to return to a normal life style. This chapter will consider these late effects of cancer chemotherapy.

GONADAL DYSFUNCTION FOLLOWING CANCER CHEMOTHERAPY

The effects of antitumor chemotherapy on testicular and ovarian function have been largely ignored until recently. This lack of attention has stemmed in part from the absence of acute or life-threatening symptomatology consequent upon gonadal injury, and in part from the rarity of chemotherapy- or radiotherapy-treated long-term cancer survivors who are now concerned about their reproductive potential. Many drugs used in the treatment of cancer have profound and often lasting effects on the testis and the ovary. Both germ cell production and endocrine function may be altered. These effects are generally related to the age, pubertal status, and menstrual status of the patient as well as to the particular drug class, dosage, or combination administered.

Chemotherapy Effects in Men

The adult testis functions as both an exocrine and an endocrine gland producing spermatozoa and testosterone. Spermatogenesis proceeds in the seminiferous tubules, which constitute over 75 per cent of the mass of the testis, while the interstitial cells of Leydig carry on the endocrine functions of the gland. The remainder of the testis consists of supporting and vascular tissues necessary for the protection and nourishment of the developing spermatozoa.

The seminiferous tubules are lined by stratified epithelium composed of two cell types: spermatogenic cells and Sertoli cells. The spermatogenic cells are arranged in an orderly fashion; spermatogonia lie directly on the basement membrane, while primary and secondary spermatocytes, spermatids, and maturing spermatozoa progress centrally toward the tubular lumen (Fig. 6–1). Sertoli cells also lie on the basement membrane. These specialized cells help to maintain the blood-testis barrier and to regulate the release of mature spermatozoa from the germinal epithelium.[5]

In any area of the seminiferous tubule, five to six generations of germ cells can be identified. These generations are not randomly distributed but occur in fixed cell associations. Thus, spermatids at a particular stage in their development are always associated with the same types of spermatocytes and spermatogonia. Six typical cell associations have been described in the human testis that synchronously evolve in the process of sperm maturation. A complete series of cell associations constitutes a cycle of the germinal epithelium, and each cell association may be considered a stage of the cycle. The entire process of spermatogenesis proceeds continuously throughout the tubule, and it has been estimated that 64 to 90 days elapse from spermatogonial stem cell mitosis to release of mature spermatozoa from the seminiferous epithelium.[6]

Spermatogenesis is a dynamic and complex process divided into three phases: (1) proliferation of spermatogonia to produce spermatocytes and to renew the germ cell pool; (2) meiotic division of spermatocytes to reduce the chromosome number in the germ cells by half; and (3) maturation of the

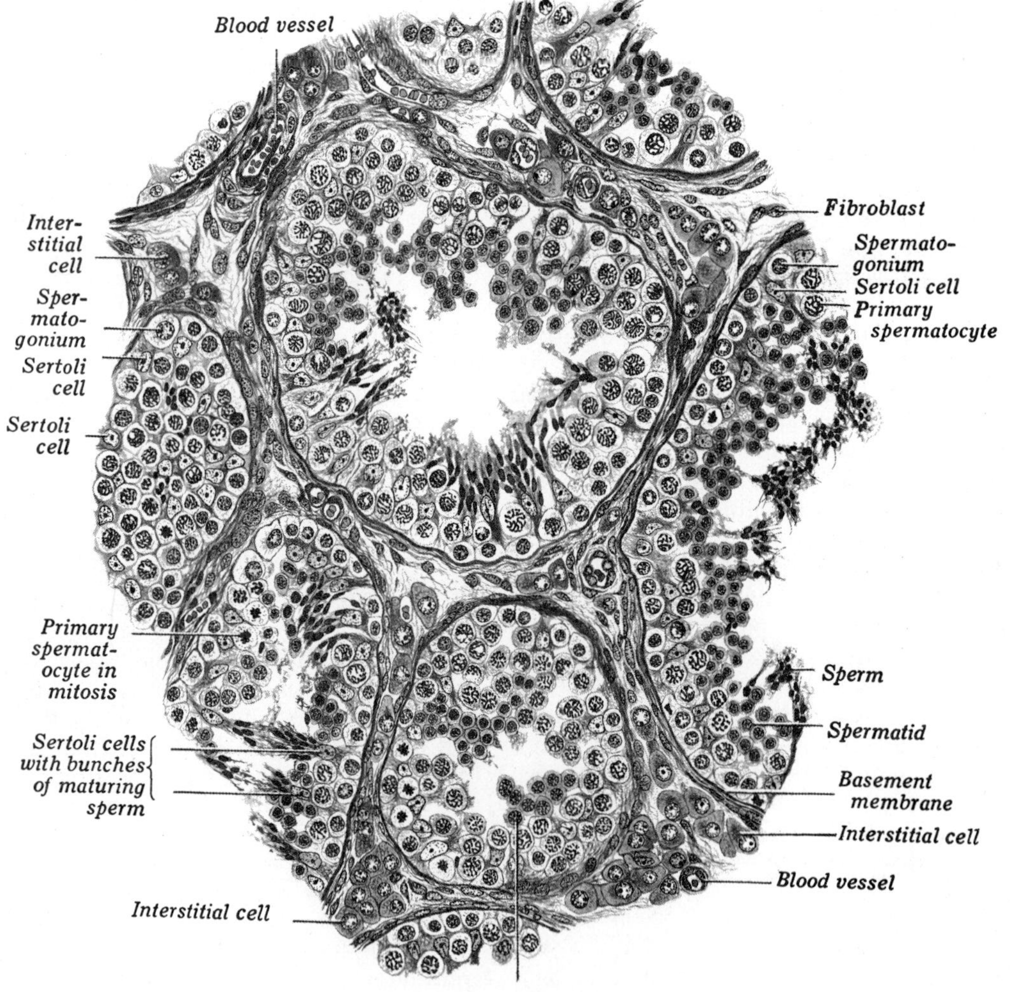

Figure 6–1. Section of normal human testis showing the various stages of spermatogenesis within the seminiferous tubule. ×170. (Reproduced with permission from Bloom W, and Fawcett DW: A Textbook of Histology. W. B. Saunders Co., Philadelphia, 1975.)

spermatids to become spermatozoa.[7] Cytotoxic agents could affect this process in a number of ways: (1) a specific cell type within the germinal epithelium might be selectively damaged or destroyed; (2) the proliferative and meiotic phases of spermatogenesis might proceed normally, but sperm maturation might be abnormal, leading to functionally incompetent mature spermatozoa; or (3) chemotherapy might damage Sertoli cells, Leydig cells, or other supportive or nutritive constituents of the testis in such a way as to alter the particular microenvironment necessary for normal germ cell production. Alterations of the kinetics of spermatogenesis are not thought to occur following cytotoxic therapy.

With knowledge of the normal histology of the germinal epithelium and of the kinetics of spermatogenesis, it is possible to estimate the specific site of a drug's effect either by examining the testis microscopically, or by performing sperm counts or mating studies at some interval after administration of the drug. The morphology of the spermatids can be used to define the stage of the germinal epithelial cycle at the time of biopsy, and the presence or absence of cells supposed to be found at that stage can be noted. Known kinetic parameters can then be used to determine precisely which spermatogenic cell was destroyed by drug administration. For example, examination of mouse testes 11 days following doxorubicin administration reveals an absence of pachytene primary spermatocytes, indicating that type A2 (primitive) spermatogonia are most sensitive to injury by this drug.[8]

Serial mating studies, whereby animals are mated at varying intervals after drug administration, and the onset of infertility is noted, can provide similar, though less precise, information. In the rat, an infertile mating occurring six to seven weeks after drug treatment implies that spermatocytes were primarily affected by the drug in question, whereas infertility occurring ten weeks after drug treatment reflects spermatogonial destruction.[9, 10] As long as the dynamics of the germinal epithelium of the species under study have been delineated, some insight into the effects of cytotoxic agents on spermatogenesis can be obtained. Table 6–1 summarizes the results of these types of investigations for several commonly used antineoplastic agents.

TABLE 6–1. Site of Toxicity of Antitumor Agents in the Germinal Epithelium

Drug	*Cell Type Affected*	*Reference*
Busulfan	Type A spermatogonia	9, 10
Cyclophosphamide	Late spermatogonia and spermatocytes	8
Doxorubicin (Adriamycin)	Primitive spermatogonia	8
Bleomycin	Intermediate spermatogonia	8
Cytosine arabinoside	Late spermatogonia spermatocytes	8

Clearly, such studies cannot be done in man and one must rely primarily on reproductive history, clinical examination, and specific laboratory tests in the evaluation of testicular function. Table 6–2 provides a summary of this type of evaluation. There appear to be common pathophysiologic changes that occur in the testis, independent of the type of drug administered but related to the total dose employed.

The primary testicular lesion caused by all antitumor agents studied thus far is depletion of the germinal epithelium lining the seminiferous tubules.[11-14] Testicular biopsy in most patients reveals complete germinal aplasia with only Sertoli cells left lining the tubular lumen. Occasionally, scattered spermatogonia, spermatocytes, or spermatids may be seen. The tubules appear atrophic and peritubular fibrosis is sometimes seen, although the interstitial cells of Leydig remain normal in appearance.

Clinically, there is a marked decrease in testicular volume noted on physical examination, severe oligospermia or azoospermia, and infertility.[15, 16] Depletion of the germinal epithelium is accompanied by a marked increase in serum follicle-stimulating hor-

TABLE 6–2. Evaluation of the Patient with Suspected Germinal Aplasia*

	Normal	*Germinal Aplasia*
Testicular size (ml)	20–30	8–15
FSH (mIU/ml)	4–25	25–90
LH (mIU/ml)	4–18	8–25
Testosterone (ng/dl)	250–1200	200–700
Sperm count (10^6/ml)	>20	0

*Adapted from Sherins RJ, and Howards SS: Male infertility. *In* Harrison JH (ed.): Campbell's Urology, 4th ed. W. B. Saunders Co., Philadelphia, 1978, pp. 715–776.

mone (FSH) levels.[17] This finding suggests that the seminiferous tubule may be the site of production of a feedback inhibitor of gonadotropin secretion. Thus, elevation of serum FSH may serve as a marker of testicular germinal aplasia.

Abnormalities of serum testosterone or changes in secondary sexual characteristics following chemotherapy have not been noted. However, subtle abnormalities of Leydig cell function may be present. Administration of luteinizing hormone (LH) releasing hormone to men following combination chemotherapy for Hodgkin's disease produces excessively high serum LH and FSH levels consistent with compensated Leydig cell failure.[18-20] This abnormality has not been correlated with any specific clinical changes in sexual function.

Among the anticancer drugs, alkylating agents have been clearly related to the development of infertility. In particular, chlorambucil and cyclophosphamide (Cytoxan) deplete the testicular germinal epithelium in a dose-related fashion. Progressive oligospermia occurs in men with lymphoma who are treated with up to 400 mg of chlorambucil.[13] Those patients receiving cumulative doses in excess of 400 mg are uniformly azoospermic. Similarly, decreased sperm counts may be noted in men treated with 50 to 100 mg of cyclophosphamide daily for courses as brief as two months, although azoospermia and germinal aplasia are infrequent until 6 to 10 gm of the drug has been administered.[11] These data suggest the presence of a threshold dose for the development of testicular germinal aplasia for each particular drug. However, prospective studies of testicular function in large numbers of men receiving a variety of antitumor agents will be necessary to provide more reliable information concerning the threshold drug dose above which severe or irreversible testicular injury occurs.

As might be expected, combination chemotherapy regimens that include alkylating agents have profound effects on spermatogenesis. Sherins and DeVita reported the effects of combination chemotherapy on the fertility of 16 men with lymphoma in complete remission two months to seven years following MOPP (nitrogen mustard, vincristine [Oncovin], procarbazine, prednisone), CVP (cyclophosphamide, vincristine, prednisone) or cyclophosphamide alone.[21] Testicular biopsy in 15 patients revealed germinal aplasia in ten, scattered spermatogonia with arrest of spermatogenesis in two, and normal spermatogenesis in three (Fig. 6–2). All but the three patients with normal biopsies had azoospermia or severe oligospermia on semen analysis. Those patients with normal ejaculates and biopsies, two of whom received MOPP and one CVP, had been off therapy for two to seven years. Subsequent studies have confirmed that at least 80 per cent of men treated with MOPP combination chemotherapy become azoospermic or severely oligospermic.[22, 23] Chapman et al.[23] found that all 74 males receiving cyclical combination chemotherapy for Hodgkin's disease were azoospermic after treatment, and only four of 74 recovered spermatogenesis after a median follow-up of 27 months. A decline in libido and decreased sexual activity also occurred during therapy, and only partially recovered after treatment. It is noteworthy that 43 per cent of males with advanced Hodgkin's disease are azoospermic *prior* to initiation of treatment, complicating the interpretation of post-treatment status.[23a]

With the completion of chemotherapy, the recovery of spermatogenesis is unpredictable for the individual patient but is likely related to the total dose of drug administered, the type of drug, and the duration of time off therapy. Complete recovery of spermatogenesis has been reported in three of five previously azoospermic patients after therapy with chlorambucil in doses ranging from 410 to 2600 mg.[16] In these patients, sperm counts were found to be normal at 33, 34, and 42 months following completion of chemotherapy. Two additional patients, who received the highest cumulative drug doses, demonstrated a partial return of spermatogenesis at 38 and 58 months after discontinuing treatment. In a similar study, 26 men treated for five to 34 months with 50 to 100 mg of cyclophosphamide daily all became azoospermic within six months of starting therapy.[24] However, serial sperm counts demonstrated a return of spermatogenesis in 12 patients a mean period of 31 months following discontinuation of cyclophosphamide. Those patients demonstrating a recovery of spermatogenesis tended to receive lower initial drug doses. These studies, along with numerous anecdotal reports,[25, 26] clearly demonstrate that the germinal epithelium can regenerate and spermatogenesis can resume following chemotherapy. Fur-

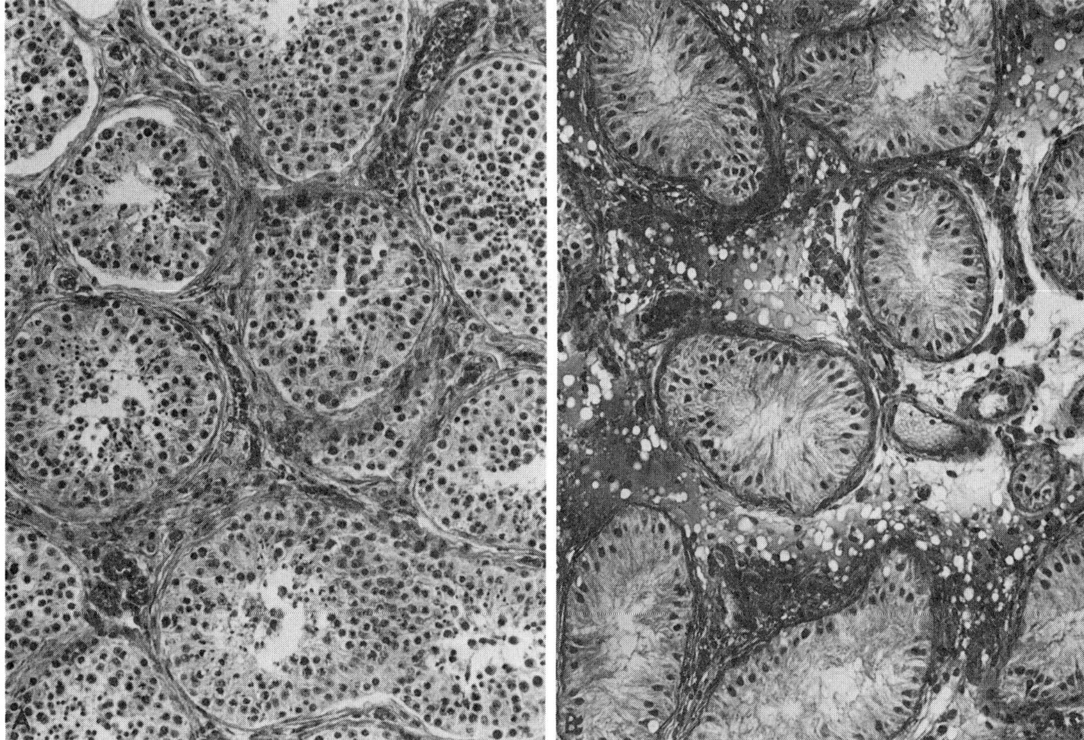

Figure 6–2. *A*, Testicular biopsy from a patient with a normal ejaculate, showing normal testicular histology. *B*, Testicular biopsy from a patient with chemotherapy-induced azoospermia showing germinal aplasia. (Reproduced with permission from Sherins RJ, and DeVita VT: Effects of drug treatment for lymphoma on male reproductive capacity. Ann. Intern. Med. 79:216–220, 1973.)

ther, the evidence suggests that the rapidity with which spermatogenesis resumes may be related to the total dose of chemotherapy administered.

Treatment with combination chemotherapy may produce more long-lasting azoospermia than does therapy with single agents. Sherins and DeVita observed azoospermia and testicular germinal aplasia in patients for as long as four years after completion of MOPP combination chemotherapy.[21] No long-term prospective data are available to assess accurately the duration of germinal aplasia and the likelihood of recovery of spermatogenesis following completion of combination chemotherapy. One group of investigators in 1978 reported the results of long-term follow-up of testicular function in patients treated with MOPP, CVP, or related regimens for Hodgkin's disease and non-Hodgkin's lymphoma.[27] Thirty-one of 32 patients developed increased serum FSH levels during their initial therapy and, of 15 studied, all had azoospermia. Sixteen patients were evaluated for recovery of testicular function. In seven of ten patients treated with CVP or a related regimen, plasma FSH levels returned to normal during 34 months of follow-up. Of four patients studied, three had normal sperm counts and the fourth was oligospermic. In contrast, only one of six patients treated with a procarbazine-containing regimen demonstrated a fall of serum FSH or rise in sperm count during 52 months of follow-up. Although the patient numbers are small, these data suggest that the use of procarbazine in combination chemotherapy regimens may be associated with more long-lasting testicular damage than that seen with alkylating agents alone. Indeed, Sieber has demonstrated that procarbazine by itself is toxic to the germinal epithelium in adult male monkeys.[28]

In summary, the testicular germinal epithelium is clearly sensitive to the cytotoxic effects of alkylating agents and procarbazine, and appears to be depleted in a progressive dose-related fashion during the course of chemotherapy. Recovery of spermatogenesis is unpredictable for the individual patient, but does occur, and may be inversely related to the total dose of chemotherapy administered and directly related to the length of time off therapy. Recent data suggest that Leydig cell function may also be affected by antitumor chemotherapy, although clinical sequelae are not apparent. Long-term prospective studies are needed to define further the patterns of testicular injury and recovery that result from cancer chemotherapy.

In contrast to the availability of at least some data for alkylating agents and procarbazine, there is a paucity of information describing the impact on the testis of newer agents such as bleomycin and *cis*-platinum. One report has touched on the effects of doxorubicin and noted that the drug appears less toxic to the human testis than to the mouse testis.[29] In the mouse model a single injection of 35 mg/m^2 produces total azoospermia, yet two patients treated with doxorubicin-containing chemotherapy regimens developed only mild oligospermia. Anecdotal reports such as these serve only to underscore the need for comprehensive studies in large numbers of patients, and to caution against the extrapolation of animal data to man.

Chemotherapy Effects in Women

The evaluation of chemotherapy effects on ovarian function is hampered by the relative inaccessibility of the ovary to biopsy. Unlike the semen analysis, no direct measurement of the female germ cell population is readily available. Further, no reliable animal model has been developed to assess the effects of cytotoxic drugs on ovarian function. Thus, one must rely primarily on menstrual and reproductive history and on determinations of serum hormone levels to assess the functional status of the ovary.

Oogenesis is the process of maturation of the primitive female germ cell to the mature ovum. This process occurs primarily during intrauterine life and involves multiple mitotic divisions to increase the number of germ cells, followed by the beginning of the first meiotic division, which will eventually reduce the diploid chromosome number to half prior to fertilization. At the time of birth the oocytes are in the long prophase of their first meiotic division, and they remain in that state until the formation of a mature follicle prior to ovulation.[30]

In the postnatal ovary, most of the ongoing cellular growth and replication is related to the growth and development of follicles. Primordial follicles develop during gestation and consist of a primary oocyte covered by a layer of mesenchymal cells called "granulosa cells." At the time of birth the ovary may contain 150,000 to 500,000 primordial follicles, many of which subsequently become atretic. From childhood to menopause follicular growth occurs as a continuous process, with ovulation occurring in a cyclic fashion.[31] The granulosa cells surrounding the primary oocyte proliferate, follicular fluid accumulates, and the ovum completes its first meiotic division to become a secondary oocyte. At this time the follicle is known as a secondary or graafian follicle. The follicle continues to enlarge until the time of ovulation. Those follicles not undergoing ovulation then become atretic and regress. During the reproductive life of a woman, only 300 to 400 oocytes mature and are extruded in the process of ovulation; the remainder undergo some form of atresia.

It is the process of follicular growth and maturation that is most likely to be affected by cytotoxic chemotherapy. Indeed, the primary histologic lesion noted in the ovaries of women receiving antineoplastic chemotherapy is ovarian fibrosis and follicle destruction.[32-34] Clinically, amenorrhea ensues and is accompanied by elevation of serum FSH and LH and by a fall in serum estradiol. Vaginal epithelial atrophy and endometrial hypoplasia occur, and patients may complain of menopausal symptoms such as "hot flashes" or of symptoms of estrogen deficiency such as vaginal dryness and dyspareunia.

The onset and duration of amenorrhea appear to be both dose- and age-related. Generally, younger patients are able to tolerate larger cumulative drug doses before amenorrhea occurs and have a greater likelihood of resumption of menses when therapy is discontinued.

Among the anticancer drugs, alkylating agents are the most frequent cause of ovarian dysfunction. During the early clinical trials of busulfan, amenorrhea was a common side effect. Several investigators noted the onset of permanent amenorrhea among patients receiving busulfan in doses varying from 0.5 to 14 mg/day for at least three months.[35, 36]

The effects of cyclophosphamide on ovarian function were first noted in the rheumatology literature, as early cessation of menses and menopausal symptoms developed in six of 33 patients treated for rheumatoid arthritis with daily cyclophosphamide for six to 40 months.[37] One of these patients had elevated serum FSH levels consistent with primary ovarian failure. Subsequently, several investigators have documented the occurrence of amenorrhea, decreased urinary estrogens, and increased urinary gonadotropins in at least 50 per cent of premenopausal women receiving 40 to 120 mg of cyclophosphamide daily for an average of 18 months.[38, 39] Ovarian biopsy in some patients has demonstrated arrest of follicular maturation and absence of ova.

More recent studies of the use of adjuvant chemotherapy for the prevention of recurrence of breast cancer suggest that the onset of amenorrhea and the resumption of menses is related to the age of the patient during chemotherapy and to the total dose administered. Amenorrhea has been reported to develop in 17 of 18 women treated with adjuvant cyclophosphamide for 13 to 14 months postoperatively.[40] Permanent cessation of menses occurred following a mean total dose of 5.2 gm in all patients 40 years and older. Amenorrhea also developed in four of five women under 40 years of age, but only after a mean cyclophosphamide dose of 9.3 gm was administered. Menses subsequently returned in two of these patients within six months of discontinuing therapy. Further, a recent prospective study of ovarian function in premenopausal women receiving melphalan alone or in combination with 5-fluorouracil has demonstrated the occurrence of amenorrhea in 22 per cent of patients younger than 39 but in 73 per cent of patients older than 40.[41] It appears, then, that alkylating agent chemotherapy accelerates the onset of menopause, particularly in the older patients, whereas younger patients may tolerate higher total doses before amenorrhea becomes irreversible.

Comparatively little information is available concerning the effects of treatment with combination chemotherapy on ovarian function. As might be expected, at least 50 per cent of women treated with combination chemotherapy become amenorrheic.[42-44] The cessation of menses is accompanied by elevations of serum FSH and LH consistent with primary ovarian failure. Apart from age, no clear differences have been noted between those women who become amenorrheic during therapy and those who do not. In one study of ovarian function in women treated with combination chemotherapy for Hodgkin's disease, patients developing amenorrhea were noted to have received an average of four times more methylhydrazine, two times more chlorambucil, and 1.4 times more vinblastine than did patients maintaining normal menses.[42] However, a subsequent study demonstrated no significant differences in cumulative drug dosages between those women becoming amenorrheic and those maintaining normal menses after MOPP chemotherapy for Hodgkin's disease.[43] In neither study, however, were the patients' ages carefully considered in analysis of the data. When patient age is considered, there appears to be a definite relationship between age and total chemotherapy dose that can be administered before amenorrhea ensues.[44] Younger patients can tolerate higher drug doses or more prolonged therapy before irreversible amenorrhea occurs.

Clearly, then, the ovary can be damaged by antineoplastic chemotherapy, and the developing follicle is likely the target of these drugs. The effects of alkylating agents have been most thoroughly investigated, but little information is available concerning the potential of drugs belonging to other classes to interfere with ovarian function. The occurrence and persistence of amenorrhea in women receiving chemotherapy is related to both the total dose of drug administered and the age of the patient. Continued, long-term prospective follow-up of women maintaining normal menses during chemotherapy is necessary to determine the degree of risk of premature ovarian failure and early menopause in these patients.

Chemotherapy Effects in Children

Any study of the effects of cytotoxic chemotherapy on gonadal function in children is particularly complex because of the variables introduced by the continuum of sexual development present in this patient population. Thus, the effects of chemotherapy can be expected to vary according to when drugs are given and when their effects are evaluated relative to puberty. The few available reports suggest differences in the sensitivity of the prepubertal, pubertal, and adult testis to alkylating-agent chemotherapy. For example, one investigator reported that 15 boys treated with cyclophosphamide when prepubertal or in early puberty had normal serum FSH, LH, and testosterone levels for their age when studied.[45] All had been off therapy for 1.5 to 5.5 years when evaluated, but most were still prepubertal or in early puberty. Testicular biopsy in one patient who received 5.7 gm of cyclophosphamide was normal, and biopsies in four other patients receiving 7.5 to 21.5 gm showed only focal tubular atrophy.

A prospective evaluation of gonadal function in 14 boys undergoing combination chemotherapy (prednisone, vincristine, methotrexate, and 6-mercaptopurine) for acute lymphoblastic leukemia has confirmed that these agents do not cause irreversible damage to the germinal epithelium.[45a] Nine patients were prepubertal, four were intrapubertal, and one was sexually mature at the start of treatment. After a median follow-up of 5½ years, all patients had normal testicular size and normal serum gonadotropin and testosterone levels. Five of six patients tested had normal semen analyses; one had a low-normal sperm count. Shalet et al.,[45b] in a study of 44 patients undergoing chemotherapy for acute lymphoblastic leukemia, found a median decrease of 51 per cent in the number of seminiferous tubules containing spermatogonia, as compared with normal age-matched controls. These findings suggest that leukemia therapy has definite, although at least partially reversible, effects on the germinal epithelium of the prepubertal and intrapubertal male.

These data suggest that the prepubertal testis may be more resistant to the effects of alkylating agents than is the adult gonad, although the time elapsed from cessation of therapy to evaluation may have been sufficient to allow recovery of a previously damaged testis. Ettledorf has demonstrated that even for the prepubertal patient a dose-toxicity relationship may exist.[46] These investigators evaluated eight boys treated with cyclophosphamide at ages 7.5 to 13 years. All had been off therapy for 6.5 to 10 years when studied. All patients receiving total cyclophosphamide doses of 6.2 to 10.5 gm, as well as one patient receiving 14.3 gm, had normal sperm counts, testicular histology, and serum gonadotropins, whereas those patients receiving 11.8 to 39.3 gm of the drug were uniformly azoospermic with germinal aplasia on biopsy. From these and other data[47,48] one can conclude that the prepubertal testis may be more tolerant of moderate doses of alkylating agents than is the adult testis, yet a threshold dose does appear to exist above which germinal epithelial injury will result.[49,50]

By contrast, chemotherapy delivered to male patients during puberty may have profound effects on both germ cell production and endocrine function. Sherins et al. in 1978 reported studies of testicular function in boys treated with MOPP combination chemotherapy for Hodgkin's disease.[51] Gynecomastia developed in nine of 13 pubertal patients a mean of 28 months after initiation of treatment. This was accompanied by elevated serum FSH and LH levels and by low normal serum testosterone levels. Testicular biopsy in six patients with gynecomastia revealed germinal aplasia. These data suggest that in pubertal patients both Leydig cells and germinal epithelium may be affected by combination chemotherapy, and that gynecomastia may be the clinical manifestation of this endocrine dysfunction.

Little information is available concerning the effects of cytotoxic chemotherapy on ovarian function in children. There appears to be no delay in menarche and no interruption of menses in girls treated with single-agent cyclophosphamide.[45,50,52,53] Further, Arneil reported normal ovarian histology at postmortem examination in six girls treated with cyclophosphamide for malignancy.[48] However, the drug dosages were not clearly specified. Other investigators have noted absence or inhibition of follicle development following cytotoxic chemotherapy in girls dying from leukemia.[54] However, a careful study of ovarian function in girls treated with combination chemotherapy for acute leukemia yielded more encouraging results. Treatment included intermittent cycles of prednisone, vincristine, methotrexate, and 6-mercaptopurine, with some receiving cyclophosphamide also. Seventeen patients were prepubertal at the time of treatment, 11 were aged 10.5 to 15.5 years but were premenarchal, and seven were postmenarchal.[55] Overall, 80 per cent of the patients demonstrated normal ovarian function when studied. Sixteen of 17 prepubertal patients either had achieved spontaneous menarche or were progressing normally through puberty. Seven of 11 patients of pubertal age at the time of treatment achieved spontaneous menarche — five while receiving chemotherapy. Three patients developed secondary amenorrhea and elevated gonadotropins consistent with ovarian failure, but menses subsequently returned in two. Although ovarian dysfunction was not prominent in this series, it is difficult to draw generally applicable conclusions because the chemotherapy administered consisted primarily of antimetabolites. It would appear that these drugs do not cause ovarian dysfunction in young girls. The effects of combination chemotherapy including alkylating agents on the prepubertal and pubertal ovary require further evaluation.

With the introduction of antineoplastic chemotherapy, lasting clinical remissions have been obtained for many patients who would otherwise have died. The long-term effects of such therapy are only now being recognized. Among them, infertility must be considered an unfortunate but acceptable side effect for many patients. Although alkylating agents appear to be primarily responsible for gonadal injury, doxorubicin,[29] cytosine arabinoside,[56] procarbazine,[28] and vinblastine[57] have also been implicated. A summary of cytotoxic drug effects on fertility is shown in Table 6–3. Virtually no data are available concerning the potential antifertility effects of other recently introduced drugs such as *cis*-platinum and bleomycin. As new effective antitumor agents are introduced into clinical practice, further screening for gonadal toxicity will become necessary. In addition, long-term prospective studies of reproductive function in patients receiving cancer chemotherapy are necessary to determine the magnitude and duration of gonadal dysfunction resulting from any therapeutic regimen.

TABLE 6–3. Drug-Related Infertility

Definite	*Probable*
Chlorambucil	Doxorubicin (Adriamycin)
Cyclophosphamide	Vinblastine
L-Phenylalanine mustard	Cytosine arabinoside
Nitrogen mustard	
Busulfan	
Procarbazine	
Unlikely	*Unknown*
Methotrexate	Bleomycin
5-Fluorouracil	*cis*-Platinum
6-Mercaptopurine	Nitrosoureas
Vincristine	

Counseling

For patients facing the problem of chemotherapy-induced sterility, sperm banking prior to therapy remains a consideration. Although the technology of freezing, preserving, and thawing human semen has advanced considerably, ultimate conception rates using preserved semen remain at only 50 to 60 per cent.[58-60] In 1973 Sherman summarized the results of artificial insemination with frozen human semen.[58] Of 621 reported pregnancies, the spontaneous abortion rate was 8 per cent and the congenital abnormality rate only 1 per cent, both less than expected for the general population. Little additional information has accumulated since that time. Most physicians practicing artificial insemination prefer fresh donor semen. Among those using frozen semen, the great majority do not store it for longer than 24 months.[60]

For patients with cancer, sperm banking and successful insemination may be even less likely because of poor-quality semen. As many as one third of male patients with Hodgkin's disease have decreased sperm counts or poor sperm motility before receiving any therapy.[23a] These findings would indicate a low probability of successful semen preservation and, ultimately, of conception. Nevertheless, sperm banking at a reliable institution can be offered to patients if they are properly informed of the cost/benefit ratio of the procedure.

Finally, patients in whom reproductive capacity returns after chemotherapy frequently have questions concerning the risks of spontaneous abortion and fetal abnormalities. Cytotoxic chemotherapy administered during pregnancy, particularly the first trimester, is teratogenic. However, the mutagenic potential of these drugs remains undefined. Anecdotal reports suggest that there is no increased incidence of spontaneous abortion or fetal abnormalities in those treated with chemotherapy in comparison with the general population.[61-63] However, a recent study suggests that women previously treated with both chemotherapy and irradiation have a greater chance of pregnancy ending in abortion or with delivery of an abnormal child than do sibling controls.[64] At present, it is impossible to define the risk of fetal wastage or abnormality in patients previously treated with cytotoxic drugs. Whether a specific fetal abnormality may occur more commonly than others or whether a specific drug class, dose, or combination is more mutagenic than others remains unknown. Additional studies carried out over many years will be required before the true risks to subsequent generations are known.

CARCINOGENESIS — A LATE COMPLICATION OF CANCER CHEMOTHERAPY

Although the potential of antineoplastic agents to induce new malignancies was suggested by Haddow in 1947 on the basis of the ability of chemical carcinogens to cause growth inhibition,[65] convincing evidence for carcinogenic effects of these agents in man has only recently been reported. The major reasons for this belated recognition of the problem are the long latent period required for expression of carcinogenicity in man (three to four years) and the brief survival of most patients treated with chemotherapy Only in the past decade has a sizable number of patients with advanced malignancy been cured by chemotherapy; thus, sufficient time has elapsed and sufficient numbers of individuals are now at risk for second tumors to begin to be seen in clinically significant numbers. Although survival benefits will undoubtedly continue to accrue from the use of these agents and will probably outweigh the risks of second neoplasms, greater concern for this complication will be required in the use of antineoplastic drugs in adjuvant programs and in non-neoplastic conditions such as renal transplantation or autoimmune disease, where long-term survival of a large fraction of the treated population is assured. In these instances the benefits and risks of alternative therapies must be carefully weighed against those of the antineoplastic agents, and carcinogenicity must be included in the equation.

Definition of the risk of carcinogenesis due to chemotherapy is a difficult task and at present only suggestive conclusions can be drawn. Prediction of carcinogenicity on the experimental level depends on test systems that examine the ability of chemicals to cause mutation of bacteria or mammalian cells, malignant transformation of mammalian cells, chromosomal aberrations, or tumors in mice or rats. Such tests are subject to interspecies variability in drug metabolism and target tissue kinetics, and to other host factors that influence tumor development; these factors make extrapolation of the quantitative risk to man a difficult if not impossible task. Second, the immune status of the patient is believed to play an important role in determining carcinogenicity, as indicated by the increased risk of lymphoid and cutaneous neoplasms in patients receiving immunosuppressive therapy; in cancer patients the immune system is suppressed both as a result of the neoplastic process and as a consequence of therapy. This immunosuppression undoubtedly influences the risk of carcinogenesis, but is not duplicated in test systems. Finally, the assessment of risk in man at present is primarily based on analysis of retrospective series or anecdotal reports, which often give incomplete information regarding key parameters of treatment (dose, duration) and which lack a control or untreated population. Such a control population would be particularly important in risk assessment since an increased incidence of second tumors, such as acute myelocytic leukemia in patients with Hodgkin's disease, may exist in the absence of treatment.

With these limitations in mind, the following section considers available information concerning the carcinogenic potential of antitumor agents. This discussion examines the common pharmacologic properties shared by antineoplastic agents and classical carcinogens, specific predictions of carcinogenicity based on nonhuman test systems, and clinical evidence for an increased risk of second neoplasms in patients receiving these agents.

The Relationship of Antineoplastic Agents to Chemical Carcinogens

The chemical induction of cancer in animals is thought to involve a multistage process with a long latency period This process can be initiated by a variety of chemical structures that have at least one common thread in their mode of action — an interaction with DNA.[66-68] One of the most carefully studied systems of tumor induction is the induction of skin cancer in mice and rabbits by alkylating agents, polycyclic hydrocarbons, or ethyl carbamate (Fig. 6–3). Repeated applications of these agents over long periods result in the development of benign or malignant tumors. However, exposure to these compounds in limited doses causes morphologic changes in the epithelium but does not result in tumors unless this stage of initiation is followed by the introduction of a promoter, such as a phorbol ester, an ingredient of croton oil. Promoters are not carcinogenic by themselves, but lead to tumor production if applied after the initiating agent. Treatment with a specific promoter before exposure to the initiating agent does not result in tumor formation. This stage of promotion occurs over weeks and months and may be reversible in its early stages. The specific chemical action of promoting compounds is not understood. Promoters such as phorbol-12-myrestate-13-acetate have a variety of biologic actions; they alter differentiation, cause changes in cell surface glycopeptides, alter various metabolic activities, and suppress immune surveillance of tumors by cytotoxic macrophages and natural killer cells.[69] Thus, carcinogenesis is a multistep process which may be arrested at intermediate stages, which requires a long latency period for induction, and which may be influenced by, if it does not require, a promoting agent.

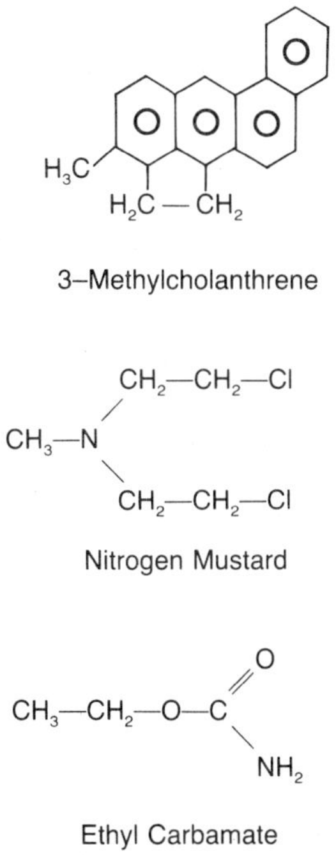

The existence or identity of an associated promoter has not been established for well-documented carcinogens in man. For cancer patients, induction of second tumors may require not only an initiator but also a promoter, a function that may be fulfilled by a second chemotherapeutic agent, by radiotherapy, or by a disease-related abnormality in metabolism or immune function. This consideration could explain the higher risk of second tumors in patients receiving a combination of drugs and irradiation.

Chemical carcinogens show a diversity of structures, but share important metabolic features. Most are inert and require microsomal metabolic activation to positively charged (or electrophilic) intermediates that react with DNA bases. The primary sites for attack of DNA are relatively negatively charged (or nucleophilic) sites such as the 7 position of guanine.[70, 71] These characteristics of carcinogens, namely microsomal metabolism to an electrophilic intermediate that attacks DNA, are shared by certain antineoplastic agents such as cyclophosphamide and mitomycin C, and are essential in the antineoplastic action of these drugs. Other agents, such as L-phenylalanine mustard and nitrogen mustard, do not require metabolic activation to form alkylating species. Carcinogenicity has also been ascribed to ionizing irradiation, which produces free radicals such as superoxide or hydroxyl radicals. A number of antitumor drugs have the same ability to promote formation of reactive oxygen intermediates; such agents include those that possess quinone functional groups (doxorubicin and mithramycin) or those that bind electron donating heavy metals (such as bleomycin and its analogues).[72] Four antineoplastic agents that are suspected carcinogens, and their probable carcinogenic intermediates, are given in Table 6–4; these structures illustrate the varied chemical features of their reactive intermediates.

H_3C ; $H_2C—CH_2$

3–Methylcholanthrene

$CH_3—N(CH_2—CH_2—Cl)_2$

Nitrogen Mustard

$CH_3—CH_2—O—C(=O)—NH_2$

Ethyl Carbamate

Figure 6–3. Chemical structures of three carcinogenic agents.

TABLE 6–4. Antineoplastic Agents with Reactive Intermediates

Parent Compound	*Reactive Intermediates*
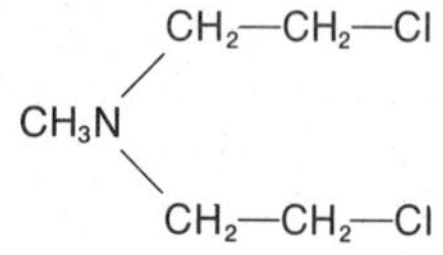 $CH_2—CH_2—Cl$ CH_3N $CH_2—CH_2—Cl$ Nitrogen mustard	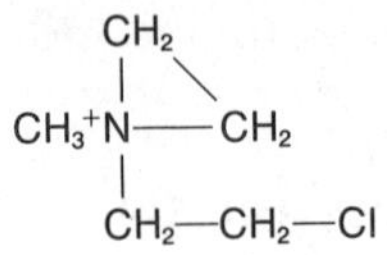 CH_2 $CH_3{}^{+}N—CH_2$ $CH_2—CH_2—Cl$
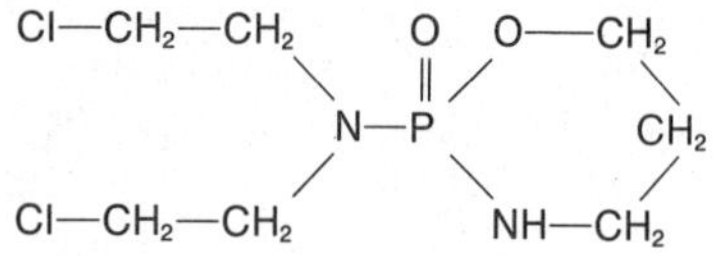 $Cl—CH_2—CH_2$ O $O—CH_2$ N—P CH_2 $Cl—CH_2—CH_2$ $NH—CH_2$ Cyclophosphamide	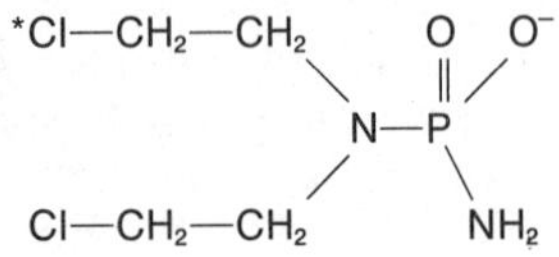 *$Cl—CH_2—CH_2$ O O^- N—P $Cl—CH_2—CH_2$ NH_2
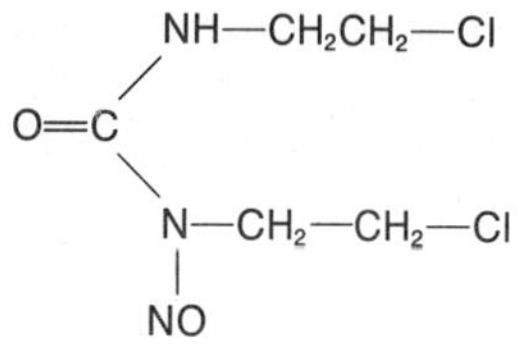 $NH—CH_2CH_2—Cl$ O=C $N—CH_2—CH_2—Cl$ NO Carmustine (BCNU)	$ClCH_2CH_2{}^{+}$
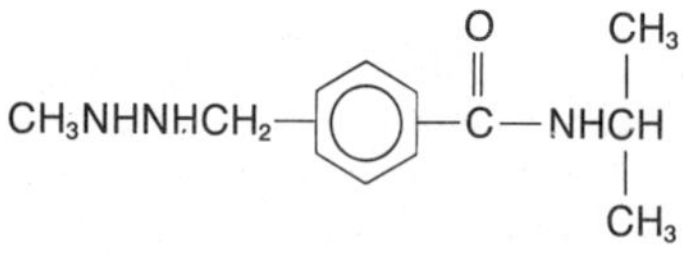 O CH_3 $CH_3NHNHCH_2$—⟨benzene ring⟩—C—NHCH CH_3 Procarbazine	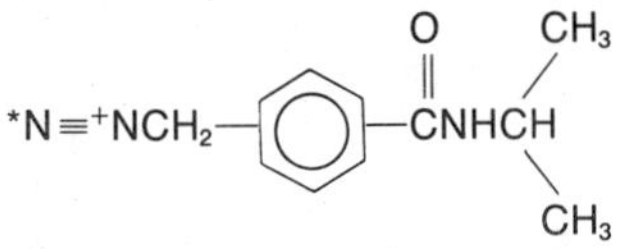 O CH_3 *$N{\equiv}{}^{+}NCH_2$—⟨benzene ring⟩—CNHCH CH_3

*One of several reactive intermediates identified.

Testing Antineoplastic Agents for Carcinogenic Potential

In view of the damaging effects of many antineoplastic agents on DNA and the suggestive clinical evidence of their carcinogenicity, it has become imperative to apply methods for determining carcinogenic potential prior to widespread use of new agents in man. An ideal test system would be simple, rapid, inexpensive, and yet specific for carcinogens and sensitive to modestly potent agents. Unfortunately, the various methods available, ranging from *in vitro* bacterial mutagenesis assays to long-term studies in rodents, all have recognized drawbacks and none has been adequately evaluated as a predictive system for man.[73] Nevertheless, the development of relatively simple mutagenesis assays by Ames and others[74] represents a considerable step forward in allowing rapid detection of potential carcinogens.

There are four main types of test systems for carcinogens. *Mutagenesis* assays attempt to quantify the frequency with which a chemical induces mutational events based on the assumption that mutagenicity correlates with the likelihood of causing cancer in animals. The underlying premise is that carcinogenesis is the product of a mutational event that can be expressed in the short term as a change in biochemical features of a test organism. *Cytogenetic* studies attempt to correlate drug-induced chromosomal aberrations such as sister chromatid exchanges (SCE), with carcinogenicity. Although certain characteristic karyotypic changes are associated with specific malignancies, such as the Ph[1] chromosome in chronic granulocytic leukemia, cytogenetic abnormalities are not proved to be either necessary or sufficient causes of neoplastic transformation. Tests of *oncogenesis in tissue culture* are based on the hypothesis that agents which produce neoplastic transformation in culture are likely to be carcinogenic in the whole animal. This system, as does the Ames assay of bacterial mutagenesis, entails the assumption that the drug concentration, duration of exposure, and metabolism of the suspected carcinogen are relevant to the *in vivo* situation, but this assumption is of uncertain validity since precise pharmacokinetic and metabolic information is not available for many of the compounds tested. Finally, *in vivo mammalian* studies are conducted usually in rodents over extended periods and at great expense. The primary drawbacks of this system are the known species-, sex-, and age-dependencies of drug metabolism in rodents and the lack of pharmacologic information that would allow an extrapolation of results from rodents to man.

Mutagenesis Assays

Among the many mutagen testing systems under study at present, the Ames test, which employs *Salmonella typhimurium,* has received the most attention and validation. This system satisfies the requirements of simplicity and a rapid return of results, and in addition appears to possess high specificity for carcinogens, although certain exceptions have been identified. This test[74] employs specific strains of *Salmonella typhimurium* that are histidine-requiring mutants. Exposure of these strains to the suspected mutagen in a histidine-free medium will lead to growth of revertant mutants if the appropriate mutation is induced. Small amounts of chemicals (less than 1 mg) can be used and results are obtained in about two days. For agents that require metabolic activation (as do many carcinogens), rat or human liver microsomes can be added to the test plates.

In extensive testing of a wide variety of previously documented carcinogens and noncarcinogens, 90 per cent of the known carcinogens were postive in the Ames assay and 87 per cent of the noncarcinogens were inactive.[75, 76] These results suggest that the system has a high degree of specificity. Many of the antineoplastic agents in use today have been examined in the Ames system[77-80] and some of the results are incorporated in Table 6–5. Several observations can be made regarding the value of this test as a screening system. It appears that a high degree of correlation exists between the Ames test results and *in vivo* studies of carcinogenesis. Most antimetabolites and the vinca alkaloids are negative in both the Ames test and *in vivo* systems, whereas alkylating agents and many antitumor antibiotics are positive in both assay systems. However, both procarbazine and actinomycin D are carcinogenic in animals but negative in the Ames test. In the case of procarbazine, this discrepancy may be due to the failure of the test system to simulate the metabolism of procarbazine as it occurs *in vivo* (see Chapter 15). 6-Mercaptopurine, which has been reported to be carcinogenic in animals, is weakly mutagenic in the *Salmonella* system.

TABLE 6–5. Results of Testing Antineoplastic Agents in Three Systems for Carcinogenicity

Agent	*Ames Test*	*Sister Chromatid Exchanges*	*Animal Studies*
Nitrogen mustard	+	+	+
Cyclophosphamide	+	+‡	+
Melphalan	+	+	+
Thio-TEPA	+	+	+
Chlorambucil	NR	+	+
Procarbazine	−	+‡	+
Lomustine (CCNU)	NR	+*	+
Doxorubicin (Adriamycin)	+	+	+
Streptozotocin	+	NR	+
Bleomycin	−	+†	−
Actinomycin D	−	±	+
Mitomycin C	+	+	+
Dacarbazine (DTIC)	NR	−*	+
cis-Platinum	+	+	NR
5-Fluorouracil	−	NR	NR
6-Mercaptopurine	+	−	+
Ara-C	−	NR	−
Vincristine	−	±	−
Vinblastine	−	NR	+
Methotrexate	−	+	−

+ = Positive result reported in at least one study; − = no positive result reported; NR = no result reported; ± = slight decrease over control which is of unknown significance; *test done on patient lymphocytes after treatment with agent; †concentration giving positive results also causes significant numbers of other chromosomal aberrations; ‡drug must be activated.

From the foregoing analysis it would appear that the Ames test is an excellent screening procedure, but one with obvious false negatives. An analysis of the Ames test results by Pinkus and Legator[81] indicates that the false-negative rate is particularly high for specific chemical classes. At least seven classes of agents known to contain carcinogenic compounds are poorly detected in the Ames system, including azo compounds as well as carbamyl, hydrazine, chlorethylene, steroid, and antimetabolite structures. In some cases, known carcinogens such as urethane probably cannot be metabolized to their carcinogenic form in the test system. Many compounds in common clinical use have not been adequately addressed at this writing.

In an effort to increase sensitivity of the assay, plasmids or R factors may be introduced into the assay test strain. However, R factors have caused a general increase in the spontaneous mutation rate of some tester strains and thus have masked the effects of at least one mutagen. Additional problems are presented by the sensitivity of the system, since minor contamination with carcinogens in the test compound formulation could result in a false-positive assay. The test system does not take into account nonmicrosomal detoxifying systems in the whole animal, such as glutathione transferases and reactive sulfhydryls, or the surveillance and destruction of tumors by the immune system. Thus, although the Ames test system is useful in screening agents, it must be followed up by other *in vitro* and *in vivo* tests before definite positive or negative conclusions can be drawn. In particular, a negative Ames result for a compound of suspicious structure or mechanism of action should be confirmed by *in vivo* testing.

Sister Chromatid Exchanges

Chromosomal damage resulting from exposure to chemical substances *in vitro* or *in vivo* has been used as an index of mutagenic or carcinogenic potential for many years, but has required significant skill in recognizing the many different possible aberrations. Sister chromatid exchange (SCE), a relatively new type of chromosomal study that detects the exchange of small DNA fragments between sister chromatid pairs, has considerable appeal because relatively few cells need to be examined, exchanges can be easily visualized, and the system is quite sensitive to small amounts of chemicals. The exchange is symmetric and does not alter the overall chromosomal morphology (Fig. 6–4). The development of differential labeling of sister strands with 5-bromo-2′-deoxyuridine (BUdR),[82] making the exchanges easily visible, has led to the use of this technique for the detection of carcinogenic agents. Cells are first exposed to a potential carcinogen and then grown in the presence of BUdR for two cell cycles. Finally, the cells are exposed to demecolcine (Colcemid) to produce metaphase arrest, and the chromosomal preparation is stained. One chromatid is substituted with BUdR in one of its spirals, and its sister strand is substituted with BUdR in

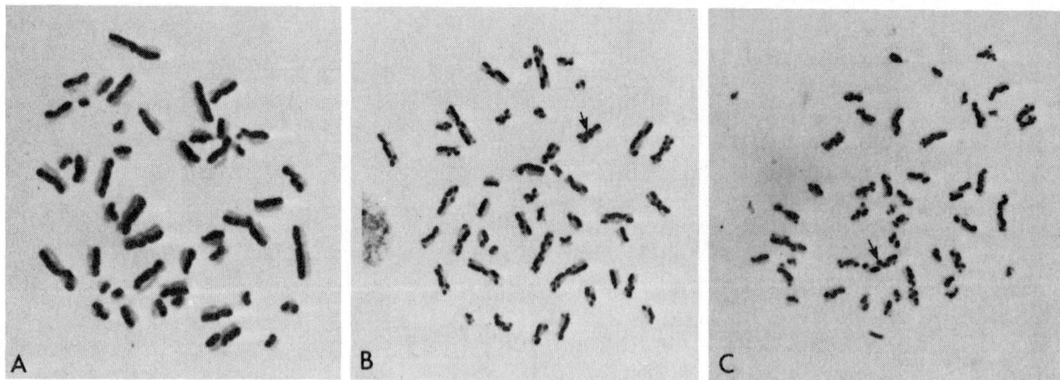

Figure 6–4. Sister chromatid exchanges (SCE). Metaphase spread of a normal human peripheral lymphocyte. *B*, Metaphase spread of a peripheral lymphocyte from a patient with Bloom's syndrome (courtesy of Dr. P. Kohn). *C*, Metaphase spread of a human peripheral lymphocyte exposed to mitomycin C (0.075 μg/ml) for 48 hours. Arrows point out one of many SCE. (Reproduced with permission from Latt et al.: *In vitro* and *in vivo* analysis of sister chromatid exchange. Pharmacol. Rev. 30: 501, 1979.)

both spirals. SCE can then be recognized as a region of juxtaposition of high and low staining density (Fig. 6–4).

The ability of various chemotherapeutic agents to induce SCE indicates that this technique might be useful as an assay for mutagenesis and ultimately carcinogenesis, but limitations of its potential have also become clear.[82, 83] Ionizing radiation, known to be a potent mutagen and carcinogen, causes only slight increments in SCE; these changes are minimal in comparison with other chromosomal damage, including breaks, deletions, and other aberrations induced at the same dose. On the other hand, ultraviolet light evokes dramatic increases in SCE frequency. Some chemicals, such as caffeine and bleomycin, do not induce significant SCE's but produce large numbers of chromosomal aberrations similar to ionizing radiation. Alkylating agents and some DNA intercalators induce a high frequency of SCE in addition to other chromosomal damage. Cyclophosphamide induces SCE's only after microsomal activation.[84] Among the antimetabolites, methotrexate, which is not carcinogenic in laboratory animals, has been reported to induce SCE, but 6-mercaptopurine, a suspected carcinogen, does not cause these chromosomal abnormalities.[85]

The use of SCE has particular appeal because the effects of chemotherapeutic agents can be assessed *in vivo* by performing this test on peripheral lymphocytes from patients receiving antineoplastic therapy. Studies of lymphocytes from patients before and at intervals after chemotherapy have shown a marked increase in SCE following the administration of lomustine (CCNU), dacarbazine (DTIC), and mitomycin C.[86-88] Whether such increases in SCE frequency reflect the likelihood of carcinogenicity is still unclear. A recent report has suggested that DNA single strand breaks, DNA-DNA interstrand crosslinks, and DNA-protein crosslinks are not necessary for SCE.[89] Thus, some of the classic mechanisms of DNA damage leading to mutations have no obvious correlation with SCE frequency. However, there is a relationship between the incidence of a specific mutation, 8-azaguanine resistance, and the frequency of SCE as examined in Chinese hamster ovary cells exposed to mitomycin C, ethyl methane sulfonate, N-ethyl-N-nitrosourea, and proflavine sulfate.[90]

Cell Culture Systems

Cell culture systems have also been advocated for the testing of carcinogenicity. Morphologic transformation of cells in culture and the ability of these cells to produce tumors when implanted in animals have been the primary criteria used for carcinogenicity. Three major test systems, which employ hamster embryo cells, fibroblasts from the ventral prostate, or 3T3-like cells, have been applied to the screening of environmental carcinogens.[91, 92] Using all three lines, it has been possible to show a good quantitative correlation between transformation *in vitro* and *in vivo* carcinogenesis, although the number of antineoplastic agents tested has been limited. However, mammalian cell culture systems are subject to many of the same problems as those of the bacterial mutagenesis assays discussed previously, including the need to activate compounds to reactive intermediates. An additional problem pertinent to these three systems is the use of cells of nonhuman and nonepithelial origin. Finally, tumors resulting from implantation of transformed cells are sarcomas and thus may not reflect the potential of the tested agent to cause tumors in epithelial cells or in man.

The results of testing antineoplastic drugs in cell transformation systems have not correlated well with tests of carcinogenicity in experimental animals.[93, 94] Carcinogenic alkylating agents (melphalan and thio-TEPA) increased the transformation frequency of C3H/10T½ cells; actinomycin D and bleomycin showed a concentration-dependent increase in transformation frequency, and these results are consistent with the known carcinogenicity of these agents. However, methotrexate also caused a concentration-dependent increase in transformation but at a relatively low frequency, whereas two other antimetabolites, 5-fluorodeoxyuridine and cytosine arabinoside, produced transformation in synchronized cells exposed during S phase of the cell cycle. None of these antimetabolites has proved to be carcinogenic in animals or man.

Animal Studies

The classic yardstick for assessing carcinogenicity has been the ability of the suspected agent to induce tumors in laboratory animals. These studies, although the most direct and reliable source of experimental information, are fraught with difficulties, including high cost (over $300,000 per compound), interspecies variability in susceptibility to carcinogens, and the long time required to obtain results. In addition, efforts must be made to design protocols of drug administration that mimic the intensity and duration of exposure found in man, a problem compounded by differences in drug metabolism and pharmacokinetics between man and rodent. A definite advantage of the bioassay system in intact animals is the preservation of the role of the immune system in determining the outcome. This factor is obviously missing in any of the *in vitro* assays. The role of immunosuppression by antineoplastic agents relative to their carcinogenic action has been addressed only in a preliminary way, and no clear relationship between these two factors has been suggested.[95]

The results of various bioassays of antineoplastic agents are recorded in Table 6–5.[96-99] Some results are conflicting and appear to depend on the age, sex, and species of animal used in the test. However, in general, most alkylating agents and antitumor antibiotics are carcinogenic in animals, whereas antimetabolites, including methotrexate, cytosine arabinoside, and hydroxyurea, are negative. Drug combinations have received only limited testing in bioassay systems.[98] The combination of prednisone and azathioprine, commonly used in organ transplantation, resulted in a decrease in time before tumor appearance as compared with azathioprine alone. With other combinations (e.g., prednisone plus CCNU; ara-C plus CCNU; and prednisone, vincristine, and cyclophosphamide), median time before tumor appearance was increased as compared with the alkylating agent alone. Of the ten combinations studied, four resulted in slightly higher tumor incidence than controls, whereas six caused fewer tumors than did the individual drugs.

In conclusion, there exist several different test systems for evaluating the ability of antitumor agents to cause cancer. Each system evaluates this question under different conditions and with a different end point; the more rapid systems, such as the Ames assay and tests of cell transformation *in vitro*, pose unresolved questions regarding their specificity for carcinogenesis and their sensitivity to all classes of carcinogens; but offer significant advantages in terms of speed and cost. The *in vivo* systems, such as long-term carcinogenesis testing in rodents and evaluation of chromosomal changes in test animals or man, allow for appropriate interaction of the test chemical with host metabolic and immune systems, but have additional problems of interspecies variability and cost. Not one system by itself fulfills the requirements for rapid and sensitive testing, although the Ames test represents a considerable step forward.

Clinical Studies Implicating Antineoplastic Agents in Carcinogenesis

Although experimental evidence for the carcinogenic potential of many antineoplastic agents is abundant, clinical evidence for this problem has been slow to surface. An extensive review of anecdotal cases of second malignancy,[100] in addition to more detailed reports of an increased incidence of second tumors in ovarian cancer, Hodgkin's disease, and multiple myeloma after drug therapy, have supplied convincing documentation of this problem. The magnitude of the risk of second neoplasms is difficult to evaluate, for several reasons.

First, most reports of second tumors in man are retrospective or anecdotal in nature and do not provide an accurate quantitation of the population at risk. Therefore, the incidence of second malignancy can be only crudely estimated. Second, retrospective reports of second malignancy are prompted by the observation of index cases, and these suffer from an inherent statistical bias. Thus, institutions not observing second tumors would be unlikely either to examine the incidence of this problem in their treated populations or to report their negative findings.

A further complication is the difficulty of obtaining reliable information on drug dosage, total amount of drug administered, and duration of therapy in the few cases and series reported, because of the retrospective nature of these studies. Information concerning the total drug administered and the duration of therapy is particularly important in establishing risk since it is likely that a total dose threshold may exist above which the risk of neoplasia rises sharply. Such thresholds have been identified in experimental carcinogenesis and in the induction of SCE's.[74, 83] Duration of treatment may also have a bearing on risk, in that the same total dose of carcinogen, given in brief but intense exposure, may be less carcinogenic than chronic low-dose exposure. In many reports, further difficulties are posed by the fact that combination treatment regimens, or regimens employing irradiation and chemotherapy, were used. Thus, the carcinogenic effects cannot be ascribed to one component of the regimen with certainty, although conclusions can be drawn regarding the carcinogenicity of the regimen as a whole.

In addition to the problems of evaluating clinical studies, there exists a further possibility of an underlying increased incidence of second malignancy in patients with multiple myeloma, Hodgkin's disease, breast cancer, and other tumors.[101-110] This increased risk further complicates the problem of estimating the additional effects of chemotherapy. It is unlikely that a true control group of untreated patients will be identified, since it would be unethical to withhold treatment from patients with many types of advanced malignancy. The assessment of risk in untreated patients in a retrospective fashion also presents problems in that such patients would likely not live as long as those receiving chemotherapy, and therefore would be at risk for a shorter time. In spite of this dilemma, an accurate assessment of risk may be forthcoming from prospective adjuvant chemotherapy trials such as the CMF trial in Stage II breast cancer,[111] since untreated controls form one arm of this study.

Finally, the critical reader of these retrospective studies must consider the statistical methods used in assessing patients at risk.[112] The use of a person–years-of-risk type of analysis assumes that the yearly incidence of second malignancies is constant for the entire follow-up period. This approach does not allow for the fact that a patient must live a certain time through the latency period before the occurrence of a second malignancy. Although such an analysis allows a reasonable estimate of the carcinogenic effects of a single therapy, its use when comparing two treatments biases results against the treatment that leads to a longer survival and a sufficiently long follow-up to allow detection of second cancers. Alternative methods exist that take into account the effect of prolonged survival and must be applied before a statistically sound conclusion can be derived.

With these limitations in mind, it is possible to categorize antineoplastic agents into three groups on the basis of their oncogenic potential in man — high-risk, low-risk, and risk-unknown (Table 6–6). The primary basis for this classification is provided by the numerous reports of second malignancy in patients treated for ovarian carcinoma, breast cancer, multiple myeloma, and the lymphomas; additional information has been forthcoming from trials of cytotoxic agents in patients with autoimmune diseases or after organ transplantation.

Advanced ovarian cancer is treated primarily with alkylating agents such as melphalan.[113] Several reports have implicated alkylating agents (particularly melphalan and cyclophosphamide used as single agents) as a causative factor in the high incidence of acute nonlymphocytic leukemia in this group of patients.[114-117] A review of 5455 cases of ovarian cancer revealed a 36.1-fold increased risk of acute leukemia in chemotherapy-treated patients when compared with the incidence of leukemia in an age-matched control group. For patients surviving at least two years after institution of therapy, the risk was 171.4-fold higher than that in the controls.[118] These results must be tempered by the fact that nine of the 13 cases of acute leukemia identified in this series also received radiotherapy; it is possible that the radiotherapy alone or its combination with alkylating agents was responsible for leukemia. Nonetheless, the markedly increased risk in this patient population is convincing and alarming.

Breast cancer is another malignancy responsive to various antineoplastic combinations[119] and is associated with an apparent increased risk of leukemia. Most patients with metastatic breast cancer receive both

TABLE 6–6. Categorization of Antineoplastic Agents According to Carcinogenic Risk in Man

High	*Low*	*Unknown*
Melphalan	Methotrexate	Bleomycin
Cyclophosphamide	Ara-C	Doxorubicin (Adriamycin)
Chlorambucil	5-Fluorouracil	Actinomycin D
Azathioprine		Vincristine
Procarbazine		Vinblastine
Thio-TEPA		*cis*-Platinum
Nitrosoureas		

radiotherapy and combination chemotherapy at some point in their disease course, complicating the analysis of the association of chemotherapy and leukemia. The relationship of drug treatment to second neoplasms in this group of patients was considered in a 1978 review,[120] which concluded that the risk of leukemia was increased sevenfold in patients with metastatic breast cancer. A second report described the development of acute leukemia in four patients who received continuous long-term cyclophosphamide chemotherapy for breast cancer.[121] Two of the four patients also had received radiotherapy, and two had received other potentially carcinogenic antineoplastic drugs. Of interest was the mean of 6.9 years from the diagnosis of breast cancer to the development of leukemia in one report[120] and 6.3 years from institution of chemotherapy in the other.[121] These observations are consistent with the expected long latency period from exposure to appearance of the second neoplasm.

Two studies dealt with the risk of second malignancy in patients receiving adjuvant chemotherapy for breast cancer. No increased risk was identified in a group of 1265 patients who received postoperative chemotherapy (thio-TEPA), with or without radiotherapy, as compared with untreated controls.[122] The authors raised the possibility of an increased risk of second tumor for patients receiving the highest cumulative doses of chemotherapy. A second report[123] offered strong evidence for the carcinogenicity of chlorambucil. Four of 13 patients developed myeloproliferative disorders (three were definite cases of acute leukemia) following long-term continuous treatment for four or more years. The actual risk of leukemia may have been distorted by the small number of patients. However, the higher frequency of cases is of particular concern in an adjuvant therapy group, some of whom are cured of their primary disease by surgery. The ongoing prospective adjuvant studies in breast cancer should be able to address this question more definitively, but only after a delay of several years.[111, 124]

Multiple myeloma, a disease commonly treated with single agent alkylators such as melphalan, has also been associated with a high incidence of acute nonlymphocytic leukemia.[125-129] Because myeloma itself involves a bone marrow element, the possibility exists that a common process may be responsible for both diseases. However, the reported incidence of leukemia in patients with myeloma not receiving alkylating therapy is not greater than expected for an age-matched population.[104, 130] This suggests that the alkylating agents have contributed to the high incidence of leukemia. This contention is supported by a prospective trial of alkylating therapy for myeloma, which found that the actuarial risk of developing acute leukemia was 17.4 per cent at 50 months — 214 times that expected.

The incidence of second malignancies among patients with malignant lymphoma was not higher than expected in the era before intensive therapy,[107] but the use of combination chemotherapy and combined radiotherapy and chemotherapy has been associated with a high incidence of second tumors, specifically acute nonlymphocytic leukemia.[131-143] Many lymphoma patients have defective immune responsiveness (delayed hypersensitivity), which may predispose to a higher risk of cancer upon exposure to an inciting agent. The use of nitrogen mustard and procarbazine in MOPP combination chemotherapy for Hodgkin's disease may further contribute to oncogenesis in these patients, since these two agents are potent carcinogens in animals.[98] Although many reports have been concerned with an increased risk of acute leukemia, solid tumors also appear to occur more frequently in patients with malignant lymphoma following intensive therapy.[132] Arseneau and colleagues reported cases of sarcoma in Hodgkin's patients after combined radiotherapy and chemotherapy, and estimated a 23-fold increased risk of second tumor in such patients.[137] The risk of second malignancies was estimated to be increased 3.8-fold with intensive radiotherapy and 3.2-fold with intensive chemotherapy. These estimates of risk are only approximations, but they raise important questions concerning the selection of treatment for Hodgkin's disease. The Stanford clinical trials have compared radiotherapy and combined radiotherapy-chemotherapy for patients with Hodgkin's disease (Stages I, II, and III).[144] The adjuvant MOPP chemotherapy increased the duration of initial freedom from relapse, but improvement in survival was minimal. However, most relapses in the radiotherapy-only arm could be induced into a second remission with chemotherapy, so that there was no apparent survival advantage for combined treatment at an early stage of follow-up. Since combined therapy exposes patients to a higher risk of neoplasm, a long-term assessment of this study will be necessary before the risks and benefits of combined modality regimens can be understood.

In addition to their primary use in the treatment of cancer, many cytotoxic agents have effectiveness in non-neoplastic diseases. Immunosuppressive agents such as azathioprine, a precursor of 6-mercaptopurine and cyclophosphamide, have been used in the treatment of rheumatoid arthritis, scleroderma, Wegener's granulomatosis, nephrotic syndrome, and glomerulonephritis, as well as in the control of rejection in renal transplantation.[145-150] The accumulated experiences with these agents suggest a different mechanism of tumor induction from that observed in patients treated for neoplastic conditions. The former group of patients develop a high incidence of lymphomas with a predilection for primary sites in the brain, in contrast to the acute nonlymphocytic leukemia seen most commonly in cancer patients. This difference may be due to long-term immunosuppression by azathioprine or cyclophosphamide resulting in decreased immune surveillance. This state resembles the chronic immunodeficiency of certain inherited disorders[151, 152] such as Wiskott-Aldrich syndrome, which is associated with a high incidence of lymphomas. Further evidence to support the contention that chronic immunosuppression contributes to neoplastic induction is found in the experience of inadvertent engraftment of human tumors in donor kidneys. In one case, immunosuppression led to the development of a tumor of donor origin, but tumor rejection occurred rapidly after cytotoxic therapy ceased.[149] Immunosuppression is not an entirely satisfactory explanation for the high incidence of lymphomas in transplant patients, since chronic alkylating agent therapy leads to nonlymphocytic leukemia in patients with multiple myeloma or ovarian carcinoma. Continued investigations into the role of immune surveillance in carcinogenesis will be necessary to define the mechanisms responsible for development of neoplasms in immunosuppressed patients.

In summary, both clinical studies and laboratory test systems have implicated alkylating agents as potent carcinogens in man on the basis of direct induction of tumors and as a consequence of chronic immunosuppression. Similar strong evidence for carcinogenicity exists for the antitumor antibiotics and procarbazine in animal test systems. Antimetabolites as a group appear to be much less hazardous in this regard, although chronic immunosuppression with azathioprine and other agents in patients undergoing organ transplantation or treatment of nonmalignant disease does lead to an increased incidence of lymphoid malignancies, perhaps by an entirely different mechanism from that producing mutagenic effects. The combined use of chemotherapy and radiotherapy appears to add to the risk of tumor induction.

These conclusions suggest that certain guidelines should be followed in the design and use of chemotherapy-containing treatments for patients with potentially curable disease. A careful surveillance must be conducted for secondary neoplasm during long-term follow-up of these patients. An attempt should be made to establish the quantitative risk of neoplasia for any regimen that proves curative, and efforts should be made to limit the use of the more highly carcinogenic agents. On the basis of present information, consideration should be given to the use of antimetabolites in adjuvant protocols in preference to alkylating agents or antitumor antibiotics, when equal therapeutic activity can be obtained. Careful prospective and retrospective studies should be aimed at establishing whether a total dose threshold exists for carcinogenicity of suspected carcinogens in man, and whether modification of the schedule of administration affects this risk. Finally, further attention should be directed at the development of substances derived from natural sources which have no mutagenic or cytotoxic actions, but which exert regulatory actions on cell growth and differentiation. Such substances would provide a welcome alternative to cytotoxic and mutagenic chemotherapy as it exists today.

References

1. DeVita VT, Canellos GP, and Moxley JH: A decade of combination chemotherapy of advanced Hodgkin's disease. Cancer 30:1495–1504, 1972.

2. George SL, Aur RJA, Mauer AM, et al.: A reappraisal of the results of stopping therapy in childhood leukemia. N. Engl. J. Med. 300:269–273, 1979.
3. Lewis JL: Current status of treatment of gestational trophoblastic disease. Cancer 38:620–626, 1976.
4. Einhorn LH, and Donohue J: *Cis*-diamminedichloroplatinum, vinblastine, and bleomycin combination chemotherapy in disseminated testicular cancer. Ann. Intern. Med. 87:293–298, 1977.
5. Walsh PC, and Amelar RD: Embryology, anatomy and physiology of the male reproductive system. *In* Amelar RD, Dubin L, and Walsh PC (eds.): Male Infertility. W. B. Saunders Co., Philadelphia, 1977, pp. 3–32.
6. Helen CG, and Clermont Y: Kinetics of the germinal epithelium in man. Recent Prog. Horm. Res. 20:545–571, 1964.
7. Clermont Y: Kinetics of spermatogenesis in mammals: seminiferous epithelium cycle and spermatogonial renewal. Physiol. Rev. 52:198–236, 1972.
8. Lu CC, and Meistrich ML: Cytotoxic effects of chemotherapeutic drugs on mouse testis cells. Cancer Res. 39:3575–3582, 1979.
9. Jackson H: The effects of alkylating agents on fertility. Br. Med. Bull 20:107–114, 1964.
10. Jackson H, Fox BW, and Craig AW: Antifertility substances and their assessment in the male rodent. J. Reprod. Fertil. 2:447–465, 1961.
11. Fairley KF, Barrie JU, and Johnson W: Sterility and testicular atrophy related to cyclophosphamide therapy. Lancet 1:568–569, 1972.
12. Kumar R, Biggart JD, McEvoy J, et al.: Cyclophosphamide and reproductive function. Lancet 1:1212–1213, 1972.
13. Richter P, Calamera JC, Morgenfeld MC, et al.: Effect of chlorambucil on spermatogenesis in the human with malignant lymphoma. Cancer 25:1026–1030, 1970.
14. Miller DG: Alkylating agents and human spermatogenesis. J.A.M.A. 217:1662–1665, 1971.
15. Qureshi MJA, Goldsmith HJ, Pennington HJ, et al.: Cyclophosphamide therapy and sterility. Lancet 2:1290–1291, 1972.
16. Cheviakoff J, Calamera JC, Morgenfeld M, et al.: Recovery of spermatogenesis in patients with lymphoma after treatment with chlorambucil. J. Reprod. Fertil. 33:155–157, 1973.
17. Van Thiel DH, Sherins RJ, Myers GH, et al.: Evidence for a specific seminiferous tubular factor affecting follicle-stimulating hormone secretion in man. J. Clin. Invest. 51:1009–1019, 1972.
18. Mecklenberg RS, and Sherins RJ: Gonadotropin response to luteinizing hormone releasing hormone in men with germinal aplasia. J. Clin. Endocrinol. Metab. 38:1005–1009, 1974.
19. Jacobson RJ, Sagel J, Distiller LA, et al.: Leydig cell dysfunction in male patients with Hodgkin's disease receiving chemotherapy. Clin. Res. 26:437A, 1978.
20. Chapman RM, Sutcliffe SB, Rees LH, et al.: Cyclical combination chemotherapy and gonadal function. Lancet 1:285–289, 1979.
21. Sherins RJ, and DeVita VT: Effects of drug treatment for lymphoma on male reproductive capacity. Ann. Intern. Med. 79:216–220, 1973.
22. Asbjornsen G, Molne K, Klepp O, et al.: Testicular function after combination chemotherapy for Hodgkin's disease. Scand. J. Haematol. 16:66–69, 1976.
23. Chapman R, Sutcliffe, SB, Rees L. et al.: Cyclical combination chemotherapy and gonadal function. Retrospective study in males Lancet 1:265, 1979.
23a. Chapman RM, Sutcliffe SB, and Malpas JS. Male gonadal dysfunction in Hodgkin's disease. A prospective study. J.A.M.A. 245:1323, 1981.
24. Buchanan JD, Fairley KF, and Barrie JU: Return of spermatogenesis after stopping cyclophosphamide therapy. Lancet 2:156–157, 1975.
25. Hinkes E, and Plotkin D: Reversible drug-induced sterility in a patient with acute leukemia. J.A.M.A. 223:1490–1491, 1973.
26. Blake DA, Heller RH, Hsu SH, et al.: Return of fertility in a patient with cyclophosphamide-induced azoospermia. Johns Hopkins Med. J. 139:20–22, 1976.
27. Roeser HP, Stocks AE, and Smith AJ: Testicular damage due to cytotoxic drugs and recovery after cessation of therapy. Aust. N. Z. J. Med. 8:250–254, 1978.
28. Sieber SM, Correa P, Dalgard DW, et al.: Carcinogenic and other adverse effects of procarbazine in nonhuman primates. Cancer Res. 38:2125–2134, 1978.
29. deCunha MF, Meistrich ML, Reid HL, et al.: Effect of chemotherapy on human sperm production. Proc. Am. Assoc. Cancer Res. 20:100, 1979.
30. Mayer DL, and Odell WD: Physiology of Reproduction. C.V. Mosby Co., St. Louis, 1971, pp. 20–27.
31. Peters H, Byskov AG, Himelstein-Braw R, et al.: Follicular growth: the basic event in the mouse and human ovary. J. Reprod. Fertil. 4:559–566, 1975.
32. Belohorsky B, Siracky J, Sandor L, et al.: Comments on the development of amenorrhea caused by Myleran in cases of chronic myelosis. Neoplasma 4:397–402, 1960.
33. Sobrinho LG, Levine RA, and DeConti RC: Amenorrhea in patients with Hodgkin's disease treated with antineoplastic agents. Am. J. Obstet. Gynecol. 109:135–139, 1971.
34. Miller JJ, Williams GF, and Leissring JC: Multiple late complications of therapy with cyclophosphamide including ovarian destruction. Am. J. Med. 50:530–535, 1971.
35. Louis J, Limarzi LR, and Best WR: Treatment of chronic granulocytic leukemia with Myleran. Arch. Intern. Med. 97:299–300, 1950.
36. Galton DAG, Till M, and Wiltshaw E: Busulfan: summary of clinical results. Ann. N.Y. Acad. Sci. 68:967–973, 1958.
37. Fosdick WM, Parsons JL, and Hill DF: Long term cyclophosphamide therapy in rheumatoid arthritis. Arthritis Rheum. 11:151–161, 1968.
38. Warne GL, Fairley KF, Hobbs JB, et al.: Cyclophosphamide-induced ovarian failure. N. Engl. J. Med. 289:1159–1162, 1973.
39. Uldall PR, Kerr DNS, and Tacchi D: Sterility and cyclophosphamide. Lancet 1:693–694, 1972.
40. Koyama H, Wada T, Nishizawa Y, et al.: Cyclophosphamide-induced ovarian failure and its therapeutic significance in patients with breast cancer. Cancer 39:1403–1409, 1977.
41. Fisher B, Sherman B, Rockette H, et al.: L-Phenylalanine mustard in the management of premenopausal patients with primary breast cancer. Cancer 44:847–857, 1979.
42. Morgenfeld MC, Goldberg V, Parisier H, et al.: Ovarian lesions due to cytostatic agents during the treatment of Hodgkin's disease. Surg. Gynecol. Obstet. 134:826–828, 1972.
43. Sherins R, Winokur S, DeVita VT, et al.: Surprisingly high risk of functional castration in women receiving chemotherapy for lymphoma. Clin. Res. 23:343, 1975.
44. Chapman RM, Sutcliffe SB, and Malpas JS: Cytotoxic-induced ovarian failure in women with Hodgkin's disease. I. Hormone function. J.A.M.A. 242:1877–1881, 1979.
45. Pennisi AJ, Grushkin CM, and Lieberman E: Gonadal function in children with nephrosis treated with cyclophosphamide. Am. J. Dis. Child. 129:315–318, 1975.
45a. Blatt J, Poplack DG, and Sherins RJ: Testicular function in boys after chemotherapy for acute lymphoblastic leukemia. N. Engl. J. Med. 304:1121, 1981.
45b. Shalet SM, Hann IM, Lendon M, et al.: Testicular function after combination chemotherapy in childhood for acute lymphoblastic leukemia. Arch. Dis. Child. 56:275, 1981.
46. Etteldorf JN, West CD, Pitcock, JA, et al.: Gonadal function, testicular histology, and meiosis following cyclophosphamide therapy in patients with nephrotic syndrome. J. Pediatr. 88:206–212, 1976.
47. Kirkland RT, Bongiovanni AM, Cornfeld D, et al.: Gonadotropin responses to luteinizing releasing factor in boys treated with cyclophosphamide for nephrotic syndrome. J. Pediatr. 89:941–944, 1976.

48. Arneil GC: Cyclophosphamide and the prepubertal testis. Lancet 2:1259–1260, 1972.
49. Rapola J, Koskimies O, Hutternen NP, et al.: Cyclophosphamide and the pubertal testis. Lancet 1:98–99, 1973.
50. Lentz RD, Bergstein J, Steffes MW, et al.: Post-pubertal evaluation of gonadal function following cyclophosphamide therapy before and during puberty. J. Pediatr. 91:385–394, 1977.
51. Sherins RJ, Olweny CLM, and Ziegler JL: Gynecomastia and gonadal dysfunction in adolescent boys treated with combination chemotherapy for Hodgkin's disease. N. Engl. J. Med. 299:12–16, 1978.
52. Chiu J, and Drummond KN: Long-term follow-up of cyclophosphamide therapy in frequent relapsing minimal lesion nephrotic syndrome. J. Pediatr. 84:825–830, 1974.
53. DeGroot GW, Faiman C, and Winter JSD: Cyclophosphamide and the prepubertal gonad: a negative report. J. Pediatr. 84:123–125, 1974.
54. Himelstein-Braw R, Peters H, and Faber M: Morphological study of the ovaries of leukaemic children. Br. J. Cancer 38:82–87, 1978.
55. Siris EJ, Leventhal BG, and Vaitukaitis JL: Effects of childhood leukemia and chemotherapy on puberty and reproductive function in girls. N. Engl. J. Med. 294:1143–1146, 1976.
56. Lendon M, Hann IM, Palmer MK, et al.: Testicular histology after combination chemotherapy in childhood for acute lymphoblastic leukaemia. Lancet 2:439–441, 1978.
57. Vilar O: Effect of cytostatic drugs on human testicular function. *In* Mancini RE, and Martini L (eds.): Male Fertility and Sterility. Academic Press, New York, 1974, pp. 423–440.
58. Sherman JK: Synopsis of the use of frozen human semen since 1964: state of the art of human semen banking. Fertil. Steril. 24:397–412, 1973.
59. Ansbacher R: Artificial insemination with frozen spermatozoa. Fertil. Steril. 29:375–379, 1978.
60. Curie-Cohen M, Luttrell L, and Shapiro J: Current practice of artificial insemination by donor in the United States. N. Engl. J. Med. 300:585–590, 1979.
61. Johnson SA, Goldman JM, and Hawkins DF: Pregnancy after chemotherapy for Hodgkin's disease. Lancet 2:93, 1979.
62. Li FP, Fine W, Jaffee N, et al.: Offspring of patients treated for cancer in childhood. J. Natl. Cancer Inst. 62:1193–1197, 1979.
63. Van Thiel DH, Ross GT, and Lipsett MB: Pregnancies after chemotherapy of trophoblastic neoplasms. Science 169:1326–1327, 1970.
64. Holmes GE, and Holmes FF: Pregnancy outcome of patients treated for Hodgkin's disease. Cancer 41:1317–1322, 1978.
65. Haddow A: Mode of action of chemical carcinogens. Br. Med. Bull. 4:331, 1947.
66. Miller JA: Carcinogenesis by chemicals: an overview — G.H.A. Clowes Memorial Lecture. Cancer Res. 30:559, 1970.
67. Farber E: Carcinogenesis — cellular evolution as a unifying thread: Presidential address. Cancer Res. 33:2537, 1974.
68. Miller EC: Some current perspectives on chemical carcinogenesis in humans and experimental animals: Presidential address. Cancer Res. 38:1479, 1978.
69. Keller R: Suppression of natural antitumour defence mechanisms by phorbol esters. Nature 282:729, 1979.
70. Singer B: Sites in nucleic acids reacting with alkylating agents of differing carcinogenicity or mutagenicity. J. Toxicol. Environ. Health 2:1279, 1977.
71. Price CC, Gaucher GM, Koneru P, et al.: Mechanism of action of aklylating agents. Ann. N.Y. Acad. Sci. 163:593, 1969.
72. Donehower RC, Myers CE, and Chabner BA: Minireview: new developments on the mechanisms of action of antineoplastic drugs. Life Sci. 25:1, 1979.
73. Bridges BA: Short-term screening tests for carcinogens. Nature 261:195, 1976.
74. McCann J, and Ames BN: A simple method for detecting environmental carcinogens as mutagens. Ann. N.Y. Acad. Sci. 271:5, 1976.
75. McCann J, Choi E, Yamasaki E, et al.: Detection of carcinogens as mutagens in the *Salmonella*/microsome test: assay of 300 chemicals. Proc. Natl. Acad. Sci. USA 72:5135, 1975.
76. McCann, J, and Ames BN: Detection of carcinogens as mutagens in the *Salmonella*/microsome test: assay of 300 chemicals: discussion. Proc Natl. Acad. Sci. USA 73:950, 1976.
77. Benedict WF, Baker MS, Haroun L, et al.: Mutagenicity of cancer chemotherapeutic agents in the *Salmonella*/microsome test. Cancer Res. 37:2209, 1977.
78. Genther CS, Schoeny RS, Loper JC, et al.: Mutagenic studies of folic acid antagonists. Antimicrob. Agents Chemother. 12:84, 1977.
79. Brundrett RB, Colvin M, White EH, et al.: Comparison of mutagenicity, antitumor activity, and chemical properties of selected nitrosoureas and nitrosoamides. Cancer Res. 39:1328, 1979.
80. Seino Y, Nagao M, Yahagi T, et al.: Mutagenicity of several classes of antitumor agents to *Salmonella typhimurium* TA98, TA100, and TA92. Cancer Res. 38:2148, 1978.
81. Rinkus SJ, and Legator MS: Chemical characterization of 465 known or suspected carcinogens and their correlation with mutagenic activity in the *Salmonella typhimurium* system. Cancer Res. 39:3289, 1979.
82. Kato H: Spontaneous and induced sister chromatid exchanges as revealed by the BUdR-labeling method. Int. Rev. Cytol. 49:53, 1977.
83. Perry P, and Evans HJ: Cytological detection of mutagen-carcinogen exposure by sister chromatid exchange. Nature 258:121, 1975.
84. Guerrero RR, Rounds DE, and Hall TC: Bioassy procedure for the detection of mutagenic metabolites in human urine with the use of sister chromatid exchange analysis. J. Natl. Cancer Inst. 62:805, 1979.
85. Banerjee A, and Benedict WF: Production of sister chromatid exchanges by various cancer chemotherapeutic agents. Cancer Res. 39:797, 1979.
86. Lambert B, Ringborg U, Harper E, et al.: Sister chromatid exchanges in lymphocyte cultures of patients receiving chemotherapy for malignant disorders. Cancer Treat. Rep. 62:1413, 1978.
87. Lambert B, Ringborg U, Lindblad A, et al.: The effects of DTIC, melphalan, actinomycin D and CCNU on the frequency of sister chromatid exchanges in peripheral lymphocytes of melanoma patients. *In* Salmon S, and Jones SE (eds.): Adjuvant Therapy of Cancer II. Grune & Stratton, New York, 1979, p. 55.
88. Ohtsuru M, Ishi Y, Takai S, et al.: Sister chromatid exchanges in lymphocytes of cancer patients receiving mitomycin C treatment. Cancer Res. 40:477, 1980.
89. Bradley MO, Hsu IC, and Harris CC: Relationship between sister chromatid exchange and mutagenicity, toxicity and DNA damage. Nature 282:318, 1979.
90. Carrano AV, Thompson LH, Lindl PA, et al.: Sister chromatid exchange as an indicator of mutagenesis. Nature 271:551, 1978.
91. Heidelberger C: Chemical oncogenesis in culture. Adv. Cancer Res. 18:317, 1973.
92. Heidelberger C: Chemical carcinogenesis. Cancer 40:430, 1977.
93. Benedict WF, Banerjee A, Gardner A, et al.: Induction of morphological transformation in mouse C3H/10T½ clone 8 cells and chromosomal damage in hamster A(T1)C1–3 cells by cancer chemotherapeutic agents. Cancer Res. 37:2202, 1977.
94. Jones PA, Benedict WF, Baker MS, et al.: Oncogenic transformation of C3H/10T½ clone 8 mouse embryo cells by halogenated pyrimidine nucleosides. Cancer Res. 36:101, 1976.
95. Schmähl D: Carcinogenic action of antineoplastic drugs

with special reference to immunosuppression. Cancer 40:1927, 1977.

96. Schmähl D, and Habs M: Experimental carcinogenesis of antitumour drugs. Cancer Treat. Rev. 5:175, 1978.
97. Weisburger JH, Griswald DP, Prjean JD, et al.: The carcinogenic potential of some of the principal drugs used in clinical cancer chemotherapy. Recent Results Cancer Res. 52:1, 1975.
98. Weisburger EK: Bioassay program for carcinogenic hazards of cancer chemotherapeutic agents. Cancer 40:1935, 1977.
99. Solcia E, Ballerini L, Bellini O, et al.: Mammary tumors induced in rats by Adriamycin and daunomycin. Cancer Res. 38:1444, 1978.
100. Sieber SM, and Adamson RH: Toxicity of antineoplastic agents in man: chromosomal aberrations, antifertility effects, congenital malformations and carcinogenic potential. Adv. Cancer Res. 22:57, 1975.
101. Berg JW: The incidence of multiple primary cancers. I. Development of further cancers in patients with lymphomas, leukemias and myeloma. J. Natl. Cancer Inst. 38:741, 1967.
102. Schoenberg BS, Greenberg RA, and Eisenberg H: Occurrence of certain multiple primary cancers in females. J. Natl. Cancer Inst. 43:15, 1969.
103. Newell GR, Krementz ET, and Roberts JD: Multiple primary neoplasms in blacks compared to whites. II. Further cancers in patients with cancer of the buccal cavity and pharynx. J. Natl. Cancer Inst. 52:639, 1974.
104. Newell GR, Krementz ET, Roberts JD, et al.: Multiple primary neoplasms in blacks compared to whites. I. Further cancers in patients with Hodgkin's disease, leukemia and myeloma. J. Natl. Cancer Inst. 52:635, 1974.
105. Reimer R, Hoover R, Fraumeni JF, et al.: Second primary neoplasms following ovarian cancer. J. Natl. Cancer Inst. 61:1195, 1978.
106. Schottenfeld D, and Berg J: Incidence of multiple primary cancers. IV. Cancers of the female breast and genital organs. J. Natl. Cancer Inst. 46:161, 1971.
107. Moertel CG, and Hagedorn AB: Leukemia or lymphoma and coexistent primary malignant lesions: a review of the literature and a study of 120 cases. Blood 12:788, 1957.
108. Moertel CG, Dockerty MB, and Baggenstoss AH: Multiple primary malignant neoplasms. Cancer 14:221, 1961.
109. Whitelaw DM: Multiple primary carcinomas associated with Hodgkin's disease. Can. Med. Assoc. J. 99:291, 1968.
110. Watson TA: Incidence of multiple cancer. Cancer 6:365, 1953.
111. Bonadonna G, Rossi A, Valagussa P, et al.: The CMF program for operable breast cancer with positive axillary nodes. Cancer 39:2904, 1977.
112. Makuch R, and Simon R: Recommendations for the analysis of the effect of treatment on the development of second malignancies. Cancer 44:250, 1979.
113. Bagley CM, Young RC, Canellos GP, et al.: Treatment of ovarian carcinoma: possibilities for progress. N. Engl. J. Med. 287:856, 1972.
114. Einhorn N: Acute leukemia after chemotherapy (melphalan). Cancer 41:444, 1978.
115. Sotrel G, Jafari K, Lash AF, et al.: Acute leukemia in advanced ovarian carcinoma after treatment with alkylating agents. Obstet. Gynecol 47:67S, 1976.
116. Morrison J, and Yon JL: Acute leukemia following chlorambucil therapy of advanced ovarian and fallopian tube carcinoma. Gynecol. Oncol. 6:115, 1978.
117. Casciato DA, and Scott JL: Acute leukemia following prolonged cytotoxic agent therapy. Medicine 58:32, 1979.
118. Reimer RR, Hoover R, Fraumeni JF, et al.: Acute leukemia after alkylating-agent therapy of ovarian cancer. N. Engl. J. Med. 297:177, 1977.
119. Carbone PP, Bauer M, Baud P, et al.: Chemotherapy of disseminated breast cancer. Cancer 39:2916, 1977.
120. Rosner F, Carey RW, and Zarrabi MH: Breast cancer and acute leukemia. Am. J. Hematol. 4:151, 1978.
121. Portugal MA, Falkson HC, Stevens K, et al.: Acute leukemia as a complication of long-term treatment of advanced breast cancer. Cancer Treat. Rep. 63:177, 1979.
122. Chan PYM, Sadoff C, and Winkley JH: Second malignancies following first breast cancer in prolonged thio-TEPA adjuvant chemotherapy. *In* Salmon S, and Jones SE (eds.): Adjuvant Therapy of Cancer. Elsevier/North-Holland Biomedical Press, Amsterdam, 1977, p. 597.
123. Lerner HJ: Acute myelogenous leukemia in patients receiving chlorambucil as long-term adjuvant chemotherapy for stage II breast cancer. Cancer Treat. Rep. 62:1135, 1978.
124. Fisher B, Glass A, Redmond C, et al.: L-Phenylalanine mustard (L-PAM) in the management of primary breast cancer. Cancer 39:2883, 1977.
125. Kyle RA, Pierre RV, and Bayrd ED: Multiple myeloma and acute myelomonocytic leukemia. N. Engl. J. Med. 283:1121, 1970.
126. Rosner F, and Grunwald H: Multiple myeloma terminating in acute leukemia. Am. J. Med. 57:927, 1974.
127. Karchmer RK, Amare M, Larsen WE, et al.: Alkylating agents as leukemogens in multiple myeloma. Cancer 33:1103, 1974.
128. Kyle RA, Pierre RV, and Bayrd E: Multiple myeloma and acute leukemia associated with alkylating agents. Arch. Intern. Med. 135:185, 1975.
129. Bergsagel DE, Bailey AJ, Langley GR, et al.: The chemotherapy of plasma-cell myeloma and the incidence of acute leukemia. N. Engl. J. Med. 301:743, 1979.
130. Sieber SM: Cancer chemotherapeutic agents and carcinogenesis. Cancer Chemother. Rep. 59 (Part I):915, 1975.
131. Brody RS, Schottenfeld D, and Reid A: Multiple primary cancer risk after therapy for Hodgkin's disease. Cancer 40:1917, 1977.
132. Arseneau JC, Sponzo RW, Levin DL, et al.: Nonlymphomatous malignant tumors complicating Hodgkin's disease. N. Engl. J. Med. 287:1119, 1972.
133. Coleman CN, Williams JC, Flint A, et al.: Hematologic neoplasia in patients treated for Hodgkin's disease. N. Engl. J. Med. 297:1249, 1977.
134. Krikorian JG, Burke JS, Rosenberg SA, et al.: Occurrence of non-Hodgkin's lymphoma after therapy of Hodgkin's disease. N. Engl. J. Med. 300:452, 1979.
135. Canellos GP, DeVita VT, Arseneau JC, et al.: Carcinogenesis by cancer chemotherapeutic agents: second malignancies complicating Hodgkin's disease in remission. Recent Results Cancer Res. 49:108, 1974.
136. Canellos GP, Arseneau JC, DeVita VT, et al.: Second malignancies complicating Hodgkin's disease in remission. Lancet 1:947, 1975.
137. Arseneau JC, Canellos GP, Johnson R, et al.: Risk of new cancers in patients with Hodgkin's disease. Cancer 40:1912, 1977.
138. Cadman EC, Capizzi RL, and Bertino JR: Acute nonlymphocytic leukemia. Cancer 40:1280, 1977.
139. Crosby WH: Acute granulocytic leukemia, a complication of therapy in Hodgkin's disease. Clin. Res. 17:463, 1969.
140. Rosner F, and Grunwald H: Hodgkin's disease and acute leukemia. Am. J. Med. 58:339, 1975.
141. Toland DM, and Coltman CA: Second malignancies complicating Hodgkin's disease. Blood 46:1013, 1975.
142. Zarrabi MH, Rosner F, and Bennett JM: Non-Hodgkin's lymphoma and acute myeloblastic leukemia: report of 10 cases and review of the literature. Blood 50:213, 1977.
143. Zarrabi MH, Rosner F, and Bennett JM: Non-Hodgkin's lymphoma and acute myeloblastic leukemia. Cancer 44:1070, 1979.
144. Rosenberg SA, Kaplan HS, Glatstein EJ, et al.: Combined modality therapy of Hodgkin's disease. Cancer 42:991, 1978.
145. Tchernia G, Mielot F, Subtil E, et al.: Acute myeloblastic

leukemia after immunodepressive therapy for primary nonmalignant disease. Blood Cells 2:67, 1976.

146. Roberts MM: Acute leukemia after immunosuppressive therapy. Lancet 2:768, 1976.

147. Carcassonne Y, Gastaut JA, and Blanc AP: Acute leukemia after prolonged immunosuppressive therapy for glomerulonephritis. Cancer Treat. Rep. 62:1110, 1978.

148. Westberg NG, and Swolin B: Acute myeloid leukemia appearing in two patients after prolonged continuous chlorambucil treatment for Wegener's granulomatosis. Acta Med. Scand. 199:373, 1976.

149. Penn I: Second malignant neoplasms associated with immunosuppressive medication. Cancer 37:1024, 1976.

150. Steinberg AD, Plotz PH, Wolff SM, et al.: Cytotoxic drugs in treatment of nonmalignant diseases. Ann. Intern. Med. 76:619, 1972.

151. Waldmann TA, Strober W, and Blaese RM: Immunodeficiency disease and malignancy. Ann. Intern. Med. 77:605, 1972.

152. Penn I: Occurrence of cancer in immune deficiencies. Cancer 34:858, 1974.

153. Latt SA, Schreck RR, Loveday KS, et al.: *In vitro* and *in vivo* analysis of sister chromatid exchange. Pharmacol. Rev. 30:501, 1979.

Section II

7 STEROID THERAPY OF CANCER

Marc E. Lippman
Charles Eil

INTRODUCTION

The rational application of any given drug requires a clear understanding of its mechanism of action and a detailed knowledge of its clinical pharmacology. In no area of antineoplastic therapy has such knowledge more impressively increased efficacy and safety than in that of steroid therapy. The mechanism by which all classes of steroid hormones induce their phenotypic effects on target tissues has permitted a precise identification of those patients who have hormone-dependent tumors. Second, the establishment of hormone-dependent cell culture systems and the derivation of hormone-independent variants or mutant sublines has focused attention on the ways in which loss of hormone responsiveness may occur. Third, an understanding of the pathways of steroid biosynthesis and peripheral metabolism, as well as central nervous system regulation of gonadal and adrenal function, has permitted pharmacologic interference with normal endocrine function.

This chapter provides an in-depth examination of the role of steroid hormones in the treatment of malignant disease.

HISTORICAL BACKGROUND

The earliest demonstration of the biologic significance of steroids came in 1849 when Berthold showed that the effects of castration on the cockscomb could be prevented by testis transplantation. Thus, the origin of endocrinology as a discipline began with androgen deprivation and restoration. Since that time the steroid hormones have been isolated, purified, and demonstrated to induce numerous and diverse biologic effects in vertebrate species. Physiologically important steroids include the bile acids, the sterols, the adrenocortical hormones, the androgens, the estrogens, and the progestins. These agents, whether from endogenous or exogenous sources, can have profound influence on both physiologic and pathologic processes.

STRUCTURE AND NOMENCLATURE

Detailed chemical descriptions and nomenclature of these compounds are available in other sources.[1-9] A brief overview of these topics will aid in comprehension of subsequent discussions.

The basic steroid nucleus is the hydrated four-ring system of cyclopentane-perhydrophenanthrene, in which the five-sided D ring is attached to the three six-sided rings of phenanthrene (Fig. 7–1). The carbon atoms of the basic ring structure are numbered 1 to 17; those of the side chain occurring in the sex hormones are 18 for the carbon atom attached to no. 13, 19 for the carbon atom attached to no. 10, and 20 and 21 for the side chain attached to no. 17 (Fig. 7–2) in the

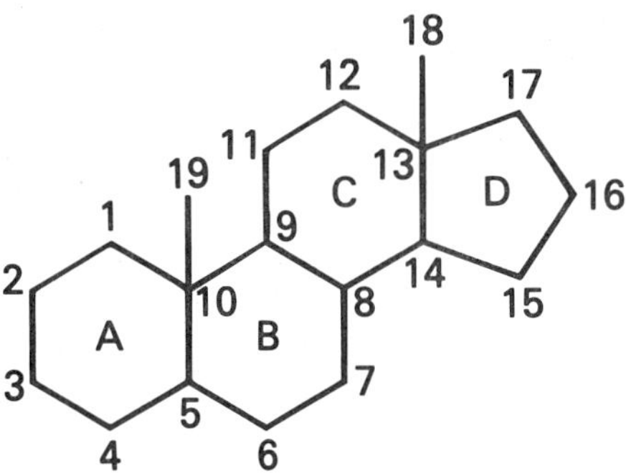

Steroid Nucleus

Figure 7–1. The structure and numbering of the cyclopentane-perhydrophenanthrene nucleus.

corticoids and progestins. The trivial (or common) and systematic names of the five major steroid hormones are also shown in Figure 7–2. Table 7–1 provides a list of the derivative names for other clinically relevant compounds.

GENERAL COMMENTS ON HORMONE BIOSYNTHESIS AND TRANSPORT

The ultimate source of all endogenous steroid molecules is cholesterol, which derives either directly from the diet or via endogenous synthesis from acetate. All tissues, except possibly those of the adult brain, can synthesize cholesterol, although quantitatively the liver is the most important source.[10] The adrenal gland synthesizes and secretes variable amounts of all five classes of the steroid hormones: glucocorticoids, mineralocorticoids, androgens, estrogens, and progestins. The testes and ovaries both synthesize and secrete androgens and estrogens in differing amounts. Progesterone, the most significant endogenous progestin, derives predominantly from the corpus luteum. However, the placenta is responsible for the increased amounts of progesterone and estrogens synthesized during pregnancy. Figure 7–3 summarizes the enzymatic steps required for the formation of all these compounds. The specific reactions and sites involved in the biosynthesis of each major class of hormones will be dealt with in separate sections devoted to each.

Although all the steroids circulate in the blood stream to reach their target tissues, they are predominantly bound to plasma proteins, i.e., albumin and specific steroid binding globulins. Cortisol and progesterone circulate bound primarily to corticosteroid binding globulin (CBG), also called transcor-

21
20

PREGNANE
(corticoids and progestins)
C_{21}

ANDROSTANE
(androgens)
C_{19}

ESTRANE
(estrogens)
C_{18}

THE FIVE MAJOR STEROID HORMONES:

TRIVIAL NAME	SYSTEMATIC NAME
CORTISOL	4-PREGNEN-11β, 17α, 21-TRIOL-3, 20-DIONE
ALDOSTERONE	4-PREGNEN-11β, 21-DIOL-18-AL-3, 20-DIONE
PROGESTERONE	4-PREGNEN-3, 20-DIONE
TESTOSTERONE	4-ANDROSTEN-17β-OL-3-ONE
ESTRADIOL	1,3,5(10)-ESTRATRIEN-3, 17β-DIOL

Figure 7–2. The structure and names of the five major steroid hormones.

TABLE 7–1. Trivial and Systematic Names for Clinically Relevant Steroids and Analogues

Adrenal Steroids and Antagonists	
Androstenedione	Androst-4-ene-3,17-dione
Betamethasone	9-Fluoro-11β,17,21-trihydroxy-16β-methylpregna-1,4-diene-3,20-dione valerate
Cortisone	17α, 21-Dihydroxy-pregn-4-ene-3,11,20-trione
Dehydroepiandrosterone	3β-Hydroxyandrost-5-en-17-one
Dexamethasone (Decadron)	9α-Fluoro-16d-methy-11β,17α,20-trihydroxypregna-1,4-diene-3,20-dione
Fluorocortisone (Florinef)	9α-Fluoro-11β,17α,21-trihydroxy-pregna-4-ene-3,20-dione
Methylprednisolone	16α-Methyl-11β,17α,21-trihydroxypregna-1,4-diene-3,20-dione
Prednisolone	11β,17α,21-Trihydroxypregna-1,4-diene-3,20-dione
Prednisone	17α,21-Dihydroxypregna-1,4-diene-3,11,20-trione
Spironolactone (Aldactone)	17-Hydroxy-7-mercapto-3-oxo-17α-pregna-4-ene-21-carboxylic acid γ-lactone, 7-acetate
Triamcinolone	9α-Fluoro-11β,16α,21-tetrahydroxypregna-1.4-diene-3,20-dione
Androgens and Antiandrogens	
STEROIDAL	
Cyproterone acetate	6-Chloro-1α,2α-methylene-4,6-pregnadien-17-ol-3,20-dione acetate
Fluoxymesterone (Halotestin)	9α-Fluoro-17α-methyl-4-androsten-4β,17-diol-3-one
Mesterolone	1α-Methyl-5α-androstan-17β-0l-3-one
Methyltestosterone	17α-Methyl-4-androstan-17-0l-3-one
Methyltrienolone (R1881)	17α-Methyl-4,9,11-androstatriene-17-0l-3-one
Nandrolone phenylpropionate	19-Nor-4-androsten-17β-0l-3-one-phenylpropionate
Oxandrolone	17α-Methyl-2-oxa-5α-androstan-17-0l-3-one
R2956	2α,2β,17α-Trimethyl-4,9,11-estratrien-17-0l-3-one
Testololactone (Teslac)	17α-Oxa-0-homo-1,4-androstadiene-3,17-dione
Testosterone enanthate	4-Androsten-17β-0l-3-one enanthate
Testosterone propionate	4-Androsten-17β-0l-3-one-propionate
NONSTEROIDAL	
Flutamide	4′-Nitro-3′-trifluorome thylisobutyranilide
Estrogens and Anti-Estrogens	
STEROIDAL	
Estradiol	1,3,5-Estratriene-3,17β-diol
Estradiol benzoate	1,3,5-Estratriene-3-17β-diol-3 benzoate
Estriol	1,3,5-Estratriene-3,16α,17β-triol
Estrone	1,3,5-Estratriene-3-0l-17-one
Ethinyl estradiol	17α-Ethinyl-1,3,5-estratriene-3,17β-diol
NONSTEROIDAL	
Clomiphene	2-[4-(2-Chloro-1,2-diphenylvinyl)phenoxy] triethylamine
Dienestrol	3,4-Di-p-hydroxyphenylhex-2,4-diene
Diethylstilbestrol	3,4-Di-p-hydroxyphenylhex-3-ene
Nafoxidine	3,4-Dihydro-6-methoxy-2-phenyl-1-pyrrolidinoethexyphenyl-neptholene
Tamoxifen	trans-1-(p-β-Dimethylaminoethoxyphenyl)-1,2-diphenylbut-1-ene
Progesterones	
ETHISTERONE	
Medroxyprogesterone acetate	6α-Methyl-4-pregnon-17-0l-3,20-dione acetate
Megestrol acetate	6-Methyl-4,6-pregnadien-17-0l-3,20-dione acetate
Norethisterone	17α-Ethinyl-18-methyl-4-pregnene 17-0l-3-one
Norgestrel	17α-Ethinyl-18-methyl-4-pregnene 17-0l-3-one
R-5020	17,21-Dimethyl-19-nor-4,9-pregnadiene-3,20-dione

tin, while the androgens and estrogens are transported via testosterone-estradiol binding globulin (TEBG) or sex steroid binding globulin (SSBG). Although aldosterone is present in the blood in far smaller amounts than most of the other steroids, binding globulins have also been described for the mineralocorticoids.[11, 12] In any case, for all the steroids, it is the unbound or free hormone that enters cells and therefore is considered biologically active. Presumably the hormone enters the cell by a non-energy-dependent process, the cell membrane providing a favorable, lipid-rich environment for passage of the hormone by diffusion. Specific uptake mechanisms (i.e., non-

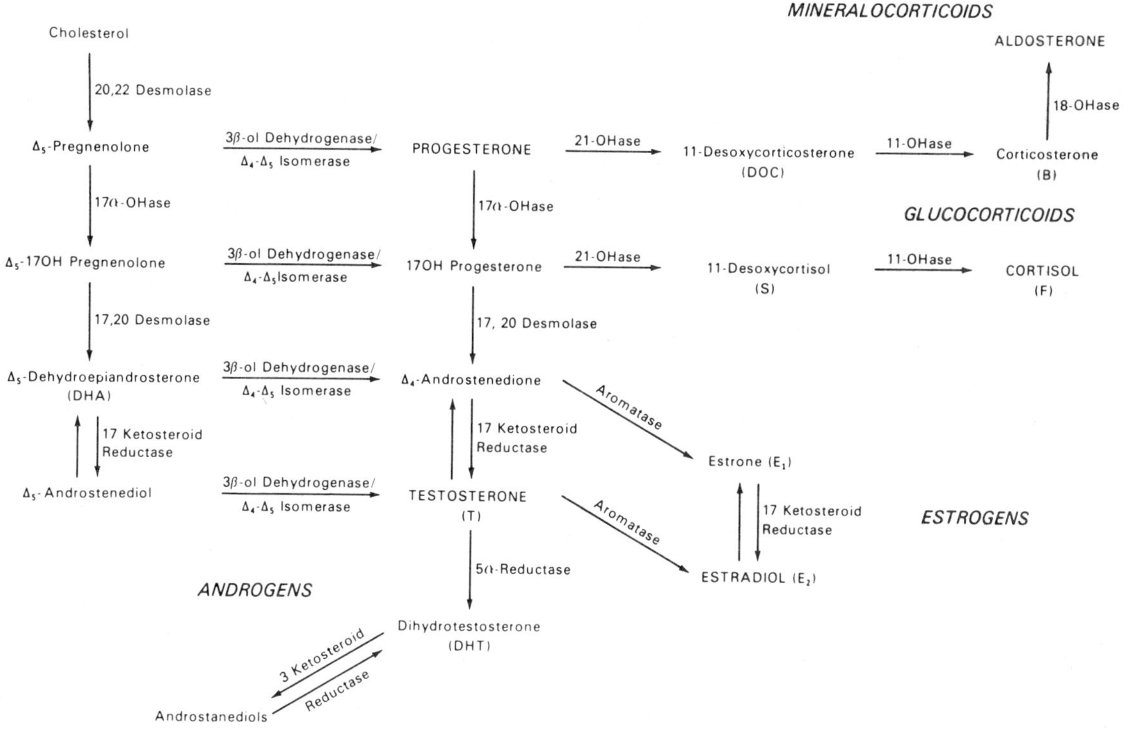

Figure 7–3. Enzymatic steps in the biosynthesis of the steroid hormones.

passive) for the hormones have been suggested by some experimental data, although evidence is generally regarded as inconclusive.[13-16]

Mechanism of Steroid Hormone Action

A knowledge of the physiologic concentrations at which the steroids circulate is critical in order to account for their mechanisms of action. Although the concentrations of total hormone in the blood range from a high of approximately 10^{-7}M for cortisol to a low of 3×10^{-11}M for estradiol, the free concentrations are even lower, depending on the extent to which the steroids are bound to serum proteins. Before the advent of radioimmunoassay or other competitive binding assays, the very low concentration of these hormones required for their biologic potency was not fully appreciated. As a consequence, it is not surprising that older reviews of steroid hormones portrayed these compounds as allosteric effectors, coenzymes, stabilizers of lysosomes *in vitro*, modifiers of mitochondrial ionic content, and inducers of various membrane effects.[17-20] This earlier work is generally disregarded because these effects were achieved only with nonphysiologic concentrations of hormone.

Over the past two decades a more uniform theory of steroid hormone action has developed, thanks in large part to the pioneering work of Jensen and Jacobsen.[21] They synthesized radiolabeled estradiol with very high specific activity, and demonstrated that estrogen was preferentially sequestered and retained by its target organs, the uterus and vagina. Cellular components were then sought that could account for this retention as well as for the structure activity relationships of other congeners. From these intense efforts emerged a unifying current concept of steroid hormone action, summarized in Figure 7–4. Although several recent thorough reviews of this topic are available,[22-28] we will provide an overview of how steroid hormones induce their diverse effects.

Receptors. The lynchpin of the current theory of steroid hormone action is the presence in the target tissues of specific hormone "receptors." Once inside the cell, steroid hormones bind to specific proteins, which are called "receptors" if they fulfill the fol-

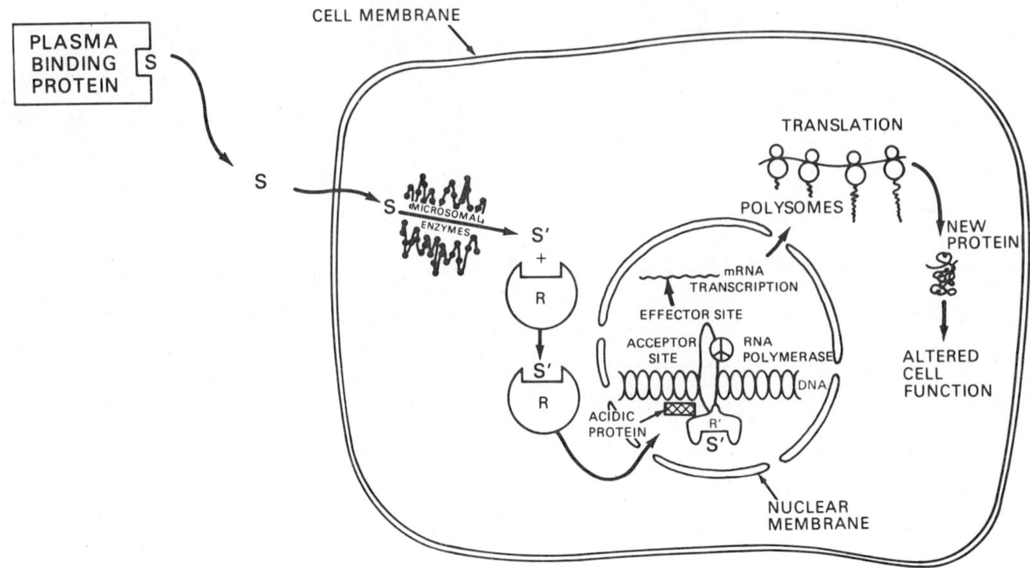

Figure 7–4. Schematic representation of the mechanisms of steroid hormone action.

lowing criteria: (1) they have limited binding capacity and high affinity for a particular hormone (binding affinities should agree with dose-response information); (2) they are generally localized in tissues that respond in some way to the hormone; (3) there exists a reasonable correlation between binding specificity and biologic effect for hormone analogues; (4) association, dissociation, and nuclear translocation of the hormone-receptor complex are consistent with the observed response data; and (5) genetic disorders of hormone action must be accounted for by deletions or alterations in the above scheme of hormone action. None of these criteria constitutes unequivocal proof for the role of receptors as mediators of steroid hormone action. Unequivocal proof of "receptor" function will derive from (and only from) *in vivo* or *in vitro* reconstitution experiments; i.e., the induction of a steroid hormone response by the addition of purified receptor to a previously unresponsive system lacking receptor.

Steroid receptors are detected classically by competitive assay with radiolabeled hormone of high specific activity, followed by some physicochemical method of separating receptor-bound from free hormone (dextran-coated charcoal, sucrose gradient centrifugation, gel chromatography, isoelectric focusing, etc.). More recently, monoclonal antibodies directed against estrogen receptor have been produced[29] and quantification of receptor by specific radioimmunoassay may soon be possible. Alternatively, histochemical techniques using fluorescent probes have shown some promise,[30-32] although none have been adequately validated. Although the numbers vary with the tissue and the hormone, there are approximately 5000 to 200,000 receptors for a given hormone per cell. The intracellular distribution of receptor between cytoplasm and the nucleus is influenced by the conditions of preparation, and possibly by free water content.[33] Glucocorticoid receptors have been found in most mammalian tissues, consistent with the ubiquity of the effects of these agents. Receptors for other steroids, however, are much more restricted in their distribution, reflecting the more limited tissue domain controlled by these hormones. Although somewhat controversial, the magnitude of the hormonal response may be governed not only by the concentration of the hormone, but also by the number of steroid hormone receptors present in the cell. For example, the condition of complete androgen insensitivity, also known as "testicular feminization," is a form of male pseudohermaphroditism in which a 46XY phenotypic female with testes makes adequate amounts of androgens, but is unable to respond to them because the target tissues completely lack androgen receptors.[34-36] Attempts have been made to characterize the syndromes of partial androgen insensitivity (incomplete "testicular feminization" and Reifenstein's syndrome), i.e., 46XY individuals with ambiguous genitalia or incomplete virilization, by decreased amounts of androgen receptors. Fibroblasts cultured from affected individuals often have fewer androgen receptors compared with androgen receptor levels in fibroblasts from normal controls.[37-39] Similar efforts have been undertaken to correlate the number of steroid receptors and antitumor response for various steroid hormone receptors in patients with leukemia, breast cancer, and prostate carcinoma, as described later in this chapter.

Activation and Translocation. In order for the steroid hormones to induce their effects, the hormone-receptor complex formed in the cytoplasm must be transferred into the nucleus. Following the initial binding of the steroid hormone to its cytoplasmic receptor, the complex undergoes activation, a poorly understood transformation of the receptor that allows it to bind to nuclear components. The process of receptor activation probably alters the affinity of the steroid-receptor complex for nuclear components, since there are no known barriers to diffusion of proteins the size of receptors through nuclear pores. The best test of the essential role of this activation process in steroid hormone action is provided by glucocorticoid-insensitive mutant sublines of leukemic lymphoblasts, which have receptors that bind hormone normally but cannot translocate it to the nucleus.[40]

Presumably, the steroid-receptor complex binds to the specific sites on the target cell genome. Although poorly defined at present, these "acceptor" sites are believed to be involved in specific gene activation elicited by binding of the appropriate hormone-receptor unit. Although the details of the molecular biology of the mechanism of action for each steroid hormone are not at the same level of knowledge, a similar process may well occur for all the hormones. For this reason, it is hoped that what is currently known about the chick oviduct progesterone receptor, the best studied of the intracellular binding proteins, applies also to the other steroid hormone receptors.

Studies of this receptor have suggested molecular heterogeneity. When target tissues are homogenized, the resultant extracts contain binding species whose size and shape appear to be sensitive to the ionic environment. At low ionic strength, for all the steroid hormones, sucrose density gradient centrifugation of cytosol often reveals a discrete peak with a sedimentation coefficient of approximately 7 to 8S. Although this peak is now known to represent aggregates,[41] this artifact of preparation is useful since it discriminates "receptor" proteins from serum binding proteins that sediment at 4S. In the presence of "high salt" (usually 0.3 to 0.4M potassium chloride) the sedimentation coefficient of the binder changes to 3 to 4S. In some instances more than one form, either structural or conformational, may exist. These differences in sedimentation coefficients are possibly accounted for by the marked asymmetric shapes of the receptor proteins, which can be altered thermally and ionically. In the case of the chick oviduct progesterone receptor, the classic 8S receptor can be shifted to a form sedimenting at 6S using intermediate ionic strength conditions and a 4S form using high salt. Schrader hypothesizes that the 6S receptor is a dimer of two dissimilar subunit molecules, termed A and B subunits, both of which have the ability to bind the hormone.[42] Both components have been purified to homogeneity. Although these subunits differ significantly in molecular weight (79,000 versus 117,000 daltons), both appear to sediment at 4S in high salt. Further structural analysis of the subunits has been hampered by the current failure to generate antibodies to completely purify the components. Functional studies with purified A and B progesterone receptor subunits show that the B subunit binds to the nonhistone protein-DNA complexes of oviduct chromatin but not to pure DNA, whereas the A subunit binds to pure DNA but poorly to chromatin.[42] Schrader and colleagues have speculated that the B subunit may be acting as a site-specific binder to localize the dimer in certain regions of chromatin, while the A subunit may alter the local structure or conformation of a segment of DNA so that altered mRNA synthesis can occur.[43]

The actual mechanism of activation (if there is a single one for all classes of steroid receptors) is not well understood. When cytosol estrogen receptors are centrifuged through sucrose gradients at physiologic ionic strength and binding performed after sedimentation, the receptor sediments mainly at about 5S, suggesting that this is the form that exists in the cytosol *in vivo* in the absence of estrogen.[44] Upon formation of the cytosol estrogen-receptor complex, the 5S receptor undergoes a change to a 4S form, which is indistinguishable by sedimentation properties from translocated receptor extracted from nuclei by high salt. Gel filtration of these forms indicates that this conversion involves the cleavage of the larger form by a calcium-dependent protease.[45] Other protein modifications, such as reversible phosphorylation as suggested by the experiments of Pratt and Nielsen,[47, 48] may also be involved in receptor activation and inactivation. Moreover, Notides has even suggested that activation may involve the addition of a subunit.[49] Finally, another hypothesis of "activation" is that the binding of the steroid to the receptor protein alters the protein conformation in such a way that a previously hindered site is exposed, promoting translocation of the complex into the nucleus and/or binding to specific sites on the chromatin. Activation, therefore, may be different for each steroid-receptor complex.

The activation process appears to be temperature-dependent. For example, when uterine cytosol is incubated at 37°C in the presence of estradiol, a receptor-estradiol complex is formed that sediments at 5S (instead of 4S) on high salt sucrose gradients. This "transformed" receptor complex binds to isolated nuclei, whereas no binding occurs when the estradiol-cytosol mixture is incubated with nuclei at 0°C. The characteristics of these "nuclear" receptors are similar to those described for the cytoplasmic forms: high binding affinity, limited binding capacity, steroid and tissue specificity, and frequent correlation with biologic response.

Both components of chromatin, the DNA and the proteins packaging the DNA, appear to influence the nuclear binding of steroid-receptor complexes. Spelsberg's data suggest that occupied receptors bind to purified DNA, but with lesser affinity and specificity as compared with their binding to chromatin.[51] Additionally, optimal receptor binding to nuclei is observed with target cell chromatin. In reconstruction experiments, specific binding of progesterone receptor to nontarget tissue chromatin is promoted by addition of component(s) of nonhistone chromosomal proteins from chick oviduct, a target tissue of this hormone.[51] The study of nuclear "acceptor" sites has been hindered by failure to demonstrate convincingly a specific nuclear protein or DNA sequence responsible for receptor binding. In many target tissues, the best estimate of the number of genes activated by the hormone is less than 20 (e.g., aldosterone binding in the toad bladder or glucocorticoid binding in HTC cells). It is difficult to rationalize this observation in light of the fact that hormone-receptor complexes bind to thousands of nuclear sites. Because the number of nuclear "acceptors" is high, in some cases even greater than the number of receptors and probably far in excess of the number of messenger RNA's regulated by the steroid, it is possible that the receptor-steroid complexes are binding to "acceptor" sites that are not physiologically relevant in some target tissues. Alternatively, occupancy of a redundant number of such sites may be a requirement for optimal direction of receptor complexes to a far smaller number of specific loci.

Postreceptor Events. In any case, the binding of receptor-steroid complexes with the nuclear chromatin results in changes in the concentration of hybridizable and translatable mRNA species in the cytoplasm. Although this increase in specific polysomic mRNA might represent an altered rate of primary transcription, many other effects could lead to the same net result. These include altered rates of message splicing (the removal of introns), effects on capping or polyadenylation, or even effects on specific mRNA half-lives. In fact, for most steroid hormone effects, the evidence that mRNA is regulated at the level of transcription is derived indirectly from antibiotic inhibition experiments. For some steroid hormone actions, such as glucocorticoid-induced inhibition or killing of lymphocytes, specific protein or RNA mediators of the effect have never been identified. Killing of normal and malignant lymphocytes in culture occurs at low concentrations of glucocorticoid that just saturate receptor sites. Killing is well correlated with binding affinity of different compounds.

There are only two bases for assuming that primary transcription by RNA polymerase is the most important site regulated by steroid hormones. First, by analogy to prokaryotic systems that lack a nuclear envelope and in which translation can occur on mRNA molecules still being transcribed, gene expression appears to be controlled at the transcription step. The second comes from preliminary data on the ovalbumin gene for which probes of primary gene transcripts have been developed.[52] In this latter system, evidence suggests that the formation of initiation sites on the DNA and the production of nonprocessed transcripts is rate-limiting for production of mature ovalbumin mRNA.[53] Secondary (but important) effects on other aspects of this system also occur, since it is known that ovalbumin mRNA is translated *in vitro* more efficiently in heterologous systems containing oviduct "translation" factors and that ovalbumin mRNA has a longer half-life in induced than in regressed oviducts.[54]

Steroid-induced effects on gene transcription lead to secondary changes in RNA translation and protein synthesis. These induced proteins are then responsible for some immediate or ultimate hormonal response. The variable control of specific messenger RNA's by hormones might account for poorly coordinated synthesis of chick egg-white proteins other than ovalbumin (namely conalbumin, ovomucoid, and lysozyme) as stimulated by estrogen.[55] Differential rates of translation, protein catabolism, or secretion could also explain these differences. Thus, the rate of synthesis of one or more of the proteins could change in relation to the others even though they were all synthesized in the same cell. Examples of specific proteins induced by steroid hormones are shown in Table 7–2.

Nonreceptor-Mediated Steroid Effects. Despite the overwhelming evidence that favors receptor mediation of steroid-hormone action, some experiments are not well explained by the currently accepted theory. For example, physiologic concentrations of estrogens catalyze transhydrogenations by purified hydroxy-steroid dehydrogenases.[56] Other effects have been described that do not require receptor mediation, among them direct steroid binding to nucleic acids.[57] Hydrocortisone binds to phenylalanyl RNA and affects amino acid incorporation into protein in *in vitro* translation systems.[58] Steroids also bind to histones and other cellular proteins,[59,60] but there is no convincing evidence for a physiologic role for such binding in either case.

Rabin et al. have provided evidence that smooth endoplasmic reticulum from rat liver of one sex preferentially binds the sex steroid of the opposite sex, albeit at supraphysiologic concentrations, and that this binding promotes the formation *in vitro* of membrane-polysome complexes.[61,62] Since different proteins may be synthesized on

TABLE 7–2. Specific Proteins Induced by Steroid Hormones

	Tissue	*Protein*
GLUCOCORTICOIDS		
	Liver and hepatoma	Tyrosine aminotransferase
		Tryptophan oxygenase
	Kidney	Phosphoenol pyruvate carboxykinase
	Mouse mammary cancer cells	Mammary tumor virus RNA
	Embryonic chick retina	Glutamine synthetase
	Rat pituicytes in culture	Growth hormone
	HeLa cells	Alkaline phosphatase
ANDROGENS		
	Rat liver	Alpha 2_u globulin
	Rat prostate	Aldolase
	Mouse liver	Major urinary protein complex
	Mouse kidney	β-glucuronidase
ESTROGENS		
	Chick oviduct	Ovalbumin
		Conalbumin, ovomucoid, lysozyme
	Chick liver	ApoVLDL-II
		Vitellogenin, transferrin
	Xenopus liver	Vitellogenin
	Rat pituitary	Prolactin
	Breast cancer cells	Progesterone receptor
PROGESTERONE		
	Chick oviduct	Avidin, ovalbumin, ovomucoid, conalbumin, lysozyme
	Rabbit uterus	Uteroglobin

free, as opposed to bound, polysomes, these findings imply that steroids could influence cellular protein production by modulating the ratio of free/bound ribosomes.

Other effects of steroids, the rapidity of which suggests a direct action rather than receptor-mediated gene activation, include: adenylate cyclase activation following five-minute exposure of human leukocytes to concentrations of cortisol less than 10^{-6}M[63]; the rapid cessation of pituitary ACTH secretion following cortisol treatment of adrenally insufficient patients[64]; and the rapid increment in uterine intravenous estrogens.[65] Unfortunately, none of these heterodox observations have received sufficient attention to allow any firm conclusions to be drawn regarding their physiologic relevance.

Mechanisms of Hormone Resistance

One can imagine a number of ways in which a target tissue may fail to demonstrate a hormonal response (see Table 7–3). First, the hormone may not be synthesized, as occurs in various forms of congenital adrenal hyperplasia and male pseudohermaphroditism due to adrenal or testicular enzyme deficiencies.[66, 67] Individuals with these conditions, however, are not resistant to exogenous hormone treatment. Second, even if the hormone is synthesized adequately, rapid metabolic clearance peripherally may prevent sufficient exposure of the target tissues. Resistance to hormone action may arise owing to a deficiency of hormone receptors, as in receptor-deficient breast cancer. Alternatively, if receptors are present they may be defective in binding the ligand (either because of a faulty receptor molecule or because of the presence of a receptor antagonist), in entering the nucleus, or in binding of the hormone-receptor complex to the chromatin. If the receptor is not defective in any of its functions, it is possible that hormone insensitivity may result from absent or abnormal chromatin components forming the "acceptor" sites required for appropriate binding of the hormone-receptor complex inside the nucleus. Finally, the responding mechanism (i.e., RNA polymerase, mRNA processing, specific message translation, and so forth) may be incapable of operating properly despite normal chromatin-hormone-receptor interactions. Mutations with such "postreceptor" defects have been postulated when apparently normal hormone receptors have been identified in cells from hormone-resistant phenotypes.[36, 68, 69] When the information is available, examples of each kind of hormone resistance will be provided in the following discussion of individual hormones.

TABLE 7–3. Potential Mechanisms of Apparent Hormone Resistance

I. Defective hormone biosynthesis

II. Rapid metabolic clearance of hormone

III. Receptor defects
- A. Complete receptor deficiency
- B. Competition by receptor antagonist
- C. Receptor with altered ligand affinity
- D. Unstable receptor
- E. Receptor unable to activate or enter nucleus
- F. Hormone-receptor complex unable to bind to chromatin

IV. Postreceptor defects
- A. Absent or abnormal "acceptor" sites
- B. Defective triggering of RNA polymerase
- C. Mutation of gene coding for mRNA responsible for physiologic effect
- D. Incomplete or aberrant mRNA translation
- E. Altered specific mRNA processing
- F. Increased mRNA degradation

GLUCOCORTICOIDS

The physiologic effects of the glucocorticoids are many and protean (Table 7–4). Insight into the role of glucocorticoid hormones in maintaining homeostasis arose early from the recognition of the pathologic conditions of glucocorticoid deficiency and excess. In 1855 Addison provided the classic description of the wasting disease associated with the destruction of the "suprarenal" glands,[70] and shortly thereafter Brown-Séquard demonstrated the essential role of the adrenal gland in sustaining life in dogs.[71] The syndrome of glucocorticoid excess was characterized in 1932 by Harvey Cushing,[72] and as a result of this description the condition bears his name.

It is now known that adrenal function is regulated in a circadian fashion by the pituitary gland. In 1926 Foster and Smith established that hypophysectomy resulted in adrenal atrophy,[73] which in 1932 was shown by several groups[74-76] to be reversed by treatment with extracts of the pituitary. The

TABLE 7–4. Major Physiologic Effects of Glucocorticoids

Metabolic Effects
- A. Carbohydrate
  1. Increased blood sugar
  2. Increased hepatic glycogenolysis and glyconeogenesis
  3. Decreased peripheral uptake of glucose by adipose, lymphoid, and connective tissue
- B. Protein
  1. Increased protein degradation and decreased protein synthesis in muscle, adipose, lymphoid, and connective tissue, providing increased amino acids for hepatic protein synthesis and glyconeogenesis
- C. Lipid
  1. Increased mobilization of free fatty acids from triglyceride

Circulatory Effects
- A. Increased cardiac output
- B. Increased sensitivity to the pressor effects of catecholamines
- C. Sodium retention by the kidney

Musculoskeletal Effects
- A. Increased capacity for work

Immune Modulation

agent in these extracts, adrenocorticotrophic hormone (ACTH), was purified by 1943,[77, 78] chemically and structurally identified by 1956,[79] and synthesized by 1963.[80]

Under the negative feedback mechanisms governing the release of ACTH, the glucocorticoids are synthesized in the fasciculata zone of the adrenal cortex from cholesterol upon binding of ACTH to the steroid synthesizing cells (see Fig. 7–3). The rate-limiting step is generally considered to be the conversion of cholesterol to Δ_5-pregnenolone, by a mechanism mediated by cyclic AMP and calcium ions, possibly requiring the synthesis of a short-lived protein.[81] The capacity of the adrenal gland for steroidogenesis is rapid (taking place within minutes) and great: the daily production of cortisol can be increased up to tenfold in periods of stress.

Once synthesized in the adrenal, cortisol enters the circulation and reaches the periphery mostly bound to plasma proteins including albumin, orosomucoid (α-acidic glycoprotein), and corticosteroid binding globulin (CBG), a glycoprotein also known as transcortin.[82] These proteins differ in their binding affinities for the corticoids (CBG having the highest and albumin the lowest) and in their plasma concentrations. At physiologic concentrations of cortisol in human plasma (approximately 10 gm/dl), 76 per cent of cortisol is bound to CBG, 13.5 per cent is bound to albumin, 10.5 per cent is unbound, and negligible amounts are bound to orosomucoid. Certain changes in endocrine status can alter the binding capacity of CBG and therefore the total blood levels of the steroids (although the amount of free hormone does not change drastically because of normal feedback control of pituitary ACTH secretion). Estrogens stimulate CBG synthesis in the liver and, as a result, total cortisol levels are markedly elevated during pregnancy. However, hypercortisolism is not evident clinically, because the transcortin-bound steroid is not biologically active.[83, 84] Corticosteroids also affect CBG levels: adrenalectomy causes a decrease in plasma CBG that is reversible with cortisol replacement.[85] Moreover, CBG activity can be significantly increased by suppression of endogenous cortisol secretion with dexamethasone,[82] an extremely potent synthetic glucocorticoid. Finally, thyroidectomy decreases, the thyroxine administration increases, CBG activity in studies done with rats.[86]

Although it was thought initially that steroid binding to plasma proteins served a transport function, it now appears that protein binding provides a storage or buffer function. Thus, large quantities of hormone circulate in a biologically inert reservoir, from which the active agent is readily available by dissociation. An additional advantage of protein binding is protection from degradation and excretion, which thereby decreases the metabolic clearance rate. Furthermore, protein binding decreases the accumulation of highly lipophilic steroids in adipose tissue, where they would be relatively inaccessible to the blood stream and ultimately the target tissues.

Free cortisol, upon dissociation from the plasma binders, then exerts its effects by entering cells and binding to an intracellular receptor. Although glucocorticoid-responsive tissues may respond in a highly tissue-specific fashion, these actions all appear to be mediated by the glucocorticoid receptor. The specificity of the response is probably accounted for by differences in specific gene activation within each tissue. The physiologic actions of glucocorticoids include the following: (1) metabolic effects — a permissive role in epinephrine and glucagon-stimulated lipolysis, gluconeogenesis, and glycogenolysis; (2) catabolic-increased protein degradation and decreased protein synthesis in muscle, adipose, lymphoid, and connective tissue to provide increased amino acids for hepatic protein synthesis and gluconeogenesis; (3) cardiac-increased contractility, cardiac output, and sensitivity to catecholamines; and (4) musculoskeletal-increased capacity for muscular work.[87] Another major glucocorticoid effect is the anti-inflammatory action that provides the basis for much of the therapeutic usefulness of the glucocorticoids. At pharmacologic levels, glucocorticoids inhibit nearly every aspect of the immune response (Table 7–5), including hormonal and cell-mediated immunity. Other deleterious effects produced by pharmacologic amounts of glucocorticoids include posterior subcapsular cataracts; inhibition of skeletal growth; impaired granulation tissue formation and wound healing; osteoporosis; alterations in mentation, including euphoria and psychosis; and the other effects listed in Table 7–5. In the mid-1950s it became apparent that glucocorticoids regulate the activity of a number of specific enzymes.[89] Since many of these enzymes are involved in the metabolic steps affected by the steroid, it was thought that glucocorticoid regulation of metabolism could be due to effects on enzyme induction. The inductions of two of these enzymes, tyrosine aminotransferase and tryptophan oxygenase, have served as excellent modes for studying the basic mechanism of glucocorticoid hormone action (as well as other steroid hormones). The reader is referred to Knox et al.[89] for further consideration of this topic. The clinical uses of glucocorticoids in various disease states (including malignancy) and the appropriate dosage schedules are available elsewhere[88] and are not dealt with here.

TABLE 7–5. Major Pharmacologic Effects of Glucocorticoids

Anti-Inflammatory and Immunosuppressive Effects
A. Decreased vascular permeability
B. Decreased polymorphonuclear leukocyte diapedesis, chemotaxis, and phagocytosis
C. Decreased mast cell histamine reaccumulation and release
D. Decreased antibody formation, especially the primary response
E. Decreased thymocyte and lymphocyte mass, and impaired delayed hypersensitivity
F. Decreased resistance to bacterial, viral, fungal, and parasitic infections
G. Decrease in Fc receptor concentration
H. Decreased response to T-cell mitogen
I. Decreased synthesis of lymphokines

Connective Tissue Effects
A. Decreased collagen formation
B. Decreased mucopolysaccharide formation
C. Impaired granulation tissue formation and wound healing
D. Osteoporosis

Musculoskeletal Effects
A. Proximal muscular weakness (steroid myopathy)

Central Nervous System Effects
A. Euphoria, mood lability, psychosis
B. Sleeplessness

Eye Effects
A. Posterior subcapsular cataracts

Developmental Effects
A. Induction of surfactant, myelin, retina proteins, pancreatic and breast proteins, etc.
B. Inhibition of skeletal growth

Miscellaneous Effects
A. Decreased intestinal calcium absorption
B. Decreased pituitary TSH secretion

Many protocols in current vogue utilize vastly suprapharmacologic concentrations of glucocorticoid. Plasma concentrations saturate receptor and induce killing of sensitive cells *in vitro*. However, on a once-daily dosage 20 or more half-lives may elapse before the next dose of drug is administered.

Because most glucocorticoid effects (at normal physiologic levels) are short-lived and because of the rapid metabolic clearance of cortisol (plasma half-life of about 60 minutes), a continuous supply of glucocorticoids is necessary to prevent the prompt appearance of symptoms of adrenal insufficiency, the large binding capacity of CBG notwithstanding. In fact, other steroids are cleared from plasma at rates of about 2000 liters per day, which corresponds to a plasma half-life of 20 minutes.[87] Cortisol is extensively metabolized in a number of tissues, such that only 1 to 2 per cent of the steroid actually ends up in the urine unaltered. By far the most important organ for metabolism is the liver. The liver also plays a crucial role in activating certain synthetic 11-keto glucocorticoids such as cortisone and prednisone, which must be converted to 11-hydroxy-metabolites in order to exert glucocorticoid against activity. Thus, patients with compromised hepatic function may not respond to these agents since they will be less able to perform the normally rapid conversion *in vivo* to 11β-OH steroids by the 11-keto reductase enzyme system. Hyperthyroidism

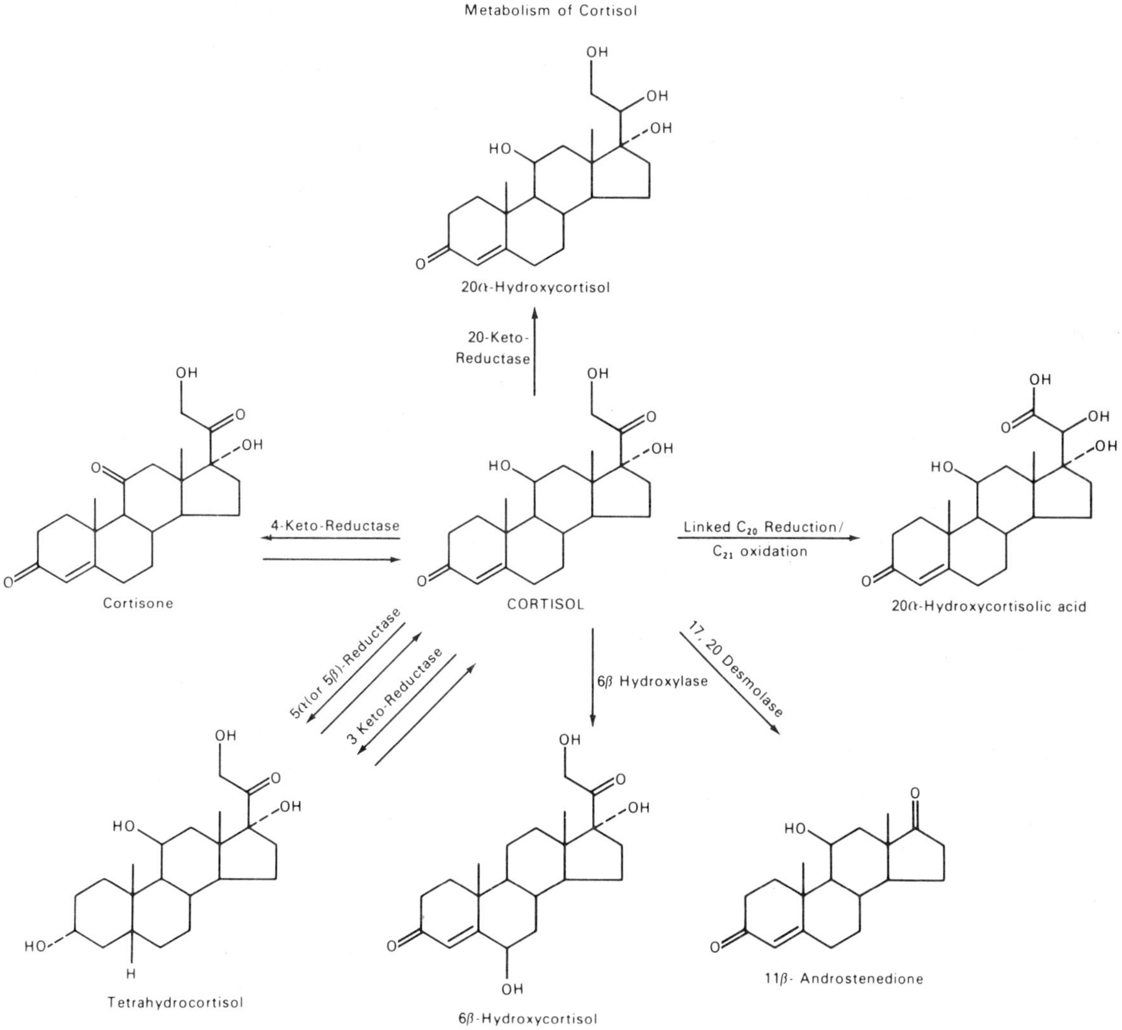

Metabolism of Cortisol

Figure 7–5. A summary of the enzymatic transformations of cortisol.

markedly shifts the equilibrium of this reaction in favor of the inactive oxidized forms, whereas hypothyroidism does the reverse.[86] Anorexia nervosa, and possibly other malnourished states, influence the equilibrium in a manner similar to the effect of hypothyroidism.[91]

At least seven enzymatic reactions that occur predominantly in the liver contribute to the metabolism of cortisol; of these, tetrahydroreduction of the A ring alone provides nearly half of the total urinary metabolites (Fig. 7–5).[92, 93] In children a considerable proportion of the urinary steroids are excreted unconjugated or "free," whereas in adults most of the steroids are conjugated to form glucuronides and, to a lesser degree, sulfates.[6] These modifications either decrease or abolish glucocorticoid activity. Because the metabolic clearance rate of cortisol is quite similar among most people, the replacement dose of hydrocortisone (approximately 12 to 15 mg/m^2/day) is fairly uniform. Because of systemic absorption from the skin and mucous membranes, topical preparations containing triamcinolone or other potent fluorinated glucocorticoid analogues may also have cushingoid consequences.

MINERALOCORTICOIDS

Adrenal extracts contain a potent, sodium-retaining factor capable of maintaining adrenalectomized animals in electrolyte balance. This factor is aldosterone, an unusual steroid possessing an 18-aldehyde group.[96, 97] Aldosterone is synthesized in the zona glomerulosa of the adrenal cortex[98] and secreted in quantities of up to 150 μg per day. Aldosterone secretion is regulated primarily by angiotensin II (via the renin system), but is increased acutely by ACTH, sodium depletion, and/or potassium loading.

Aldosterone is bound by CBG and possibly other specific binding proteins.[11, 12, 99] It is cleared from the circulation rapidly, mainly by the liver and kidney. Aldosterone is reduced in the liver to tetrahydroaldosterone and conjugated with glucuronic acid to form the major urinary metabolite.[100, 101] The kidney synthesizes an acid-labile conjugate of aldosterone,[100] and a small proportion of hormone is excreted in the urine unchanged.

The target organs for aldosterone are principally the kidney,[102] the gastrointestinal tract to a lesser degree,[103, 104] and other tissues including the sweat glands.[105-108] Aldosterone is bound in the target organs by specific cytoplasmic and nuclear proteins, and thereupon induces protein synthesis. One of these proteins increases the net flux or the rate of sodium from the cell.

Conditions of mineralocorticoid excess are manifested by mild hypertension, hypokalemia, and sodium retention. Treatment of this condition, whether it arises from primary hyperaldosteronism or from secondary causes (e.g., congestive heart failure, cirrhosis of the liver) is often facilitated by the use of spironolactone, which blocks the aldosterone receptor. This compound is effective, but also has antiandrogenic properties and in high doses can cause gynecomastia in males.[107]

Forms of resistance to aldosterone have been known since the original description in 1958 by Cheek and Perry.[110-126] This condition (known as pseudohypoaldosteronism) is characterized by congenital renal salt loss in association with hyponatremia and hyperkalemia. Adrenal and renal function are normal. Affected patients have a dramatic clinical response to saline administration, but are insensitive to mineralocorticoids.

ANDROGENS

Although the first androgenic effect (growth of the capon comb) was demonstrated by Berthold in 1849, it was not until 1931 that Butenandt isolated a crystalline androgen, androsterone, from 15,000 liters of male urine.[127] Active testicular extracts were first prepared in 1927 by Loewe,[128] but the identification and synthesis of testosterone was not accomplished until 1935.[129]

A great many other steroids with androgenic activity soon became known; some were isolated from ovarian and adrenal sources as well as the testes, and numerous analogues and derivatives were prepared. Thus far, no nonsteroidal androgen has been discovered. A summary of the effects of androgens in humans is presented in Table 7–6. Efforts have been made to find so-called anabolic steroids, i.e., compounds that promote general body growth without masculinization. A complete dissociation of the two effects has not been achieved. However, several impeded androgens (calusterone and danazol) appear to have approximately equivalent activity to classical androgens in metastatic breast cancer, with substantially less virilizing activity.

As is true for the glucocorticoid secretion, the secretion of testosterone from the testes is under the regulation of the pituitary gland via a trophic hormone, luteinizing hormone (LH) (Fig. 7–3). A small amount of testosterone (about 0.1 mg day) is also secreted from the adrenal glands in both males and females via synthesis along the Δ_5 pathway involving Δ_5-pregnenolone, 17-hydroxypregnenolone, and dehydroepiandrosterone. As with ACTH, LH appears to regulate the first step of the five-step pathway: conversion of cholesterol to Δ_5-pregnenolone by 20α-hydroxylation (Fig. 7–3). The LH effect is mediated by cyclic AMP and requires protein synthesis.[120]

Testosterone is secreted at a steady rate

TABLE 7–6. Physiologic Effects of Androgens

1. Male sexual differentiation *in utero*
2. Enlargement of male internal and external genitalia
3. Pubertal expression of male secondary sex characteristics
   A. Growth of pubic and axillary hair
   B. Deepening of voice
   C. Beard growth
   D. Increase in muscle mass
4. Onset and maintenance of spermatogenesis (with FSH)
5. Increased growth velocity and epiphyseal closure
6. Awakening and maintenance of libido
7. Suppression of breast development and growth
8. Increase in red cell mass

throughout the day in amounts totaling about 7 mg per day, reaching blood levels of about 500 ng/dl. Circulating hormone is more than 95 per cent bound to TEBG and albumin.[131] At puberty the hypothalamic-pituitary axis becomes less sensitive to sex steroid inhibition, resulting in an increased testosterone production rate owing to increased gonadotropin secretion. There is no decrease in testosterone clearance.[132] Moreover, TEBG levels, which are augmented by estrogens and lowered by androgens, fall during puberty.[133]

Free testosterone has a plasma half-life of about 15 minutes, but little if any is excreted unchanged in the urine. The three major metabolic pathways for clearance of testosterone are: (1) conversion of testosterone back to androstenedione via the reversible 17-keto reductase step (equilibrium tends to favor androstenedione slightly); (2) reduction of the double bond at the 5 position to form the potent androgen, dihydrotestosterone; and (3) reduction of the 3-ketone to an alcohol. The products are weakly androgenic 5α-androsterone (20 per cent) and its inactive 5β-isomer, etiocholanolone (26 per cent), which are excreted in the urine largely as sulfates and glucuronides. Hydroxylations also occur at the 6β, 11β, 16, and 18 positions.[8] When ^{14}C-androstenedione or testosterone is given to humans, about 90 per cent of the dose is excreted in the urine within two days and about 6 per cent in the feces.[8] As would be expected, the extent to which testosterone is bound influences its metabolic clearance rate.[134] Small amounts of testosterone are converted to estradiol by aromatase in muscle and adipose tissue. Although the percentage conversion is small, the contribution to the total urinary estrogen is substantial. This important area is discussed more fully in the section on estrogens.

The physiologic effects of androgens (summarized in Table 7–6) include intrauterine mediation of normal male sexual differentiation; induction of the male secondary sex characteristics at puberty, such as deepening of the voice, growth spurt, enlargement of the genitalia, the appearance of acne, beard growth, and awakening of the libido; and the onset and maintenance of spermatogenesis, epiphyseal closure of the bones, and increased muscle mass. Androgens also promote a moderate increase in red cell mass and are responsible for the suppression of breast development in males *in utero* and at puberty. When gynecomastia does occur it is the result of increases in estrogens relative to androgens, such as might occur because of increased peripheral aromatization of androstenedione to estrone and of testosterone to estradiol.

TABLE 7–7. Disorders of Androgen Action

Androgen Insufficiency
A. Male pseudohermaphroditism
B. Ambiguous genitalia (i.e., varying degrees of hypospadias) in males
C. Gynecomastia
D. Male infertility
E. Impotence

Androgen Excess
A. Ambiguous genitalia (i.e., clitoromegaly) in females
B. Hirsutism in females
C. Acne
D. Premature epiphyseal closure in children
E. Precocious puberty
F. Increased muscle mass and male habitus in females
G. Prostatic hypertrophy
H. ? Prostate carcinoma

Disorders of androgen action are shown in Table 7–7. Androgen deficiency, or hypogonadism, is treated best by intramuscular injections of long-acting preparations such as testosterone enanthate every two to three weeks. However, to avoid peripheral aromatization to estrogens, 5α-reduced compounds, such as fluoxymesterone, are available in oral form. Disorders of androgen excess can be counteracted by progestins or antiandrogens such as cyproterone acetate. However, significant side effects, such as altered adrenal function, limit their use.[36]

The therapeutic use of androgens is occasionally associated with other, nonvirilizing effects. Water retention and resultant weight gain are common sequelae to androgens. Edema may occur when large doses are given as in the treatment of neoplastic diseases.[137] Cholestatic jaundice is not uncommon (10 to 20 per cent incidence) in patients receiving steroids with a 17α-methyl substituent,[138] such as fluoxymesterone (Fig. 7–6), or with other steroids substituted in the 17 position, such as norethandrolone.[139] Hepatic adenocarcinomas have been reported in patients with aplastic anemia receiving 17-alkyl derivatives for one to seven years.[140-142] The 17α-methyl compounds are also associated with creatinuria.[143]

Of all the forms of hormone resistance, unresponsiveness to androgen action is the best understood with regard to genetics,

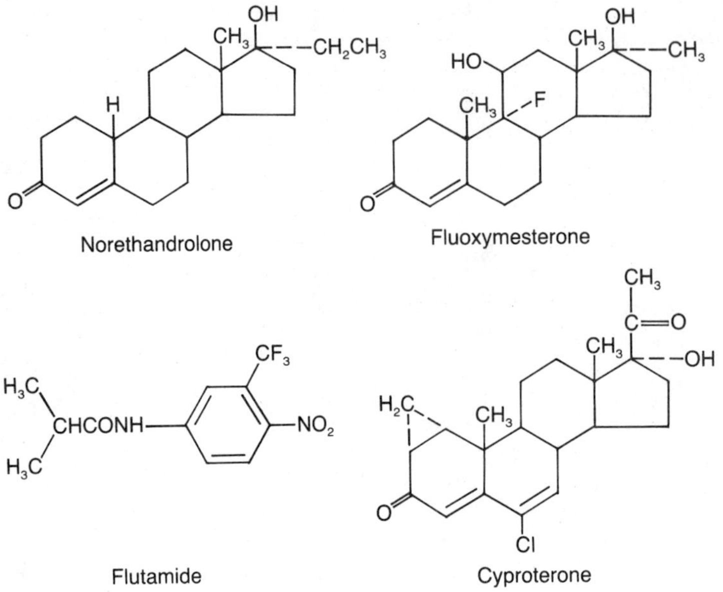

Norethandrolone

Fluoxymesterone

Flutamide

Cyproterone

Figure 7–6. Synthetic androgens and antiandrogens.

pathophysiology, molecular biology, and clinical manifestations. This is partly because these disorders of sexual differentiation are encountered frequently in a broad range of animal species,[144-150] including man. In humans the syndrome of complete testicular feminization occurs with a frequency of approximately one in 50,000 male newborns.[151] Resistance to androgens arises in at least five ways: (1) failure of active hormone formation at the target, such as occurs in the syndrome of 5α-reductase deficiency[152-154]; (2) complete receptor deficiency as judged by failure to detect androgen receptor binding (proof of gene deletion or lack of receptor protein synthesis awaits a means of androgen receptor identification other than hormone binding)[34-36]; (3) defective receptor (i.e., decreased affinity or increased thermolability)[39]; (4) postreceptor defects, thought to be responsible for complete male pseudohermaphroditism in patients having normal quantities of cytosolic and nuclear androgen receptors[67]; and (5) rapid metabolic conversion of hormone to other (and inactive or antagonistic) substances such that the target tissues are inadequately exposed to the active agent. This latter type of defect is believed to be responsible for failure of androgenic action in the Sebright bantam rooster, in which testosterone is rapidly aromatized in the skin to estradiol.[155] An analogous situation has been demonstrated in one obese male who presented with florid gynecomastia.[156] Estradiol has some antiandrogenic properties since it is able to compete at high physiologic levels for androgen receptor binding.[157] All the above defects except the last could conceivably be involved in resistance of human prostatic cancer to hormone manipulation, although thus far only loss of binding activity has actually been described. In the sections on leukemia and breast cancer, other nonreceptor defects are described.

ESTROGENS

The demonstration by Knauer in 1900[158] that ovarian transplants prevented the uterine atrophy and loss of sexual function accompanying ovariectomy established the hormonal nature of ovarian function in regulating reproductive function. With the development by Allen and Doisy in 1923 of a rat bioassay for assessing changes in the vaginal smear induced by ovarian extracts, Frank et al. in 1925[160] were able to demonstrate a female sex hormone in the blood of various species. Loewe and Lange in 1926[161] then discovered such a hormone in the urine of menstruating women, the concentration of which varied with the phase of the cycle. Zondek reported in 1928[162] the presence of large amounts of estrogen in the urine during pregnancy. This finding quickly led to the isolation and crystallization of an active substance,[163, 164] later to be identified and synthesized as estradiol.

As is true of the adrenal glands and the testes, the ovarian follicles are capable of synthesizing and secreting estrogens. This process is regulated in the ovary by two pituitary gonadotropins, follicle-stimulating hormone (FSH) and luteinizing hormone (LH). What sets female apart from male gonadal function is the cyclic nature of ovarian steroidogenesis, which corresponds to the cyclic secretory patterns of FSH and LH as established by gonadotropin-releasing hormone (GnRH or LHRH) from the arcuate nucleus of the hypothalamus. As with the other hormone synthesizing glands, steroidogenesis in the ovary is initiated by peptide hormone (LH) binding to specific cell surface membrane receptors on target cells, the theca interna cells. The binding of all the peptide hormones that regulate steroid biosynthesis activates a membrane-bound adenylate cyclase resulting in the formation of cyclic AMP. Increases in this nucleotide give rise to the phosphorylation of certain protein(s) owing to the activation of protein kinase, an enzyme regulated by cyclic AMP. These phosphoproteins are believed to initiate the synthesis of critical proteins — whether they are enzymes or structural, regulatory, or transport proteins is not clear — that promote the conversion of cholesterol to pregnenolone, the rate-limiting step in the pathway. In contrast to androgens and progesterone, which are synthesized by a single cell type in the target organ, ovarian estrogens are synthesized by the cooperators action of two cell types. Androgens (either androstenedione or testosterone) are synthesized by ovarian thecal cells and converted to estrogens in the neighboring granulosa cells. This conversion is effected by an enzyme complex known as aromatase, resulting in the loss of the methyl group at the 19 position residing on C 10 of the precursor and aromatization of the A ring to yield a phenolic hydroxyl at C 3[165] (see Fig. 7–7). Both in the ovaries and the testes, aromatase is probably regulated by FSH. In women there are certain pathologic conditions, such as polycystic ovary disease (Stein-Leventhal syndrome), in which the aromatase reactions appear to be defective[166] and the androgenic precursors escape into the circulation, resulting in hirsutism and other signs of virilism. Estradiol is readily oxidized to esterone, which can also be formed directly by aromatization of androstenedione. Further hydroxylation at the 16 position results in the formation of estriol, the other biologically important estrogen in humans. These compounds are shown in Figure 7–8. Estrogen metabolism occurs primarily in the liver, where there is free interconversion between estrone and estradiol.[167] Equilibrium slightly favors estrone, which probably serves as the main precursor for the hydroxylated estrogen metabolites in urine.[168] During pregnancy, estrogens are synthesized in large quantities by the placenta, and apparently by the same enzymatic reactions as in the ovary.

As with the androgens, circulating estrogens are bound to TEBG, although the exact extent of binding is not agreed upon.[169, 171] Total blood concentrations of estradiol range from a low of approximately 10 pg/ml (5×10^{-11}M) in early follicular phase to as high as 500 pg/ml (2.5×10^{-9}M) during midcycle. This peak is quite sharp and usually precedes the ovulatory gonadotropin surge.[172] A second rise in serum estrogen occurs during the luteal phase and is lower but more prolonged. At the target tissues the estrogens are responsible, in concert with other hormones, for the development and maintenance of female sexual organs and secondary sexual characteristics, and also for the maintenance of the menstrual cycle and pregnancy (see Table 7–8).

The major role of estrogens is to control the growth and function of the uterus, as well as the vagina and the fallopian tubes. These hormones are necessary for the enlargement of the breasts through development of the ductal and secretory systems, the accumulation of breast fat, and for the increase in the size and pigmentation of the

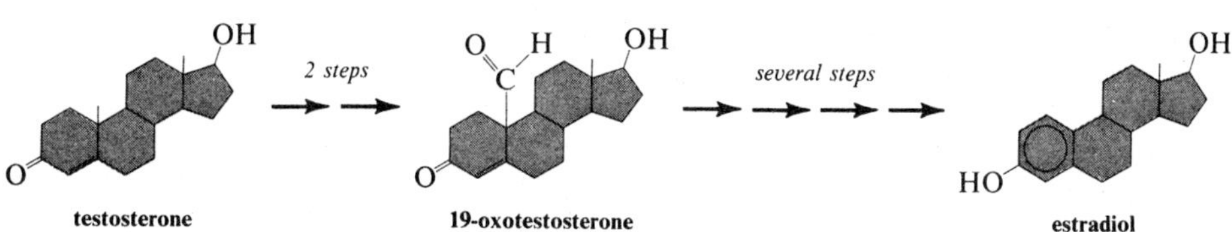

Figure 7–7. Aromatase reaction sequence. (Reproduced with permission from McGilvery RW: Biochemistry: A Functional Approach, 2nd ed. W. B. Saunders Co., Philadelphia, 1979, p. 729.)

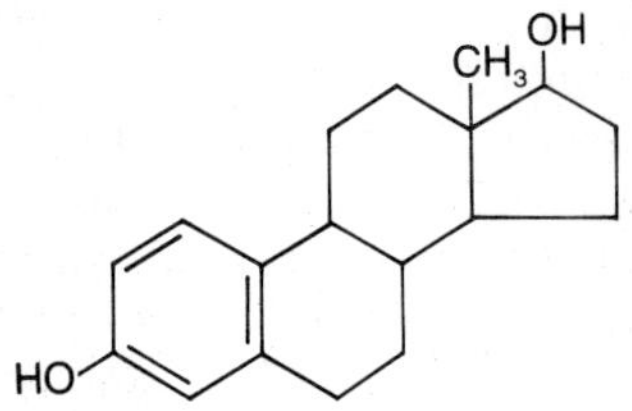

Estradiol

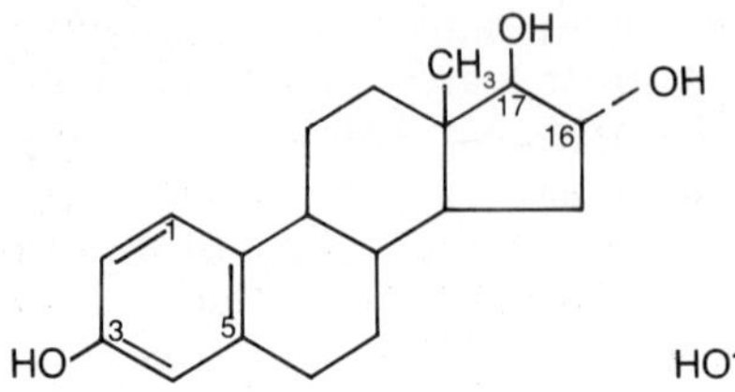

Estriol

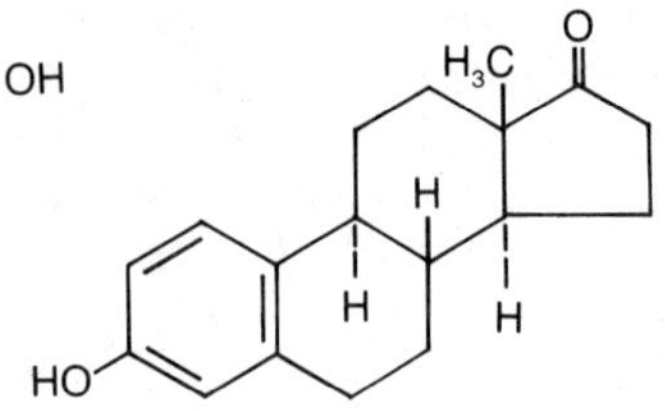

Estrone

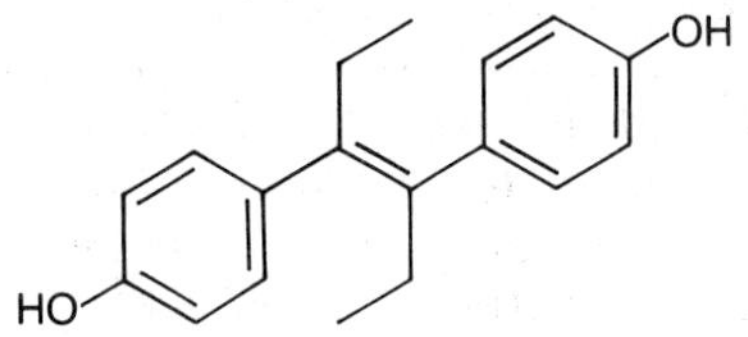

Diethylstilbestrol

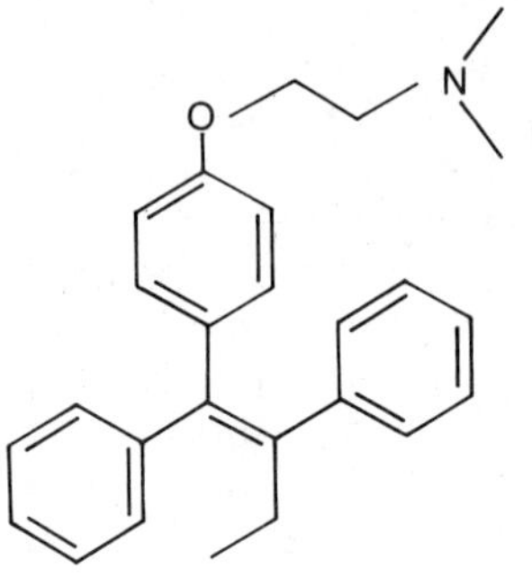

Tamoxifen

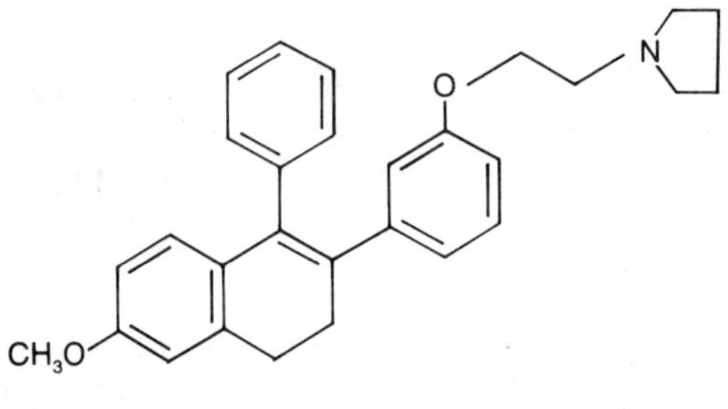

Nafoxidine

Figure 7–8. Estrogens and estrogen antagonists.

skin of the nipples and areolae. Additional but less well understood effects include molding the body contours by alterations in body fat deposition and by shaping the skeleton to give rise to the typical female appearance. Other female pubertal changes, such as growth spurt, epiphyseal closure, growth of pubic and axillary hair, and pigmentation of the external genital skin, may be due in part to estrogens, but more likely are induced by androgens either from the ovaries or the adrenals. Finally, the estrogens influence psyche formation; promote a soft, fine skin texture; and are responsible for mild sodium retention, which occurs in its extreme immediately before menses. Estrogens in pharmacologic doses have a wide range of side effects.

TABLE 7–8. Physiologic Effects of Estrogens

1. Growth and maintenance of female genitalia
2. Pubertal expression of female secondary sex characteristics
   A. Breast enlargement
   B. Increase in size and pigmentation of nipple and areolae
   C. Molding of body contour with alterations in subcutaneous fat deposition
   D. Promotion of female psyche formation
   E. Alterations in skin texture
3. Maintenance of pregnancy (in concert with progestins)
4. Sodium retention

Administration of estrogens postmenopausally has been associated with hypertension, glucose intolerance, thromboembolic diseases, and cholelithiasis[173]; of greater concern, however, are reports linking estrogens to neoplasms. Large doses of diethylstilbestrol (DES), a potent synthetic estrogen, during pregnancy clearly predispose female fetuses to subsequent development of adenocarcinoma of the vagina,[174] Unopposed estrogens are also thought to favor endometrial carcinoma,[175-176] and hepatic adenomas occur with increased frequency in women who use oral estrogenic contraceptives.[177] Finally, oral contraceptives or DES continued during pregnancy increases the incidence of congenital malformation in the off-spring.[178-180] These mutagenic and carcinogenic side effects are discussed more fully below.

All three of the endogenous estrogens are excreted in the urine predominantly as glucuronides and sulfates, although numerous other water-soluble metabolites have been identified. Estrogens undergo enterohepatic recirculation. Over half the estrogen metabolites and one third of the progesterone metabolites are excreted in the bile shortly after the administration of radioactive hormone; eventually, 50 to 80 per cent of an administered dose is excreted as metabolites into the urine within four to six days, and up to 18 per cent may be found in the feces. In the liver, two systems for sulfation exist, one for the estrogens and the other for 3β-hydroxy steroids. Glucuronides are formed from diphosphoglucuronic acid by the microsomal enzyme glucuronyl transferase.

Another class of estrogen metabolites, the cathechol estrogens, discovered by Fishman et al. in 1960,[181] is currently receiving increased attention. Estrone and estradiol can both serve as substrates for enzymes in the liver, the gonads, the placenta, the kidney, and the brain, which add hydroxyl groups at the 2 and 4 positions of the A ring.[182] Because these compounds have extremely rapid metabolic clearance rates — probably 100 times faster than that of the other steroids[183] — it is not clear whether these compounds have physiologic significance as hormones at the site of local production, particularly in the hypothalamus and other regions of the limbic system, or whether they are simply degradation products. The catechol estrogens themselves, like the catecholamines, are rapidly converted to methyl derivatives and conjugated by the enzyme catechol-O-methyltransferase (COMT), present in the liver and red blood cells.[183] Interestingly, the 2-methoxyestrogens have an affinity for TEBG greater than estradiol itself,[184] suggesting that the catechol estrogens may enhance estradiol activity by displacing the latter hormone from its binding globulin.

Resistance to the action of estrogens has not been described in animal species, possibly because estradiol may be essential for early embryonic development.[26] Recent studies into mechanisms of resistance to estrogens have employed mutants of the estrogen-dependent MCF-7 breast cancer cells cloned in tissue culture in the presence of the antiestrogen tamoxifen. Preliminary results indicated that insensitivity to estrogens may arise at a site distal to initial binding of hormone. The experiments will be considered more fully below.[185]

PROGESTINS

As early as 1897 Beard[186] postulated that the corpus luteum served a necessary function during pregnancy. Support for this concept was provided by Fraenkel in 1905[187] who showed that destruction of the corpora lutea in pregnant rabbits causes abortion, a phenomenon that could be prevented by injection of luteal extracts.[188]

Although progesterone, the active principal in the extracts, was isolated in 1929 from the corpora lutea of sows by Corner and Allen, the limited amounts of the hormone that were available hampered further studies until the 1950s, when newer progestational agents with prolonged activity were introduced. Since that time, the number of progestins has increased dramatically and, most important, these agents are widely used as oral contraceptives.

Progesterone is secreted mainly by the corpus luteum of the ovary during the second half of the menstrual cycle. Progesterone secretion begins just prior to the time of ovulation coincident with the LH surge,[178] and derives from the follicle that becomes the corpus luteum once the ovum is released. Progesterone is synthesized from cholesterol and pregnenolone in all the steroid-producing tissues: the ovary, testis, adrenal cortex, and placenta. Although the luteotroph varies with the species, in humans LH is the primary stimulator of progesterone synthesis and secretion in the corpus luteum in a cyclic AMP-dependent process.[189] If the ovum is fertilized, seven days later, upon implantation, the developing trophoblast begins to secrete its own luteotroph, chorionic gonadotropin (hCG), into the maternal circulations, further sustaining the life of the corpus luteum. During the second and third month of pregnancy, as hCG synthesis falls dramatically, the corpus luteum becomes less of a contributor of progesterone for maintenance of pregnancy. Thereafter, and up to the time of delivery, the developing placenta assumes this role and begins to secrete estrogen and progesterone in large amounts. The production rate of progesterone varies from a few milligrams per day during the follicular phase to 10 to 20 mg per day during the luteal phase (reaching blood levels of 10 ng/ml), and increases to several hundred milligrams daily during the latter parts of pregnancy.[190] Rates of from 1 to 5 mg per day have been measured in males and are comparable to the values in females during the follicular phase of the cycle.[190]

Once secreted into the blood stream, progesterone is either bound to corticosteroid binding globulin (with an affinity roughly equal to that of cortisol) or is rapidly cleared from the circulation within a few minutes, predominantly by the liver, where glucuronidation or sulfation occurs prior to excretion in the urine. The isomers of pregnanediol are the principal metabolites.[191, 192] In total, 50 to 60 per cent of the ^{14}C-progesterone given is excreted in the urine. A small, and probably physiologically insignificant, proportion is stored in body fat from which it is slowly released. The enhanced biologic potency of such synthetic progestins as medroxyprogesterone acetate (6α-methyl, 17α-OH progesterone acetate) may be explained both by a lower metabolic clearance rate than progesterone[193] and by the greater affinity of medroxyprogesterone acetate for the progesterone receptor.[194]

The primary and essential biologic role of progesterone is the maintenance of pregnancy. It appears to be the only naturally occurring progestational agent. It also appears to be an antiandrogen (sometimes weakly androgenic) and antimineralocorticoid on the basis of its ability to interact with the receptors for those hormones. The principal target organ for progesterone is the uterine endometrium. It causes the development of secretory epithelium, provided the tissue has previously been exposed to estrogen. Progesterone promotes the establishment of a thick epithelium richly supplied with blood and glycogen-optimal conditions for implantation and nourishment of a fertilized ovum. An abrupt decline in the secretion of progesterone from the corpus luteum at the end of the normal cycle is the main determinant of the onset of menses. During pregnancy the major effects of progesterone are reduction in the muscle tone of the uterus, possibly by direct diffusion from the placenta where it is synthesized, thereby rendering the smooth muscle unresponsive to oxytocin[8] as well as maintenance of the placenta.

Progesterone also affects the secretions of the endocervix and the vaginal epithelium, changing the abundant watery secretion of the estrogen-stimulated epithelium to a scant, viscid material. Progestins also induce flattening and nuclear shrinkage of vaginal epithelium. If adequate quantities of estrogen are acting on the vagina, the cytologic response to a progestin can be used to assess its biologic potency.

Aside from these physiologic effects of the progestins, the effects on the mammary glands are also listed in Table 7–9. During pregnancy and to a lesser extent during the luteal phase of the cycle, progesterone acting in conjunction with estrogen brings about a proliferation of the acini. Toward the end of pregnancy the acini fill with secretion, and vascularization of the glands increases. Only after parturition, however, when estrogen and progesterone are withdrawn, does lactation begin. The main extragenital effect of progesterone is on body temperature. If the body temperature is measured each day throughout the normal menstrual cycle, preferably at the same time each morning, an increase of about 1°F may be noted at midcycle, and this can be used as a simple and precise means of assessing the occurrence and time of ovulation. The temperature rise

TABLE 7–9. Physiologic Effects of Progestins

1. Establishment and maintenance of pregnancy
2. Promotion of development of secretory epithelium of uterine endometrium following estrogen priming
3. Alterations in vaginal epithelium causing change from abundant watery secretions to scant viscid material.
4. Proliferation and engorgement of mammary acini (in concert with estrogens)
5. Thermogenesis
6. Weakly antiandrogenic
7. Weakly antimineralocorticoid

persists for the remainder of the cycle until the onset of menstruation. If conception occurs, the body temperature remains raised until about midpregnancy when it declines to normal, possibly owing to the antagonist action of the estrogens. Since the thermogenic phenomenon can be caused by exogenous administration of as little as 5 mg of progesterone to non-ovulating women or to men,[191] it seems clear that this effect is mediated by the hormone although the mechanism is not known. Finally, because of the protection of the fetus from the material immune system, progesterone, among other factors, has been suspected of having immunosuppressive activity although only limited data are available to support this concept.[195, 196]

Some of the undesirable side effects of the progestins, specifically cholostatic jaundice, increased clotting and thrombosis, and hepatic neoplasms, have already been referred to in the sections on androgens and estrogens. In some cases where the toxic effects result from use of oral contraceptives, it is not clear in some instances whether the effects were due to the estrogenic component of the regimen. Other deleterious effects of synthetic progestins appear to be related to fetal development. Preliminary studies have indicated that use of oral contraceptives before pregnancy results in a higher incidence of female offspring.[197] Also, teratogenic malformations and hypospadias, possibly due to antagonism of androgen-mediated fetal male sexual differentiation, have been reported as a consequence of continuation of oral contraceptives during pregnancy.[198, 199] Finally, decreased hepatic microsomal activity is found in women taking norethindrone.[200]

As in the case of androgens, but not estrogens, progesterone resistance has been implicated as a cause of sex organ dysfunction.[208] In one reported case a 23-year-old woman failed to have cyclic changes in endometrial histology; there was no evidence of decidual reaction on sequential endometrial biopsies,[20] despite normal changes in serum sex hormones and gonadotropins. Moreover, exogenous progesterone did not reverse the abnormality. Progesterone receptors measured in the cytosol of the biopsied endometrial material were found to be 50 per cent lower than those obtained from normal subjects, suggesting a target tissue defect. The inheritance of the disorder is not known.

SELECTION OF PATIENTS FOR ENDOCRINE THERAPY ON THE BASIS OF HORMONE RECEPTOR ANALYSIS

General Considerations

Succeeding sections of this chapter amply document the benefits of endocrine therapy in some human malignancies. These therapies are often less hazardous and less toxic than alternative means of treatment. Nonetheless, only a minority of patients with breast or endometrial cancer will show objective responses to hormone treatment. Although prostatic cancer more frequently responds to orchiectomy, a substantial minority of patients fail to benefit. Finally, although a varying proportion of patients with leukemia and lymphoma respond to glucocorticoids, these steroids are usually administered in combination with other cytotoxic therapy in repeated induction courses, making it difficult if not impossible to determine when specific resistance to hormone treatment has emerged. Furthermore, all endocrine therapies are associated with morbidity and potential mortality, as discussed elsewhere. Even if nontoxic, a trial of an ineffective therapy may, on the basis of delay alone, seriously undermine a patient's chance of benefit by some alternative means of palliation. Thus, it is critical to attempt to select treatment on as rational a basis as possible. A clearer understanding of the basic mechanism of steroid hormone action has already substantially improved selection of specific endocrine therapies for breast cancer patients, and also yielded promising results for leukemia and lymphoma, endometrial cancer, prostatic tumors and other malignancies. In this section a few general comments concerning receptor analyses will be made, and then some specific information concerning their usefulness in individual disease states will be discussed.

As already mentioned, the first step in steroid hormone action is the binding of the hormone to specific cytoplasmic receptor proteins. Thus, it follows that presence of receptor is a necessary, albeit insufficient, condition for a hormone-dependent tissue. There are many reasons why a one-to-one correlation between the presence of binding activity and hormonal response does not occur. A consideration of these permits a more accurate understanding of the usefulness of these tests and their limitations.

False-Positive Receptor Assays

First, we will examine situations in which binding activity is obtained but the tissue in question fails to reveal hormone dependency.

Receptor Defects. The ability to bind hormone is only one function of receptor. Clearly, inability to activate or bind to appropriate nuclear sites or initiate nuclear events may occur. Nontranslocating, receptor-maintaining, hormone-independent cells have been derived from certain parental cell lines inhibited by glucocorticoids.[202] In addition, limited proteolysis of almost all steroid receptors yields a low molecular weight fragment — termed the Mero receptor by Sherman[203] — that binds hormone normally, but apparently cannot initiate other receptor-related functions. Recent data developed by Schrader and colleagues[204] have suggested that the chick oviduct progesterone receptor may be a dimer of two different proteins with substantial sequence homology. Both bind hormone. Both are required for functionality. Hence, loss of one subunit would leave a receptor-positive, hormone-independent cell. Such an explanation might account for the observation of Wittliff[205] that the response rate is substantially lower in human breast cancers that contain estrogen receptor, which sediments solely at a 4S position as opposed to the more typical 8S or 8S/4S patterns.

It has now become possible to obtain hormone-independent variants of estrogen-responsive human breast cancer cells in long-term tissue culture.[206] Nawata et al. report that two of these variants bound hormone in a perfectly normal fashion. Receptor quantity and affinity were normal. Characteristic 8S/4S sucrose density gradient behavior was seen. Nuclear translocation occurred. However, analysis of receptor by DNA cellulose chromatography revealed a markedly different pattern from that seen in the wild-type, hormone-dependent cell line. Similar defects have been described in glucocorticoid binding components from fresh human leukemic myeloblasts. Several patterns of DNA cellulose binding to receptor were reported.[207] It was postulated that only those patients with a normal chromatographic pattern of receptor were likely to be hormone-dependent. Thus, receptor defects at sites other than the ligand binding site are plausible.

In addition, it is possible that receptor activity may be regulated within the cell.[208] For example, a role for reversible phosphorylation or limited proteolysis as a means of receptor regulation might result in functional inactivation of receptor under certain circumstances. Much more work is needed in the area of post-translational regulation of receptors.

Postreceptor Defects. Very little is known with certainty about the exact steps that lie between binding of hormone to receptor and increased synthesis of functional gene product. Many workers have hypothesized that there are specific acceptor sites for steroid receptor complexes located in the chromatin, though their unequivocal identification has not been accomplished. In fact, all the glucocorticoid-independent mutant leukemic cell lines thus far identified appear to have receptor defects, even those in which receptor is present but nuclear binding of the hormone-receptor complex is defective. The commonality of receptor defects is best shown by somatic cell hybridization studies in which fusion of cells lacking receptor with cells failing to show nuclear transfer of steroid receptor complexes never results in complementation, i.e., a hormone-dependent synkaryon.[209] Each parental cell line is presumed to have a single defect: no receptor in one, receptor but abnormal translocation in the other. If these defects were in different proteins, the hybrid phenotype should result in restoration of the hormone-responsive state. Therefore, the failure to show complementarity is strong evidence that both phenotypes of hormone-independence are due to a defect in a common protein: i.e., receptor. Nonetheless, cells in which postreceptor defects occur remain a possibility. For example, if glucocorticoids induce the synthesis of a substance lethal to the cell (as is postulated to occur in glucocorticoid-sensitive lymphocytes), a defect in this gene product would result in a hormone-independent cell that contains receptor. Substantial data exist showing that estrogen regulation of uterine growth may be regulated by a single intermediary protein "IP".[210] A defective "IP" would lead to an unresponsive target tissue.

Hormone Metabolism. Although the potential to respond to a given hormone may exist in a target tissue, rapid metabolism of the ligand to inactive metabolites at the target site may impair the expression of all the potential biologic effects. Similarly, rapid metabolic clearance peripherally may result in less biologic effect. Thus, the synthetic fluorinated glucocorticoids such as dexamethasone have substantially greater biologic activity owing to their three- to fourfold longer plasma half-lives. Similarly, estriol, when kept continuously in contact with target tissue, has been shown to be a complete estrogen, fully capable of inducing all responses typical of more potent estrogens.[211] However, estriol bound to estrogen receptor has a much shorter nuclear occupancy time. Thus, when given as a single pulsed dose it is less effective than estradiol, and when given concurrently with estradiol it can antagonize estradiol effect. Antagonism occurs because both estradiol and estriol have similar affinities for the estrogen receptor and compete for unoccupied receptor. The unbound estradiol is then cleared while the bound estriol, whose estrogenic effects are shorter-lasting, occupies receptor sites.

Methodologic Defects in Receptor Assays. Receptors are recognizable as high-affinity binders of their own homologous hormones, but other receptors and nonreceptor proteins that bind the ligand with high affinity may masquerade as receptor unless great care is taken during the assay procedure. For example, progesterone will bind not only to its own receptor but also to glucocorticoid and androgen receptor.[212] In addition, progesterone binds as tightly to the plasma transport protein corticosteroid binding globulin, CBG, as does cortisol. To a variable extent, plasma transport proteins contaminate all tumor samples used for receptor assays. Thus, a ligand unable to distinguish between binding to a high-affinity receptor and binding to a high-affinity plasma transport protein is useless. The synthetic progestin R5020 has virtually no affinity for CBG, although it binds about ten times more tightly to progesterone receptor than progesterone.[213] Similarly, 5-dihydrotestosterone (DHT), the active metabolite of testosterone, binds not only to androgen receptor but to some extent to progesterone receptor also. DHT also binds tightly to testosterone-estradiol binding globulin (TEBG). Finally, DHT is rapidly metabolized in many tissues to the androstanediols. Thus, DHT is a poor ligand for androgen receptor assays. The synthetic androgen R1881 (methyltrienolone) is superior because it binds more tightly to androgen receptor while having essentially no affinity for TEBG.[213] On the other hand, this ligand binds tightly to progesterone receptor; thus, concurrent blockade of progesterone receptor with another steroid such as triamcinolone acetonide, which has little interaction with the androgen receptor, is required for accurate assay of the androgen receptor with R1881. The point is that false-positive receptor results will certainly occur unless exquisite care is exercised in the choice of ligand and competitor. A suggested set of ligands and competitors is shown in Table 7–10.

Tissue Heterogeneity. An additional source of error in receptor analyses arises because of the heterogeneity of cell types in any biopsy sample. This heterogeneity may be of two types: differences between tissue in the biopsy sample, and differences between tumor cell types. In the first case, a falsely positive assay result occurs when other receptor-containing cells are intermingled in the biopsy sample. For example,

TABLE 7–10. Preferred Ligand and Competitor for Steroid Hormone Receptor Analyses

Receptor	*Radiolabeled Ligand*	*Unlabeled Competitor**	*Unlabeled Blocker†*
Mineralocorticoid	[^{3}H]Aldosterone	Aldosterone 9-Fluorocortisol	– –
Glucocorticoid	[^{3}H]Dexamethasone	Dexamethasone	
Androgen	[^{3}H]R1881	R1881	Triamcinolone acetonide
Progesterone	[^{3}H]R5020	R5020	Cortisol
Estrogen	[^{3}H]Estradiol [^{3}H]R2858	Estradiol, DES Tamoxifen Nafoxidine	5 DHT

*Unlabeled competitor used to determine specific and nonspecific binding of radiolabeled ligand.
†Blocker used to inhibit binding of radiolabeled ligand to other proteins besides the receptor being assayed.

normal prostate or benign prostatic hypertrophy are both rich in androgen receptor. A biopsy containing these cells plus receptor-negative prostatic cancer may well be reported as positive. Virtually all tissues in the body are glucocorticoid targets and, as such, contain glucocorticoid receptors. Unless physical separation of tumor from stroma or surrounding cells is achieved, false-positive results are inevitable. Even if only tumor cells are examined, errors may occur. Morphologic, chromosomal, biochemical, and clonogenic data all suggest that important differences may exist between individual tumor cells in a sample. Steroid receptor analyses are very sensitive. If only a few cells in a sample contain receptor, a positive assay may result while insufficient hormone-dependent cells are present to allow an objective response to endocrine therapy. Some support for this concept derives from the fact that there is a strong quantitative relationship between the quantity of receptor present in a tumor and the likelihood of observing an objective response to endocrine therapy.

Receptor-Therapy Mismatches. A completely different explanation for failure of hormonal therapy of a receptor-positive tumor may lie in inadequate therapy rather than the assessment of hormonal responsiveness. For example, the endocrine manipulation may not alter the hormonal milieu sufficiently to induce a response. About 35 per cent of patients with estrogen receptor-positive breast cancer will fail to respond to oophorectomy. Of these failures, about 15 per cent do respond to subsequent adrenalectomy. Clearly, these patients do have hormone-dependent tumors. Data exist that suggest that postmenopausal (oophorectomy) concentrations of estrogen in plasma are still sufficient to stimulate the growth of some human breast cancer cells.[214] Subsequent adrenalectomy, by removing a source of androgens that can serve as a substrate for peripheral aromatization to estrogens, induces a further reduction in ambient estrogen concentration; on this basis the receptor assay would be deemed falsely positive if based on the oophorectomy results alone. Similarly, some endocrine therapies, such as administration of pharmacologic doses of estrogens, progestins, or androgens in breast cancer, or estramustine in prostatic cancer, may not depend for their effect on the presence of tumor hormone receptors. *A priori*, these therapies need not work directly through a given receptor system such as estrogen receptor in breast cancer or androgen receptor in prostatic cancer.

False-Negative Receptor Assays

A second anomalous situation requiring discussion occurs when a receptor assay is purportedly negative but an objective response to endocrine therapy is induced.

Methodologic Flaws. Steroid receptor proteins are unstable, thermolabile proteins. A host of circumstances can lead to destruction of binding activity, including incorrect sample transport or storage; assay of adjacent nontumorous tissue; faulty selection of ligand concentrations; ligand metabolism; or incorrect pH or ionic conditions. In addition, in most laboratories, "positive" versus "negative" receptor values are selected somewhat arbitrarily. Samples that are correctly quantitated may nonetheless be incorrectly assigned to a negative receptor status, since the cutoff between "negative" and "positive" samples is an arbitrary decision supported by the treatment experience of an institution.

Dilution Errors. Clearly, any biopsy is made up of an admixture of tumor cells plus a variable proportion of normal cells and stroma. It may be a simple matter for the pathologist to detect a few malignant cells scattered throughout a tumor biopsy when the overwhelming majority of the tissue is nonmalignant. A receptor assay on such a sample will yield a negative or extremely low result when binding is normalized against total homogenate or cytosol protein. In at least one situation, dilutional errors are actually advantageous. Because normal breast tissue is predominantly fat and connective tissue, estrogen receptor analyses on these specimens yield negative or very low values. Thus, estrogen receptor-rich tumors are easily detected against this low background. Prostatic tumors are far less easily evaluated because the background matrix of normal prostate is also androgen receptor-rich. Thus, unless meticulous care is taken to ascertain that only tumor tissue is assayed, a false-positive result may ensue.

Sampling Errors. Careful histopathologic confirmation of biopsy specimens is mandatory. Samples submitted for receptor analysis may not include the tumor, and thus produce a false-negative result.

A much more interesting source of lack of clinical and laboratory correlation may result when metastatic sites differ in their receptor status. In breast cancer this occurs 10 to 15 per cent of the time.[215] Obviously, sampling of the one receptor-negative tumor in a mixed population would yield a false-negative result. Similarly, if any tumor nodule in a heterogeneous group of metastases is receptor-negative it will be hormone-independent and continue to grow in the face of endocrine therapy. If a receptor-containing metastasis is sampled a false-positive result will ensue. There are important predictions that derive from this situation. If for approximately 15 per cent of the time there is a failure of concordance between any pair of samples, and only one sample is assessed for receptor content, it follows that with increasing numbers of sites of metastatic involvement the predictive accuracy of the test will diminish. We have shown that, as the number of sites involved with metastatic tumor increases, the objective response rate (50 per cent or greater regression in all sites) to endocrine therapy decreases. If the assayed lesion is estrogen receptor-positive, the likelihood of an objective response of cell lesions to endocrine therapy diminishes. On the other hand, if the signal lesion is estrogen receptor-negative, the accuracy of prediction of no response to endocrine therapy increases with increased numbers of involved sites. A mathematical model based solely on these concordance rates closely approximates the observed data.[216]

Therapy Inappropriate for Receptor Analyzed. A response, or a lack of response that fails to correspond to receptor status, may occur because the endocrine therapy chosen may not act through the receptor analyzed. For example, the mechanisms of action of many antineoplastic endocrine therapies, including androgens, progestins, L-dopa, and hypophysectomy in breast cancer and estrogens and estramustine in prostatic cancer, are not conclusively known. There is no *a priori* reason for these therapies to act via estrogen receptor in breast cancer or androgen receptor in prostatic cancer. Thus, if breast tumor contains androgen receptor (known to exist in about one third of breast cancer samples),[217, 218] some estrogen receptor-negative tumors may respond to androgen therapy.

Occupancy. Most commonly employed methodologies for receptor quantification measure cytosolic receptors under conditions that do not permit detection of either occupied sites or endogenously translocated sites. Under several circumstances, occupancy or translocation can lead to an underestimation of receptor concentration sufficient to yield a falsely negative result. The higher circulating levels of estrogen in premenopausal women may mask estrogen receptor sites, and may account for the finding that such women have lower concentrations of estrogen receptor and are less frequently estrogen receptor-positive. Saez and colleagues have shown that progesterone receptor is undetectable in premenopausal breast cancer specimens during the luteal phase of the menstrual cycle,[219] presumably owing to occupancy and nuclear translocation by endogenous hormone. The occupancy problem also arises if attempts are made to quantify estrogen receptor concentrations for subsequent endocrine therapy in women discontinuing tamoxifen therapy. Recent data have shown that tamoxifen and its active metabolites have prolonged plasma half-lives in the range of 10 to 14 days.[220] Thus, prolonged periods may be required for regeneration of unoccupied receptor sites. In theory, these problems can be circumvented by exchange assays or assays performed on receptor extracted from the nucleus. In practice, these assays are technically difficult or (in the case of progesterone and androgen receptor) simply not successful. However, exchange assays, even if available, may fail because chronic exposure to hormone leads to substantial loss of total cellular receptor due to "processing."[221] Finally, some experiments suggest that, even in the absence of high hormone concentrations, a fraction of unoccupied receptor sites may be localized in the nucleus.[222] Thus, assay of cytosol components may fail to detect receptor.

Failure to Induce Receptor. Receptor assays are usually performed to identify hormone-dependent tumors. In breast cancer, progesterone receptor is induced by estrogen.[223] Receptor assays are usually performed to identify hormone-dependent tumors, since the presence of progesterone receptor is a predictor of response to estrogen and its presence may strongly influence selection of patients for endocrine therapy. In some postmenopausal patients, endogenous estrogen concentrations may be too low to induce progesterone receptor fully. Bloom and Degenshein (personal communication) have shown that progesterone receptor activity can be induced in at least some of these women by a short course of estrogen therapy. In addition, the antiestrogen tamoxifen can increase progesterone receptor concentration in some women. Although the progesterone receptor assay in the setting of low estrogen levels does not yield a truly "false"-negative result (since the progesterone receptor is not present without induction), the assay result is an inaccurate reflection of the biologic potential of the tumor and will lead to a falsely negative clinical interpretation unless this potential error is appreciated.

Heterodox Explanations. As previously discussed, some evidence suggests that all steroid hormone effects may not be mediated by classical receptor mechanisms.[13-16] Steroids have been shown to influence directly many enzymatic activities under *in vitro* assay conditions. Steroids also have important detergent effects on cell membranes, particularly lysosomal membranes. This, in turn, may influence transport of other drugs or physiologic substances. One must always keep an open mind. Some hormonal effects may not be receptor-mediated. If this is true, receptor obviously will not correlate with response.

EPIDEMIOLOGY AND ENDOCRINOLOGY OF CANCER AS IT RELATES TO STEROID HORMONE-DEPENDENT TUMORS OF MAN

We turn next to a presentation of the specific hormone-dependent neoplasias, beginning with breast cancer. Each of these sections begins with a consideration of the epidemiology of the disease as it pertains to endocrinologic considerations. Although the literature in this area is vast and at times confusing, it seems highly appropriate to summarize this work here, for several reasons. First, this field has largely been the province of epidemiologists and endocrinologists rather than oncologists. An organized presentation geared toward clinical oncologists seems useful. Second, there can be no doubt that for the hormone-dependent neoplasias of man, endocrine factors are critical in their expression. At present, a variety of "prophylactic" interventions are being proposed, including delayed puberty and estrus in breast cancer, oral contraceptives in endometrial and ovarian cancer, and so on. To understand and evaluate these proposals, an understanding of the endocrinology underlying these diseases is critical. Finally, by understanding the hormones thought to be involved in tumor promotion, a more strategically sound approach to pharmacologic alteration of the hormonal milieu is possible.

Breast Cancer

Epidemiologic studies of breast cancer have provided information concerning multiple risk factors such as sex, age, age at menarche and menopause, age at first birth, geographic area of residence, dietary factors, family history of breast cancer, and a variety of indicators related to steroid hormone concentrations in blood or urine.[224, 225] Many of these risk factors are interdependent; some may be related to endocrine status. Unfortunately, no risk factor, either alone or in combination (with the exception of certain very rare, high-risk kindreds) is sufficiently discriminatory at present to identify women in whom prophylactic therapeutic intervention is warranted. The importance of these epidemiologic factors lies in the potential for altering causative influences to diminish the risk of breast cancer.

Those risk factors in which endocrine influences are significant can be grouped under four headings: international variation, reproductive history, familial clustering, and hormonal milieu.

International Variation

There is a striking variation in rates of breast cancer in various areas of the world. In 50-year-old individuals, the incidence of breast cancer is about six times higher in the United States than in Japan or Taiwan. This difference was once attributed to genetic factors, but Chinese descendants living in Hawaii for several generations have the same rate of breast cancer as do the Caucasians, and first and second generation Japanese in Hawaii have rates higher than do those in

Japan.[226] The incidence of breast cancer is now increasing in Japan. Obviously, environmental factors must be considered.

The relation of breast cancer incidence rates to age have interesting and differential characteristics. In countries with a high incidence of breast cancer, there is a continued increase with age. However, in "low-risk" countries, the rate of development of breast cancer decreases after the menopause. DeWaard[227] has suggested that these data imply two different etiologic types of breast cancer. Breast cancer incidence in countries of lower socioeconomic status correlates strongly with such factors as increased food consumption, increased fat and meat intake, and higher rates of obesity, all of which generally are associated with industrialization. As described below, the mediator of these environmental factors may well be hormonal.

Reproductive History

Reproductive history strongly influences breast cancer risk. If a relative risk of one is assigned to nulliparous women, there is nearly a threefold alteration in risk of breast cancer, varying from 0.5 for those having their first child before age 20 to 1.4 for those giving birth after age 37. The protective effect of early age at first birth is maintained throughout life, even among women aged 75 and older.[228]

The protective effect of early pregnancy could be due either to a permanent, pregnancy-induced alteration in the mammary gland or to a chronic postpartum alteration in circulating hormone levels. Explanation of this finding is critical because identification of the source of this substantial protection against breast cancer risk provided by early first birth might allow prophylactic endocrine manipulations in young women. Lactation *per se* does not appear to be particularly protective.[229, 230] However, a recent study in Oriental women who nursed their children on only one breast showed a highly significant reduction in breast cancer on that side.[231]

Family History

Family history is an important risk factor in breast cancer. Petrakis[232] has reviewed the evidence supporting a genetic component in breast cancer. Strong familial incidence, clustering of both male and female cases, relatively stable incidence rates, as well as stable racial differences, all support the role of genetic factors. Weak associations of breast cancer with HL-A antigens[233] and cerumen type[234] constitute additional evidence. Although genetic factors could be expressed at a variety of levels, heritable differences in the endocrine milieu are a likely locus. Thus, a comparison of high-risk individuals (by family history) with an appropriate control group might yield important insights into hormonal background for development of breast cancer. Two such studies, though well designed, have been disappointing.[235, 236] Thus far, no significant differences have been reported in prolactin, gonadotropin, estrone, estradiol, or estriol concentrations in serum from high- and normal-risk subjects. These results are different from similar studies in male breast cancer,[237] and suggest that genetic effects may be mediated either nonhormonally or via chronic subtle changes in the endocrine milieu that have not been appreciated.

Hormonal Milieu

It has long been supposed that the hormonal environment may influence the risk of development of breast cancer and the rate of progression of established cancer. This concept has experimental support from studies of induction of mammary cancer in rodents, in which the preparative or promotional role of estrogens can be clearly demonstrated. However, initial measurement of urinary estrogens revealed no differences between women with breast cancer and those in the normal population. These studies suffer from the criticism that estrogens should have been measured at the time of carcinogenesis rather than at a late stage of clinical disease. In addition, the large fluctuations of estrogens during the menstrual cycle and the alterations in route of metabolism with disease or with drugs further complicate interpretation of these results.

Nevertheless, ovarian activity is a clear risk factor in breast cancer. Surgical menopause is protective against breast cancer in proportion to the reduction in years of menstrual life.[238] Age at menarche and age at natural menopause are also risk factors in breast cancer; longer menstrual life is associated with a higher risk of breast cancer. This excess risk exists even for very elderly women, an observation consistent with a long latent period for some human breast cancers. It seems probable that ovarian estrogen is the predominant causative factor, since the protective effects of early ovariectomy are negated by administration of estrogen.[239] In addition, estrogen treatment of men who either have prostatic cancer[240] or are undergoing transsexual operations[241] also increases the risk of breast cancer. A strong case can be made for disturbance in endogenous estrogen production or metabolism as an etiologic factor in most cases of male breast cancer.[242]

Women with a high urinary excretion of estriol have a decreased risk of breast cancer. For example, Japanese women (a low-risk group) have a higher urinary estriol excretion than do Australian women,[243] possibly because estriol is an antagonist under certain circumstances.[244] However, this explanation is inconsistent with other experimental findings. First, estriol acts as an estrogen only when given intermittently combined with estradiol.[245] When given continuously, it is a potent estrogen and acts as a promotor of mammary gland carcinogenesis in experimental systems. Second, urinary estriol has no direct relationship to plasma estriol concentrations or production rates.[246] Finally, the ratio of estriol to estrone plus estradiol in urine is not related to differences between estrogen blood levels and production rates in normal women or in women with breast cancer.

Studies of plasma estrogen concentrations and production rates have not shown differences between women with early breast cancer and control populations.[246, 247]

Androgens

Initial interest in androgen metabolites and breast cancer was spurred by Bulbrook, who developed discriminant functions for breast cancer risk and response to treatment based primarily on androgen excretion.[248] He has shown that a higher excretion of androgen metabolites was correlated with a greater likelihood of response to adrenalectomy or hypophysectomy. This discriminant function is little used at present because of the much higher reliability of estrogen receptors.

Of greater interest was the finding of lower urinary excretion of etiocholanolone (an androgen metabolite) in women who later develop breast cancer.[249] Urinary testosterone excretion[250] and plasma testosterone levels[251] tend to be higher in women with early breast cancer. However, conflicting and overlapping data do not support these observations.

Most data on androgens relate to hormones present in plasma or in urine. However, Adams and colleagues[252] reported that human breast cancer tissue could metabolize dehydroepiandrosterone to androstenedione, and possibly to estriol. Cholesterol was converted to C-19 steroids, and breast cancer tissue could further convert androgenic precursors to estrone and estradiol. Thus, breast tissue may have the potential to create its own microenvironment and thereby defeat efforts to lower estradiol levels in the surrounding medium. Some breast cancers have the capacity to add sulfate to various steroids, thereby inactivating estrogens: it has been noted that the absence of the sulfokinase enzyme correlates with the lack of response to adrenalectomy.[253] Thus, hormone metabolic activity may play an important role in determining eventual hormonal response.

Benign Breast Disease

Although most benign breast diseases are not considered to be premalignant, there is strong evidence to suggest that women with benign breast disease have a substantially increased risk (up to four times in one well studied series[46]) of developing breast cancer. It is likely, therefore, that benign and malignant breast disease share common etiologic factor(s) possibly related to the endocrine milieu. Thus, an examination of the effects of exogenous sex hormones on benign breast disease is of interest. Both retrospective analyses[254-258] and prospective studies[259, 260] strongly suggest that oral contraceptive use diminishes the risk of benign breast disease. Generally, these studies show a greater protective effect for cystic disease as compared with fibroadenoma. Protection is greater in "long-term users" than in "ever users," an important point in favor of a causal relationship. The study conducted by the Royal College of General Practitioners[159] showed the incidence rates for benign breast disease to be inversely related to the amount of progestagen in the preparation. This observation is supported by surveys of women using noncontraceptive estrogen preparations without progestagens in which no protection against benign breast disease was demonstrated.[256, 261]

Certain forms of benign breast disease, such as intraductal papilloma and fibrosing adenosis as well as severe atypia of the ductular lining cells, have been associated with a high likelihood of subsequent malignancy.[262, 263] Effects of oral contraceptives on women with these specific histologic features have not been assessed. Because of this and the studies mentioned below, it should not be concluded that a reduction in benign breast disease is equivalent to a protection against breast cancer. It may be that, in particular subsets of women with benign breast disease, estrogen use increases the risk of breast cancer.

Malignant Breast Disease

There was a small but significant increase in the incidence of breast cancer during the decade 1960 to 1970, a period in which the use of oral contraceptives and postmenopausal estrogens increased sharply.[264] Many other factors could contribute to these findings, making it difficult to conclude that exogenous estrogens increase breast cancer risk.[264, 265] Multiple, retrospective case control studies have failed to reveal a significant overall increase in risk among oral contraceptive users.[254, 257, 266, 267] Several observations prevent a totally sanguine view of this conclusion. In general, the time required for tumor promotion in humans is long and a sufficient observation period as yet may not have elapsed. Two studies in younger women show a relative risk ratio of 1.7 for users of oral contraceptives for more than eight and five years, respectively,[268, 269] although this increase was not statistically significant. Two other studies failed to show an increase in risk with duration of use.[257, 266] However, in one of these studies,[266] oral contraceptives were associated with a higher incidence of breast cancer in three subsets of patients: nulliparous women, women using the pill prior to the birth of their first child, and women with a history of benign breast disease. Prospective trials of oral contraceptives are negative at this point,[259, 266] and in fact may suggest a reduction in risk. Longer follow-up studies are required before the risk can be adequately assessed.

Several retrospective analyses of women using estrogens after the menopause fail to show a significant association between use and breast cancer risk.[261, 267-269] A relative risk ratio of 1.3 (borderline statistical significance) was found for estrogen users in one large retrospective study.[239] Risk was related to duration of use, with a doubling of this risk ratio after 12 years of use. No follow-up of oral contraceptive users of this duration is available. The risk was greater in women taking the highest-strength preparation, but not related to duration of use. Finally, as in the study of oral contraceptives,[257] the risk of development of breast cancer was twice as great in women with a history of benign breast disease, and increased sevenfold in women who developed benign breast disease after starting on estrogens.

Hormone Receptors and Endocrine Therapy of Breast Cancer

The fact that some human breast cancers might respond to endocrine manipulations has been appreciated since George Beatson induced tumor regressions in patients following bilateral oophorectomy nearly a century ago.[270] Unequivocally, patients who respond to such endocrine therapies not only have palliation of their illness, but have substantially longer survivals than do nonresponders. Despite the clear-cut benefits to responders, only about one third of unselected patients can be expected to have objective tumor regressions following hormonal therapy. With the advent of effective chemotherapy alternatives, a more precise selection of different treatment modalities is necessary.

A variety of empirically derived clinical guidelines (long disease-free interval, soft-tissue or bone involvement, and so on) as well as a few biochemical tests (high excretion of androgen metabolites, presence of steroid sulfation) have been suggested as being of value in selecting patients with hormone-responsive tumors. Unfortunately, none of these approaches is sufficiently reliable for widespread adoption.

As described elsewhere in this chapter, the first step in steroid hormone action is the binding of the hormone to specific receptors. Jensen found specific estrogen binding activity in human breast cancers, and established a correlation between the presence of estrogen receptor and the likelihood of response to endocrine therapy.[272] Since these pioneering studies, a great deal of information has accumulated concerning the value of these receptor determinations.[273] In brief, about two thirds of primary breast cancers contain detectable concentrations of estrogen receptor, and a somewhat smaller proportion of metastatic samples are positive for estrogen receptor in untreated patients. Premenopausal patients have tumors that are less frequently estrogen receptor-positive and contain, on average, lower concentrations of receptor than in cancer occurring after the menopause. These observations are only partially explained by the fact that the higher concentrations of endogenous estrogen in plasma of premenopausal women mask binding sites. Estrogen receptors are detectable in about 90 per cent of male breast cancers, although no clear correlation between receptor concentration and response to endocrine therapy has been established.[274]

Overall, there is a highly significant association between the presence of estrogen receptor and the likelihood of response to endocrine therapy. Overall predictive accuracy for the test is about 85 per cent. Absolute receptor concentration above the minimal value for "positivity" further correlates with response. Patients with higher concentrations of estrogen receptor have a higher response rate, and are more frequently progesterone receptor-positive also.[273]

As already mentioned, a progesterone receptor determination is of value because, as an estrogen-inducible function, it provides a better correlation with hormone dependency. If the tumor is estrogen and progesterone receptor-positive, objective response rates approach 80 per cent. Interestingly, estrogen receptor-positive, progesterone receptor-negative tumors respond to endocrine therapy only 30 per cent of the time. Many of these latter tumors are not truly progesterone receptor-negative. During the luteal phase of the menstrual cycle in premenopausal women, high progesterone concentrations make detection of progesterone receptor impossible by standard techniques. Furthermore, in some postmenopausal patients, endogenous estrogen concentrations are insufficient to induce progesterone receptor synthesis by hormone-dependent tumors. Thus, not only does progesterone receptor add to the accuracy of determination of hormone dependence but, with careful attention to the above situations in which ambient hormone concentrations influence receptor detection, even better results are possible.

Receptor determinations may have other important uses. Patients with estrogen receptor-positive primary breast cancers have a substantially prolonged disease-free interval independent of other known prognostic variables, including menopausal status, tumor size, histologic grade, or axillary lymph node status.[275-277] Thus, estrogen receptor determinations may aid in the selection of receptor-negative patients at higher risk of early recurrence who may benefit from adjuvant therapy. In addition, receptor status of the primary tumor may even aid in the choice of the adjuvant therapy employed. Bubay and colleagues have shown that ER-positive patients treated with CMF plus tamoxifen have a significantly lower disease-free interval than do patients treated with CMF alone.[278]

Two studies have suggested that estrogen receptor-negative tumors have a substantially higher response rate to cytotoxic chemotherapy.[279, 280] This observation is consistent with the finding that less well differentiated tumors, which are more often estrogen receptor-negative, tend to have shorter disease-free intervals and higher growth fractions and rates of DNA synthesis. Since most cytotoxic drugs are more effective against rapidly dividing cells, one might expect adjuvant chemotherapy to be more effective in patients with estrogen receptor-negative tumors. Although this hypothesis seems reasonable, several other studies fail to confirm the correlation of negative estrogen receptors and a high rate of response to chemotherapy.[281, 282]

In rodent mammary carcinoma, prolactin has an important role in the genesis and stimulation of growth of neoplastic cells.[283] A relationship between prolactin receptor content and response has been suggested. As with estrogen receptors, tumors are heterogeneous for prolactin receptor content. Prolactin receptors are present in human breast cancer,[284] but early studies do not suggest responses to therapies that alter prolactin levels.[285] Epidemiologic data suggest that prolonged use of prolactin-releasing drugs such as the phenothiazines does not increase the incidence of breast cancer in humans and may actually be protective.[286]

Endocrine Therapy of Breast Cancer

It is convenient to divide the endocrine management of breast cancer into two phases: early-stage disease and advanced (metastatic) disease.

Early Breast Cancer. Patients presenting with a breast mass require therapy that not only is sufficient for local control of disease, but at the same time is as attentive to cosmetic outcome as possible. This is an area of active investigation comparing radical surgery, limited surgery, and biopsy followed by radiotherapy. In addition, patients require adequate staging of extent of disease, including assessment of axillary lymph node involvement with tumor. Part of this pretreatment evaluation must include estrogen and progesterone receptor determination. An important link between early-stage breast cancer and epidemiologic considerations has recently emerged. Obesity has been established as a risk factor for early relapse and worse prognosis. This is presumably based on the conversion of adrenal precursors to estrone in peripheral tissues, most notably fat.

Based on this evaluation, adjuvant therapy regimens may be considered in patients at high risk of relapse. Chemotherapy has clearly been established as having a substantial impact on disease-free survival in patients with Stage II (axillary node-positive) breast cancer, but the role of hormonal therapy is less clear.

Several studies have failed to demonstrate any overall survival benefit in breast cancer patients treated with prophylactic oophorectomy[287] or ovarian irradiation.[288, 289] However, these studies were completed before the availability of estrogen receptor analyses. A minority of premenopausal patients are strongly estrogen receptor-positive. Thus, an advantage in a small subset of patients might have been "washed out" by the preponderance of patients in whom no benefit could be expected. Furthermore, in one prospective randomized trial, hormonal therapy was successful in prolonging overall patient survival.[290] In this study, following mastectomy, patients were randomized to receive either no further therapy, ovarian irradiation, or ovarian irradiation plus oral prednisone for five years. After ten years of follow-up, premenopausal patients over 45 years old who were treated with both ovarian irradiation and prednisone had a significant improvement in both disease-free survival and overall patient survival compared with the control group. The addition of glucocorticoid presumably provided some additional suppression of adrenal steroidogenesis. Thus, the role of adjuvant hormonal therapy needs further careful evaluation, particularly in conjunction with estrogen receptor analysis. Combination chemotherapy combined with hormonal therapy in the adjuvant setting requires further investigation. Preliminary results of a trial using adjuvant chemotherapy and tamoxifen appear quite encouraging in the subset of patients who are estrogen receptor-positive.[278]

Advanced Breast Cancer. About one third of unselected patients with metastatic breast cancer achieve a partial or complete response with endocrine therapy. By appropriate selection according to steroid receptor and clinical status, substantial improvement in response rates can be achieved. Obviously, other factors must be weighed in such decision making, including performance status, sites of involvement, and the relative impact of various treatment modalities on life style. Furthermore, there is substantial latitude in the choice of a given endocrine or chemotherapy, since the superiority of particular regimens may still be in question. In the next few sections, we provide information concerning specific endocrine therapies, with emphasis on newer modalities such as antiestrogens and inhibitors of endogenous steroidogenesis.

Oophorectomy

Since the pioneering work of Beatson more than 80 years ago, the removal of the ovaries of premenopausal patients has been known to be an effective treatment for some women with inoperable breast cancer.[270] Using rigid criteria, the regression rate is 25 to 30 per cent,[291, 292] and the median duration of remission is nine months. Surgery is the usual method of choice, since radiation may require several weeks to ablate ovarian endocrine activity and may do so incompletely.

An accurate assessment of ovarian status is essential prior to oophorectomy. A high plasma FSH is a reliable indication of loss of follicles and consequent cessation of estradiol secretion. Low plasma estradiol ($<$ 20 pg/ml) is also characteristic of cessation of ovarian function. The vaginal smear is unreliable for assessing ovarian endocrine function. In perimenopausal and postmenopausal patients, the regression rate from oophorectomy is too low to consider ovarian ablation as the primary endocrine therapy.[293]

Adrenalectomy and Hypophysectomy

Estrogens persist in blood and urine after ovariectomy. The adrenal cortex secretes a small amount of estrone,[294] but the main source of estrone after castration is the transformation of androstenedione, secreted by the adrenal cortex, to estrone in peripheral tissues.[295] The positive correlation between the presence of estrogen receptor in tumor tissue and adrenalectomy response additionally supports this concept. The low concentrations of estradiol and estrone in postmenopausal patients are sufficient to support the growth of endocrine-sensitive tumors.[211] Estrogen concentrations as low as 2×10^{-11}M stimulate the growth of human breast cancer cells in continuous tissue culture responses; these concentrations are approximately equal to those in the plasma of postmenopausal women.

Criteria that assist the selection of patients for adrenalectomy or hypophysectomy include: (1) the presence of estrogen receptor in tumor tissue, a factor associated with a 60 per cent response rate; (2) a prior response to castration, which increases the likelihood of response to 50 per cent; and (3) a long disease-free interval between mastectomy and development of metastatic disease.

Adrenalectomy and hypophysectomy produce approximately equal[296] response rates, although some studies favor hypophysectomy.[297] The mean duration of remission appears longer after hypophysectomy. The choice of operation must usually be based on more pragmatic considerations, such as the surgical skills available and the age of the patient.

Androgen Therapy

Androgen therapy in women with metastatic cancer was initiated 30 years ago. The Cooperative Breast Cancer Group surveyed the response of 521 patients treated with testosterone propionate and reported a remission rate of 21 per cent.[298] Response rate was influenced by menopausal status and site of involvement. The remission rate was less than 10 per cent within one year of the menopause and was highest five years after the menopause. Soft tissue metastases responded most favorably and visceral metastases least. The median period of remission was eight months. Any androgen given in large amounts produces about the same rate of regression. Long-acting preparations such as testosterone enanthate should be avoided, since it then becomes impossible to stop therapy should the disease accelerate, as in the case of the sudden development of severe hypercalcemia. Results of trials with many androgens do not yield differences in responses attributable to the steroid.

Attempts have been made to find steroids less androgenic than testosterone, since virilization is severe and often distressing. Synthetic androgen analogues such as testololactone or calusterone have essentially no virilizing activity and have been reported to produce regression of disease.[299] Moreover, these compounds appear to have some weak antiandrogenic properties. Although the incidence of remissions is low, their occurrence is evidence that antitumor effect may be a reflection of the drug's antiandrogenicity, as well as of its known ability to block aromatization of testosterone to estradiol.

Typical schedules of androgen administration are 100 mg of testosterone propionate intramuscularly three times a week, or fluoxymesterone 10 mg orally twice a day (Fig. 10–6). No schedule differences in response have been reported. The major side effects of virilization (nearly universal) and cholestatic jaundice (up to 20 per cent) may require discontinuation of the drug. Hypercalcemia is uncommon (less than 10 per cent) but must always be considered, particularly in patients with osseous disease. When it occurs it can usually be managed by drug discontinuation and hydration; rarely, mithramycin may be required. Hypercalcemia occurring early in therapy may be a sign of hormone dependency. Therefore, therapy should be reinstituted at 25 per cent doses and escalated at 25 per cent per week, with careful follow-up. If hypercalcemia recurs the patient should probably be treated with an alternative endocrine therapy.

Estrogen Therapy

The observation that some patients with breast cancer respond to pharmacologic estrogen therapy was not predictable, nor was it based on data from animal models. Following the initial observations, however, remission rates of 30 to 37 per cent were reported in two large series[300, 301] when estrogen was used as initial therapy. In a randomized trial of steroid therapy, estrogen (diethylstilbestrol, 5 mg t.i.d.) produced a 29 per cent remission rate compared with 10 per cent for androgens.[302] The duration of response to estrogen has generally been longer than the duration of response to androgen in most series. Response rates to pharmacologic doses correlated with the number of years after the menopause. As with androgen and ablative procedures, the longer the disease-free interval, the higher is the probability of response to estrogen. Although often more toxic in premenopausal patients, pharmacologic doses of estrogens can induce tumor regressions in younger patients also. Antiestrogens should usually be tried before additive therapy in younger women.

When estrogens are used in patients who have relapsed from previous endocrine therapy, remission rates are low, the chances of response usually being less than 10 per cent. Also, estrogen administration is generally ineffective following hypophysectomy or adrenalectomy.

The most commonly used estrogen is the nonsteroidal compound diethylstilbestrol (DES) (Fig. 7–8): most patients receive 5 mg orally three times a day. Patients should be started on full doses, as lower concentrations may stimulate hormone-dependent neoplasia. Slightly higher response rates may occur with substantially more toxicity in patients treated with even higher doses. If no response is seen with DES, there is no point in treating with any other estrogen such as ethinyl estradiol.

Toxicity from estrogens at high doses is not insignificant. Endometrial hyperplasia and breakthrough bleeding occur in 15 to 20 per cent of patients and can usually be managed by giving a progestogen, followed by a short period of cessation of hormone therapy to permit sloughing of the endometrium. Salt and water retention, particularly in the elderly, may occur with any estrogen. Of greatest consequence, however, is hypercalcemia. This can occur abruptly in any patient, but most commonly is seen shortly after the institution of therapy. Hypercalcemia is rare in patients ten or more years after the menopause. Extensive bone involvement with metastatic tumor should prompt particularly close observation of the patient during the institution of therapy. Hypercalcemia is managed by hydration and withdrawal of estrogen. Often, on reinstitution of therapy, a regression is obtained without recurrence of hypercalcemia. The overall response rate is higher in patients who develop hypercalcemia.

An objective response may also be seen following withdrawal of estrogen, or less commonly of androgen.[303] Thus, new attempts at therapy generally should not be started until at least one month after stopping steroids. Rapidly advancing disease, of course, may constitute an exception to this suggestion.

The mechanism by which patients respond to pharmacologic concentrations of estrogens is not known. Physiologic doses of hormone stimulate receptor-positive tumor cell growth both *in vitro* and *in vivo*. The usual order of stimulation is RNA, then protein synthesis, and finally, after 24 hours, DNA. Since the presence of estrogen receptor is positively associated with the response to estrogen therapy, it is plausible that the effect is mediated through the same receptor mechanism responsible for tumor stimulation. Conceivably, higher concentrations of hormone interact with recently identified lower-affinity, Type II estrogen receptors found in some estrogen target tissues, or impede receptor processing.

Progestin Therapy

A variety of progestogens have been used in patients with breast cancer. These include both the C-21,17-acetoxysteroids, such as medroxyprogesterone (Fig. 7–9), and the 19-carbon steroids, such as norethisterone. In general, remission rates have clustered about 20 per cent,[304] the same as those noted with androgens. Response to progestins is correlated with estrogen receptor; information as to correlation with progesterone receptor is not available. The response rate to progestins may not be influenced by previous response to castration, estrogen, or androgen. Thus, progestogens may be given a trial in patients who fail to respond to other therapeutic modalities. Progestins usually have been given orally (e.g., 40 mg megestrol acetate four times a day). Some experience has accumulated with extremely high-dose

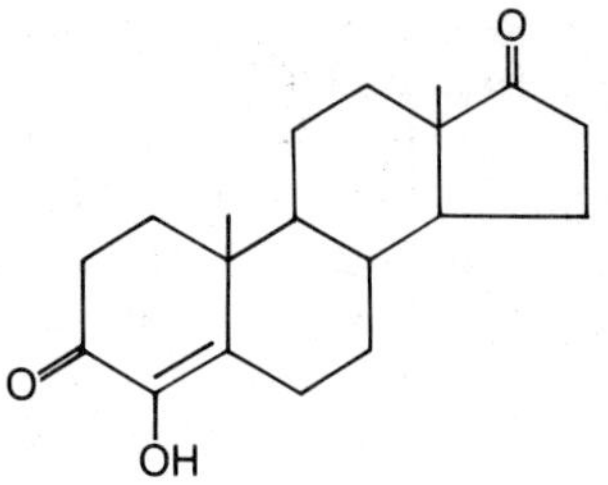

4-Hydroxy-androstenedione

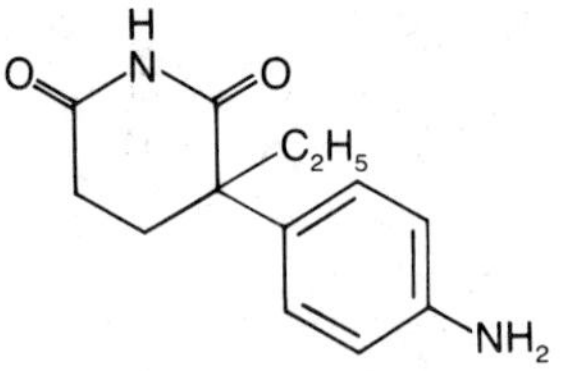

Aminoglutethimide

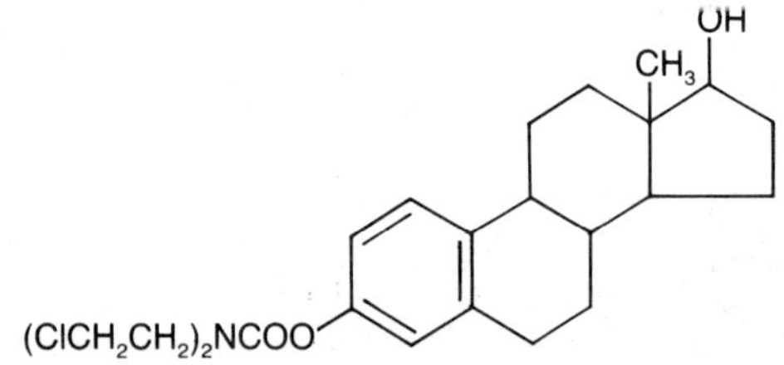

Estramustine

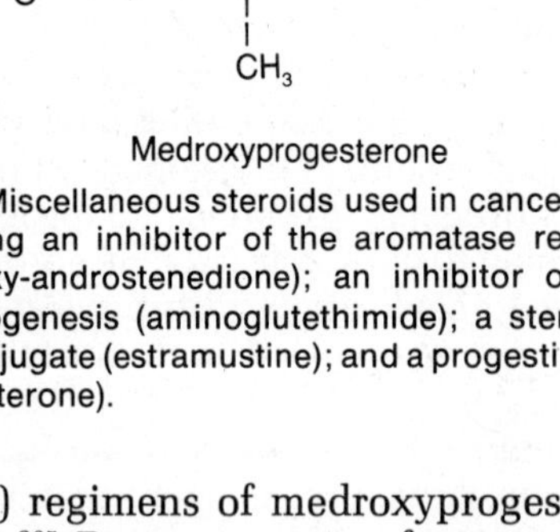

Medroxyprogesterone

Figure 7–9. Miscellaneous steroids used in cancer therapy, including an inhibitor of the aromatase reaction (4-hydroxy-androstenedione); an inhibitor of adrenal steroidogenesis (aminoglutethimide); a steroid-alkylator conjugate (estramustine); and a progestin (medroxyprogesterone).

(1500 mg/day) regimens of medroxyprogesterone acetate.[305] Response rates of over 40 per cent were reported. No comparisons of standard with high-dose progestins have been made. Additional clinical data will be needed to delineate the effectiveness of progestins at these doses. One of the potential attractions of progestins is their very minimal toxicity. Gluteal abscesses may occur after high-dose medroxyprogesterone injection. Generally, less than 10 per cent of patients have fluid retention or weight gain. Hypercalcemia, virilization, and phlebites are very unusual.

Glucocorticoid Therapy

Large doses of any glucocorticoid (equivalent to 200 to 300 mg of cortisol daily) can occasionally induce regression of metastatic breast cancer. Remissions are short-lived, but the rapid onset of action of the glucocorticoids makes them useful in rapidly advancing disease. A response to glucocorticoids is not predictive of response to other endocrine modalities. Glucocorticoids are also of value in managing acute emergencies such as hypercalcemia (in part by blocking intestinal calcium absorption) and intracranial metastases.

Antiestrogen Therapy

Antiestrogens may be defined as any substances that antagonize the action of estrogens. Many compounds that would fit this definition include a variety of nonspecific inhibitors of protein and RNA synthesis. However, with the possible exception of certain weak, short-acting agonists, such as estriol, all such compounds of current clinical relevance are derivatives of triphenylethylene (Fig. 7–8). These include nafoxidine, clomiphene, and tamoxifen. These compounds compete with estradiol for binding to specific estrogen receptor sites. However, the explanation for their biologic activity is far more complicated. Detailed information on this subject has been presented.[306, 307] It is likely that antiestrogenic compounds, after binding to estrogen receptors, translocate these receptors to nuclear sites. It is uncertain whether these nuclear sites are[308] or are not[309, 310] identical to nuclear sites occupied by estrogen receptor complexes. In fact, there is some suggestion that separable tamoxifen cytoplasmic binding sites may exist that do not bind estrogens.[311] All such studies are hampered by a failure either to purify or unequivocally to identify the specific nuclear "acceptor site" (if it exists at all) responsible for estrogenic effect. However, estrogen receptor does predict for response to antiestrogen.

Pharmacokinetic information is critical in the design of clinical dosage and schedules of antiestrogen therapy. Tamoxifen and its biologically active hydroxylated or demethylated metabolites all have plasma half-lives of 10 to 14 days.[220, 320] Thus, peak drug levels may not occur until two months following initiation of daily therapy, unless a loading dose schedule is used. In addition, receptor determinations performed for many weeks after discontinuation of therapy may be erroneous, either because of receptor occupancy or because of receptor processing secondary to tamoxifen.

Antiestrogens have proved extremely useful in the management of postmenopausal breast cancer.[312-314] Premenopausal patients appear to have a response rate equal to that of postmenopausal patients,[315] and may either continue to have normal menstrual cycles or show menopausal symptoms while exhibiting objective tumor regressions.[316] Antiestrogens have considerable effects that must be termed "estrogenic." In mice, nafoxidine and tamoxifen are complete estrogens. The vaginal epithelium of postmenopausal women usually shows an estrogenic effect. In addition, some women have a brief "flare" of tumor growth following the institution of antiestrogen therapy,[317] although very careful attempts to quantify the incidence of this phenomenon have not been successful.[318] Withdrawal responses to antiestrogens have been reported anecdotally. As mentioned previously, there is at present no proved role for antiestrogens in the adjuvant setting, although important trials in this area are ongoing. Animal studies suggest that continued administration of antiestrogen may be required to prevent appearance of DMBA-induced tumors in rats.[319] Most trials involving antiestrogens in the adjuvant setting continue the drug for two years or less. Under these conditions it will be important to observe whether antiestrogens simply prolong the disease-free interval or whether recurrences are prevented.

Antiestrogens thus are of proved value in male and female breast cancer.[242, 313, 314] About one third of unselected patients benefit from antiestrogen therapy, and these drugs therefore are at least as efficacious as other forms of endocrine manipulation. A particular advantage of antiestrogens is their almost complete lack of serious toxicity. Tamoxifen administration is not associated with significant myelosuppression, or renal, hepatic, or CNS toxicity. Transient and usually mild falls in platelet count may occur. Retinopathy induced by particularly high doses of tamoxifen (~100 mg/m^2 administered for over six months) has been reported.[321] The retinopathy, characterized by macular degeneration, has not been reversible.* Particularly encouraging, and of theoretical interest, is that an appreciable response rate has been seen following relapse after successful adrenalectomy.[322] This result is consistent with *in vitro* studies of human breast cancer, which have suggested that antiestrogens are capable of receptor-mediated tumor inhibition even in the absence of ambient estrogen.[323] Needless to say, the mechanism of action and cytoxicity of tamoxifen and their antiestrogen are poorly understood; further work is required to delineate the optimal utilization of antiestrogens in breast cancer and other neoplasms.

Pharmacologic Interference with Endogenous Steroidogenesis

Although major ablative endocrine therapies are unquestionably effective for some patients, the morbidity and occasional mortality associated with surgery has prompted efforts to achieve similar results pharmacologically. Transient palliative responses may be seen in some patients with metastatic breast cancer following glucocorticoid administration. Although glucocorticoids can directly inhibit human breast cancer cells in long-term tissue culture,[324] it is likely that the *in vivo* response is the result of partial suppression of adrenal androgen production and subsequent estrogen synthesis in peripheral tissues. In 1973 Griffiths and colleagues proposed the use of aminoglutethimide (Fig. 7–9), an inhibitor of cholesterol conversion to pregnenolone,[325] combined with dexamethasone to suppress adrenal function.[326] This regimen was effective in some women, but it was found that aminoglutethimide substantially shortened the plasma half-life of dexamethasone by increasing its hepatic metabolism,[327] and as a result pituitary ACTH secretion resumed and overrode the adrenal blockade imposed

*Nafoxidine (Fig. 7–8) has largely been supplanted in clinical use by tamoxifen because the former is associated with significant side effects (photophobia and ichthyosis).

by aminoglutethimide. By substituting hydrocortisone (whose metabolism was not altered by aminoglutethimide), it was possible to derive a fixed-dose regimen that gave adequate adrenal suppression in most patients.[328] The effectiveness of aminoglutethimide-hydrocortisone has been confirmed.

Over 90 per cent of patients show adequate suppression of adrenal steroidogenesis when treated with a fixed-dose regimen of 250 mg of aminoglutethimide four times a day orally, plus hydrocortisone 25 mg orally twice a day. Adequate suppression of the adrenal can be documented by measurements of plasma dehydroepiandrosterone and its sulfate. Both should fall below 25 ng/ml by three weeks. If suppression is inadequate, aminoglutethimide can be increased at the rate of 250 mg per week up to 2 gm. In the unusual patient not adequately suppressed, difficulty with gastrointestinal absorption or patient compliance should be investigated.

Although dehydroepiandrosterone levels declined in patients so treated, there is also an initial rise in Δ_4-androstenedione, the immediate precursor of estrone, and a fall in estrone and estradiol. These findings are consistent with an additional action of aminoglutethimide: blockade of peripheral aromatization of androstenedione to estrone. This inhibition has been substantiated by *in vitro* measurements in which aminoglutethimide blocked androgen aromatization by human placenta, and by additional studies of estrogen metabolism in aminoglutethimide-treated patients.[329]

Minor adverse reactions are extremely common with aminoglutethimide. A generalized macular skin rash, usually pruritic, but rarely associated with fever, may occur in over one third of treated patients and usually disappears with continued therapy. In addition, a variety of central nervous system reactions may occur including lethargy, somnolence, and ataxia. Reduction in drug dosage usually relieves these symptoms, but occasional patients cannot tolerate the drug.

Direct comparisons of antisteroidogenic regimens with ablative surgery are under way. Preliminary results suggest that these nonsurgical modalities may be as effective as surgical means for achieving suppression of plasma estrogen concentrations[330] and inducing clinical responses. It is possible that combinations of aminoglutethimide with an antiestrogen, antiandrogen, or a gonadotropin inhibitor such as danazol or progestin, will lead to greater effectiveness than single agents.

In an effort to decrease the conversion of androgens to estrogens in the ovary and in many peripheral tissues, including tumors, inhibitors of the aromatase reaction sequence shown in Figure 7–7 have been synthesized. Several weak androgens inhibit this reaction, including 4-hydroxyandrostenedione (Figure 7–9), a compound that decreases circulating estrogens in rats bearing DMBA-induced breast carcinomas and induces a high rate of remissions.[330A] This compound and others of similar structure have not been evaluated clinically at this time.

Endometrial Cancer

Endocrinology of Endometrial Cancer

Uterine endometrium is a classic example of a hormone-dependent tissue, its growth and morphology changing cyclically in response to estradiol and progesterone throughout menstrual life. The identification of the specific uterine cytosol receptor for estradiol in 1960[331] initiated the "receptor" era of endocrinology. Estrogen receptor concentration of the endometrium varies throughout the menstrual cycle; it is highest in the proliferative phase and is decreased in the luteal phase or by administration of progestins.[332, 333] Progesterone receptor concentration is highest at the time of the estradiol peak[332] and can be induced by estrogens. Estrogen receptor persists in most endometrial carcinomas.[332] Cytosolic progesterone receptor concentration[332, 334] and nuclear progesterone receptors are highest in well-differentiated cancer.[332] The enzyme 17β-hydroxysteroid dehydrogenase, which catalyzes the conversion of estradiol to estrone, is induced by progesterone[335] and can serve as an index of progestational effect.

A variety of steroid- and peptide-mediated abnormalities have been implicated in the etiology of the disease, including chronic abnormal estrogen stimulation, disordered anterior pituitary function, diabetes mellitus, obesity, and infertility.[336] Biologic, clinical, and epidemiologic data strongly suggest that prolonged or unopposed estrogenic stimulation increases the risk of developing endometrial carcinoma. The longer the endometrium is stimulated, as with the use of postmenopausal estrogen or in patients with late menopause, the greater is the risk of endometrial cancer.[337] The increase in endometrial cancer among women with estrogen-secreting tumors and the polycystic ovary syndrome[338] who have no luteal phase emphasizes the role of progesterone-induced endometrial sloughing as a protective mechanism. A higher incidence of endometrial cancer is also seen with several other ovarian abnormalities, such as cortical stromal hyperplasia and persistent stromal thecal cells. In each case, estrogen secretion probably is not excessive. It is, however, continuous, since there are no ovulatory cycles with their accompanying progesterone secretory periods and subsequent endometrial sloughing. Recent reports of endometrial cancer in women with Turner's syndrome treated with estrogens alone is further evidence for this concept. The causal role of continued, unopposed, estrogenic stimulus is supported by the high incidence of a history of irregular menses in women with endometrial cancer.[338] The resumption of cyclic ovarian function in response to ovarian wedge resection in the Stein-Leventhal syndrome[339] results in regression of endometrial hyperplasia. Progesterone has also been shown to reverse estrogen-induced endometrial hyperplasia.

Obesity is a risk factor for endometrial carcinoma. In premenopausal women, the association of obesity with anovulatory cycles and amenorrhea may provide the physiologic basis for the association. In postmenopausal women, the etiologic pathway may be traced more clearly. After the menopause, the predominant blood estrogen is estrone, derived almost entirely from aromatization of androgen precursor in peripheral tissues. The rate of this conversion increases with age[340] and weight,[341] leading to increased plasma estrogen concentrations with increasing weight.[342] Since fat tissue can aromatize androgens, obesity is directly linked to greater exposure to estrogens and increased risk of endometrial carcinoma. This therapy has been difficult to confirm by measurement of estrogen levels in blood. Plasma estrone production rates[341] and concentrations[342] are the same in women with endometrial cancer as in weight- and age-matched controls, but the higher incidence of obesity in the women with cancer suggests that as a group there is greater exposure in obese women to estrogen, perhaps owing to alterations in the concentrations of sex steroid binding globulin and free estrogens or to elevations of estrogens not being measured.

Estrogen use by postmenopausal women is associated with a four- to ninefold increased risk of endometrial cancer.[336] Risk increases with duration of use. This is consistent with a two-stage carcinogenesis model in which the estrogen functions as a classical promotor. Feinstein has suggested that these estimates of excess risk are spurious because of an increased rate of discovery of early endometrial cancer, owing to the vaginal bleeding that may accompany estrogen therapy or to closer surveillance of patients on estrogen therapy.[343] This argument has been refuted by additional data and theoretical considerations.[337] It is now widely accepted that the use of estrogen after the menopause is an important risk factor for endometrial cancer. However, in all studies of estrogen use in postmenopausal women, greater than physiologic doses of estrogen have been used and progestin-induced withdrawal bleeding has not generally been part of the regimens. Attention to both of these factors might appreciably reduce the risk.

Therapy

In 1961 Kelley and Baker reported that progestogens could cause regression in about one third of patients with metastatic endometrial cancer.[344] This has been confirmed in large series of patients treated at many centers.[345] Objective response rates to therapy do not strongly depend on patient age, site of metastasis, or previous or concurrent therapy. However, women with slowly growing or more differentiated tumors and pulmonary metastases respond better than those with aggressive cancers. Duration of life after initiation of therapy was 27 months in those who responded and only seven months in those who did not. These combined data have been duplicated in other reports. Neither the progestogen used nor the dose administered appears critical,[346] although large doses are generally required. Despite many clinical studies,[347] clear establishment of clinical or pharmacologic guidelines for therapy are lacking. Neither loading dose versus daily dose schedules nor intramuscular versus oral regimens have shown any advantage. Part of these difficulties may reflect problems in evaluation of these patients. Effective regimens include megestrol acetate, 40 mg orally four times a day or medroxyprogesterone acetate, 1 gm intramuscularly twice a week. In the absence of a major impact of chemotherapy in this disease, a trial of progestogens should be initiated in any patient with metastatic disease.

Trials of antiestrogen therapy in endometrial cancer have revealed some antitumor activity,[347, 348] not a suprising finding since normal endometrium is clearly an estrogen-responsive tissue.

Just as estrogen receptor determinations have revolutionized patient selection in breast cancer, it now appears that progesterone receptors can similarly aid in selection of patients for progestogen therapy.[349-352] Progesterone receptor is always detectable in high concentrations in the proliferative phase of normal human endometrium, and nearly as often, but at lower concentrations, in secretory endometrium. A variety of endometrial hyperplasias (almost invariably responsive to progestogen therapy) are usually progesterone receptor-positive.[349] Endometrial adenocarcinomas are less often progesterone receptor-positive. As shown in Table 7–11, there is a good correlation between grade and progesterone receptor concentration. Although response data are far more preliminary, positive correlations between progesterone receptor and response rate to progestogen therapy have emerged.[349] If chemotherapy for endometrial cancer proves to be a rational alternative to endocrine therapy,[353] progesterone receptor determinations will assume an even greater importance in treatment planning.

TABLE 7–11. Progesterone Receptor Activity in Normal, Hyperplastic, and Malignant Endometria*

Tissue	*No. of Assays*	*PR*†‡	*PR Activity ± SEM*
Normal			
Proliferative	15	100%	596 ± 325
Secretory	15	94%	326 ± 346
Endometrial Hyperplasia			
All types	19	79%	514 ± 421
Endometrial polyps	6	83%	282 ± 210
Endometrial adenocarcinomas			
Grade I	19	84%	430 ± 584
Grade II	17	47%	61 ± 54
Grade III	16	25%	62 ± 127
All grades	52	58%	

*Modified from Young and Ehrlich.[349]
†≥50 fmols/mg protein.

The mechanism of action of progestogens is not known.[354] In the normal estrogen-primed uterus, progesterone causes specific maturational changes, followed by atrophy when a progestogen is continued for long periods. Following administration of progestogens to women with endometrial cancer, changes in the tumor occur that mimic those induced in normal endometrial epilthelium. Mitotic activity ceases, there is increased glandular differentiation, and an increase in cytoplasm:nucleus ratio is seen. Atrophy is also noted. These morphologic changes are accompanied by a host of changes in many enzyme systems.[354] These include induction of glycogen synthesis followed by induction of glycogen-metabolizing enzymes. Estradiol 17β-dehydrogenase (the enzyme catalyzing the conversion of estradiol to estrone) is induced.[355] This enzyme may be a marker for progestational responses in endometrial cancer. These enzymatic changes occur concurrently with suppression of nucleoside incorporation into nucleic acid.[354, 356]

Carcinoma of the Prostate

Endocrinology of Prostate Cancer

Cancer of the prostate is the second most frequent cancer in males in the United States, more than 60 per cent of cases occurring in men over 70 years of age. The death rate is significantly higher in American blacks than in whites. American black males have an age-standardized incidence rate about six times that of Nigerian black males,[357] although the incidence of latent carcinoma is the same.[358] In this same study, it was reported that the fat intake of patients with carcinoma of the prostate exceeded that of matched controls. Fat intake and possibly testosterone levels may act as conditioning factors in the progression of latent to clinical cancer. The role of environmental factors in the etiology of clinical cancer of the prostate has been further supported by the finding that Japanese males living in Hawaii have a higher incidence of clinical cancer of the prostate than do Japanese males in Japan, although once again the incidence of latent carcinoma is the same.[359]

Prostate is the target tissue on which virtually all studies of androgen action have been performed. It should be appreciated that studies of the hormone dependency of benign prostatic hypertrophy may not be applicable to the problem of prostate cancer. Benign prostatic hypertrophy, for example, arises from the central zone of the prostate, whereas carcinoma originates in the periphery. Both diseases respond to withdrawal of androgen.

The pioneering work of Huggins[360, 361] established the role of androgen in maintenance of the prostate and gave rise to the concept of androgen dependence. The subsequent demonstration that castration caused regression of prostatic cancer in man[362] initiated the era of hormonal management of cancer of the prostate.

It is almost certain that, in man and many other species, the active intracellular androgen is dihydrotestosterone, a metabolite of testosterone.[363] Studies of prostate in organ culture suggest that a metabolite of dihydrotestosterone, 5α-androstane-3,17β-diol, specifically stimulates prostatic secretion, whereas dihydrotestosterone induces growth.[364] Although both testosterone and androstenedione are precursors of intracellular dihydrotestosterone, high plasma concentrations of testosterone are apparently necessary, since prostate weight is not maintained after castration. However, interference with adrenal androstenedione production can occasionally produce temporary improvement in a few patients with metastatic prostatic cancer. Plasma androgens are the same in males with prostatic cancer as in the normal population.[365-367]

Prolactin plays a role in the prostatic growth of rodents and other species. Hypophysectomy causes a more profound atrophy of the rat prostate than does castration,[368] and endogenous prolactin synergizes with testosterone in maintaining the male mouse sexual accessory glands. Injection of a prolactin antiserum inhibits prostate growth in rabbits.[369] The prostate has specific prolactin binding sites and these are androgen-dependent.[370] Thus, there may be steroid and peptide hormone interaction in prostate carcinogenesis.

Therapy

Based on information extensively described elsewhere in this chapter, one would predict that since prostatic carcinoma is a hormone-dependent cancer, androgen receptor studies might be of value in selecting patients for endocrine manipulation. As pointed out in an earlier section on receptors and in two excellent reviews,[371, 372] there are many difficulties in the quantification of androgen receptors. The tissue contains many proteolytic enzymes; the surrounding stroma of normal prostatic or benign prostatic hypertrophy is strongly androgen receptor-positive; plasma contains a high-affinity binder for dihydrotestosterone and prostate is capable of rapid metabolism of radiolabeled androgen to nonbinding metabolites.

Despite these many difficulties, androgen receptors can be detected in human prostatic cancer.[371-375] Although these receptors are detectable in prostatic cancer, it has been possible to correlate androgen receptor activity with response to endocrine therapy in only a few cases.[376] In truth, this correlation is of limited importance because, unlike the situation in breast and endometrial cancers, there are no effective alternatives at present to endocrine therapy. In addition, secondary endocrine therapies employed after failure of estrogens or orchiectomy have less than 10 per cent response rates. Thus, selective tests would have little impact on therapy even were they as accurate as receptor determinations in breast cancer. However, if complete faith is placed in an androgen receptor negative assay, orchiectomy or estrogens might be avoided in 20 per cent of patients.

The endocrine therapy of prostatic cancer has been based on a simple premise. If, as originally proposed by Huggins, it is necessary to decrease plasma androgens to a low level, orchiectomy should suffice. Estrogen can inhibit the effect of androgen on prostatic secretion in the absence of the pituitary gland.[377] These and other data have implied a direct effect of estrogen on the prostate in addition to its suppression of LH. Thus, a rationale can be cited for the simultaneous use of orchiectomy and estrogen.

In large, collected series of patients with metastatic disease,[378, 379] three- and five-year survival rates of treated patients with Stages III (locally extensive) and IV (metastatic) disease were always better than those of untreated patients. Differences between castration, estrogen therapy, or combined treatment were not significant at three and five years. In a prospective trial reported in 1967, no difference was found among the three regimens;[380] however, the daily use of 5 mg of diethylstilbestrol was associated with increased mortality from cardiovascular disease.[380] These data have been confirmed in a study of treatment of patients with coronary artery disease. In a subsequent study, 1 mg of diethylstilbestrol daily was as effective as the 5-mg dose,[381] even though plasma testosterone concentrations were not as completely suppressed.[382] The lower dose was not associated with increased cardiovascular mortality. Diethylstilbestrol did not improve the survival curve of Stages I and II patients (carcinoma confined to the prostate). There is no evidence that one estrogen is better than another, although individual patients may have fewer gastrointestinal reactions to one or another. When patients have responded to either estrogen or orchiectomy, the subsequent use of the other modality has generally proved ineffective. This would argue against a direct effect of estrogen on the prostate, independent of effects on androgen secretion.

Remission of disease has usually been defined as a significant lowering of acid phosphatase and relief of pain. Since bone metastases are usually osteoblastic, sufficient remodeling to permit diagnosis of response is not easy. Nevertheless, regression rates associated with either orchiectomy or estrogen have been 50 to 80 per cent, varying with grade and stage of disease and to some extent a function of the criteria used to evaluate response. The average duration of remission has been 15 months, although remissions may last over five years.

In some patients 17-ketosteroid excretion eventually rises following orchiectomy. This may be associated with reactivation of disease. Androstenedione and testosterone plasma concentrations are higher in some patients with prostatic cancer than might be anticipated following orchiectomy.[383] Suppression of the adrenal androgen production by exogenous glucocorticoids reduces these levels and might be beneficial in this group. Trials of glucocorticoid have been inconclusive, although some clinical improvement has been recorded. Aminoglutethimide has not been extensively evaluated in prostatic cancer, though preliminary results are encouraging.[384]

Because of residual androgen production by the adrenal cortex and the possible role of prolactin in maintaining prostate growth and adrenal androgen secretion, adrenalectomy and hypophysectomy have been performed in patients who have relapsed after primary therapy with estrogen or orchiectomy. In general, responses to adrenalectomy have been less satisfactory than those to hypophysectomy.[385] In three preliminary studies the remission rate for hypophysectomy has been surprisingly high, varying between 40 and 63 per cent.[385, 386] Hypophysectomy often produced clinical remission as defined by decrease in pain and improved sense of well-being.[387] Responders survived considerably longer than nonresponders. Further evaluation of the role of hypophysectomy and antiprolactin drugs (the ergoline derivatives) is certainly warranted, since patient selection and varying response criteria may substantially influence the proportion of responding patients. In none of the series was there a consistent decrease in acid phosphatase accompanying the decrease in pain. It is thus premature to recommend these ablature procedures routinely for the patient in relapse.

Progestational agents have been used in treatment since they suppress LH and can also act as antiandrogens, competing directly with testosterone for the prostate androgen receptors. Remissions have also been reported in response to cyproterone acetate, an effective antiandrogen.[388, 389] The agent was effective only when given prior to castration or estrogen. For further details, the reader is referred to an excellent review on antiandrogen pharmacology.[390]

Another antiandrogen, the nonsteroidal androgen antagonist flutamide (Fig. 7–6) produced substantial regression of disease in untreated patients and had some activity in patients who relapsed following stilbestrol therapy.[391] The drug does not cause a loss of libido, and in the experimental animal its antiandrogenic activity seems to be limited to prostate and seminal vesicles.[392]

An important area of pharmacologic interest has been the use of cytotoxic agents linked to hormones. A review of this field has appeared.[393] Estramustine phosphate (an alkylator linked to estradiol (Fig. 7–9) was developed to promote selective concentration of the alkylating activity in receptor-positive tumor cells. However, the compound has little affinity for the estrogen receptor[394] and, in addition, no antitumor activity in advanced breast cancer.[395, 396] On the other hand, although this is controversial, some activity has been reported in advanced prostatic cancer.[397-399] A possible rational basis for this discrepancy may lie in the discovery in 1978 that estramustine phosphate does bind with high affinity to an androgen-induced prostate cytosol protein,[400] thus conferring additional target tissue specificity on the molecule. It must be hoped that more clearly defined hormone-cytotoxic conjugates that take proper cognizance of the binding requirements of the hormone will lead to further developments in this area.

Cancer of the Kidney

Endocrinology

The kidney is not usually considered an endocrine-responsive tissue with respect to cellular proliferation, although androgen administration in the rat causes hypertrophy of the kidney. An androgen receptor has been identified in mouse kidney.[401] There are few experimental models of adenocarcinoma of the kidney, the best being the estrogen-induced renal cell adenocarcinoma in the hamster, which closely resembles human adenocarcinoma.[402] These tumors can be transplanted to male hamsters only after pretreatment with estrogen,[403] but cannot be induced in females except after oophorectomy, suggesting that ovarian progesterone inhibits induction. An estrogen antagonist decreases the growth rate of a transplantable tumor.[404] The growth of the tumors can be suppressed by cortisone and medroxyprogesterone given concurrently, but not by either agent alone. Specific androgen receptors have been demonstrated in the normal kidney and in estrogen-dependent hamster carcinoma.[405] Both estrogen and progesterone receptors may be present in primary hamster tumors.[406, 407]

Evidence that studies of this unique system are relevant to the treatment of human kidney cancer is sparse and depends chiefly on the observation that hormonal therapy, particularly with progesterone, occasionally causes regression of disease in humans. Renal cell cancer occurs twice as commonly in men as in women,[408] thereby minimizing a role for estrogens in tumor induction. In human renal cell carcinoma, almost two thirds of the specimens had either estrogen or progesterone receptors.[409] Higher receptor content is claimed to be predictive of response to progestational agents.

Therapy

Bloom has summarized his data on patients treated with endocrine therapy for renal cell carcinoma.[410] Of 80 patients with metastatic disease, 55 per cent underwent remissions (mean duration of 11.5 months). All were treated initially with high doses of medroxyprogesterone and a few secondarily with testosterone. Remissions were rare in women. The results reported in this series are much better than those given in other series.[411] The sex difference among responses recorded by Bloom has not been confirmed. An occasional good response to testosterone has also been recorded.

The use of medroxyprogesterone acetate (Fig. 7–9) is associated with few side effects. Although this steroid, in high doses, has a low glucocorticoid potency, neither adrenal atrophy nor Cushing's syndrome has been reported in adults on long-term therapy. The agent causes loss of libido in men via its suppressive effect on LH.[412] At present, given the lack of alternatives, a trial of a progestational therapy may be considered, but hopes for a clinical remission should not be overly sanguine.

Leukemia and Lymphoma

Glucocorticoids influence the growth, differentiation, and function of virtually every tissue and organ system of the body.[22] Among these diverse effects, inhibitory actions on lymphoid tissue have long been appreciated.[413, 414] Glucocorticoids produce marked lymphocytopenia and thymic atrophy in experimental animals. Thus, these steroids were initially used with great enthusiasm when it was discovered that they could also kill some leukemic lymphoblasts in humans.[415, 416] Despite this important observation, several difficulties prevented their more effective use. First, variable response rates were observed in patients with differing histologic types of acute and chronic leukemia and lymphoma. Thus, the subset of patients likely to benefit from glucocorticoid therapy has not been defined. Second, patients in whom clinical disease is controlled by glucocorticoid therapy eventually relapse, and inevitably they become unresponsive to glucorticoid therapy. Thus, although initial response rates in pediatric acute lymphoblastic leukemia range between 45 and 65 per cent, the rate of subsequent remission induction with glucocorticoids alone falls to 25 per cent after primary relapse.

Furthermore, glucocorticoid administration is associated with many complications. These include immunosuppression with concomitant nosocomial infections, Cushing's syndrome, diabetes mellitus, poor wound healing, psychosis, and other problems.[22] Since most patients with leukemia die of infectious complications rather than leukemia *per se*, it is likely that glucocorticoids may be a significant detriment to survival in some cases. This particular difficulty is amplified by the fact that most patients with leukemia and lymphoma are currently managed by combinations of agents that include glucocorticoids along with cytotoxics. Thus, possibly harmful components in the drug combination, such as the glucocorticoid, may be continued long after they have ceased to be of benefit.

It is therefore of value to select patients for glucocorticoid therapy on a rational basis. One obvious approach is to measure glucocorticoid sensitivity *in vitro* using some type of cytotoxic or inhibitory end point. Unfortunately, such methods have not proved useful for leukemic therapy. First, it is difficult to culture leukemic cells reliably. Second, studies on circulating leukemic cells may not correlate with effects on proliferating neoplastic cells in the marrow.

Studies performed in breast cancer and other malignancies supported the notion that quantification of specific steroid receptors is useful in predicting response to endocrine therapy. Based on these observations, plus a clearer understanding of the mechanism of action of glucocorticoids, several groups have specific glucocorticoid receptors in various populations of human leukemic and lymphoid cells.[417-419]

Glucocorticoid receptors can be demonstrated in normal peripheral blood lymphocytes as well as in partially purified subpopulations of lymphocytes and monocytes.[420, 421] These receptor proteins are similar to the glucocorticoid receptors more extensively characterized in liver and rat thymocytes. Agents that induce blastic transformation of human lymphoid cells, such as phytohemagglutinin or concanavalin A, lead to several-fold increases in intracellular glucocorticoid receptor activity,[420, 422] from $2–4 \times 10^3$ receptors per cell in mature circulating cells to $4–12 \times 10^3$ receptor molecules per cell in activated cells. These lymphoblasts are similar morphologically, and in glucocorticoid receptor content, to human leukemic lymphoblasts.

Early studies in human acute lymphoblastic leukemia suggested that quantitative glucocorticoid receptor analyses would be clinically relevant.[417, 419, 423] Glucocorticoid receptors are readily detectable by assay of either cytoplastic extracts or intact whole cells in most previously untreated patients with acute lymphoblastic leukemia. There is good agreement between concentrations of glucocorticoids that fully occupy receptor sites and concentrations that inhibit cellular processes. Further data in acute lymphoblastic leukemia suggest that a reasonable correlation may exist between loss of glucocorticoid receptor activity and *in vitro* resistance to glucocorticoids.[419] Furthermore, there are substantial differences in receptor content of the various types of acute lymphoblastic leukemia of childhood — so called T-cell leukemias having substantially fewer receptor sites than Null cell leukemia (usually less than 3000 compared with more than 5000).[423] The concentration of receptor in acute lymphoblastic leukemic cells correlates well with initial complete remission duration,[417] independent of known prognostic factors such as cell type, initial white blood cell count, or sex. Thus, in acute lymphoblastic leukemia, pretreatment analyses of glucocorticoid receptors has significant prognostic value.

Other workers have produced somewhat contradictory data. Duval[424] and Crabtree[418] and their colleagues have suggested that correlations between receptor content and *in vitro* response to therapy were imperfect. In their hands, most leukemic cells showed some *in vitro* inhibition of macromolecular synthesis by glucocorticoids. Very few samples were totally receptor-negative. These studies did not attempt to correlate receptor content with *in vivo* response. Direct confirmation of the predictive value of receptor determinations in a second lymphoproliferative malignancy state was reported by

Bloomfield et al.,[425] who found that quantity of glucocorticoid receptor was directly correlated with likelihood of response to single-agent glucocorticoid therapy in patients with non-Hodgkin's lymphoma.

Glucocorticoid receptors have also been identified in other hematologic malignancies, including acute myelogenous leukemia,[418, 426] chronic myelogenous leukemia in blast crisis,[418] chronic lymphocytic leukemia,[427, 428] and the Sézary syndrome. In none of these illnesses have significant correlations between receptor content and either clinical parameters or prognosis been reliably documented. Clearly "receptorology" as it pertains to glucocorticoid-responsive neoplasia is in an early stage of development and, with the possible exception of acute lymphoblastic leukemia and some lymphomas, should be regarded as experimental.

Many schedules of glucocorticoid administration have been employed ranging from low-dose daily oral therapy (e.g., 20 to 40 mg of prednisone orally per day) to massive intravenous therapy (1 gm of prednisolone per square meter of body surface area). Plasma concentrations with the latter regimen approach 1000 times those required to saturate receptor. However, since 15 to 20 plasma half-lives may elapse (between doses) with daily intravenous administration, there is a rationale for such massive doses. Also, as previously stated, it is possible that at least some effects of glucocorticoids may not require receptor. There are no data, however, to suggest that such massive doses have any benefit over conventional oral regimens. It is worth mentioning that utilization of glucocorticoids with no mineralocorticoid activity, e.g., dexamethasone, may reduce toxicity as compared with that of prednisone.

Ovarian Cancer

Several observations suggest possible endocrine dependence in some forms of ovarian cancer. Ovarian cancer occurs at a higher rate in women with breast cancer[429] and endometrial cancer.[430] Second-generation Japanese women in America show increases in rates of ovarian cancer as well as of breast cancer.[431] In at least one study, the use of estrogen by postmenopausal women has been correlated with a higher risk of ovarian cancer.[432] Although these data suggest an association of estrogen and ovarian cancer, correlation does not necessarily imply causation.

Estrogen receptors have been demonstrated in the ovary and in ovarian cancers.[433] Although progestins have been reported to induce response rates of up to 38 per cent in ovarian cancer,[434] clinical experience of many gynecologic oncologists has not confirmed such a high response rate. Many of the responding tumors have been reported to be "endometrioid," and it is possible that at least some are misdiagnosed endometrial carcinomas. Prospective trials, with full reporting of clinical findings, histologic data, and response criteria, will be required before the exact role of progestational therapy in ovarian cancer is established.

Laryngeal Carcinoma

The larynx is a target organ for androgens, as manifested by the hypertrophy of the vocal cords at puberty in the male. Androgen administration to females induces vocal changes that mimic the pubertal changes seen in males. The majority of laryngoepitheliomas occur in males, although alternative epidemiologic data such as smoking and ethanol intake may be important. Androgen receptors have been demonstrated in the human larynx, and similar receptors are present in epithelial cancers of the larynx.[435, 436] Estrogen has been reported to produce remission in several patients with metastatic disease. Three out of 13 patients achieved objective responses, including one complete response.[435] These early encouraging studies are in accord with the theme of this chapter, namely, that cancer derived from a hormone-sensitive tissue may regress following withdrawal of the hormone or following treatment with an agent that antagonizes that hormone. Certainly, further exploration of this area may be worthwhile.

References

1. Klyne W: The Chemistry of the Steroids. Methuen, London, 1957.
2. Fieser LF, and Fieser M: Steroids. Reinhold, New York, 1959.
3. Shoppee CW: Chemistry of the Steroids. Butterworth, London, 1964.
4. Dorfman RI, and Ungar F: Metabolism of Steroid Hormones. Academic Press, New York, 1965.
5. IUPAC Commission on the Nomenclature of Organic Chemistry and IUPAC-IUB Commission on Biochemical Nomenclature. Revised tentative nomenclature of steroids. Biochem. J. 113:5, 1969.

6. Hakin HLJ, and Trafford DJH: The Chemistry of the Steroids. Clin. Endocrinol. Metab. 1:333–360, 1972.
7. Briggs MH, and Brotherton J: Steroid Biochemistry and Pharmacology. Academic Press, London, 1970.
8. Brotherton J: Sex Hormone Pharmacology. Academic Press, London, 1976.
9. Briggs MH and Christie GA: eds. Advances in Steroid Biochemistry and Pharmacology. Academic Press, London, 1977.
10. Danielson H, and Tchen TT: Steroid Metabolism. *In* Greenberg DM (ed.): Metabolic Pathways, Vol. II. Academic Press, New York, 1968, Chap. 11, p. 128.
11. Richardson KC, Nowaczynski W, and Genest J: Specific aldosterone-binding proteins in human plasma: partial characterization. J. Steroid Biochem. 8:951, 1977.
12. Katayama S, and Yamaji T: A novel binding protein for aldosterone in human plasma. 60th Annual Meeting of the Endocrine Society, Miami, 1978, p. 230 (abstr.).
13. Szego CM: Steroid-protein binding from circulating blood to target cell nucleus. Gynecol. Invest. 7:251, 1976.
14. Harrison RW, Fairfield S, and Orth DN: Evidence for glucocorticoid transport into AtT-20/D-1 cells. Biochemistry 14:1304, 1975.
15. Pietras R, and Szego C: Specific binding sites for oestrogen at the outer surfaces of isolated endometrial cells. Nature 265:69, 1977.
16. Muller RE, Johnston TC, and Wotiz HH: Binding of estradiol to purified uterine plasma membranes. J. Etiol. Chem. 254:7895, 1979.
17. Willmer EN. Steroids and cell surfaces. Biol. Rev. 36:368, 1961.
18. Tomkins GN, and Maxwell ES: Some aspects of steroid hormone action. Annu. Rev. Biochem. 12:677, 1963.
19. Williams-Ashman HG: New facets of the biochemistry of steroid hormone action. Cancer Res. 25:1096, 1965.
20. Grant JK: Actions of steroid hormones at cellular and molecular levels. Essays Biochem. 5:1, 1969.
21. Jensen EV, and Jacobsen HI: Basic guides to the mechanism of estrogen action. Recent Prog. Horm. Res. 18:387, 1962.
22. Thompson EB, and Lippman ME: Mechanism of action of glucocorticoids. Metabolism 23:159, 1974.
23. Chan L, and O'Malley BW: Mechanism of action of the sex steroid hormones. N. Engl. J. Med. 294:1322, 1430, 1976.
24. Chan L, and O'Malley BW: Steroid hormone action: recent advances. Ann. Intern. Med. 89:694, 1978.
25. Baxter JD, and Rousseau GG: Glucocorticoid hormone action: an overview. *In* Baxter JD, and Rousseau GG (eds.): Glucocorticoid Hormone Action. Springer-Verlag, New York, 1979, p. 1.
26. Verhoeven GF, and Wilson JD: The syndromes of primary hormone resistance. Metabolism 28:253, 1979.
27. Baxter JD, and Funder JW: Hormone receptors. N. Engl. J. Med. 301:1149, 1979.
28. Griffin JE, and Wilson JD: The syndromes of androgen resistance. N. Engl. J. Med. 302:198, 1980.
29. Greene GL, Fitch FW, and Jensen EV: Monoclonal antibodies to estrophilin: probes for the study of estrogen receptors. Proc. Natl. Acad. Sci. USA 77:157, 1980.
30. Nenci I: Receptor and centriole pathways of steroid action in normal and neoplastic cells. Cancer Res. 38:4204, 1978.
31. Pertschuk LP, Tobin EH, Gaetjeus E, et al.: Histochemical assay of steroid hormone receptors. *In* Eresciani F (ed.): Perspectives in Steroid Receptor Research. Raven Press, New York, 1980, p. 299.
32. Mercer WD, Wahl TM, Carlson CA, et al.: Techniques for the detection of steroid hormone in breast cancer cells. Cancer 12:2859, 1980.
33. Sheridan PJ, Buchanan JM, Anselmo VC, et al.: Equilibrium: the intracellular distribution of steroid receptors. Nature 282:579, 1979.
34. Keenan BS, Meyer WJ III, Hadjian AJ, et al.: Syndrome of androgen insensitivity in man: absence of 5α-dihydrotestosterone binding protein in skin fibroblasts. J. Clin. Endocrinol. Metab. 38:1143, 1974.
35. Griffin JE, Punyashthiti K, and Wilson JD: Dihydrotestosterone binding by cultured human fibroblasts: comparison of cells from control subjects and from patients with hereditary pseudohermaphroditism due to androgen resistance. J. Clin. Invest. 57:1342, 1976.
36. Kaufman M, Straisfeld C, and Pinsky L: Male pseudohermaphroditism presumably due to target organ unresponsiveness to androgens: deficient 5α-dihydrotestosterone binding in cultured skin fibroblasts. J. Clin. Invest. 58:345, 1976.
37. Amhein JA, Klingensmith GJ, Walsh PC, et al.: Partial androgen insensitivity: the Reifenstein syndrome revisited. N. Engl. J. Med. 297:350, 1977.
38. Griffin JE, and Wilson JD: Studies on the pathogenesis of the incomplete forms of androgen resistance in man. J. Clin. Endocrinol. Metab. 45:1137, 1977.
39. Griffin JE: Testicular feminization associated with a thermolabile androgen receptor in cultured human fibroblasts. J. Clin. Invest. 64:1624, 1979.
40. Sibley C, and Tomkins GM: Mechanisms of steroid hormone resistance. Cell 2:221, 1974.
41. Vedekis WV, Schrader WT, and O'Malley BW: The chick oviduct progesterone receptor. *In* Litwack G (ed.): Biochemical Actions of Hormones, Vol. 5. Academic Press, New York, 1978, p. 32.
42. Schrader WT, and O'Malley BW: Progesterone-binding components of chick oviduct. IV. Characterization of purified subunits. J. Biol. Chem. 247:51, 1976.
43. O'Malley BW, and Schrader WT: The receptors of steroid hormones. Sci. Am. 234:32, 1976.
44. Chamness GC, and McGuire WL: Estrogen receptor in the rat uterus. Physiologic forms and artifacts. Biochemistry 11:2466, 1972.
45. Puca GA, Nola E, Sica V, et al.: Estrogen-binding proteins of calf uterus. Molecular and functional characterization of the receptor transforming factor: a calcium-activated protease. J. Biol. Chem. 252:1358, 1977.
46. Kelsey JL: Oral contraceptives and breast disease. Am. J. Epidemiol. 107:236, 1978.
47. Nielsen CJ, Sando JJ, Vogel WM, et al.: Glucocorticoid receptor inactivation under cell-free conditions. J. Biol. Chem. 252:7568, 1977.
48. Sando JJ, Nielsen CJ, and Pratt WB: Reactivation of thymocyte glucocorticoid receptors in a cell-free system. J. Biol. Chem. 252:7579, 1977.
49. Notides AC, and Nielson S: The molecular mechanism of the 4S to 5S transformation of the uterine estrogen receptor. J. Biol. Chem. 249:1866, 1974.
50. Spelsberg TC, Webster R, Pickler G, et al.: Nuclear binding sites ("acceptors") for progesterone in avian oviduct: characterization of the highest affinity sites. Ann. N.Y. Acad. Sci. 286:43, 1977.
51. Spelsberg TC, Steggles AW, Chytil F, et al.: Progesterone-binding components of chick oviduct. V. Exchange of progesterone binding capacity from target to non-target tissue chromatins. J. Biol. Chem. 1247:1368, 1972.
52. McReynolds LA, Catterall JF, and O'Malley BW: The ovalbumin gene: cloning of a complete cDNA in a bacterial plasmid. Gene 2:217, 1977.
53. Schwartz RJ, Tsai M-J, Tsai SY, et al.: Effect of estrogen on gene expression in the chick oviduct. V. Changes in the number of RNA polymerase binding and initiation sites in chromatin. J. Biol. Chem. 250:5175, 1975.
54. Comstock JP, Rosenfeld GC, O'Malley BW, et al.: Estrogen-induced changes in translation and specific messenger RNA during oviduct differentiation. Proc. Natl. Acad. Sci. USA 69:1377, 1972.
55. Palmiter RD: Regulation of protein synthesis in chick oviduct. I. Independent regulation of ovalbumin, conalbumin, ovomucoid, and lysozyme induction. J. Biol. Chem. 247:6450, 1972.
56. Williams-Ashman HG, and Reddi AH: Action of vertebrate sex hormones. Annu. Rev. Physiol. 33:31, 1971.
57. Cohen P, and Kidson C: Interactions of hormonal steroids with nucleic acids. I. A specific requirement for guanine. Proc. Natl. Acad. Sci. USA 63:458, 1969.
58. Chin RC, and Kidson C: Selective associations of hormonal

steroids with aminoacyl transfer RNAs and control of protein synthesis. Proc. Natl. Acad. Sci. USA 68:2448, 1971.
59. Sluyser M: Interaction of steroid hormones and histones. *In* Smellie RMS (ed.): The Biochemistry of Steroid Action. Biochem. Soc. Symp. No. 32. Academic Press, New York, 1971, p. 31.
60. Gardner RS, and Tomkins GM: Steroid hormone binding to a macromolecule from hepatic tissue culture cells. J. Biol. Chem. 244:4761, 1969.
61. Rabin BR, Blyth CA, Doherty D, et al.: The effects of steroid hormones and carcinogens on the interactions of membranes with polysomes. *In* Rabin BR, and Freedman RB, (eds.): Effects of Drugs on Cellular Control Mechanisms. Macmillan, London, 1971, p. 27.
62. Blyth CA, Cooper MB, Roobol A, et al.: The binding of steroid hormones to degranulated microsomes from rat-liver endoplasmic reticulum. Eur. J. Biochem. 29:293, 1972.
63. Logsdon PJ, Middleton E Jr, and Coffey RG: Stimulation of leukocyte adenyl cyclase by hydrocortisone and isoproterenal in asthmatic and non-asthmatic subjects. J. Allergy Clin. Immunol. 50:45, 1972.
64. Irvine WJ, and Barnes EW: Adrenocortical insufficiency. Clin. Endocrinol. Metab. 1:549, 1972.
65. Szego CM: The lysosomal membrane complex as a proximate target for steroid hormone action. *In* McKerns KW (ed.): The Sex Steroid. Appleton-Century-Crofts, New York, 1971, p. 1.
66. Bongiovanni AM: Congenital adrenal hyperplasia and related disorders. *In* Stanbury JB, Wyngaarden JB, and Fredrickson DS (eds.): The Metabolic Basis of Inherited Disease, 4th ed. McGraw-Hill Book Co., New York, 1978, p. 868.
67. Griffin JE, and Wilson JD: Hereditary male pseudohermaphroditism. Clin. Obstet. Gynecol. 5:457, 1978.
68. Amrhein JA, Meyer WJ III, Jones HW Jr, et al.: Androgen insensitivity in man: evidence for genetic heterogeneity. Proc. Natl. Acad. Sci. USA 73:891, 1976.
69. Collier ME, Griffin JE, and Wilson JD: Intranuclear binding of [3H]dihydrotestosterone by cultured human fibroblasts. Endocrinology 103:1499, 1978.
70. Addison T: On the Constitutional and Local Effects of Disease of the Suprarenal Capsules. Samuel Highley, London, 1855.
71. Brown-Séquard GG: Researches experimentals sur la physiologie et la pathologie des capsule surrenele. C. R. Acad. Sci (D) (Paris) 3:422, 1856.
72. Cushing H: The basophil adenomas of the pituitary body and their clinical manifestations. Bull. Johns Hopkins Hosp. 50:137, 1932.
73. Foster GL, and Smith PE: Hypophysectomy and replacement therapy in relation to basal metabolism and specific dynamic action in the rat. J.A.M.A. 87:251, 1926.
74. Collip JB, Anderson EM, and Thompson DL: The adrenotropic hormone of the anterior pituitary lobe. Lancet 2:347, 1933.
75. Evans HM: Present position of our knowledge of anterior pituitary function. J.A.M.A. 101:425, 1933.
76. Houssay BA, Biasotti A, Mazzoco P, et al.: Accion del extracto antero-hipofirio soabre las glandulas adrenales. Revista. Soc. Argent. Biol. 9:262, 1933.
77. Li CH, Evans HM, and Simpson ME: Adrenocorticotrophic hormone. J. Biol. Chem. 149:413, 1943.
78. Sayers G, White A, and Long CNH: Preparation and properties of pituitary adrenocorticotrophic hormone. J. Biol. Chem. 149:425, 1943.
79. Bell PH, Howard KS, Shepherd RG, et al.: Studies with corticotrophin. II. Pepsin degradation of β-corticotrophin. J. Am. Chem. Soc. 78:5059, 1956.
80. Schwyzer R, and Seibert P: Total synthesis of adrenocorticotrophic hormone. Nature 199:172, 1963.
81. Ontjes DA: Minireview: The pharmacologic control of adrenal steroidogenesis. Life Sci. 26:2023, 1980.
82. Westphal U: Binding of corticosteroids by plasma proteins. *In* Greep RO, Astwood EB, Blaschko H, et al. (eds.): Handbook of Physiology Section I: Endocrinology, Vol. VI, Adrenal Gland. American Physiological Society, Washington, DC, 1975, p. 117.
83. Slaunwhite WR, and Sandberg AA: Transcortin: a corticosteroid-protein of plasma. J. Clin. Invest. 38:384, 1959.
84. Sandberg AA, and Slaunwhite WR Jr: Transcortin: a corticosteroid-binding protein of plasma. II. Levels in various conditions and the effects of estrogens. J. Clin. Invest. 38:1290, 1959.
85. Westphal U, Williams WC Jr, Ashley BD, et al.: Steroid protein interactions. X. Protein binding der Corticosteroide in serum adrenalektomierter und hypophyektomierter Ratten. Z. Physiol. Chem. 332:54, 1963.
86. Gordon GG, and Southren AL: Thyroid-hormone effects on steroid-hormone metabolism. Bull. N.Y. Acad. Med. 53:241, 1977.
87. Loriaux DL, and Cutler GB Jr: Diseases of the adrenal glands. *In* Kohler PO (ed.): Basic Clinical Endocrinology. John Wiley & Sons, New York, 1981.
88. Azarnoff DL (ed.): Steroid Therapy. W. B. Saunders Co., Philadelphia, 1975.
89. Knox WE, Auerback UH, and Lin ECC: Enzymatic and metabolic adaption in animals. Physiol. Rev. 36:164, 1956.
90. Baxter JD, and Rousseau GG (eds.): Glucocorticoid Hormone Action. Springer-Verlag, New York, 1979.
91. Boyer RM, Hellman LD, Roffwarg H, et al.: Cortisol secretion and metabolism in anorexia nervosa. N. Engl. J. Med. 296:190, 1977.
92. Peterson RE: Metabolism of adrenal corticol steroids. *In* Christy NP (ed.): The Human Adrenal Cortex. Harper & Row, New York, 1971, p. 87.
93. Bradlow AL, Zumoff E, Monder C, et al.: Isolation and identification of four new carboxylic acid metabolites of cortisol in man. J. Clin. Endocrinol. Metab. 37:811, 1973.
94. Vingerhoeds ACM, Thijssen JHH, and Schwarz F: Spontaneous hypercortisolism without Cushing's syndrome. J. Clin. Endocrinol. Metab. 43:1128, 1976.
95. Brown GM, Grota LJ, Penney DP, et al.: Pituitary-adrenal function in the squirrel monkey. Endocrinology 86:519, 1970.
96. Simpson SA, et al.: Isoleirung eines neuen kristallisierten Hormons ans Nebennieren mit besonders hohes Wicksamkeit auf den Minerstoffwechsel. Experientia 9:333, 1953.
97. Simpson SA, et al.: The structure of aldosterone. Helv. Chem. Acta 37:1200, 1954.
98. Ayres PJ, et al.: The *in vitro* demonstration of differential corticosteroid production within the ox adrenal gland. Biochem. J. 63:19, 1956.
99. Richardson KSC, Nowaczynski W, and Genest J: Specific aldosterone binding proteins in human plasma: partial characterisation. J. Steroid Biochem. 8:951, 1977.
100. Luetscher JA, Mills IH, Biglieri EG, et al.: Conjugation of 1,2-3H-aldosterone in human liver and kidneys and renal extraction of aldosterone and labeled conjugates from blood plasma. J. Clin. Endocrinol. Metab. 25:628, 1965.
101. Brown JJ, Fraser R, Lever AF, et al.: Aldosterone: physiological and pathophysiological correlations in men. Clin. Endocrinol. Metab. 1:397, 1972.
102. Bartte FC, et al.: Studies on the control and physiological action of aldosterone. Recent Prog. Horm. Res. 15:311, 1959.
103. Shields R, Mulholland AT, and Elallie PG: Action of aldosterone upon the intestinal transport of potassium, sodium and water. Gut 7:686, 1966.
104. Edmonds CJ, and Marriott JC: The effects of aldosterone and adrenalectomy on the electrical potential difference of the rat colon and on the treatment of potassium chloride and bicarbonate. J. Endocrinol. 39:517, 1967.
105. McConahay TP, Robinson S, and Newton JL: D-Aldosterone and sweat electrolytes. J. Appl. Physiol. 19:575, 1964.
106. May CD: Electrolyte excretion by sweat glands and kidneys. Am. J. Dis. Child. 109:2, 1965.

107. Bott E, Blair-West JR, and Coghlan JP: Action of aldosterone on the lachrymal gland. Nature 210:102, 1966.
108. Adler S: An extrarenal action of aldosterone on mammalian skeletal muscle. Am. J. Physiol. 218:616, 1970.
109. Loriaux DL, Menard R, Taylor A, et al.: Spironolactone and endocrine dysfunction. Ann. Intern. Med. 85:630, 1976.
110. Cheek DB, and Perry JW: A salt-wasting syndrome in infancy. Arch. Dis. Child 33:252, 1958.
111. Donnell GN, Litman N, and Roldan M: Pseudohypoadrenalcorticism. Renal sodium loss, hyponatremia, and hyperkalemia due to a renal tubular insensitivity to mineralocorticoids. Arch. Dis. Child. 97:813, 1959.
112. Raine DN, and Roy J: A salt-losing syndrome in infancy. Arch. Dis. Child. 37:548, 1962.
113. Corbeel L: Diabete salin du nourrisson sans insuffisance surrenalienne. Pediatrie 18:557, 1963.
114. Royer P, Bonnette J, Mathieu H, et al.: Pseudohypoaldosteronisme. Ann. Pediatr. 2612:596, 1963.
115. Polonovski C, Zittoun R, and Mary F: Hypocorticisime global hypoaldosteronisme et pseudo-hypoaldosteronisme du nourrisson. Arch. Fr. Pediatr. 22:1061, 1965.
116. Rosler A, Theodor R, Boichis H, et al.: Metabolic responses to the administration of angiotensin II, K and ACTH in two salt-wasting syndromes. J. Clin. Endocrinol. Metab. 44:292, 1977.
117. Pham Huu Trung C, Piussan C, Rodary C, et al.: Etude du faux de secretion de l'aldosterone et de l'activite de la renine plasmatique d'un cas de pseudo-hypoaldosteronisme. Arch. Fr. Pediatr. 27:603, 1970.
118. Poesmans W, Geussens H, Corbeel L, et al.: Pseudohypoaldosteronism. Am. J. Dis. Child. 126:510, 1973.
119. Postel-Vinay MC, Alberti GM, Ricour C, et al.: Pseudohypoaldosteronism. Persistence of hyperaldosteronism and evidence for renal tubular and intestinal responsiveness to endogenous aldosterone. J. Clin. Endocrinol. Metab. 39:1038, 1974.
120. Barthe P, Thai VK, Bouissou F, et al.: A propos d'un cas de pseudohypoaldosteronisme. Arch. Fr. Pediatr. 31:973, 1974.
121. Harayama N, Kato S, and Shimisu S: A male with pseudohypoaldosteronism. Clin. Endocrinol. (Tokyo) 23:581, 1975.
122. Perez AC, Govantes JM, Hinojosa CL, et al.: Pseudohipoaldosteronismo. An. Esp. Pediat. 8:443, 1975.
123. Roy C: Pseudohypoaldosteronisme familial. Arch. Fr. Pediatr. 34:37, 1977.
124. Rampini S, Furrer J, Keller HP, et al.: Congenital pseudohypoaldosteronism: case report and review. Effect of indomethacin during sodium chloride depletion. Helv. Paediatr. Acta 33:153, 1978.
125. Anand SK, Froberg L, Northway JD, et al.: Pseudohypoaldosteronism due to sweat gland dysfunction. Pediatr. Res. 10:677, 1976.
126. Oberfield SE, Levine LS, Carey RM, et al.: Pseudothypoaldosteronism: multiple target organ unresponsiveness to mineralocorticoid hormones. J. Clin. Endocrinol. Metab. 48:228, 1979.
127. Butenandt A: Uber die chemische Untersuchung der Sexualhormons. Z. Angew. Chem. 44:905, 1931.
128. Loewe S, and Voss HE: Der Stand der Erfassung des manlichen Sexualhormons (Androkinins). Klin. Wochenschr. 9:481, 1930.
129. Ruzicka L, Wettstein A: Synthetische Darstellung des Testishormons. Testosteron (Androst-3-17-o1). Helv. Clin. Acad. 18:1264, 1935.
130. Marsh JM: The role of cyclic AMP in gonadal function. *In* Greengold P, and Robinson GA (eds.): Advances in Cyclic Nucleotide Research, Vol. 6. Raven Press, New York, 1975, p. 137.
131. Nisula BC, and Dunn JF: Measurement of the testosterone binding parameters for both testosterone-estradiol binding globulin and albumin in individual serum samples. Steroids 34:771, 1979.
132. Robert A, and Delost P: Peripheral metabolism of testosterone during puberty in the male guinea pig. J. Reprod. Fertil. 53:273, 1978.
133. Bartsch W, Horst H-J, and Derwahl K-M: Interrelationships between sex hormone-binding globulin and 17β-estradiol, testosterone, 5α-dihydrotestosterone, thyroxine, and triiodothyronine in prepubertal and pubertal girls. J. Clin. Endocrinol. Metab. 50:1053, 1980.
134. Vermeulen A, and Ando S: Metabolic clearance rate and interconversion of androgens and the influence of the free androgen fraction. J. Clin. Endocrinol. Metab. 48:320, 1979.
135. Bird CE, Finnis W, Eoroomand K, et al.: Kinetics of testosterone metabolism in normal postmenopausal women and women with breast cancer. Steroids 32:323, 1978.
136. Girard J, Baumann JE, Buhler U, et al.: Cyproterone acetate and ACTH adrenal function. J. Clin. Endocrinol. Metab. 47:581, 1978.
137. Murad F, and Gilman AG: Androgens and anabolic steroids. *In* Goodman LS, and Gilman A (eds.): The Pharmacologic Basis of Therapeutics. Macmillan Co., Toronto, 1975, p. 1451.
138. Feldman EE, and Carter AC: Endocrinologic and metabolic effects of 17α-methyl-19-nortestosterone in women. J. Clin. Endocrinol. Metab. 20:842, 1960.
139. Kory RC, Bradley MH, Watson RN, et al.: A six-month evaluation of an anabolic drug, norethandrolone, in underweight persons. II. Bromsulphalein (BSP) retention and liver function. Am. J. Med. 76:243, 1959.
140. Bernstein MS, Hunter RL, and Yachnin S: Hepatoma and peliosis hepatitis in Fanconi's anemia. N. Engl. J. Med. 284:1135, 1971.
141. Johnson FL, Feagler JR, Lerner KG, et al.: Association of androgenic-anabolic steroid therapy with development of hepatocellular carcinoma. Lancet 2:1273, 1972.
142. Henderson JT, Richmond J, and Sumerling MD: Androgenic anabolic steroid therapy and hepatocellular carcinoma. Lancet 1:934, 1973.
143. Wilkins L, and Fleischmann W: Studies on the creatinuria due to methylated steroids. J. Clin. Invest. 24:21, 1945.
144. Schultz MG: Male pseudohermaphroditism diagnosed with aid of sex chromatin technique. J. Am. Vet. Med. Assoc. 140:241, 1962.
145. Bardin CW, Bullock L, Schneider G, et al.: Pseudohermaphrodite rat: end organ insensitivity to testosterone. Science 167:1136, 1970.
146. Lyon MF, and Hawkes SG: X-linked gene for testicular feminization in the mouse. Nature 227:1217, 1970.
147. Nes, N.: Testikulaer feminisering hos storfe. Nørd. Vet. Med. 18:19, 1966.
148. Mullen HS, and Hawe, RS: Male pseudohermaphroditism in a guinea pig (cana porcellanus). Vet. Med/Small An. Clin. 74:1801, 1979.
149. Kieffer NM, Burns SJ, and Judge NG: Male pseudohermaphroditism of the testicular feminizing type in a horse. Equine Vet. J. 8:38, 1976.
150. Eil C, Merriam GR, Bown J, et al.: Testicular feminization in the chimpanzee. Clin. Res. 28:624A, 1980.
151. Wilson JD, and MacDonald PC: Male pseudohermaphroditism due to androgen resistance: testicular feminization and related syndromes. *In* Stanbury JB, Wyngaarden JB, and Frederickson DS (eds.): The Metabolic Basis of Inherited Disease. McGraw-Hill Book Co., New York, 1978, p. 894.
152. Nowakowski H, and Lenz W: Genetic aspects in male hypogonadism. Recent Prog. Horm. Res. 17:53, 1961.
153. Walsh PC, Madden JD, Harrod MJ, et al.: Familial incomplete male pseudohermaphroditism, type 2: decreased dihydrotestostone formation in pseudovaginal perineoscrotal hypospadias. N. Engl. J. Med. 291:944, 1974.
154. Imperato-McGinley J, Guerrero L, Gautier T, et al.: Steroid 5α-reductase deficiency in man: an inherited form of male pseudohermaphroditism. Science 186:1213, 1974.
155. George FW, and Wilson JD: Pathogenesis of the henny feathering trait in the Sebright bantam chicken. J. Clin. Invest. 66:57, 1980.
156. Hemsell DL, Edman CD, Manks JF, et al.: Massive extraglandular aromatization of plasma androstenedione

resulting in feminization of a prepubertal boy. J. Clin. Invest. 60:455, 1977.

157. Eil C, Lippmann ME, and Loriaux DL: A dispersed-whole cell method for the determination of androgen receptors in cultured skin fibroblasts. Steroids 34:389, 1980.
158. Knauer E: Die Ovarien-Transplantation. Arch. Gynaekol. 60:322, 1900.
159. Royal College of General Practitioners Oral Contraceptives Study: Effective on hypertension and benign breast disease of progestagen component in combined oral contraceptives. Lancet 1:624, 1977.
160. Frank RT, Frank ML, Gustavson RG, et al.: Demonstration of the female sex hormone in the circulating blood. I. Preliminary report. J.A.M.A. 85:510, 1925.
161. Loewe S, and Lange F: Der Gehalt des Frauenharns an brunsterzengenden Stoffen in Abhangigkeit von ovariellen Zylkus, Klin. Wochenschr. 5:1038, 1926.
162. Zondek B: Darstellung des weiblichen Sexualhormon aus dem Harn. Klin. Wochenschr. 7:485, 1928.
163. Butenandt A: Uber "Progynon" ein crystallisiertes, weibliches Sexualhormon. Naturwissenschaften 17:879, 1929.
164. Doisy EA, Veler CD, and Thayer SA: The preparation of the crystalline ovarian hormone from the urine of pregnant women. J. Biol. Chem. 86:499, 1930.
165. Bagget B, Engel LL, Savard K, et al.: The conversion of testosterone 3-C^{14} to C^{14}-estradiol-17β by human ovarian tissue. J. Biol. Chem. 221:931, 1956.
166. Mahesh VB, and Greenblatt RB: Steroid secretions of the normal and polycystic ovary. Recent Prog. Horm. Res. 20:341, 1964.
167. Ryan KJ, and Engel LL: The interconversion of estrone and estradiol by human tissue slices. Endocrinology 52:287, 1953.
168. Pundel JP: Die androgen Abstrichbilder. Archiv. Gynaekol. 188:577, 1957.
169. Vigersky RA, Kono S, Sauer M, et al.: Relative binding of testosterone and estradiol to testosterone-estradiol-binding globulin. J. Clin. Endocrinol. Metab. 49:899, 1979.
170. Hammond GL, Nisker JA, and Siiteri PK: Estradiol binding in serum under physiological conditions. Abstract 760, presented at 62nd Annual Meeting of Endocrine Society, Washington, DC, 1980, p. 264.
171. Dunn JF, Nisula B, and Rodbard D: Transport of steroid hormones, binding of 21 endogenous steroids to both testosterone binding globulin and corticosteroid binding globulin in human plasma. Submitted for publication.
172. Speroff L, and Vande Wiele RL: Regulation of the human menstrual cycle. Am. J. Obstet. Gynecol. 109:234, 1971.
173. Boston Collaborative Drug Surveillance Program: Surgically confirmed gallbladder disease, venous thromboembolism, and breast tumors in relation to postmenopausal estrogen therapy. N. Engl. J. Med. 290:15, 1974.
174. Herbst AL, Ulfelder H, and Poskanzer C: Adenocarcinoma of the vagina: association of maternal stilbestrol therapy with tumor appearance in young women. N. Engl. J. Med. 284:878, 1971.
175. Smith DC, Prentia R., Thompsen DJ, et al.: Association of exogenous estrogen and endometrial carcinoma. N. Engl. J. Med. 293:1104, 1975.
176. Ziel HK, and Finkle WD: Increased risk of endometrial carcinoma among users of conjugated estrogens. N. Engl. J. Med. 293:1167, 1975.
177. Ameriks JA, Thompson NM, Frey CF, et al.: Hepatic cell adenomas, spontaneous liver rupture, and oral contraceptives. Arch. Surg. 110:548, 1975.
178. Saunders FJ, and Elton RL: Effects of ethynodiol diacetate and mestranol in rats and rabbits, on conception, on the outcome of pregnancy and on the offpsring. Toxic. Appl. Pharmacol. 11:229, 1967.
179. Janerich DT, Piper JM, and Glebatis DM: Oral contraceptives and congenital limb-reduction defects. N. Engl. J. Med. 291:697, 1974.
180. Bibbo M, Gill WB, Azizi F, et al.: Follow-up study of male and female offspring of DES-exposed mothers. Obstet. Gynecol. 49:1, 1977.
181. Fishman J, Cox RI, and Gallagher TF: 2-Hydroxyestrone: a new metabolite of estradiol in man. Arch. Biochem. Biophys. 90:318, 1960.
182. Merriam GR: Catechol estrogens: a brief review. J. Am. Med Wom. Assoc. 34:363, 1979.
183. Merriam GR, Brandon DD, Kono S, et al.: Rapid metabolic clearance of the catechol estrogen 2-hydroxyestrone. J. Clin. Endocrinol. Metab. 51:1211, 1980.
184. Dunn JF, Merriam GR, Eil C, et al.: Testosterone-estradiol binding globulin binds to 2-methoxyestradiol with greater affinity than to testosterone. J. Clin. Endocrinol. Metab. 51:404, 1980.
185. Nawata HJ, Bronzert D, and Lippman ME: Isolation and characterization of a tamoxifen-resistant cell line derived from MCF-7 human breast cancer cells. J. Biol. Chem. 256:5616, 1981.
186. Beard J: The Span of Gestation and the Cause of Birth. G. Fisher, Jena, 1897.
187. Fraenkel L: Die Funktion des Corpus Luteum. Arch. Gynaekol. 68:483, 1905.
188. Corner GW, and Allen WM: Physiology of the corpus luteum. II. Production of a special uterine reaction (progestational proliferation) by extracts of the corpus luteum. Am. J. Physiol. 88:326, 1929.
189. Williams MT, Clark MR, Ling WY, et al.: Role of cyclic AMP in the action of luteinizing hormone on steroidogenesis in the corpus luteum. *In* George WJ, and Ignarro LJ (eds.): Advances in Cyclic Nucleotide Research, Vol. 9. Raven Press, New York, 1978, p. 573.
190. Vande Wiele RL, Gurpide E, Kelly WG, et al.: The secretory rate of progesterone and aldosterone in normal and abnormal late pregnancy. Acta Endocrinol. Copenh. 34: Suppl. 51, 159, 1960.
191. Murad F, and Gilman AG: Estrogens and progestins. *In* Goodman LS, and Gilman A (eds.): The Pharmacologic Basis of Therapeutics. Macmillan Co., Toronto, 1975, p. 1423.
192. Fotherby K, and James F: Metabolism of synthetic steroids. Adv. Steroid Biochem. Pharmacol. 3:67, 1972.
193. Gupta C, Osterman J, Santen R, et al.: In vivo metabolism of progestins. V. The effect of protocol design on the metabolic clearance rate and volume of distribution of medroxyprogesterone acetate in women. J. Clin. Endocrinol. Metab. 48:816, 1979.
194. Janne O, Kontula K, Luukkainen T, et al.: Oestrogen-induced progesterone receptor in human uterus. J. Steroid Biochem. 6:501, 1975.
195. Mendelsohn J, Mutter MM, and Bernheim JL: Inhibition of human lymphocyte stimulation by steroid hormones: cytokinetic mechanisms. Clin. Exp. Immunol. 27:127, 1977.
196. Wyle FA, and Keat JR: Immunosuppression by sex steroid hormones. I. The effect upon PHA- and PPD-stimulated lymphocytes. Clin. Exp. Immunol. 27:407, 1977.
197. Keseru TL, Maraz A, and Szabo J: Oral contraceptives and sex ratio at birth. Lancet 1:369, 1974.
198. Andrew FD, Christensen HD, Williams TL, et al.: Comparative teratogenicity of contraceptive steroids in mice and rats. Teratology 7:A11, 1973.
199. Aarskog D: Maternal progestins as a possible cause of hypospadias. N. Engl. J. Med 300:75, 1979.
200. Field B, Lu C, and Hepner GW: Inhibition of hepatic drug metabolism by norethindrone. Clin. Pharmacol. Ther. 25:196, 1979.
201. Keller DW, Wiest WG, Askin FB, et al.: Pseudocorpus luteum insufficiency: a local defect of progesterone action on endometrial stroma. J. Clin. Endocrinol. Metab. 48:127, 1979.
202. Yamamoto KR, Stampfer MR, and Tomkins GM: Receptors from glucocorticoid-sensitive lymphoma cells and two classes of insensitive clones: physical and DNA-binding properties. Proc. Natl. Acad. Sci. USA 71:3901, 1974.
203. Sherman MR, Tuazon FB, and Miller LK: Estrogen receptor cleavage and plasminogen activation by enzymes in

human breast tumor cytosol. Endocrinology 106:1715, 1980.

204. Coty WA, Schrader WT, and O'Malley BW: Purification and characterization of the chick oviduct progesterone receptor: a subunit. J. Steroid Biochem. 10:1, 1979.

205. Wittliff JL, and Savlov ED: Biochemical basis for the selection of hormonal manipulation in the patient with breast carcinoma. Int. J. Radiat. Oncol. Biol. Phy. 4:463, 1978.

206. Nawata H, Chong MT, Bronzert D, et al.: Estradiol independent growth of a subline of MCF-7 human breast cancer cells in culture. J. Biol. Chem. 256:6895, 1981.

207. McCaffrey R, Lillquist A, and Bell R: Biochemical and biophysical characterization of glucocorticoid receptors in normal lymphoid tissue. Blood, in press.

208. Litwack G, Schmidt TJ, Mackovic RD, et al.: Activation and DNA binding of the glucocorticoid receptor. *In* Bresciani F (ed.): Perspectives in Steroid Receptor Research. Raven Press, New York, 1980, p. 113.

209. Bourgeois S, and Newby RF: Correlation between glucocorticoid receptor and cytolytic response of murine lymphoid cell lines. Cancer Res. 39:4749, 1979.

210. Kaye AM, and Reiss N: The uterus "estrogen-induced protein" (IP): purification, distribution and possible function in steroid-induced uterine proteins. *In* Beato M (ed.). Elsevier/North-Holland, Amsterdam, 1980, p. 3.

211. Lippman ME, Monaco ME, and Bolan G: Effects of estrone, estradiol and estriol on hormone-responsive human breast cancer in long-term tissue culture. Cancer Res. 37:1001, 1077.

212. Lippman ME, Huff K, Bolan G, et al.: Interactions of R5020 with progesterone and glucocorticoid receptors in human breast cancer and peripheral blood lymphocytes *in vitro*. McGuire WL, et al. (eds.). Raven Press, New York, 1977, p. 193.

213. Ojasoo T, and Raynaud JP: Unique steroid congeners for receptor studies. Cancer Res. 38:4186, 1978.

214. Lippman ME, Bolan G, and Huff K: The effects of estrogens and antiestrogens on hormone-responsive human breast cancer in long-term tissue culture. Cancer Res. 36:4595, 1976.

215. Allegra JC, Barlock A, Huff KK, et al.: Changes in multiple or sequential estrogen receptor determinations in breast cancer. Cancer 45:792, 1980.

216. DeWys WD, Allegra JC, Simon R, et: A proposed model for the prediction of response to endocrine therapy in breast cancer from the estrogen receptor status of one site and the number of metastatic sites. Cancer Res. 40:2423, 1980.

217. Allegra JC, Lippman ME, Thompson EB, et al.: Distribution, frequency and quantitative analysis of estrogen progesterone, androgen and glucocorticoid receptors in human breast cancer. Cancer Res. 39:1447, 1979.

218. Maass H, Engel B, Trams G, et al.: Steroid hormone receptors in human breast cancer and the clinical significance. J. Steroid Biochem. 6:743, 1975.

219. McGuire WL: Hormone receptors: their role in predicting prognosis and response to endocrine therapy. Semin. Oncol. 4:428, 1978.

220. Fabian C, and Sternson L: Clinical pharmacology of tamoxifen in patients with breast cancer: comparison of traditional and loading dose schedules. Cancer Treat. Rep. 64:765, 1980.

221. Horwitz KB, and McGuire WL: Estrogen control of progesterone receptor in human breast cancer. J. Biol. Chem. 253:2223, 1978.

222. Garola RE, and McGuire WL: An improved assay for nuclear estrogen receptor in experimental and human breast cancer. Cancer Res. 37:3333, 1977.

223. Horwitz KB, and McGuire WL: Specific progesterone receptors in human breast cancer. Steroids 25:497, 1975.

224. MacMahon B, Cole P, and Brown J: Etiology of human breast cancer: a review. J Natl. Cancer Inst. 50:21, 1973.

225. Miller AB: An overview of hormone-associated cancers Cancer Res. 38:3985, 1978.

226. Haenzel W, and Kurihara M: Studies of Japanese migrants' mortality from cancers and other diseases among Japanese in the United States. J. Natl. Cancer Inst. *40*:43, 1968.

227. DeWaard F: The epidemiology of breast cancer: review and prospects. Int. J. Cancer 4:577, 1969.

228. MacMahon B, Cole P, Lin TM, et al.: Age at first birth and breast cancer risk. Bull. WHO 43:209, 1970.

229. MacMahon B, and Feinleib M: Breast cancer in relation to nursing and menopausal history. J. Natl. Cancer Inst. 24:733, 1960.

230. Abramson JM: Breastfeeding and breast cancer. Isr. J. Med. Sci. 2:457, 1966.

231. Ing R, Ho JHC, and Petrakis NL: Unilateral breast-feeding, breast cancer. Lancet 2:124, 1977.

232. Petrakis NL: Genetic factors in the etiology of breast cancer. Cancer 39:2709, 1977.

233. Lynch HT, Thomas RJ, Terasaki PI, et al.: HLA in cancer family "N." Cancer 36:1315, 1975.

234. Petrakis NL: Cerumen genetics and human breast cancer. Science 173: 347, 1971.

235. Pike MC, Casagrande JT, Brown JB, et al.: Comparison of urinary and plasma hormone levels in daughters of breast cancer patients and controls. J. Natl. Cancer Inst. 59:1351, 1977.

236. Fishman J, Fukishima D, O'Connor J, et al.: Plasma hormone profiles of young women at risk for familial breast cancer. Cancer Res. 38:4006, 1978.

237. Everson RB, Fraumeni JF, Wilson RE, et al.: Familial male breast cancer. Lancet 1:0, 1976.

238. Feinleib M: Breast cancer and artificial menopause: a cohort study. J. Natl. Cancer Inst. 41:315, 1968.

239. Hoover R, Gray LA, Cole P, et al.: Menopausal estrogens and breast cancer. N. Engl. J. Med. 295:401, 1980.

240. Wilson SE, and Hutchinson WB: Breast masses in males with carcinoma of the prostate. J. Surg. Oncol. 8:105, 1976.

241. Symmers WS: Carcinoma of breast in trans-sexual individuals after surgical and hormonal interference with the primary and secondary sex characteristics. Br. Med. J. 2:83, 1968.

242. Everson RB, and Lippman ME: Male breast cancer. *In* McGuire WL (ed.): Breast Cancer: Advances in Research and Treatment. Plenum Medical Book Co., New York, 1979, p. 239.

243. MacMahon B, and Cole P: Oestrogen profiles of Asian and North American women. Lancet 2:900, 1971.

244. Leman HM, Wotiz HH, Parsons L, et al.: Reduced estriol excretion in patients with breast cancer prior to endocrine therapy. J.A.M.A. 196:1128, 1966.

245. Anderson JN, Peck EF, and Clark JF: Estrogen-induced uterine responses and growth: relationship to receptor estrogen binding by uterine nuclei. Endocrinology 96:160, 1975.

246. Longcope C, and Pratt JN: Relationship between urine plasma estrogen ratios. Cancer Res. 38:4025, 1978.

247. Kirschner MA, Cohen FB, and Ryan C: Androgen-estrogen production rates in postmenopausal women with breast cancer. Cancer Res. 38:4029, 1978.

248. Bulbrook RD: Endocrine status of women with an enhanced risk of breast cancer. *In* Heuson JC, et al. (eds.): Breast Cancer: Trends in Research and Treatment. Raven Press, New York, 1976, p. 271.

249. Bulbrook RD, Hayward JL, and Spicer CC: Relation between urinary androgen and corticoid excretion and subsequent breast cancer. Lancet 2:395, 1971.

250. Grattarola R, Secreto G, and Recchione C: Androgens in breast cancer: breast cancer recurrences years after mastectomy and increased androgenic activity. Am. J. Obstet. Gynecol. 121:169, 1975.

251. McFaden IJ, Prescott RJ, Groom GV, et al.: Circulating hormone concentrations in women with breast cancer. Lancet 1:1100, 1976.

252. Adams JB, Archibald L, and Clarke C: Adrenal dehydroepiandrosterone and human mammary cancer. Cancer Res. 38:4036, 1978.

253. Dao TL, and Libby PR: Conjugation of steroid hormones by normal and neoplastic tissues. J. Clin. Endocrinol. Metab. 28:1431, 1968.
254. Kelsey JL: Oral contraceptives and breast disease. Am. J. Epidemiol. 107:236, 1978.
255. Royal College of General Practitioners Oral Contraceptive Study: Effect on hypertension and benign breast disease of progestagen component in combined oral contraceptives. Lancet 1:624, 1977.
256. Numura A, and Comstock GW: Benign breast tumor and estrogenic hormones: a population-based retrospective study. Am. J. Epidemiol. 103:439, 1976.
257. Paffenbarger RS, Fasal E, Simmons ME, et al.: Cancer risks as related to use of oral contraceptives during fertile years. Cancer 39:1887, 1977.
258. Vessey MP, Doll RS, and Sutton PM: Oral contraceptives, breast neoplasia: a retrospective study. Br. Med. J. 3:719, 1972.
259. Org H, Cole P, MacMahon B, et al.: Oral contraceptives and reduced risk of benign breast diseases. N. Engl. J. Med. 294:419, 1976.
260. Vessey MP, Doll R, Peto R, et al.: A long-term follow-up study of women using different methods of contraception: an interim report. J. Biosoc. Sci. 8:373, 1976.
261. Boston Collaborative Drug Surveillance Program: Surgically confirmed gallbladder disease venous thromboembolism and breast tumor in relation to postmenopausal estrogen therapy. N. Engl. J. Med. 290:15, 1974.
262. Black MM, Barclay THC, Cutler SJ, et al.: Association of typical characteristics of benign breast lesions with subsequent risk of breast cancer. Cancer 29:338, 1972.
263. Kodlin D, Winger EE, Morgenstern NL, et al.: Chronic mastopathy and breast cancer. Cancer 39:2603, 1977.
264. Armstrong B: Recent trends in breast cancer incidence and mortality in relation to changes in possible risk factors. Int. J. Cancer 17:204, 1976.
265. Vessey MP, Doll R, and Jones K: Oral contraceptives and breast cancer. Lancet 1:941, 1975.
266. Boston Collaborative Drug Surveillance Program: Oral contraceptives and venous thromboembolic disease surgically confirmed gallbladder disease and breast tumours. Lancet 1:1399, 1973.
267. Sartwell PE, Arthes FG, and Tonascia JA: Exogenous hormones, reproductive history and breast cancer. J. Natl. Cancer Inst. 59:1589, 1977.
268. Casagrande J, Gerkins V, Henderson BE, et al.: Brief communication: Exogenous estrogens and breast cancer in women with natural menopause. J. Natl. Cancer Inst. 56:839, 1976.
269. Craig MJ, Comstock GW, and Geiser PB: Epidemiologic comparison of breast cancer patients with early and late onset of malignancy and general population controls. J. Natl. Cancer Inst. 53:1577, 1974.
270. Beatson GT: The treatment of inoperable cases of carcinoma of the mamma: suggestions for a new method of treatment with illustrative cases. Lancet 2:104, 1896.
271. Folca PJ, Glascock RF, and Irvine WT: Studies with tritium labelled hexoestrol in advanced breast cancer. Lancet 2:796, 1961.
272. Jensen EV, DeSombre ER, and Jungblut PW: Estrogen-receptors in hormone-responsive tissues and tumors. *In* Wissler RW, et al. (eds.): Endogenous Factors Influencing Host-Tumor Balance. University of Chicago Press, Chicago, 1967, p. 68.
273. Lippman ME, and Thompson EB: Steroid Receptors and the Management of Cancer. CRC Press, Boca Raton, FL, 1979.
274. Everson RB, Lippman ME, Thompson EB, et al.: Steroid receptors in male breast cancer. Cancer Res. 40:991, 1980.
275. Knight WA, Livingston RB, Gregory EJ, et al.: Estrogen receptor as an independent prognostic factor for early recurrence in breast cancer. Cancer Res. 37:4669, 1977.
276. Maynard PV, Blamey RW, Elston CW, et al.: Estrogen receptor assay in primary breast cancer and early recurrence of the disease. Cancer Res. 38:4292, 1978.
277. Allegra JC, Lippman ME, Simon R, et al.: Association between steroid receptor status and disease-free interval in breast cancer. Cancer Treat. Rep. 63:1271, 1979.
278. Hubay CA, Pearson OH, Marshall JS, et al.: Antiestrogen, cytotoxic chemotherapy and bacillus Calmette-Guerin vaccination in stage II breast cancer: a preliminary report. Surgery 87:494, 1980.
279. Lippman ME, Allegra JC, Thompson EB, et al.: The relationship between estrogen receptors and response rate to cytotoxic chemotherapy in metastatic breast cancer. N. Engl. J. Med. 298:1223, 1978.
280. Jonat W, and Maass H: Some comments on the necessity of receptor determinations in human breast cancer. Cancer Res. 38:4305, 1978.
281. Kiang DT, Frenning DH, Goldman AI, et al.: Estrogen receptors and response of breast cancer to chemotherapy. N. Engl. J. Med. 229:1330, 1978.
282. Rubens RD, King RJB, Senton S, et al.: Oestrogen receptors and response to cytotoxic chemotherapy in advanced breast cancer. Cancer Chemother. Pharmacol. 4:43, 1980.
283. Welsch CW: Prolactin and the development and progression of early neoplastic mammary gland lesions. Cancer Res. 38:4054, 1978.
284. Holdaway IM, and Friesen HG: Hormone binding by human mammary carcinoma. Cancer Res. 37:1946, 1977.
285. European Breast Cancer Group: Clinical trial of 2-bromoergocryptine (CB154) in advanced breast cancer. Eur. J. Cancer 8:155, 1972.
286. Wagner S, and Mantel N: Breast cancer at a psychiatric hospital before and after the introduction of neuroleptic agents. Cancer Res. 38:2703, 1978.
287. Ravdin RG, Lewison EF, and Slack NH: Results of a clinical trial concerning the worth of prophylactic oophorectomy for breast cancer. Surg. Gynecol. Obstet. 131:1055, 1970.
288. Cole MP: Suppression of ovarian function in primary breast cancer. *In* Forrest APM, and Kunkler PB (eds.): Prognostic Factors in Breast Cancer. Livingstone Press, Edinburgh, 1968, p. 146.
289. Nissen-Meyer R: Prophylactic endocrine treatment of carcinoma of the breast. Clin. Radiol. 15:152, 1964.
290. Meakin JW: Is there a place for adjuvant endocrine therapy of breast cancer? *In* Henningsen E, Linder F, and Steichele C (eds.): Endocrine Treatment of Breast Cancer. Springer-Verlag, Berlin, 1980, p. 178.
291. Papac RJ, Jacobs EM, Foye LV Jr, et al.: Systemic therapy with Amethopterin in squamous carcinoma of head and neck. Cancer Chemother. Rep. 31:47, 1963.
292. Vincent TN, Satterfield JV, and Ackerman LV: Carcinoma of the lung in women. Cancer 18:559, 1965.
293. Fracchia AA, Farrow JH, DePalo AJ, et al.: Castration for primary inoperable or recurrent breast carcinoma. Surg. Gynecol. Obstet. 128:1226, 1969.
294. Saez JM, Morera AM, Dazord A, et al.: Adrenal, testicular contribution to plasma oestrogens. J. Endocrinol. 55:41, 1972.
295. Grodin JM, Siiteri PK, and MacDonald PC: Source of estrogen production in postmenopausal women. J. Clin. Endocrinol. 36:207, 1973.
296. Joint Committee on Endocrine Ablative Procedures in Disseminated Mammary Carcinoma. J.A.M.A. 175:787, 1968.
297. Dao TL: Ablation therapy for hormone-dependent tumors. Annu. Rev. Med. 23:1, 1972.
298. Maddox WD, Winkelman RK, Harrison EG Jr, et al.: Multiple nevoid basal cell epitheliomas, jaw cysts and skeletal defects. J.A.M.A. 188:106, 1964.
299. Goldenberg IS: Clinical trial of testololactone (NSC 23759), medroxy progesterone acetate (NSC 26386) and oxylone acetate (NSC 47438) in advanced female mammary cancer. Cancer 23:109, 1969.
300. Kennedy BJ: Hormone therapy in inoperable breast cancer. Cancer 24:1345, 1969.
301. Stoll BA: Castration and oestrogen therapy. *In* Stoll BA

(ed.): Endocrine Therapy in Malignant Disease. W. B. Saunders Ltd., London, 1972, p. 139.
302. Kennedy BJ: Diethylstilbestrol versus testosterone propionate therapy in advanced breast cancer. Surg. Gynecol. Obstet. 120:1246, 1965.
303. Kaufman RF, and Escher GC: Rebound regression in advanced mammary carcinoma. Surg. Gynecol. Obstet. 113:635, 1961.
304. Stoll BA: Correspondence: Cyclophosphamide in disseminated malignant disease. Br. Med. J. 2:337, 1962.
305. Pannoti F, Martoni A, DiMarco AR, et al.: Prospective randomized clinical trial of two different high dosages of medroxyprogesterone acetate in the treatment of metastatic breast cancer. Eur. J. Cancer 15:593, 1979.
306. Mouridsen H, Palshof T, Patterson J, et al.: Tamoxifen in advanced breast cancer. Cancer Treat. Rev. 5:131, 1978.
307. Heel RC, Erogden RN, Speight TM, et al.: Tamoxifen: a review of its pharmacological properties and therapeutic use in the treatment of breast cancer. Drugs 16:1, 1978.
308. Katzenellenbogen BS, Ferguson ER, and Lan NC: Fundamental differences in the action of estrogens and antiestrogens on the uterus: comparisons between compounds with similar duration of action. Endocrinology 100:1252, 1977.
309. Rinehart JS, Ruh TS, and Ruh MF: Anti-oestrogen action: uterine nuclear retention of the CI-628 anti-oestrogen receptor complex in vitro. Acta Endocrinol. 84:367, 1977.
310. Ruh TS, and Baudenstiel LJ: Different nuclear binding sites for antiestrogen and estrogen receptor complexes. Endocrinology 100:420, 1977.
311. Sutherland RL, and Foo MS: Differential binding of antiestrogens by rat uterine and chick oviduct cytosol. Biochem. Biopsy Res. Commun. 91:183, 1980.
312. Legha S, and Carter SK: Antiestrogens in the treatment of cancer. Cancer Treat. Rev. 3:205, 1976.
313. Heuson JC: Current overview of EORTC clinical trials with tamoxifen. Cancer Treat. Rep. 60:1463, 1976.
314. Kiang DT, and Kennedy BJ: Tamoxifen therapy in advanced breast cancer. Ann. Intern. Med. 87:687, 1977.
315. Pritchard KI, Thomson DB, Myers RE, et al.: Tamoxifen therapy in premenopausal patients with metastatic breast cancer. Cancer Treat. Rep. 64:787, 1980.
316. Manni A, Trujillo J, Marshall JS, et al.: Antiestrogen induced remissions in stage IV breast cancer. Cancer Treat. Rep. 60:1421, 1976.
317. McIntosh IH, and Thynne GS: Tumour stimulation by anti-estrogens. Br. J. Surg. 64:900, 1977.
318. Tormey DC, Simon RM, Lippman ME, et al.: Evaluation of tamoxifen dose in advanced breast cancer: progress report. Cancer Treat. Rep. 60:1451, 1976.
319. Jordan VC, Allen KE, Dix CJ, et al.: The pharmacology of tamoxifen in laboratory animals. Cancer Treat. Rep. 64:745, 1980.
320. Fromson JM, Pearson S, and Brama SM: The metabolism of tamoxifen (ICI 46,474). II: In female patients. Xenobiotica 3:711, 1973.
321. Kaiser-kupfer MI, and Lippman ME: Tamoxifen retinopathy. Cancer Treat. Rep. 62:315, 1978.
322. Jain J, Samal B, Singhakowinta A, et al.: Clinical trial of nafoxidine in adrenalectomized patients with advanced breast cancer. Cancer 40:2063, 1977.
323. Allegra JC, and Lippman ME: The effects of 17β-estradiol, tamoxifen on the ZR-75-1 human breast cancer cell line in defined medium. Eur. J. Cancer 16:1007, 1980.
324. Lippman ME, Bolan G, and Huff K: The effects of glucocorticoids and progesterone on hormone-responsive human breast cancer in long-term tissue culture. Cancer Res. 36:4610, 1976.
325. Griffiths CT, Hall TC, Saba Z, et al.: Preliminary trial of aminoglutethimide in breast cancer. Cancer 32:31, 1973.
326. Fishman LM, Liddle GW, Island DP, et al.: Effects of aminoglutethimide on adrenal function in man. J. Clin. Endocrinol. Metab. 27:481, 1967.
327. Santen RJ, Lipton A, and Kendall J: Successful medical adrenalectomy with aminoglutethimide. Role of altered drug metabolism. J.A.M.A. 230:1661, 1974.
328. Santen RJ, Samojlik E, Lipton A, et al.: Kinetic hormonal and clinical studies with aminoglutethimide in breast cancer. Cancer 39:2948, 1977.
329. Samojlik E, Santen RJ, and Wells SA: Adrenal suppression with aminoglutethimide on plasma androstenedione and estrogen levels. J. Clin. Endocrinol. 45:480, 1977.
330. Santen RJ, and Wells SA: The use of aminoglutethimide in the treatment of patients with metastatic carcinoma of the breast. Cancer 36:1066, 1980.
330A. Brodie AMH, Schwartel WC, Shaikh AA, and Brodie HJ: The effect of an aromatase inhibitor, 4-hydroxy-4-androstene-3,17-dione, on estrogen-dependent processes in reproduction and breast cancer. Endocrinology 100:1684, 1977.
331. Jensen EV, and Jacobsen HI: Basic guides to the mechanism of estrogen action. Recent Prog. Horm. Res. 18:387, 1962.
332. Pollow K, Lubbert H, Boquoi E, et al.: Characterization and comparison of receptors for 17-estradiol and progesterone in human proliferative endometrium and endometrial carcinoma. Endocrinology 96:319, 1975.
333. Bayard F: Cytoplasmic and nuclear estradiol and progesterone receptors in human endometrium. J. Clin. Endocrinol. Metab. 46:635, 1978.
334. Young PC, Ehrlich CE, and Cleary RE: Progesterone binding in human endometrial carcinomas. Am. J. Obstet. Gynecol. 125:353, 1970.
335. Gurpide E: Estradiol binding and metabolism in human endometrial hyperplasia and adenocarcinoma. J. Steroid Biochem. 7:891, 1976.
336. Dunn LJ, and Bradbury JT: Endocrine factors in endometrial carcinoma. Am. J. Obstet. Gynecol. 97:465, 1967.
337. Antunes CME, Stolley PD, Rosenshiem DB, et al.: Endometrial cancer and estrogen use. N. Engl. J. Med. 300:9, 1979.
338. Nisker JA, Ramzy I, and Collins JA: Adenocarcinoma of the endometrium and abnormal ovarian function in young women. Am. J. Obstet. Gynecol. 130:546, 1978.
339. Kaufman RH, Abbott JP, and Wall JA: The endometrium before, after wedge resection of the ovaries in the Stein-Leventhal syndrome. Am. J. Obstet. Gynecol. 77:1271, 1959.
340. Hemsell DL, Grodin JM, Brenner PF, et al.: Plasma precursors of estrogen. II. Correlation of the extent of conversion of plasma androstenedione to estrone with age. J. Clin. Endocrinol. Metab. 38:476, 1974.
341. MacDonald PC, Edman CD, Hemsell DL, et al.: Effect of obesity on conversion of plasma androstenedione to estrone in postmenopausal women with or without endometrial cancer. Am. J. Obstet. Gynecol. 130:448, 1978.
342. Judd HL, Lucas WE, and Yen SS: Serum 17β-estradiol, esterone levels in post-menopausal women with or without endometrial cancer. J. Clin. Endocrinol. Metab. 43:272, 1976.
343. Feinstein AR, and Horwitz RI: A critique of the statistical evidence associating estrogens with endometrial cancer. Cancer Res. 38:4001, 1978.
344. Kelley RM, and Baker WH: Progestational agents in the treatment of carcinoma of the endometrium. N. Engl. J. Med. 264:216, 1961.
345. Reifenstein EC: Hydroxyprogesterone caproate therapy in advanced endometrial cancer. Cancer 29:485, 1971.
346. Malkasian GD Jr, Decker DG, Mussey E, et al.: Progesterone treatment of endometrial carcinoma. Am. J. Obstet. Gynecol. 110:15, 1971.
347. Bonte J: Developments in endocrine therapy of endometrial and ovarian cancer. Reviews on Endocrine Related Cancer 3:11, 1979.
348. Wall JA, Franklin RR, and Kaufman RH: The effects of clomiphene citrate on the endometrium. Am. J. Obstet. Gynecol. 93:842, 1965.
349. Young PC, and Ehrlich CE: Progesterone receptors in human endometrial cancer. *In* Thompson EB, and Lipp-

man ME (eds.): Steroid Receptors and the Management of Cancer. CRC Press, Boca Raton FL, 1979, p. 135.

350. Rao RB, Wiest WG, and Allen WM: Progesterone receptor in human endometrium. Endocrinology 95:1275, 1974.

351. Pollow K, Lubbert H, Boquoi E, et al.: Characterization and comparison of receptors for 17-estradiol and progesterone in human proliferation endometrium and endometrial carcinoma. Endocrinology 96:319, 1975.

352. Pollow K, Schmidt-Grollwitzer M, and Nevinnig-Stickel J: Progesterone receptors in normal human endometrium and endometrial carcinoma. *In* McGuire WL, Raynaud JP, and Baulieu EE (eds.): Progesterone Receptors in Normal and Neoplastic Tissue. Raven Press, New York, 1977, p. 313.

353. Donovan JF: Non-hormonal chemotherapy of endometrial adenocarcinoma: a review. Cancer 34:1587, 1974.

354. MacLaughlin DT, and Richardson GS: The specificity of the endometrial response to estrogens and progestins. *In* Thompson EB, and Lippman ME (eds.): Steroid Receptors and the Management of Cancer. CRC Press, Boca Raton, FL, 1979, p. 161.

355. Tseng L, and Gurpide E: Induction of human endometrial estradiol dehydrogenase by progestins. Endocrinology 97:825, 1975.

356. Nordqvist SRB: *In vitro* effects of progestins or DNA synthesis in metastatic endometrial carcinoma. Gynecol. Oncol. 2:415, 1974.

357. Kori J, and Heshmat MY: Incidence of cancer in Negroes in Washington D.C. and selected African cities. Am. J. Epidemiol. 96:401, 1972.

358. Jackson MA: Characterization of prostatic carcinoma among blacks: a continuation report. Cancer Treat. Rep. 61:167, 1977.

359. Akazakis K, and Stennerman GN: Cooperative study of latent carcinoma of the prostate among Japanese in Japan and Hawaii. J. Natl. Cancer Inst. 50:1137, 1973.

360. Huggins C, and Clark PJ: Quantitative studies of prostatic secretion. J. Exp. Med. 72:747, 1940.

361. Huggins C: Quantitative studies of prostatic secretion: characterization of normal section and testis extirpation and androgen substitution on the prostatic output. J. Exp. Med. 10:543, 1939.

362. Huggins C, and Hodges CV: Studies of prostatic cancer: the effect of castration on estrogen and androgen injection and serum phosphatases of the prostate. Cancer Res. 1:293, 1941.

363. Wilson JD: Recent studies on the mechanism of action. N. Engl. J. Med. 287:1284, 1972.

364. Baulieu EE: Metabolism of testosterone and action of metabolites on prostate glands grown in organ culture. Nature 219:1155, 1968.

365. Habib FK, Lee IR, Stitch SR, et al.: Androgen levels in the plasma and prostatic tissue of patients with benign hypertrophy carcinoma of the prostate. J. Endocrinol. 71:99, 1976.

366. Sciarra F, Sorcini G, Silver FD, et al.: Testosterone and 4-androstene concentration in peripheral and spermatic venous blood of patients with prostatic adenocarcinoma: effects of diethylstilbestrol and cyproterone acetate therapy. J. Steroid Biochem. 2:313, 1971.

367. Hammond GL, Kontturim, Vikko P, et al.: Serum steroids in normal males and patients with prostatic diseases. Clin. Endocrinol. 9:113, 1978.

368. Grayback JT: Pituitary factors influencing growth of the prostate. Natl. Cancer Inst. Monograph 12:189, 1963.

369. Asano M, Murayama T, Komatsu H, et al.: Mesonephric adenocarcinoma of the urethra in a woman: report of a case. J. Urol. 120:500, 1978.

370. Argoma C, Bohnet HG, and Freisen HG: Localization of prolactin binding in prostate and testis: the role of serum prolactin concentration on the testicular LH receptor. Acta Endocrinol. 84:402, 1977.

371. Mainwaring WIP: Androgen receptors in the future management of carcinoma of the prostate. *In* Thompson EB, and Lippman ME (eds.): Steroid Receptor and the Management of Cancer. CRC Press, Boca Raton, FL, 1979, p. 99.

372. Geller J: Hormone dependency of prostate cancer. *In* Thompson EB, and Lippman ME (eds.): Steroid Receptors and the Management of Cancer. CRC Press, Boca Raton, FL, 1979, p. 113.

373. Mobbs BG, Johnson IE, and Connolly JG: Hormonal responsiveness of prostatic carcinoma. *In vitro* technique for prediction. Urology 3:105, 1974.

374. Hawkins EF, Nijs M, and Brassine C: Steroid receptors in the human prostate. Detection of tissue-specific androgen binding in prostate cancer. Clin. Chem. Acta 75:303, 1977.

375. Ekman P, Snochowski M, Dahlberg E, et al.: Steroid receptors in metastatic carcinoma of the human prostate. Eur. J. Cancer 15:257, 1979.

376. Gustafsson JN, Ekman P, Snochowski M, et al.: Correlation between clinical response to hormone therapy and steroid receptor content in prostatic cancer. Cancer Res. 38:4345, 1978.

377. Goodwin DA, Rasmussen-Taxdal DS, Ferreira AA, et al.: Estrogen inhibition of androgen-maintained prostatic secretion in the hypophysectomized dog. J. Urol. 80:134, 1961.

378. Nesbit RM, and Baum WC: Endocrine control of prostatic carcinoma. J.A.M.A. 174:143, 1950.

379. O'Conor VJ, Chiang SP, and Grayhack JT: Is subcapsular orchiectomy a definitive procedure? Studies of hormone excretion before and after orchiectomy. J. Urol. 89:236, 1963.

380. Veterans Administration Cooperative Urological Research Group: Treatment and survival of patients with cancer of the prostate. Surg. Gynecol. Obstet. 124:1011, 1967.

381. Blackard CE: The Veterans Administration Cooperative Urological Research Group studies of carcinoma of the prostate: a review. Cancer Chem. Rep. 59:225, 1975.

382. Shearer RJ: Plasma testosterone: an accurate monitor of hormone treatment in prostatic cancer. Br. J. Urol. 45:668, 1973.

383. Sciarra F, Sorcini G, Silvero F, et al.: Plasma testosterone and androstenedione after orchiectomy in prostatic adenocarcinoma. Clin. Endocrinol. 2:101, 1973.

384. Sandord EJ, Drago JR, Rohner TJ, et al.: Aminoglutethimide medical adrenalectomy for advanced prostatic carcinoma. J. Urol. 115:174, 1976.

385. Murphy CP, Reynoso G, Schoomees R, et al.: Hypophysectomy, adrenalectomy for disseminated prostatic carcinoma. J. Urol. 1054:817, 1971.

386. Wintermitz WW, and Norrett H: Cryohypophysectomy in the management of advanced prostatic cancer. Cancer 28:322, 1971.

387. Silverberg GD: Hypophysectomy in the treatment of disseminated prostate carcinoma. Cancer 39:1727, 1977.

388. Geller J, Freechtman E, Newman H, et al.: Effect of progestational agents on carcinoma of the prostate. Cancer Chemother. Rep. 51:41, 1967.

389. Rafla S, and Johnson R: The treatment of advanced prostatic carcinoma with medroxyprogesterone. Curr. Ther. Res. 16:261, 1974.

390. Neumann F: Pharmacology and potential use of cyproterone acetate. Hormone Metab. Res. 9:1, 1977.

391. Aurhart RA, Barnett TF, Sullivan JW, et al.: Flutamide therapy for carcinoma of the prostate. South Med. J. 71:798, 1978.

392. Neri R, Florance K, Koziol P, et al.: A biological profile of a nonsteroid antiandrogen, SCH 13521 (4-nitro-3'-trifluoromethy-lisobutyranilide). Endocrinology 91:427, 1972.

393. Lippman ME, Heuson JC, and Muggia FM: Problems in the development of cytotoxic moieties linked to hormones. Cancer Treat. Rep. 62:1255, 1978.

394. LeClercq G, Heuson JC, and Deboel MC: Estrogen receptor interaction with estrayl and degradation products: a biochemical study on a potential agent in the treatment of breast cancer. Eur. J. Drug Metab. Phar. 2:77, 1976.

395. Group European du Cancer du Sein: Essai clinique du phenol bis (2-chloro-ethyl)-carbamde d'oestradiol dans le cancer mammaire en phase avance. Eur. J. Cancer 5:1, 1969.

396. Shapira D, Hall TC, Bennet JM, et al.: A phase II study of oestradiol mustard (NSC-112259) by the Eastern Cooperative Oncology Group. Cancer Clin. Trials 5:236, 1978.
397. Jonsson G, Hogberg E, and Nilsson T: Treatment of advanced prostatic carcinoma with estramustine phosphate (Estrcyt). Scand. J. Urol. Nephrol. 11:231, 1977.
398. Mittelman A, Shukla SK, and Murphy GP: Extended therapy of state D carcinoma of the prostate with oral estramustine phosphate. J. Urol. 115:409, 1976.
399. VonHoff DD, Rosenberg M, Slavik M, et al.: Estramustine phosphate: a specific chemotherapeutic agent. J. Urol. 117:464, 1977.
400. Forsgren B, Högberg E, Gustafsson JA, et al.: Binding of estramustine, a nitrogen mustard derivative of oestradiol 17, in cytosol from rat ventral prostate. Acta Pharm. Suec. 15:23, 1978.
401. Bullock LP, Bardin CW, and Ohno S: Androgen insensitive mouse: absence of intranuclear androgen retention in the kidney. Biochem. Biophys. Res. Commun. 44:1537, 1971.
402. Horning ES, and Whittick JW: The histogenesis of stilboestrol-induced renal tumours in the male golden hamster. Br. J. Cancer 8:451, 1954.
403. Horning ES: Observations in hormone-dependent renal tumours in the golden hamster. Br. J. Cancer 10:678, 1956.
404. Bloom HJG: Sex hormones and renal neoplasia. Cancer 20:2118, 1967.
405. Li JJ, Cutherbertson TL, and Li SA: Specific androgen binding in the kidney and estrogen-dependent renal carcinoma of the Syrian hamster. Endocrinology 101:1006, 1977.
406. Li JJ, Talley DJ, Li SA, et al.: Receptor characteristics of specific estrogen binding in the renal adenocarcinoma of the golden hamster. Cancer Res. 36:1127, 1976.
407. Lin YC, Talley DJ, and Villee CA: Progesterone receptor levels in estrogen-induced renal carcinomas after serial passage beneath the renal capsule of Syrian hamsters. Cancer Res. 38:1286, 1978.
408. Wagle DG, and Scal D: Renal cell carcinoma: a review of 256 cases. J. Surg. Oncol. 2:23, 1970.
409. Concolino G, Marocchi C, Tenaglia R, et al.: Human renal cell carcinoma as a hormone-dependent tumor. Cancer Res. 38:4340, 1978.
410. Bloom HJG: Medroxyprogesterone acetate (Provera) in the treatment of metastatic renal cancer. Br. J. Cancer 25:250, 1971.
411. Wagle DG, and Murphy GP: Hormone therapy in advanced renal cell carcinoma. Cancer 28:318, 1971.
412. Gordon GG, Southern AL, Tochimoto S, et al.: Effect of medroxyprogesterone acetate (Provera) on the metabolism and biological activity of testosterone. J. Clin. Endocrinol. 30:449, 1970.
413. Baxter JD, and Forsham PH: Tissue effects of glucocorticoids. Metabolism 23:159, 1974.
414. Selye H: Studies on adaptation. Endocrinology 21:169, 1937.
415. Claman HN: Corticosteroids and lymphoid cells. N. Engl. J. Med. 267:388, 1972.
416. Golden A, Sandberg JS, Henderson ES, et al.: The chemotherapy of human and animal acute leukemia. Cancer Chemother. Rep. 55:309, 1971.
417. Lippman ME: Clinical implications of glucocorticoid receptors in human leukemia. Cancer Res. 38:4251, 1978.
418. Crabtree GR, Smith KA, and Munck A: Glucocorticoid receptors and sensitivity of isolated human leukemia and lymphoma cells. Cancer Res. 36:4268, 1978.
419. Lippman ME: Glucocorticoid binding proteins in acute lymphoblastic leukemic breast cells. J. Clin. Invest. 52:1715, 1973.
420. Neifeld JP: Steroid hormone receptors in normal human lymphocytes: induction of glucocorticoid receptor activity by PHA stimulation. J. Biol. Chem. 252:2972, 1977.
421. Lippman ME, and Barr R: Glucocorticoid receptors in purified subpopulations of human peripheral blood lymphocytes. J. Immunol. 118:000, 1977.
422. Smith KA: Glucocorticoid receptors and glucocorticoid sensitivity of mitogen stimulated and unstimulated human lymphocytes. Nature 267:523, 1977.
423. Konior GS: Glucocorticoid receptors in subpopulations of childhood acute lymphocytic leukemia. Cancer Res. 37:2688, 1977.
424. Homo F, Duval D, Meyer P, et al.: Chronic lymphatic leukaemia: cellular effects of glucocorticoids *in vitro*. Br. J. Haematol. 38:491, 1978.
425. Bloomfield C, Smith KA, Peterson BA, et al. *In vitro* glucocorticoid studies for predicting response to glucocorticoid therapy in adults with malignant lymphoma. Lancet 1:952, 1980.
426. Lippman ME: Glucocorticoid binding proteins in myeloblasts of acute myelogenous leukemia. Am. J. Med. 59:224, 1975.
427. Homo F, Duval D, Harousseau JL, et al.: Glucocorticoid receptors in normal and neoplastic human lymphoid cells. Progress in cancer research and therapy. Cancer Res. 33:2653, 1978.
428. Terenius L, Simonsson B, and Nilsson K: Glucocorticoid receptors, DNA synthesis, membrane antigens and their relation to disease activity in chronic lymphatic leukemia. J. Steroid Biochem. 7:905, 1976.
429. Schottenfeld D, and Berg J: Incidence of multiple primary cancers. IV. Cancers of the female breast and genital organs. J. Natl. Cancer Inst. 46:161, 1971.
430. Lynch HT, Krush AJ, Farsen AL, et al.: Endometrial carcinoma: multiple primary malignancies, constitutional factors and heredity. Am. J. Med. Sci. 252:381, 1966.
431. Haenszel W, and Kurihara M: Studies of Japanese migrants. 1. Mortality from cancers and other diseases among Japanese in the United States. J. Natl. Cancer Inst. 40:43, 1968.
432. Hoover R, Gray LA Sr, and Fraumeni JF Jr: Stilboestrol (diethylstilboestrol) and the risk of ovarian cancer. Lancet 2:533, 1977.
433. Kiang DT, and Kennedy BJ: Estrogen receptor assay in the differential diagnosis of adenocarcinomas. J.A.M.A. 238:32, 1977.
434. Tobias JS, and Griffiths TC: Management of ovarian cancer. N. Engl. J. Med. 294:818, 1976.
435. Saez S, and Sakai F: Androgen receptors in human pharyngo-laryngeal mucosa and pharyngo-laryngeal epithelioma. J. Steroid Biochem. 7:919, 1976.
436. Saez S, Martin PM, and Gignoux B: Androgen receptors in the normal mucosa in epithelium of human larynx and pharynx. *In* Thompson EB, and Lippman ME (eds.): Steroid Receptors and the Management of Cancer. CRC Press, Boca Raton, FL, 1979, p. 205.

PYRIMIDINE ANTAGONISTS 8

Bruce A. Chabner

FLUORINATED PYRIMIDINES

Despite many efforts to synthesize antineoplastic drugs on a rational basis, few such agents have fulfilled the expectations of biochemical, pharmacologic, and clinical activity. An exception to this generality are the fluorinated pyrimidines synthesized by Heidelberger and colleagues.[1]

The impetus for synthesis of this series of compounds came from the observation that rat hepatomas more avidly utilize radiolabeled uracil than do nonmalignant tissues.[2] This finding implies that the enzymatic pathway for utilization of uracil, or possibly analogues of uracil, resides in malignant but not normal cells, and this difference represents a possible exploitable target for antimetabolite chemotherapy.

These drugs have not only shown predicted biochemical action, but have also become useful in the treatment of human solid tumors, including breast cancer, ovarian cancer, and gastrointestinal adenocarcinomas.

STRUCTURE AND MECHANISM OF ACTION

The chemical structures of 5-fluoropyrimidines of clinical interest are shown in Figure 8–1. The simplest derivative, 5-fluorouracil (5-FU), incorporates a fluorine atom at the 5 position in place of hydrogen. The fluorine atom, which is slightly bulkier than hydrogen, does not impede the conversion of 5-FU or the other 5-fluoropyrimidines to nucleotides; indeed, this conversion is essential to the antitumor activity of this class of compounds. Multiple types of antimetabolic action are exerted by the various fluoropyrimidine nucleotides, and the precise mechanism of antitumor action remains uncertain.

At least two primary mechanisms of action appear capable of causing cell injury: (1) inhibition of thymidylate synthetase, and (2) incorporation into RNA. The first occurs through the generation of 5-FdUMP (Fig. 8–2), which binds tightly to thymidylate synthesis and prevents formation of dTMP (Fig. 8–2). dTMP is the essential precursor of dTTP, one of four deoxynucleotides required for DNA synthesis. The second mechanism results from the incorporation of 5-FUTP into RNA and the effects of this incorporation on RNA function. Initial evidence for inhibition of thymidylate synthesis was forthcoming from experiments that demonstrated that 5-FU, 5-FUdR, and 5-FUR blocked the incorporation of formate into DNA.[3] Formate serves as a source of the methyl group donated by $N^{5\text{-}10}$-methylenetetrahydrofolic acid in the conversion of dUMP to dTMP (Fig. 8–2). Subsequent work has clarified that mechanism of inhibition of thymidylate synthesis. 5-FdUMP competes with the natural substrate dUMP for the catalytic site on thymidylate synthetase and, in the presence of the folate cofactor, attaches to the enzyme covalently through a bond from the 6-carbon of the inhibitor to a free sulfhydryl group at the enzyme's active site[4, 5] (Fig. 8–3). Peptide fragments of bacterial thymidylate synthetase containing covalently bound 5-FdUMP have been isolated. In the methylation of dUMP, transfer of the folate methyl group to dUMP is made possible by elimination of the 5-H. This elimination does not occur with the more tightly bound fluorine atom in the 5 position of the inhibitor, and the enzyme is trapped and inactivated in a dead-end complex. The

R = H in 5-Fluorouracil

R = furanyl in Ftorafur

— 5-Fluorouracil Base

R = deoxyribose (HOH_2C, OH) in 5-Fluorodeoxyuridine

R = 5′-deoxyribose (CH_3, OH OH) in 5′-deoxy-5-Fluorouracil

Figure 8–1. 5-Fluoropyrimidines currently in clinical trial.

"thymine-less state" created by this inhibition is toxic to actively dividing cells; toxicity can be circumvented by salvage of circulating thymidine in cells that contain thymidine kinase, but the circulating concentrations of thymidine appear to be insufficient (approximately 1×10^{-7}M) to allow this route of escape in normal tissues and in at least some tumor cells.

The presence of a reduced folate cofactor is required for tight binding of the inhibitor to the thymidylate synthetase. The natural substrate for the thymidylate synthetase reaction, $N^{5\text{-}10}$-methylenetetrahydrofolic acid, binds through its methylene group to the C-5 position of 5-FdUMP. Methotrexate (see Chapter 10) and various naturally occurring folates can also promote 5-FdUMP binding to the enzyme, but probably in a looser complex than that formed with the physiologic cofactor. An exception may be the polyglutamates of dihydrofolic acid, which accumulate in cells exposed to methotrexate and which promote extremely tight binding of 5-FdUMP to the enzyme.[6] In cell-free experiments, methotrexate was found to substitute poorly for $N^{5\text{-}10}$ methylenetetrahydrofolic acid and to decrease the rate of formation of ternary complex(es) among 5-FdUMP, folate, and enzyme.[7] Similarly, in tissue culture, methotrexate-induced depletion of intracellular-reduced folates causes a marked reduction in the rate of formation of ternary-inhibited complex.[8]

The kinetics of formation and dissociation of the ternary complex have been studied using the enzyme from *L. casei*.[9] The bacterial enzyme has two subunits of 35,000 molec-

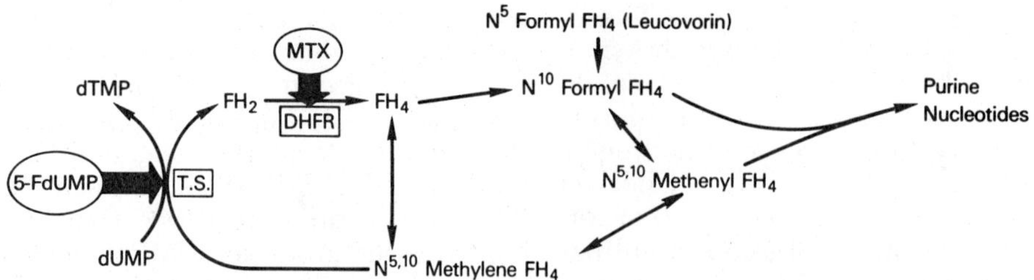

Figure 8–2. Site of action of 5-FdUMP, a potent inhibitor of thymidylate synthetase (T.S.). Also shown is the inhibition of dihydrofolate reductase (DHFR) by methotrexate (MTX). As explained later in this chapter, block of the T.S. reaction preserves the intracellular folate pool in the reduced (FH_4) state and negates the effect of DHFR inhibition by MTX. (Reproduced with permission from Donehower et al.: Minireview. New developments on the mechanism of action of antineoplastic drugs. Life Sci. 24:1–14, 1979.)

COVALENT TERNARY COMPLEX

FdUMP: METHYLENE FH_4: TS

Figure 8–3. Ternary complex formation with FdUMP-thymidylate synthetase-N^{5-10}-methylenetetrahydrofolic acid.

ular weight, each subunit having a binding site for 5-FdUMP. However, only one site is accessible for binding in the free enzyme; the second site becomes exposed only after occupancy of the first site by inhibitor and folate. There is disagreement as to the equivalency of these two sites. At least one study found that the two binding sites are nonequivalent in terms of their dissociation constants,[10] with KD's of 1.1×10^{-11} and 2×10^{-10}M.

The measurable dissociation of 5-FdUMP from bacterial thymidylate synthetase was unexpected in view of the formation of a covalent bond between inhibitor and enzyme. It is uncertain whether the binding of 5-FdUMP to mammalian thymidylate synthetase has the same characteristics as binding to the bacterial enzyme. The bacterial and mammalian enzymes differ in molecular weight and amino acid composition, and preliminary evidence indicates a less avid binding of inhibitor to the mammalian enzyme. Washtein and Santi[11] observed a dissociation half-life of 6.2 hours for the enzyme-inhibitor complex, indicating the inhibition of the mammalian enzyme is at least slowly reversible.

Despite the high specificity and potency of thymidylate synthetase inhibition by 5-FdUMP, and the well-established lethality of thymidylate depletion by other agents such as methotrexate, there are other observations not easily explained by invoking this lesion as the cause of 5-FU toxicity. If 5-FU toxicity is due to dTTP depletion, thymidine should reverse the toxic effects. However, thymidine shows variable effectiveness in rescuing cells exposed to 5-FU.[12-15] Maybaum and co-workers[12] found that mouse lymphoma cells (the S-49 cell line) experienced two phases of drug toxicity when exposed to 5-FU (Fig. 8–4). An early phase of inhibition of cell growth, lasting 24 hours, was reversed by adding thymidine to the culture medium, but a later phase of inhibition — in the period after the initial 24 hours — was not reversible. The early phase of toxicity had the characteristics of S-phase specificity and a hold-up of cells in S phase that one would associate with a DNA-directed lesion, such as dTTP depletion; however, this DNA-directed toxicity was self-limiting, in that accumulation of dUMP behind the enzymatic block led to substrate competition with the inhibitor and reversal of inhibition. Addition of thymidine prevented the S-phase block induced by thymidylate depletion and abolished the early phase of growth inhibition. The later phase of 5-FU inhibition of growth had much different characteristics. After 24 hours of incubation with 5-FU, approximately equal to one cell cycle time for these cells, the lethal lesion was no longer reversible with thymidine, and was now maximal for cells exposed to the drug during the G_1 phase of the cell cycle. The authors hypothesized that the second phase

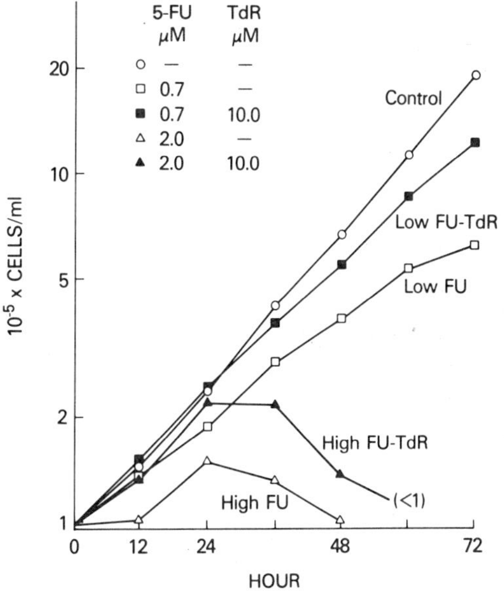

Figure 8–4. Growth inhibition of S-49 cells by 5-FU with or without thymidine. Asynchronously growing cells in log phase were diluted to 10^5/ml, and the agents were added at Time 0. (Reproduced with permission from Maybaum et al.: Regulation of RNA- and DNA-directed actions of 5-fluoropyrimidines in mouse T-lymphoma (S-49) cells. Cancer Res. 40:4209–4215, 1980.)

of inhibition was caused by progressive incorporation of 5-FU into RNA and the subsequent effects of that incorporation on RNA processing and function, as described below.

There is additional evidence to support the hypothesis that 5-FU inhibition of growth can result from at least two mechanisms. Evans and colleagues[13] found that a three-hour incubation with 5-FU at low concentrations (5 to 20 μM) produced a thymidine-reversible toxicity, whereas higher concentrations of 5-FU produced toxicity not reversible by thymidine. An interesting difference in susceptibility to the two mechanisms of toxicity was observed in comparing three mouse and three human cell culture lines. The human cells were not affected by low concentrations of 5-FU, because of their higher innate thymidylate synthetase activity and their ability to generate high concentrations of dUMP behind the blocked reaction. They were, however, sensitive to inhibition by high concentrations of 5-FU (50 to 200 μM). Mouse cell lines were sensitive to both low and high concentrations of 5-FU. The authors found a reasonably close correlation between 5-FU incorporation into RNA and growth inhibition at high concentrations. The 50 per cent inhibitory dose for the various cell lines was associated with incorporation of 6.5 to 17 nmol FU per mg RNA.

Additional experimental evidence from *in vivo* studies supports the contention that 5-FU toxicity is at least partially, if not wholly, independent of its effect on thymidylate synthetase. Coadministration of 5-FU and thymidine *prevents* the early inhibition of DNA synthesis, but markedly *increases* 5-FU toxicity to normal tissues in the whole animal,[16] increases the antitumor effect of 5-FU against various animal tumors,[16, 17] and increases 5-FU incorporation into the RNA of normal and malignant cells.[18] Other pharmacologic measures that increase 5-FU incorporation into RNA also increase its toxicity; these include coadministration of phosphono-N-acetyl-L-aspartic acid (PALA), an inhibitor of *de novo* pyrimidine synthesis,[19] or various pyrimidine nucleosides, which presumably delay 5-FU catabolism and thereby increase intracellular 5-FUTP and incorporation into RNA.[16]

It should be remembered, however, that examples of complete protection from 5-FU cytotoxicity by thymidine have been reported[14, 20] in *in vitro* experiments. It is possible that both mechanisms (thymidylate depletion and RNA incorporation) can have lethal consequences, and the importance of each may vary from one tumor to the next and may depend also on drug concentration, duration of tumor exposure, and the presence of thymidine. The evidence described in the preceding discussion suggests that the RNA incorporation mechanism would probably be favored by high concentrations of 5-FU and longer durations of exposure, and would be enhanced by the presence of thymidine, whereas the opposite conditions would favor thymidylate depletion.

Incorporation of 5-FU into RNA has profound consequences for the processing and function of RNA.[21-23] Under conditions of exposure to high concentrations of 5-FU, a maximum of 2 per cent of uracil in RNA will be replaced by 5-FU[13]: this despite the fact that 5-FUTP is the predominant nucleotide formed from 5-FU.[24] In contrast to the effects of 5-FU, when cells are incubated with the deoxyribonucleotide 5-FUdR they form little 5-FUTP; the toxicity of this agent appears to be explained satisfactorily by the action of 5-FdUMP.

Incorporation of 5-FU into RNA inhibits the processing of nuclear RNA to lower molecular weight ribosomal RNA (the transition from 45s to 28s and 18s units) (Fig. 8–5).[21] Polyadenylation of RNA, a process thought to confer stability on messenger RNA species, is also inhibited at relatively low concentrations of 5-FU,[25] whereas methylation of RNA bases is blocked at high drug concentrations.[26] The functional effects of these changes in RNA synthesis and processing have been assessed in *in vitro* experiments, with inconclusive results. 5-FU does cause errors in base pairing during transcription of DNA by RNA polymerase in isolated rat nuclei.[27] Glazer and Legraverend[27] found an increased frequency of GMP and AMP next to AMP, and a decreased frequency of AMP next to GMP and UMP. However, an examination of proteins produced in a cell-free system by poly A-RNA containing 5-FU failed to disclose a qualitative difference in the electrophoretic profile, although the overall rate of protein synthesis was stimulated as compared with the rate of synthesis using control RNA.[25] A more detailed explanation of possible subtle effects on protein

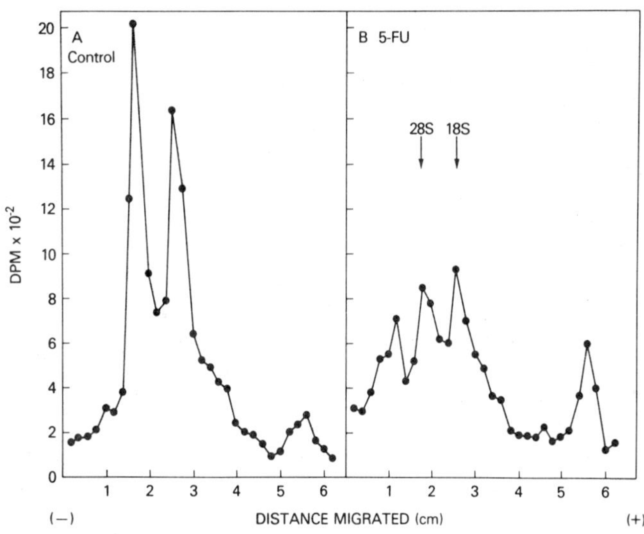

Figure 8–5. Agarose-urea gel electrophoresis of rRNA from control and 5-FU–treated animals. rRNA was isolated from liver polysomes of partially hepatectomized rats treated with either 0.9 per cent NaCl solution (*A*) or 20 mg of 5-FU per kg (*B*) at one and 16 hours after operation. [^{3}H]orotic acid was administered at 16 hrs to label RNA, and rats were killed at 18 hrs. (Reproduced with permission from Carrico CK, and Glazer RI: The effect of 5-fluorouracil on the synthesis and translation of poly (A) RNA from regenerating liver. Cancer Res. 39:3694–3701, 1979.)

structure and function will be required before the effects of 5-FU incorporation into RNA are fully understood.

Although 5-FU is readily incorporated into RNA, it has not been found in DNA. Two enzymatic activities are responsible for excluding 5-FU from DNA.[28] dUTPase hydrolyzes 5-FdUTP, preventing its accumulation intracellularly. Any fluoropyrimidine that is incorporated is removed by uracil-DNA glycosylase. Thus, multiple mechanisms are able to prevent incorporation of uracil or its analogues into DNA.

While most of the actions of 5-FU are explained by inhibition of the thymidylate pathway or by altered RNA function, the drug also produces effects on other cellular processes. 5-FU treatment decreases the surface charge and transmembrane potential of tumor cells,[29] decreases fucose incorporation into membrane proteins,[30] and decreases protein synthesis.[30] It is not known whether these effects represent primary metabolic actions or simply secondary consequences associated with cell injury.

In summary, both thymidylate synthetase inhibition, as seen in "pure" form with 5-FUdR treatment, and 5-FU incorporation into RNA, as reflected in "pure" form by the effects of 5-FU:thymidine, are capable of producing lethal effects on cells. The relative importance of these two actions has not been clarified at this time, and may vary among different normal tissues and different tumor types. Both mechanisms must be considered in any prospective study of the determinants of responses to 5-FU.

CELLULAR PHARMACOLOGY

The transmembrane transport of 5-FU is difficult to characterize in kinetic terms because of the rapidity of drug permeation and its rapid intracellular conversion to nucleotides. In the Novikoff hepatoma cell line, maximal accumulation of free intracellular 5-FU occurs within 200 seconds.[30A] Total intracellular 5-FU continues to increase thereafter owing to the formation of nucleotides and their incorporation into RNA. The estimated kinetic features of 5-FU transport in Novikoff hepatoma cells are a K_m of 16 mM and a V_{max} of 286 pmol/μl cell water/sec. 5-FU appears to share the same transport system as uracil. This conclusion is based on competitive inhibition experiments and countertransport studies (cells preloaded with one base will transport the second at an increased rate).[29] 5-FU permeation is quite pH-dependent in that ionization of the 4-OH group, which has a pK of 8.0, markedly depresses the transmembrane passage of drug. The 5-FU transport system has not been proved to be temperature- or energy-dependent, and thus cannot be classified as an "active" uptake process (see Chapter 2). The transport system for 5-FU clearly differs from that utilized by pyrimidine nucleosides, in that it is not inhibited by *p*-nitrobenzylthioinosine, a potent inhibitor of both pyrimidine and purine nucleoside uptake.

5-Floxuridine (5-FUdR) utilizes the pyrimidine nucleoside transport system and, like 5-FU, rapidly gains entry into cells.[31] In

Ehrlich ascites cells, intracellular 5-FUdR reaches equilibrium with extracellular drug within 15 seconds. Total intracellular drug continues to accumulate thereafter, owing to formation of 5-FdUMP and other nucleotides. Thus, the phosphorylation process is rate-limiting in the continued formation of intracellular nucleotides, in comparison with the rapid process of membrane transport.

Activation of 5-FU to the nucleotide level may occur through one of several pathways, as outlined in Figure 8–6. These include: (1) direct transfer of a ribose phosphate to 5-FU from PRPP as catalyzed by orotic acid phosphoribosyl transferase; or (2) a two-step sequence involving addition of a ribose by uridine phosphorylase or addition of a deoxyribose by thymidine phosphorylase, followed by phosphorylation by an appropriate nucleoside kinase. It is not certain which of these activation pathways is most important in producing active 5-FU nucleotides in either normal or malignant cells. The first pathway, catalyzed by orotic acid phosphoribosyltransferase, appears to be of primary importance for 5-FU activation in normal tissues since its inhibition by allopurinol nucleotides diminishes toxicity to bone marrow and gastrointestinal mucosa, without compromising the antitumor effect in a few murine tumors studied.[32]

The orotic acid phosphoribosyl transferase pathway *is* the dominant route of 5-FU activation in many murine leukemias,[33-35] including L5178Y, L1210, P1534, P388, and sarcoma 180, while other cell lines, such as the Novikoff hepatoma, Walker 256, HeLa, and two human colon carcinomas grown in nude mice, probably activate the drug by the action of uridine phosphorylase and uridine kinase.[32, 34, 36, 37] However, some of these conclusions are derived indirectly from drug interactions affecting the availability of PR and PRPP (substrates for the various activation pathways) and do not represent direct measurement of enzyme activities.[37, 38] A comprehensive analysis of activation mechanism in human tumors would add greatly to our understanding of 5-FU metabolism.

In contrast to 5-FU, 5-FUdR is converted to the active product 5-FdUMP by a single enzyme, thymidine kinase. The simplicity of this pathway constitutes a strong rationale for the use of this agent in preference to 5-FU, but 5-FUdR lacks effects on RNA and, unfortunately, has not yielded consistently superior therapeutic results.

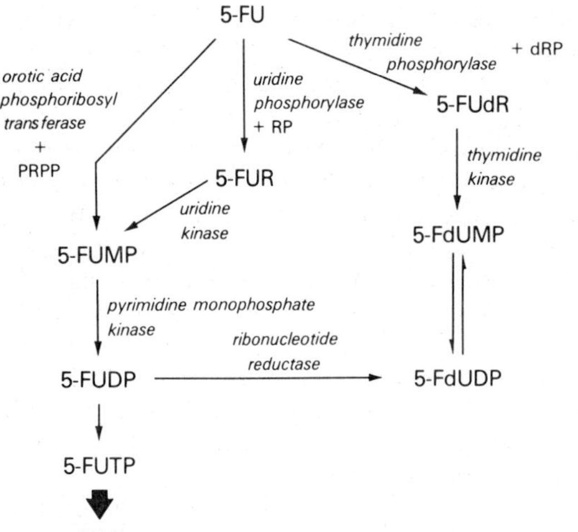

Figure 8–6. Activation pathways for 5-FU. Enzymes are italicized.

DETERMINANTS OF SENSITIVITY TO 5-FLUOROPYRIMIDINE

Because of the multiple sites of biochemical action and the multiple routes of nucleotide formation of the fluoropyrimidines, it has not been possible to specify one unique feature that distinguishes sensitive from resistant tumor cells. Many investigators have addressed the question of target cell determinants in experimental or clinical studies, but none has examined the broad range of enzymes and nucleotide pools that might influence response. Thus, most of these studies provide only a narrow perspective, and at their best provide evidence for an association rather than a causal link between one or more factors and tumor responsiveness. Table 8–1 lists the most important determinants of response and references for their measurement.

The classic approach of biochemical pharmacology has been to seek quantitative differences in enzymatic activities that might explain response. Deletion of the various possible activating enzymes has been described in murine tumors resistant to 5-FU; these missing enzymes include orotic acid phosphoribosyl transferase,[47, 48] uridine phosphorylase,[49] and uridine kinase.[50] It is not clear why the absence of any single activating enzyme would lead to resistance, since at least one alternative pathway for activation would exist. In addition to the

TABLE 8–1. Determinants of Sensitivity To 5-FU*

Biochemical Parameter	*Technique*	*Detection Limit*	*Ref.*
5-FdUMP	Enzyme inhibition	1 pmole	57
	Competitive ligand binding assay	0.01 pmole	10, 59
Thymidylate synthetase	Spectrophotometric assay	0.5 pmole†	40
	Tritium release assay	0.03 pmole†	41
	Binding assay	0.003 pmole	57
Ternary complex	[6-^{3}H]FUdR; gel filtration	Depends on specific activity	11
dUMP	Enzyme-induced change in absorbance	2000 pmoles	57
	^{14}C radiochemical synthesis	20 pmoles	59
FU incorporated into RNA	Isotope administration	Depends on specific activity	
Thymidine kinase	Radiochemical assay	0.005 pmole†	42
Thymidine content	HPLC	0.02 pmole	43
Ability to form nucleotides	*In vitro* evaluation with tumor homogenates	Depends on specific activity	60
	Assay of uridine and thymidine phos-	0.3 pmole†	44
	phorylases, and pyrimidine	0.3 pmole†	45
	phosphoribosyl transferase	0.07 pmole†	46

*Reproduced with permission from Moran RG, and Heidelberger C: Determinants of 5-fluorouracil sensitivity in human tumors. Bull. Cancer (Paris) 66:79–83, 1979.

†Approximate values based on an assumed turnover number of 500 and representative K_m values.

clear importance of these activating enzymes, the availability of ribosome phosphate (RP) or phosphoribosyl pyrophosphate (PRPP) may influence activation and response. Thus, in Novikoff hepatoma cells, inosine inhibits consumption of RP in the salvage of purine and augments 5-FU activation,[37] while, in L1210 cells, methotrexate blocks *de novo* purine synthesis, increases intracellular PRPP, and enhances 5-FU nucleotide formation.[38]

Metabolic steps past the initial formation of monophosphate are less clearly important determinants of resistance. Ardalan has described a resistant subline of P388 that has greatly decreased concentrations of pyrimidine monophosphate kinase.[51] However, this enzyme is found in 10- to 100-fold higher concentrations than the nucleoside kinases in most tumor cells,[52] and thus is unlikely to be rate-limiting for 5-FUMP phosphorylation except in unusual tumors. Finally, thymidine kinase — an enzyme that allows utilization of circulating thymidine to bypass the block in thymidylate synthetase — is deficient in some resistant cells.[24] It is unclear whether circulating thymidine concentrations (about 0.1 μM) are sufficient to replete intracellular pools, since this concentration of thymidine is insufficient to rescue cells from the toxicity of methotrexate (also an inhibitor of thymidylate biosynthesis).

Cells that become resistant to fluorinated pyrimidines may also develop alterations in the target enzyme thymidylate synthetase; thus, Heidelberger and colleagues found a decreased binding affinity for 5-FdUMP in the enzyme from 5-FU–resistant cells,[53] and increased enzyme activity was identified in 5-FUdR–resistant neuroblastoma cells[54] and mouse hepatoma cells.[55]

As an alternative to the search for enzymatic determinations of response, other investigators have directed their attention to the formation of 5-fluoropyrimidine nucleotides within target cells. It is apparent from the preceding discussion that either 5-FdUMP or 5-FUTP formation, or both, may be the important indicator of responsiveness. Accumulation of total intracellular nucleotides (both ribo- and deoxyribo- forms) correlates with responsiveness in murine tumors, but specific derivatives were not fractionated in this early study.[56] Other experiments have disagreed on the importance of 5-FdUMP formation,[24, 37, 51] but in general the results encompass only a few cell types and the methodology of measurement of 5-FdUMP may not have been sufficiently sensitive to allow accurate assessment of this parameter.

Myers and co-workers[57] were the first to examine the kinetic profile of 5-FdUMP formation and disappearance in normal and malignant tissues *in vivo*, using a sensitive and highly specific enzymatic assay for 5-FdUMP. They found that blockade of thymidylate synthetase leads to a gradual expansion of the intracellular dUMP pool; resumption of DNA synthesis thereafter is a function of two factors: (1) the rate of fall of intracellular 5-FdUMP, and (2) the rate of increase in dUMP, its competitive substrate. Different patterns of change in nucleotide pools were observed in bone marrow, intestinal epithelium, and tumor cells. In bone marrow, recovery was related to 20-fold expansion of the dUMP pool, and in the intestine recovery of DNA synthesis correlated with a more rapid fall in 5-FdUMP. In the 5-FU–sensitive P1534 leukemia, free intracellular 5-FdUMP persisted for up to seven days and was opposed by only a modest increase in free dUMP concentration.

In similar studies it was found that 5-FdUMP accumulated rapidly in both the responsive L1210 leukemia and the resistant Walker 256 carcinoma, but the more rapid recovery of DNA synthesis in the Walker carcinoma correlated with a more accelerated decline in intracellular free 5-FdUMP concentration.[58] More sensitive techniques that measure 5-FdUMP by competitive binding to thymidylate synthetase have confirmed that a more rapid decline in 5-FdUMP concentration may be characteristic of resistant neoplasms.[10] Thus, the defect in resistant cells may relate to the rate of nucleotide inactivation rather than to slower formation of the active product. Extremely sensitive assays for dUMP, thymidylate synthetase, the ternary-inhibited complex, and free 5-FdUMP are now possible and await application to clinical studies of the determinants of response.[59]

As mentioned previously, 5-FU incorporation into RNA may also determine response in some tumors.[16,19] The extent of this incorporation depends on the formation of 5-FUTP and the size of the competitive pool of UTP. In a few studies with experimental tumors, both 5-FUTP and 5-FdUMP have been measured at the same time points in the same tumor; the authors have arrived at conflicting conclusions as to the relative importance of 5-FdUMP and FUTP formation in determining response.[24, 37, 51] Preliminary studies[24] have not found a correlation between responsiveness of human xenografts and 5-fluoropyrimidine incorporation into RNA. Clearly, new prospective investigations of 5-FUTP formation and its incorporation into RNA are needed to verify the value of these parameters as predictors of response. A simple assay system — one that utilizes homogenates of human tumors with added RP, PRPP, and ATP and tests the ability of the homogenates to form nucleotides — may allow prospective clinical evaluation of these parameters.[60]

CLINICAL PHARMACOLOGY ASSAY METHODS

Initial studies of the pharmacokinetics of 5-FU in man employed radiolabeled drug or microbiologic assays. These approaches have since been replaced by more sensitive and useful chromatographic methods that have the necessary sensitivity and specificity for detection of 5-FU in clinical specimens. The current preferred method appears to be high-pressure liquid chromatography using either a normal-phase[61] or a reverse-phase[62] column. Buckpitt and Boyd[62] have devised a preliminary clean-up procedure in which plasma is applied to a Dowex AG 1 × 2 resin and the parent compound is eluted with 1N acetic acid. The lyophilized residue is then redissolved in a small quantity of buffer and applied to a C_{18} Bondapak column, and the 5-FU is eluted with phosphate buffer. In this method, ^{3}H-5-FU is added to each clinical sample to allow an internal correction for recovery of each sample, and the 5-FU content is calculated on the basis of the ratio of peak height to counts per minute in the peak tube. This method allows detection of 5-FU concentrations in plasma of 50 nM or greater, a sensitivity that equals that of the more cumbersome mass-spectrophotometric assays[63] and exceeds that of gas chromatography.[64]

The same HPLC assay, as described above, can also be used for measurement of 5-FUdR.[62, 65] An alternative method for 5-FUdR, employing rabbit antibodies to drug-bovine serum albumin complex, has been devised by Schreiber and Raso,[66] and is sensitive to approximately 0.5 μM concentrations in plasma. This lower limit of sensitivity may be insufficient to allow its application to clinical pharmacokinetics in view of the small doses of 5-FUdR employed in man.

CLINICAL PHARMACOKINETICS

The pharmacokinetics of 5-fluorouracil have become an important consideration in cancer chemotherapy because of the wide choice of routes and schedules of administration that face the clinician in use of this drug. These various routes and schedules each have advantages in terms of differing toxicity, and some offer the selective exposure of specific tumor-bearing sites to high local concentrations of drug. In the understanding and assessment of these alternatives, pharmacokinetic studies have played an important role.

Absorption and Distribution

5-Fluorouracil is usually administered by the intravenous route. Bioavailability by the oral route is erratic,[67-70] and usually less than 75 per cent of a dose reaches the systemic circulation. After oral administration, peak plasma concentrations reach a maximum of 5 to 200 μM within one hour of drug administration, although in selected patients absorption may be greatly delayed or nonexistent.[71] Two of 12 patients studied by Christophidis and co-workers[69] had no measurable 5-FU in their plasma following oral 5-FU administration. Bioavailability appears to increase with increasing dose, suggesting a saturable first-pass elimination process in the liver.[72] Thus, after a dose of 4 mg/kg, bioavailability was 25 per cent of the dose, whereas a larger dose of 15 mg/kg increased the amount reaching the systemic circulation to 40 per cent. After the lower dose, 56 per cent of the drug was removed in its first pass through the liver, whereas only 26 per cent was removed at the higher dose. Bioavailability by the oral route cannot be predicted by pretreatment liver function tests.[68] As might be expected, the clinical response rate to oral 5-FU is lower than the response rate to intravenous drug[73]; therefore, this route is rarely used in current chemotherapy protocols.

In selected clinical situations (discussed in greater detail later in this chapter), the drug may be administered by hepatic arterial infusion or by intraperitoneal instillation,[74] but the predominant route of administration is by intravenous bolus or infusion. Once access is gained to the systemic circulation, 5-FU readily penetrates the extracellular space, as well as cerebrospinal fluid and extracellular "third-space" accumulations such as ascites or pleural effusions.[75] Conventional doses of intravenous 5-FU yield cerebrospinal fluid concentrations above 10^{-8}M for 12 hours.[75] The volume of distribution for 5-FU has been estimated to be 12 to 38 per cent of total body weight, with a medial of 22 per cent, a figure slightly in excess of extracellular fluid space.[68-70, 76, 77]

Plasma Pharmacokinetics

Following intravenous infusion of conventional bolus doses of 400 to 600 mg per m^2 (10 to 15 mg/kg), peak plasma concentrations reach 0.1 to 1.0 mM (Fig. 8–7). Thereafter, rapid metabolic elimination leads to a fall in plasma concentrations with a primary half-life of six to 20 minutes, as determined by gas-liquid or high-pressure liquid chromatography (Table 8–2). All observers who have determined 5-FU pharmacokinetics have noted considerable interindividual variation in 5-FU half-life. Plasma clearance rates vary from 500 to 1500 ml/min, and thus equal or exceed hepatic blood flow in some patients.

In the dose range of 400 to 600 mg/m^2, drug concentrations exceed 1 μM, the approximate threshold for exerting cytotoxic effects on normal tissue, for approximately six hours.[70] The characteristics of later phases of drug elimination have not been clearly elucidated. A slow terminal phase has been detected using a mass spectrophotometric assay,[63] but drug concentrations during this phase of disappearance from plasma are well below the level required for biologic activity. Cano et al.[78] have found a markedly nonlinear relationship between dose and plasma concentrations of 5-FU in comparing bolus intravenous doses and prolonged intravenous infusions. For standard bolus doses, 5-FU plasma clearance was 0.5 to 1.4 liters per minute, while clearance values were 10- to 60-fold higher during prolonged intravenous infusion studies. This nonlinearity likely represents saturation of a metabolic or transport process at higher drug concentrations, and implies that it may be difficult to predict drug concentrations in plasma, or toxicity for higher-dose regimens.

Continuous intravenous infusion of 5-FU (1100 mg/m^2/day) produces plasma concen-

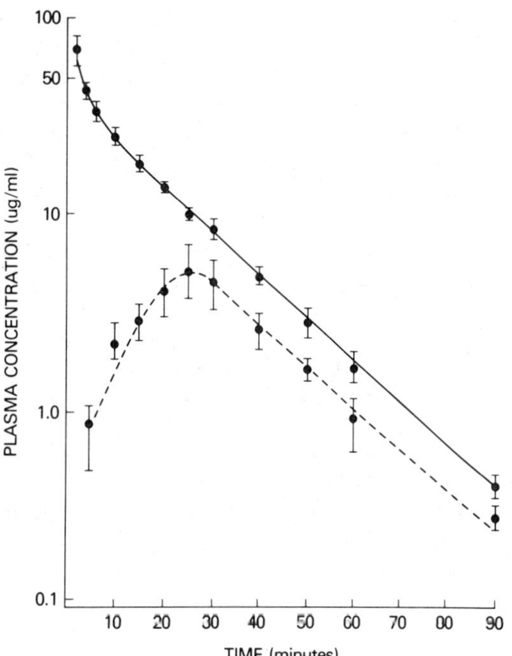

Figure 8–7. Mean plasma levels (± SEM) of 5-FU (μg/ml) on logarithmic scale versus time (min) after intravenous bolus administration of 9 to 16 mg/kg (———) and oral administration (— — —) of the same dose in 12 patients. (Reproduced with permission from Christophidis et al.: Fluorouracil therapy in patients with carcinoma of the large bowel: a pharmacokinetic comparison of various rates and routes of administration. Clin. Pharmacokinet. 3:330–336, 1978.)

trations of 0.5 to 2.5 μM, a level associated with mucositis and intestinal symptoms but little myelosuppression.[71] Fraile and colleagues[71] found that the 5-FU content of whole bone marrow sonicates relative to simultaneous plasma 5-FU was much lower after intravenous infusion than after intravenous bolus doses. This finding could explain the decreased myelotoxicity of schedules that employ continuous infusion of 5-FU.

The pharmacokinetics of 5-FU administered by intrahepatic arterial infusion have received considerable attention in an effort to maximize the infusion dose while limiting systemic toxicity. Ensminger and colleagues[65] found that 19 to 51 per cent of infused 5-FU was cleared in the first pass of drug through the liver. 5-FUdR clearance by the liver during hepatic perfusion was more complete and exceeded 94 per cent in the first pass. However, because of limited sensitivity of their assay methods, these workers used drug doses far above those employed in usual clinical trials, and the actual percentage clearance at usual infusion rates may be higher than reported in this study.

Monitoring of systemic 5-FU levels during intra-arterial therapy offers the potential benefit of allowing an increase in the infusion rate to achieve maximal-tolerated concentrations in the peripheral blood. Intrahepatic arterial infusion of 30 mg per kg per 24 hours of 5-FU produces plasma levels in the range of 0.13 to 0.35 M,[77] thus explaining the lack of myelosuppression resulting from this type of treatment. The systemic threshold for producing myelosuppression or gastrointestinal mucosal injury is not known, but probably lies in the vicinity of 1 μM, based on concentrations detected during the few reported pharmacokinetic studies of this type of treatment.

5-Fluorouracil may also be administered by the intraperitoneal route in order to exploit certain pharmacokinetic advantages.

TABLE 8–2. Plasma Pharmacokinetics of Bolus Intravenous 5-FU: Representative Studies

*Analytical Method**	*Dose† (mg/m²)*	*Primary t½ (min)*	*V_D‡ (% body weight)*	*Clearance (ml/min)*	*Ref.*
HPLC	460–525	7.8	–	–	79
HPLC	300	6.0	–	–	80
HPLC	500	9.4	24	1211	72
HPLC	340–480	11.4	25	1265	76
HPLC	not given	20.3	89	–	61
GLC	400–600	11.4	18	821	78
GLC	300	8.3	19	1040	68
	600	12.7	18	650	
GLC	360–640	18.9	38	776	69
GLC	600	10	12	588	70

*HPLC = high-pressure liquid chromatography.
GLC = gas-liquid chromatography.
†Converted from mg/kg by assuming that average patient weighs 70 kg and has body surface area of 1.7 m².
‡Volume of distribution.

Low-molecular-weight compounds injected into the peritoneal cavity are absorbed primarily through the portal circulation, passing through the liver before reaching the systemic circulation. The rate of absorption and, therefore, clearance from the peritoneal cavity depends on the lipid solubility of the drug and its molecular weight, as well as the surface of the peritoneum (which may be altered by tumor, adhesions, or other pathologic changes). Drug that enters the portal circulation will be subject to first-pass clearance by the liver, owing to metabolic conversion to dihydro-5-FU. Direct intraperitoneal administration of 5-FU has received only limited clinical evaluation. In the initial trial reported thus far,[74] dialysate concentrations of 5-FU of 5 mM or less, maintained by intermittent exchanges of fluid for up to 32 hours, produced little systemic toxicity and caused regression of intraperitoneal malignancy in two of eight patients. The mean clearance rate of drug from the peritoneal cavity was 14 ml per hr (corresponding to a half-life of 1.6 hours), as compared with the systemic clearance rate of 0.9 to 15 liters per min. The 5-FU concentration in plasma varied from 0.1 to 1 per cent of simultaneous intraperitoneal concentration (Fig. 8–8), thus explaining the limited bone marrow and gastrointestinal toxicity. Higher intraperitoneal drug concentrations (above 5 mM) saturated hepatic clearance mechanisms, leading to sharply increased systemic levels and significant myelosuppression. Although the pharmacokinetic predictions on which this regimen are based appear to be valid, the therapeutic efficacy of this approach remains to be proved.

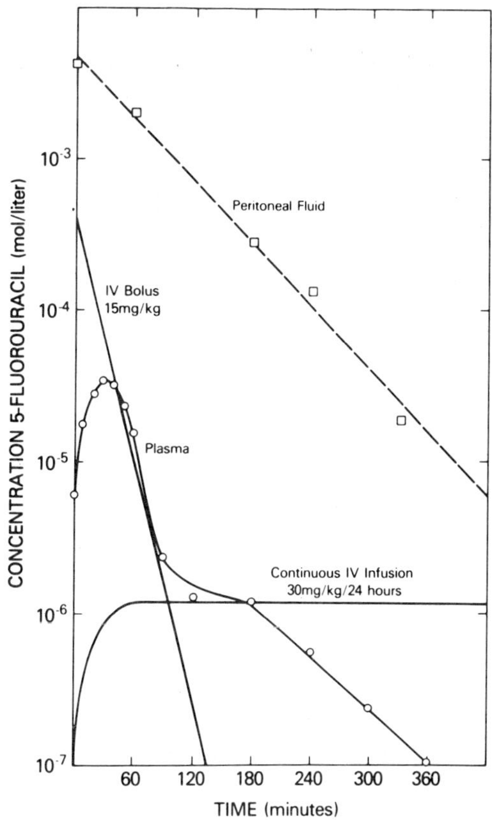

Figure 8–8. 5-FU concentrations in a patient after 2 liters of dialysate with a 4 mM concentration was instilled. □, peritoneal fluid; ○, plasma. Values for IV bolus derived from the literature; values for continuous IV infusion from the literature. (Reproduced with permission from Speyer et al.: Phase I and pharmacologic studies of 5-fluorouracil administered intraperitoneally. Cancer Res. 40:567–572, 1980.)

Pharmacokinetic Models for 5-Fluorouracil

Collins and co-workers[81] have proposed a two-compartment physiologic model for 5-FU pharmacokinetics that accurately describes the observed plasma concentrations and disappearance rates following intravenous bolus doses or infusions and following oral or intraperitoneal administration. This model assumes that 5-FU is eliminated primarily by a saturable metabolic process, with a dissociation constant of 15 μM. This saturability is indicated by the nonlinear relationship between dose and clearance rate. Second, based on experimental and clinical data, these authors conclude that the clearance of 5-FU at low drug concentrations equals or exceeds cardiac output (5 liters per minute) and therefore must take place in sites exposed to the entire cardiac output, either the blood or the lungs. Since there is no evidence for metabolism of 5-FU by plasma or blood-formed elements, the authors assume that the lungs must be responsible for the bulk of 5-FU clearance. Despite the saturability of 5-FU metabolic processes, drug disappearance curves in plasma are essentially linear over a broad range of concentrations, with half-life values between 10 and 20 minutes. In order to explain the paradox of a linear disappearance curve for a drug eliminated by a saturable process, the authors have proposed a two-compartment model composed of a well-perfused compartment — including liver, lungs, and possibly kidneys — in which saturable metabolism occurs, and a second, metabolically inactive compartment composed of fat and muscle. Re-entry of drug from the second compartment back into plasma could then account for the linear plasma disappearance curve, rather than the convex curve expected for drugs undergoing saturable metabolic elimination. The reader is referred to this analysis for more complete details of the model's application to the pharmacokinetics following various routes of administration.

Mechanisms of Drug Elimination

Approximately 90 per cent of conventional doses of 5-FU is eliminated by metabolism, while less than 5 per cent undergoes renal excretion.[80] The metabolic breakdown of 5-FU is believed to involve an initial reduction of the pyrimidine ring by dihydrouracil dehydrogenase, yielding 5,6-dihydro 5-FU.* This step is followed by an opening of the pyrimidine ring and further degradation to yield a fluoro-β-alanine, urea[82] and CO_2. The liver is known to contain dihydrouracil dehydrogenase, as do other tissues such as the gastrointestinal mucosa; the enzyme has not been demonstrated in neoplastic tissues. Although a significant fraction of 5-FU metabolism occurs in the liver, the total body clearance of 5-FU during continuous intravenous infusion exceeds hepatic blood flow by several-fold (approximately 5 liters per min versus 1 liter per min).[76] This observation suggests that the bulk of 5-FU metabolism occurs in extrahepatic tissue, and confirms the clinical impression that 5-FU doses do not have to be modified in the presence of hepatic dysfunction.

In contrast to the parent compound, the intracellular nucleotides FdUMP and FUTP have prolonged half-lives and persist in a profile characteristic of individual tissues.[57-59] The enzymes responsible for their degradation and their importance in determining response have not been defined.

*A method for measurement of 5,6-dihydro 5-FU by gas-liquid chromatography has recently been devised, but this compound has not been measured in human plasma to date (see McDermott BJ, van den Berg HW, and Murphy RF: Gas-liquid chromatographic analysis of 5-fluorouracil and its metabolite 5-fluorodihydrouracil in plasma. Biochem. Soc. Trans. 7:65–66, 1979).

The clinical pharmacokinetics and metabolism of 5-FUdR administered by intravenous infusion have not been carefully defined as yet. 5-FUdR is degraded to 5-FU by the action of phosphorylases in plasma and is further metabolized to inactive products upon passage through the liver. Greater than 95 per cent clearance of 5-FUdR occurs during the first passage of drug through the liver when the drug is administered by hepatic arterial infusion.[65]

CLINICAL TOXICITY

The main toxic effects of 5-FU and 5-FUdR are exerted on rapidly dividing tissues, primarily the gastrointestinal mucosa and bone marrow. There is considerable variation in the incidence and severity of these toxicities among individual patients and with various schedules of treatment (Table 8–3). The most commonly used schedules employ (1) a five-day loading course of daily intravenous bolus doses of 10 to 15 mg/kg, followed by single weekly doses; or (2) single weekly doses of the same magnitude. With these schedules the primary toxicity is myelosuppression, but the incidence of serious complications is considerably higher with the regimen that employs the five-day loading course.

In mice, 5-FU causes greater weight loss and myelosuppression, and a higher mortality in female animals than in males. Testosterone enanthate given for each of two days prior to 5-FU (130 mg/kg) significantly reduces myelosuppression and provides protection against toxicity, reducing mortality from 50 to 20 per cent.[83] The antitumor activity of 5-FU against a spontaneous mammary carcinoma is not diminished by androgen pretreatment.

An alternative regimen employing a continuous intravenous infusion of 5-FU (20 to 30 mg/kg/day for five days) appears to yield at least equivalent therapeutic results with only mild myelosuppression and mild-to-moderate gastrointestinal toxicity.[84] Higher doses, up to 14 gm per 24 hours, are well tolerated if the infusion duration is reduced to 24 hours.[85] The practical use of this regimen is limited by the need for careful attention to the rate of drug infusion. Automatic infusion devices may make this schedule a more practical alternative.

In patients with metastases confined to the

TABLE 8–3. Relationship of Route and Schedule to Toxicity of 5-FU

Route–Schedule–Dose	*Toxicity* MARROW SUPPRESSION	MUCOSITIS/ DIARRHEA	OTHER
Intravenous: bolus, daily × 5, then weekly, 12–15 mg/kg/day	Major	Major	Alopecia, conjunctivitis
Intravenous: bolus, weekly, 12–15 mg/kg/dose	Major	Minor	Conjunctivitis
Intravenous: constant infusion for 4–5 days, 20–30 mg/kg/day	Minor	Major	–
Oral: 15–20 mg/kg/day once weekly or daily × 5, q3w	Erratic	Erratic	–
Hepatic intra-arterial: constant infusion, 10–21 days, 20–30 mg/kg/day	Minor	Major	Catheter-related
Intraperitoneal: repeated exchanges with up to 5 mM 5-FU for 32 hrs	Minor	Moderate	Sterile or bacterial peritonitis
Topical: 5% cream	Rare	Rare	Local tissue inflammation when applied to diseased skin

liver, intrahepatic arterial infusion of 5-FU or 5-FUdR is often used to provide high local drug concentrations; the high fraction of first-pass clearance of drug by the normal hepatic parenchyma (>50 per cent for 5-FU, >95 per cent for FUdR) allows little drug to escape into the systemic circulation. The response rates reported for treatment of hepatic metastases of colon carcinoma reach 50 per cent in most studies,[86-88] and exceed the response rate of patients treated with peripheral intravenous infusion. Toxicity of intrahepatic arterial infusion of 5-FU resembles that of continuous intravenous infusion, and includes oral mucositis or gastrointestinal symptoms such as nausea, vomiting, and diarrhea. Myelosuppression is less frequent. Catheter-related complications may result from long-term infusion and include thrombosis of the extremity artery used for percutaneous catheterization, hemorrhage or infection at the arterial puncture site, or accidental slippage of the catheter into the arterial supply of the duodenum or stomach, with necrosis of the intestinal epithelium, hemorrhage, and perforation.[89] This latter catastrophe is usually heralded by epigastric pain or vomiting; these symptoms should alert the clinician to undertake prompt reassessment of the catheter position to rule out the possibility of catheter slippage. In some patients it may not be possible to use intrahepatic arterial infusion because of difficulties in placing the catheter in the appropriate branch of the hepatic arterial tree.

An alternative to arterial perfusion is hepatic portal venous perfusion. Although most large metastases obtain their blood supply predominantly from the arterial circulation, small metastases may be fed by the portal circulation. In one preliminary study, portal perfusion with 5-FU was associated with a decreased incidence of hepatic metastases in patients at high risk of relapse following resection of primary colon cancers.[90]

5-Fluorouracil may also produce acute neurologic symptoms, including somnolence, cerebellar ataxia, and upper motor neuron signs; these symptoms are seen primarily in patients receiving intracarotid arterial infusions for epithelial head and neck tumors. This syndrome is believed to be caused by fluorocitrate, a neurotoxic metabolite of the parent compound.[91]

5-Fluorouracil is suspected of causing cardiac toxicity on the basis of isolated case reports of chest pain in association with its administration. In at least three patients, chest pain recurred with subsequent administration of the drug, and in several instances was accompanied by electrocardiographic and serum enzyme changes consistent with myocardial necrosis.[91, 92] Some, but not all, reported episodes of chest pain occurred in patients who had previously received chest irradiation. The mechanism of this toxic reaction is unclear.

Long-term treatment with 5-FU has also been reported to cause conjunctivitis, tear duct stenosis, and ectropion.[93] Excessive lacrimation was the most frequent symptom noted. Conjunctivitis is reversible with discontinuation of 5-FU at an early point in the patient's course, but progression of the inflammatory response may require surgical correction of dacryostenosis and ectropion.

DRUG INTERACTIONS

A number of important interactions have been demonstrated between 5-FU and other antineoplastic drugs or normal metabolites in both experimental and clinical investigations (summarized in Table 8–4). These interactions include effects on 5-FU pharmacokinetics, modulation of its binding to thymidylate synthetase, and alteration of its incorporation into RNA. Drugs that increase the metabolic activation of 5-FU (including PALA and methotrexate), decrease the competing pool of normal uridine nucleotides (PALA), or inhibit its metabolic breakdown (thymidine, cytidine, or uridine) all enhance its cytotoxicity in experimental systems. The range of these interactions is illustrated by the potentiating effect of a long list of purine (inosine) and pyrimidine (uridine, cytidine, thymidine) nucleosides on 5-FU killing of AKR leukemia cells *in vivo*,[94] although the biochemical basis for most of these interactions is not completely understood.

Methotrexate–5-FU

The interaction of 5-FU with methotrexate has particular importance because of the frequent use of these drugs in the combination therapy of breast cancer and ovarian cancer. As reviewed in Chapter 10, both drugs inhibit the synthesis of thymidylate: 5-FU through the binding of its nucleotide 5-FdUMP to thymidylate synthetase and methotrexate through its depletion of intracellular reduced folates (see Fig. 8–2). Several possible interactions on the biochemical level are suggested by the common focus (thymidylate synthesis) of their individual mechanisms of action. The reduced folate, N^{5-10}-methylenetetrahydrofolate, is required for binding of 5-FdUMP to thymidylate synthetase in order to form a covalent ternary complex. This reduced folate is oxidized to dihydrofolate in the thymidylate synthetase reaction and cannot be resynthesized in the presence of methotrexate. Thus, pretreatment of cells with methotrexate would be expected to deplete this cofactor and prevent 5-FdUMP binding to thymidylate synthetase. This prediction has been confirmed in tissue culture experiments in which cells grown in folate-free media and then exposed to methotrexate were unable to form the ternary complex.[8] However, it should be noted that methotrexate pretreatment does not interfere with FUTP incorporation into RNA. Secondly, dihydrofolate polyglutamates, which accumulate in the presence of antifolates, may substitute for methylenetetrahydrofolate in the ternary complex with 5-FdUMP and thymidylate synthetase.[6] In addition, Cadman et al.[38] have shown that methotrexate may have beneficial effects on 5-FU activation. Methotrexate, which blocks *de novo* purine synthesis when used in concentrations above 1 + 10^{-7}M, causes an expansion of the intracellular pool of PRPP; this substrate is then available for promoting the conversion of 5-FU to 5-FdUMP by orotic acid phosphoribosyl transferase. This sequence of events has been clearly demonstrated in L1210 cells and is reflected in the cytotoxic synergism of the two agents given in the sequence: methotrexate preceding 5-FU (Fig. 8–9). 5-FU activation is promoted in a similar manner by methotrexate in human tumors, although longer periods of incubation with methotrexate may be required to produce expansion of the PRPP pools.[36] This interaction depends on the presence of the orotic acid phosphoribosyl transferase pathway, which is not found in all tumors. For example, enhanced activation of 5-FU by methotrexate pretreatment was not observed in a human breast cancer cell line studied by Donehower et al.[95]

The reverse sequence of drug administration (5-FU preceding methotrexate) has been repeatedly shown to produce the least favorable results in treating experimental tumors in tissue culture[38, 95, 96] and *in vivo*.[97] The antagonism of these two agents given in this sequence is thought to be the consequence of antagonism of the antipurine effects of methotrexate by 5-FU (Fig. 8–10). Ongoing thymidylate synthesis is required to deplete the cellular pool of reduced folates. Pretreatment with 5-FU inhibits the thymidylate synthetase reaction, and the conversion of reduced folates to dihydrofolate is blocked. As a result, the reduced folate pool is spared for purine synthesis.[98] The unfavorable result of the 5-FU-methotrexate sequence contrasts with the beneficial results of initial treatment with methotrexate, in which case

TABLE 8–4. Drug Interactions with 5-FU

Interaction	*Biochemical Basis*
WITH PYRIMIDINE NUCLEOSIDES	
1. 5-FU:Thymidine	a. Increased 5-FU incorporation into RNA b. Decreased rate of catabolism of 5-FU
2. 5-FU:Cytidine	Exchange of ribose yields 5-FUR
WITH PURINE BASES AND NUCLEOSIDES	
1. 5-FU:Hypoxanthine	Decreased toxicity to tumor cells due to PRPP consumption
2. 5-FU:Inosine	Inosine raises ribose phosphate concentration, increases 5-FU activation to FUR
3. 5-FU:Allopurinol	Decreased toxicity to normal tissue due to block in orotic acid phosphoribosyl transferase by oxypurinol ribose phosphate
WITH OTHER ANTIMETABOLITES	
1. Methotrexate:5-FU	Methotrexate pretreatment blocks purine synthesis, elevates PRPP, increases 5-FU activation
2. 5-FU:Methotrexate	5-FU blocks thymidylate synthesis, prevents consumption of reduced folate pool, antagonizes antipurine effect of methotrexate
3. PALA:5-FU	PALA blocks *de novo* pyrimidine synthesis, increases 5-FU incorporation into RNA

ongoing thymidylate synthesis leads to depletion of reduced folates and allows establishment of the block in purine biosynthesis.

In summary, despite potential interference with ternary complex formation (FdUMP–thymidylate synthetase–reduced folate), sequences employing methotrexate prior to or simultaneous with 5-FU have consistently produced more favorable results than regimens employing 5-FU first. The results of clinical trials employing various sequences may provide insight into the importance of scheduling these two agents.[99]

5-FU–Thymidine

Although thymidine (TdR) is known to reverse the cytotoxicity of low concentrations of 5-FU *in vitro*, high concentrations of 5-FU (above 10^{-5}M) are not effectively countered by thymidine, and a consistent enhancement of 5-FU potency by thymidine has been observed in the whole animal.[15] The enhancement of 5-FU toxicity by thymidine can be explained on the basis of the following pharmacologic and biochemical interactions (Fig. 8–11):

1. Thymine (a metabolic product of thy-

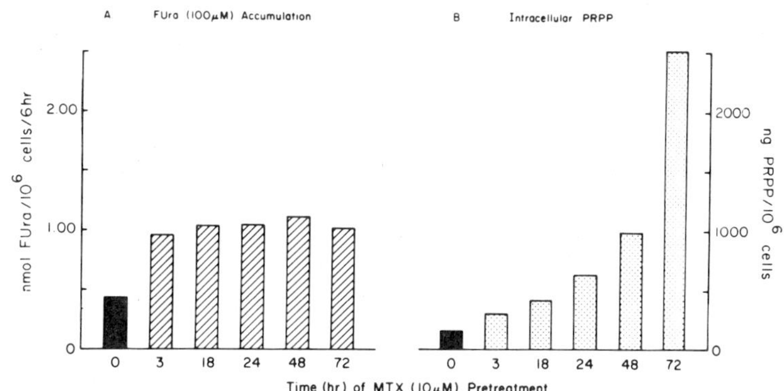

Figure 8–9. The effect of exposure time to 10 μm MTX on total intracellular 5-FU (100 μM) accumulation (*A*) and PRPP pools (*B*) in human colon carcinoma cells. (Reproduced with permission from Benz C, and Cadman E: Modulation of 5-fluorouracil metabolism and cytotoxicity by antimetabolite pretreatment in human colorectal adenocarcinoma HCT-8. Cancer Res. 41:994–999, 1981.)

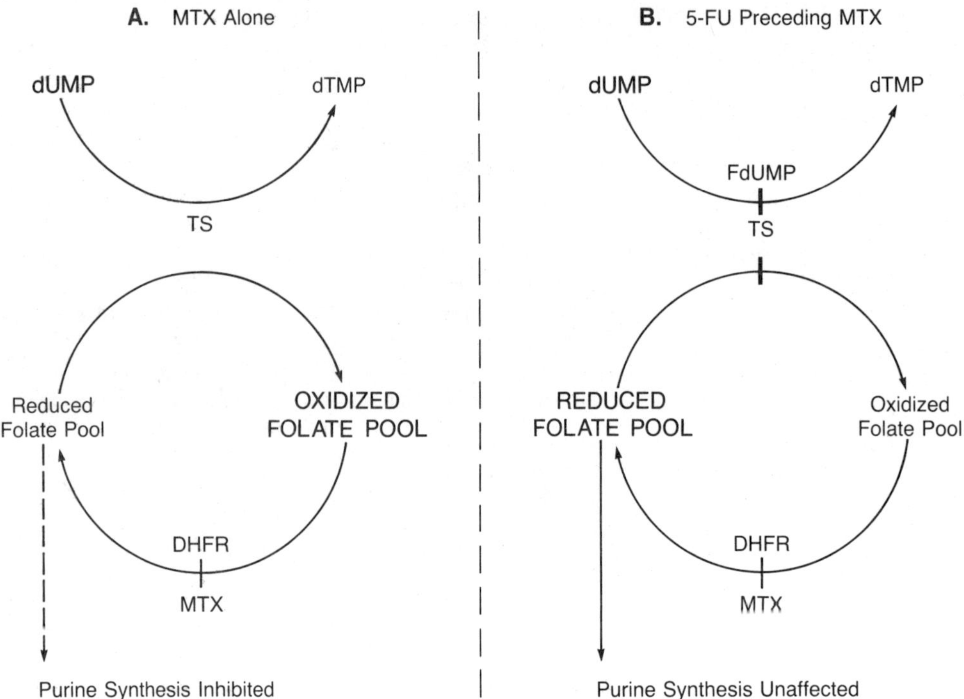

Figure 8–10. 5-Fluorouracil antagonism of the antipurine effects of MTX.

midine) inhibits 5-FU degradation by dihydrouracil dehydrogenase, thus prolonging the plasma half-life of 5-FU.

2. Thymidine is converted to TTP, which acts as a feedback inhibitor of ribonucleotide reductase. Inhibition of the latter enzyme prevents 5-FUDP conversion to 5-FdUMP and enhances formation of 5-FUTP, and ultimately increases 5-FU effects on RNA.[28]

3. Thymidine can act as a donor of a deoxyribose group to promote the conversion of 5-FU to FUdR by pyrimidine phosphorylase.

Preliminary clinical trials of the 5-FU-thymidine combination have confirmed the enhancement of 5-FU toxicity. Patients treated with 8 gm thymidine by continuous infusion experience severe myelosuppression and mucositis at 5-FU doses of 10 to 15 mg/kg/day for five days[100]; this dose of 5-FU would be tolerated with moderate toxicity in the absence of thymidine. Woodcock and colleagues estimated that the pretreatment of patients with thymidine (7.5 to 45 gm) one hour prior to 5-FU increased the biologic effects of 5-FU by five- to eightfold, producing severe thrombocytopenia, leukopenia, mucositis, and diarrhea.[80] They found that 15 gm thymidine followed one hour later by 7.5 to 10 mg/kg 5-FU given once every 21 to 28 days[80] produced a tolerable level of clinical toxicity. This schedule should be com-

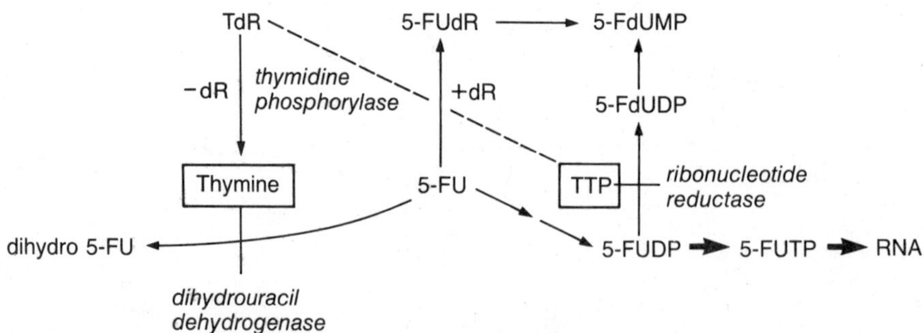

Figure 8–11. Interaction of thymidine (TdR) and 5-FU. Thymidine increases 5-FU conversion to 5-FUdR; TTP blocks formation of 5-FdUMP; and thymidine blocks degradation of 5-FU.

pared with the conventional regimens that employ 5-FU, 10 to 15 mg/kg/day for five days.

Thymidine markedly alters 5-FU plasma pharmacokinetics. For example, a 15-gm dose of thymidine one hour prior to 5-FU prolonged the primary 5-FU half-life from six minutes (without thymidine) to 188 minutes (with thymidine) and markedly inhibited its metabolism.[80] Patients receiving ^{14}C-2-5-FU with thymidine showed a nearly total reduction in the excretion of respiratory $^{14}CO_2$. Instead, renal excretion, a minor route of 5-FU elimination in the absence of thymidine, became the primary route of 5-FU clearance (Fig. 8–12). In an interesting sidelight, Woodcock and co-workers observed the formation of 5-FUdR in plasma, apparently occurring through transfer of the deoxyribose from thymidine to 5-FU by the enzyme thymidine phosphorylase. The plasma concentration of 5-FUdR reaches 10 to 100 μM in plasma in patients receiving 7.5 to 45 mg thymidine with 5-FU. However, since thymidine reverses the effects of 5-FUdR by replenishing the thymidylate pool, the formation of 5-FUdR probably has no toxic effect.

The pharmacokinetics of thymidine have also been determined by HPLC analysis in these studies. The nucleoside has a plasma half-life of seven to 98 minutes for thymidine doses of 3 to 45 gm. It is rapidly converted to thymine, which undergoes reduction and ring cleavage. Bolus thymidine doses of 15 gm per m^2 produce peak plasma concentrations of 1 mM, while continuous infusion of 8 gm per day gives steady-state plasma concentrations of 1 mM or slightly higher, as compared with pretreatment serum thymidine concentrations of approximately 0.2 mM.

Although the combination of thymidine and 5-FU has provoked much interest and there is evidence for pharmacologic and biochemical interaction, the clinical results thus far do not indicate a differential effect on tumor cells as opposed to host. The combination produces a consistent enhancement of myelosuppression and gastrointestinal toxicity, such that 5-FU must be reduced by 50 per cent or more from conventional regimens.[79, 100] In the most extensive series to date, the combination yielded only two partial remissions from a group of eight previously untreated patients with adenocarcinoma of the colon,[100] and one partial response from 17 patients with the same diagnosis who had previously failed to achieve remission with 5-FU alone.[80] More favorable clinical results will have to be obtained before the additional expense and care required for administration of this combination can be considered justified.

5-FU and Inhibitors of De Novo Pyrimidine Biosynthesis

A number of inhibitors of the *de novo* synthesis of pyrimidines have received extensive preclinical evaluation and Phase I clinical trial, including pyrazofurin, an inhibitor of orotidylate decarboxylase; 6-azauridine, an inhibitor of the same enzyme;

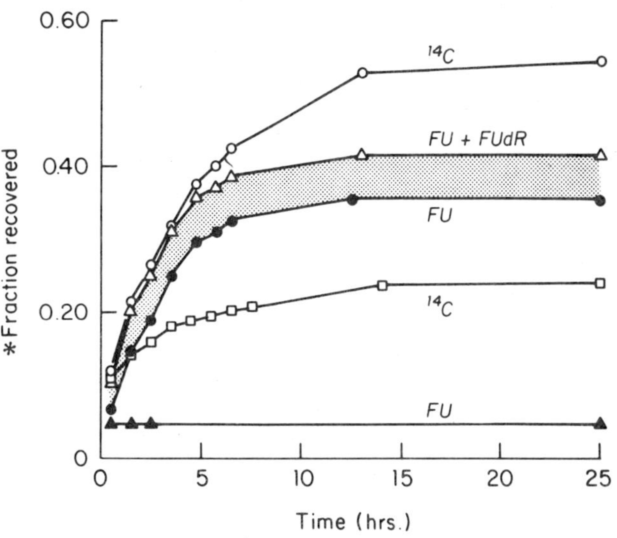

Figure 8–12. Cumulative urinary excretion of ^{14}C-2-5-FU and metabolites following 7.5 mg/kg 5-FU, with and without prior TdR. Urine was analyzed for ^{14}C, and for 5-FU and 5-FUdR by HPLC. Control: ^{14}C recovered (□). 5-FU recovered (▲). After pretreatment with 15 gm TdR: ^{14}C recovered (○), total 5-FU and 5-FUdR recovered (△), 5-FU recovered (●). Shading represents 5-FUdR. *Molar fraction of administered 5-FU dose recovered. (Reproduced with permission from Woodcock et al.: Clinical trials with thymidine and fluorouracil: a phase I and clinical pharmacologic evaluation. Cancer 45: 1135–1143, 1980.)

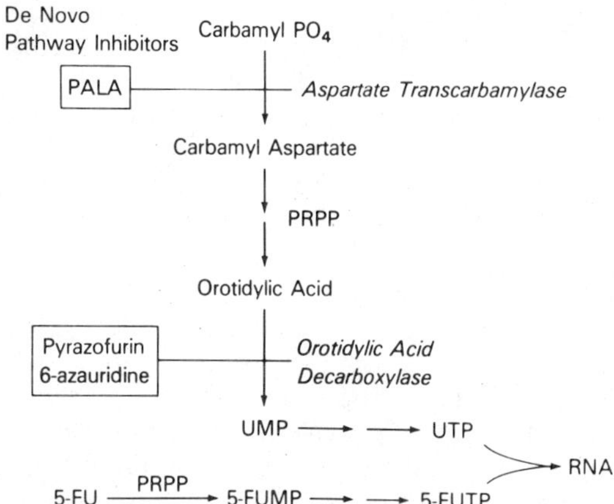

Figure 8–13. 5-FU interaction with inhibitors of *de novo* pyrimidine synthesis. PALA inhibition conserves PRPP pool for use in the activation of 5-FU.

and PALA (phosphono-N-acetyl-L-aspartic acid), an inhibitor of aspartate transcarbamylase. All these compounds, by inhibiting specific steps in the *de novo* pathway, promote utilization of preformed pyrimidines such as 5-FU (Fig. 8–13). However, the orotic acid decarboxylase inhibitors have the unfortunate side effect of elevating intracellular levels of orotic acid.[32] Orotic acid competitively inhibits the conversion of 5-FU to nucleotide form by the enzyme orotic acid phosphoribosyl transferase. PALA, which blocks a step in pyrimidine synthesis prior to the formation of orotic acid, would not have this negative effect, but in contrast enhances 5-FU nucleotide formation.[101] In addition, PALA blocks consumption of the intracellular PRPP pool through its effect on the early step in the *de novo* pyrimidine synthesis pathway. Expansion of the PRPP pool increases the activation of 5-FU and enhances its incorporation into RNA.[19] The combination of PALA with 5-FU has not shown clinical synergism in initial clinical trials.[101a]

5-FU Interaction with Purines

Differences between host and tumor in the prevalence of the various 5-FU activation pathways have been exploited by the combined use of 5-FU and allopurinol. As discussed previously, allopurinol when converted to a nucleotide inhibits OMP decarboxylase and causes a build-up in the pool of orotic acid; the latter blocks 5-FU activation by OPRT'ase.[32] Since host tissues — but not all tumors — depend on this activation pathway, toxicity to the host is reduced consistently, but antitumor responses are still seen. Thus, Fox and colleagues have reported that patients receiving 5-FU by continuous infusion are able to tolerate doses of 2.2 gm per m^2 per day if given with allopurinol, as opposed to doses of 1.1 gm per m^2 when 5-FU is given alone. In this study, six of 12 patients responded to high-dose 5-FU with allopurinol. These initial results are encouraging with respect to host toxicity reduction, but not definitive with respect to antitumor activity.[102]

OTHER FLUOROPYRIMIDINES

FTORAFUR

A new fluoropyrimidine, ftorafur [1-(2-tetrahydrofuranyl)-5-fluorouracil], has had limited clinical trial in the United States.[103] This furan nucleoside, shown in Figure 8–1, was originally synthesized and tested in the Soviet Union, and attracted interest because of its lack of myelosuppressive toxicity. Ftorafur is believed to function as a depot form of 5-FU in that its toxicity resembles that of 5-FU given by constant infusion. Low plasma concentrations (less than 1 mg/ml) of 5-FU have been detected in patients receiving ftorafur,[104, 105] but disagreement exists as to whether these levels are sufficiently high to explain the antitumor activity of this compound. This finding raises the possibility that the conversion of ftorafur to 5-FU takes place within target cells, and circulating concentrations of 5-FU may not reflect the extent of this conversion. The parent compound ftorafur has a prolonged plasma half-life of six to 16 hours. It is eliminated primarily by conversion to hydroxylated metabolites and by cleavage of the furan group from the pyrimidine base[105-107] (Fig. 8–13).

Au and Sadee have found evidence that

ftorafur is converted to 5-FU by metabolic cleavage at the N-1–C-2′ bond, yielding 5-FU and gamma-hydroxybutyrate of its lactone, gamma-butyrolactone (GBL).[107] Acid extraction of plasma from patients or from rabbits treated with ftorafur yields large quantities of GBL. The same metabolite and 5-FU are produced by incubation of ftorafur with supernatant fractions of rabbit liver. Liver microsomes also produce 5-FU from ftorafur, but do not produce GBL as a side product, suggesting the presence of pathways for 5-FU production involving a microsomal oxidation of the furan group at the 3′, 4′, or 5′ site. Small amounts of the 3 - and 4′-OH derivatives have been isolated from urine, as well as a dehydrofuran metabolite. The 4′-OH and dehydrofuran metabolites could undergo enzymatic or spontaneous cleavage to form 5-FU, but are not believed to be the primary intermediates in this reaction since they are found in only small quantities in tissue incubation mixtures that produce 5-FU from ftorafur. Rather, the 5′-OH derivative is a more likely candidate for being an intermediate in the enzymatic pathway of 5-FU formation (Fig. 8–14). Pathways for 5-FU generation from ftorafur in tumor cells have not been defined.

Ftorafur is usually administered intravenously in doses of 1.5 gm per m^2 per day for five days. The primary clinical toxicities produced by this regimen are gastrointestinal symptoms (diarrhea, cramps, vomiting, oral mucositis) and neurologic side effects (altered mental status, cerebellar ataxia, and rarely coma). The neurotoxic side effects resemble those of intracarotid infusion of 5-FU and have been attributed to the high concentrations of parent drug found in the cerebrospinal fluid.[103] The hydrolysis product of ftorafur cleavage — butyrolactone — has anesthetic properties and may also contribute to this neurotoxicity.

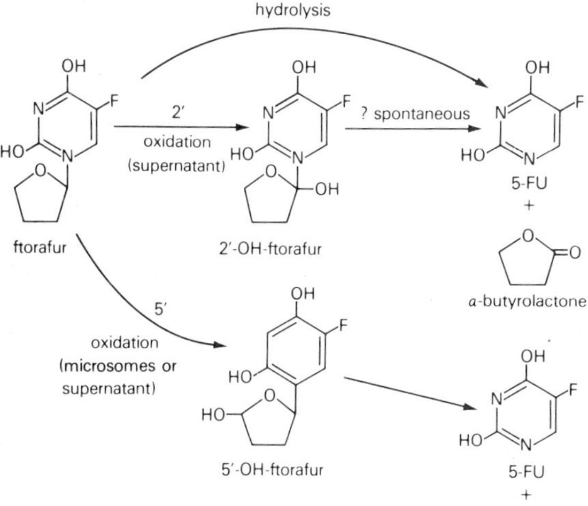

Figure 8–14. Pathways of 5-FU formation in subcellular fractions of mouse liver. (Adapted with permission from Au JL, and Sadee W: Activation of ftorafur (R,S-1-tetrahydro-2-furanyl)-5-fluorouracil to 5-fluorouracil and butyrolactone. Cancer Res. 40:2814–2819, 1980.)

The clinical activity of ftorafur relative to 5-FU has not been thoroughly evaluated.[108] If equivalent activity is demonstrated, ftorafur would have significant advantages over 5-FU because of its lack of myelosuppression.

5′-DEOXY-5-FLUOROURIDINE

A new fluoropyrimidine, 5′-deoxy-5-fluorouridine, has been synthesized[109] and has shown promising antitumor activity and increased specificity for tumor cells as compared to normal tissues[110] (Fig. 8–1). This nucleoside analogue is blocked from further activation to a phosphorylated derivative by the absence of an OH group at the 5′ position. Instead, it is converted to the base, 5-FU, by intracellular enzymatic hydrolysis. The responsible enzyme, a nucleoside phosphorylase (K_m= 0.633 mM), is found in many normal tissues and in responsive tumors,[111] but appears to be present in higher activity in neoplastic cells. The 5′-deoxy analogue has an improved therapeutic index, as compared with traditional fluoropyrimidines, in tests against a broad range of murine and rat tumors.[110, 111] Thus, in tests against CF-1 mice inoculated with Ehrlich ascites tumor cells, 5′-deoxy-5-fluorouridine produced 45-day survival in 89 per cent of animals, with a 3-gm increase in weight. 5-FU produced at best a 37.5 per cent 45-day survival, but at doses that caused a mean 1-gm weight loss. In other experiments, the ratio of the LD_{50} (50 per cent lethal dose) to the dose producing 67 per cent inhibition of sarcoma 180 growth in Swiss albino mice was 13 for the new compound, as compared with 1.3 for 5-FU and 4.2 for FUdR. Thus, the new compound appears to have lower toxicity for a given level of therapeutic effect.

The mechanism of action of the new derivative is probably identical to that of 5-FU.

Once converted to the latter compound, it is readily activated to the same intracellular nucleotides, including 5-FUTP[111] and 5-FdUMP.

In addition to its theoretical and experimental advantages in comparison to 5-FU, the new derivative is active by the oral route. Pharmacokinetic studies have not been reported and the drug has not yet undergone clinical testing.

5-AZACYTIDINE

The success of cytosine arabinoside (see Chapter 18) as an antileukemic agent has encouraged the search for other cytidine analogues, particularly those that would not require activation by deoxycytidine kinase (the enzyme deleted in many ara-C–resistant tumors). It was logical to consider ribonucleosides with structural changes in the basic pyrimidine ring, since these would be activated in all likelihood by uridine-cytidine kinase, an entirely separate enzyme. Considerable enthusiasm greeted the introduction of 5-azacytidine, an analogue of cytidine synthesized by Sorm and colleagues in 1963,[112] and later isolated as a product of fungal cultures.[113] The compund was found to be toxic for both bacterial and mammalian cells. However, in clinical trials its only important cytostatic action was exerted against acute myeloblastic leukemia,[114-116] and this is the only disease for which it is commonly used. Although occasional responses to 5-azacytidine have been reported in patients with various solid tumors, including carcinoma of the breast or colon and malignant melanoma, the clinical activity has been too meager and the toxicity too significant to warrant further clinical trials in these tumors.[117]

STRUCTURE AND MECHANISM OF ACTION

5-Azacytidine differs from cytidine in the presence of a nitrogen at the 5 position of the heterocyclic ring (Fig. 8–15). This substitution renders the ring chemically unstable and leads to spontaneous decomposition of the compound in neutral or alkaline solution, with a half-life of approximately four hours. The product of this ring opening, N-formylamidino-ribofuranosylguanylurea (Fig. 8–16), may recyclyze to form the parent compound, but is also susceptible to further spontaneous decomposition to ribofuranosylurea.[118] This spontaneous chemical instability has importance for the drug's usage in two ways: (1) the ultimate antitumor activity of the drug has been attributed to this incorporation into nucleic acids and subsequent spontaneous cleavage; and (2) the preparation formulated for clinical application must be administered within several hours of its dissolution in dextrose and water or saline.[119] In buffered solutions such as Ringer's lactate and at acidic pH, the agent is considerably more stable, with a half-life of 65 hours at 25°C and 94 hours at 20°C.[120]

The mechanism of 5-azacytidine action has not been firmly established, although the balance of evidence suggests that, after conversion to a triphosphate, it competes with CTP for incorporation into RNA.[121] This incorporation into RNA appears to be the primary event that leads to a number of different effects on RNA processing and function. These effects include an inhibition of the formation of ribosomal 28s and 18s RNA from higher molecular weight species (Fig. 8–17),[122] defective methylation[123] and acceptor function of transfer RNA,[124] disassembly of polyribosomes,[125] and a marked inhibition of protein synthesis.[126]

However, other effects of 5-azacytidine have been described that may be relevant to its antitumor activity. This analogue is also incorporated into DNA,[127, 128] although to a much lesser extent than its incorporation into RNA. In cultured L1210 cells exposed to 5-azacytidine, the time course of DNA synthesis inhibition paralleled that of RNA synthesis inhibition and was greater in magnitude.[127] In addition, the drug has greatest cytotoxicity for cells in the DNA synthetic phase of the cell cycle, a finding consistent with a cytotoxic lesion related to DNA synthesis.[129]

It has also been suggested that the toxicity of 5-azacytidine in bacteria may be due to its deamination product, 5-azauridine. The potential toxicity of this metabolite has not

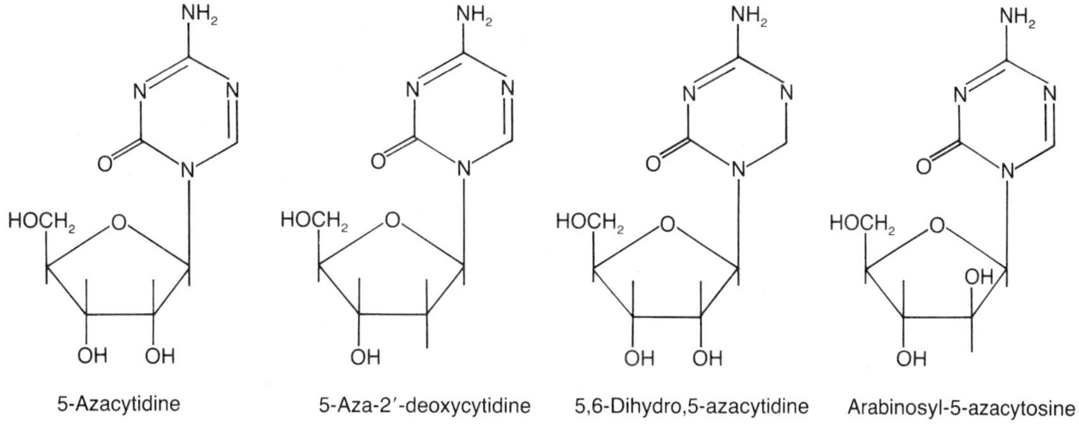

5-Azacytidine 5-Aza-2′-deoxycytidine 5,6-Dihydro,5-azacytidine Arabinosyl-5-azacytosine

Figure 8–15. Structures of 5-azacytidine and closely related cytotoxic cytidine analogues.

been examined directly owing to its extreme chemical instability, but bacteria lacking cytidine deaminase activity are known to be resistant to the drug.[131]

Finally, 5-azacytidine monophosphate inhibits orotidylate decarboxylase, leading to decreased synthesis of pyrimidines by the *de novo* pathway.[132]

Several nucleosides closely related to 5-azacytidine have been synthesized and possess antitumor activity (Fig. 8–15). 2′-Deoxy-5-azacytidine was synthesized in Czechoslovakia at the same time as 5-azacytidine.[133] Investigations of its mechanism of action revealed that it competes with deoxycytidine for incorporation into DNA. It is phosphorylated by deoxycytidine kinase (as compared with the uridine kinase activation of 5-azacytidine), but is deaminated by cytidine deaminase, the same enzyme responsible for degradation of cytosine arabinoside and 5-azacytidine. Cells resistant to 5-azacytidine retain sensitivity to 2′-deoxy-5-azacytidine, but the reverse may not be true, since mouse leukemia cells resistant to 5-azacytidine showed deletion of both uridine and deoxycytidine kinases, and were thus resistant to the 2′-deoxy analogue.[121] 2′-Deoxy-5-azacytidine has not received a clinical trial at this time.

A second related analogue, 5,6-dihydro-5-azacytidine, was synthesized in an effort to obtain a chemically stable antimetabolite.[134] However, this compound has lesser antileukemic activity in mice, and is a poorer substrate for uridine kinase and (unfortunately) a better substrate for cytidine deaminase than 5-azacytidine.[135] The arabinosyl nucleoside of 5-azacytosine has recently been synthesized[136] and has antitumor activity against L1210. Little is known concerning the metabolism or mechanism of action of this compound, although on the basis of structure one would expect predominant effects on DNA synthesis.

CELLULAR PHARMACOLOGY

5-Azacytidine readily enters mammalian cells by a facilitated nucleoside transport mechanism shared with the physiologic nucleosides, uridine and cytidine.[128] The initial step in its activation consists of conversion to a monophosphate by uridine-cytidine kinase (Fig. 8–16), which is found in low concentration in human acute myelogenous leukemia cells.[137] This enzyme has markedly lower affinity for 5-azacytidine (Km = 0.2 to 11 mM) than for uridine or cytidine (Km = 0.05 mM),[137, 138] and likely represents the rate-limiting step in 5-azacytidine activation. Either uridine[139] or cytidine is capable of preventing 5-azacytidine toxicity in the whole animal and in tissue culture,[140] probably by competitively inhibiting its phosphorylation. Deletion of uridine-cytidine kinase has been observed in mutant Novikoff hepatoma cells resistant to 5-azacytidine,[128] as well as other resistant cell types.[141] Cytidine deaminase, which is found in 10- to 30-fold higher concentration than uridine-cytidine kinase in leukemic cells, degrades 5-azacytidine to 5-azauridine. The role of this enzyme in resistance to 5-azacytidine has not been defined.

Further activation of 5-azaCMP to a triphosphate probably occurs by the enzymes dCMP kinase and nucleoside diphosphate kinase. One hour after exposure of cells to the

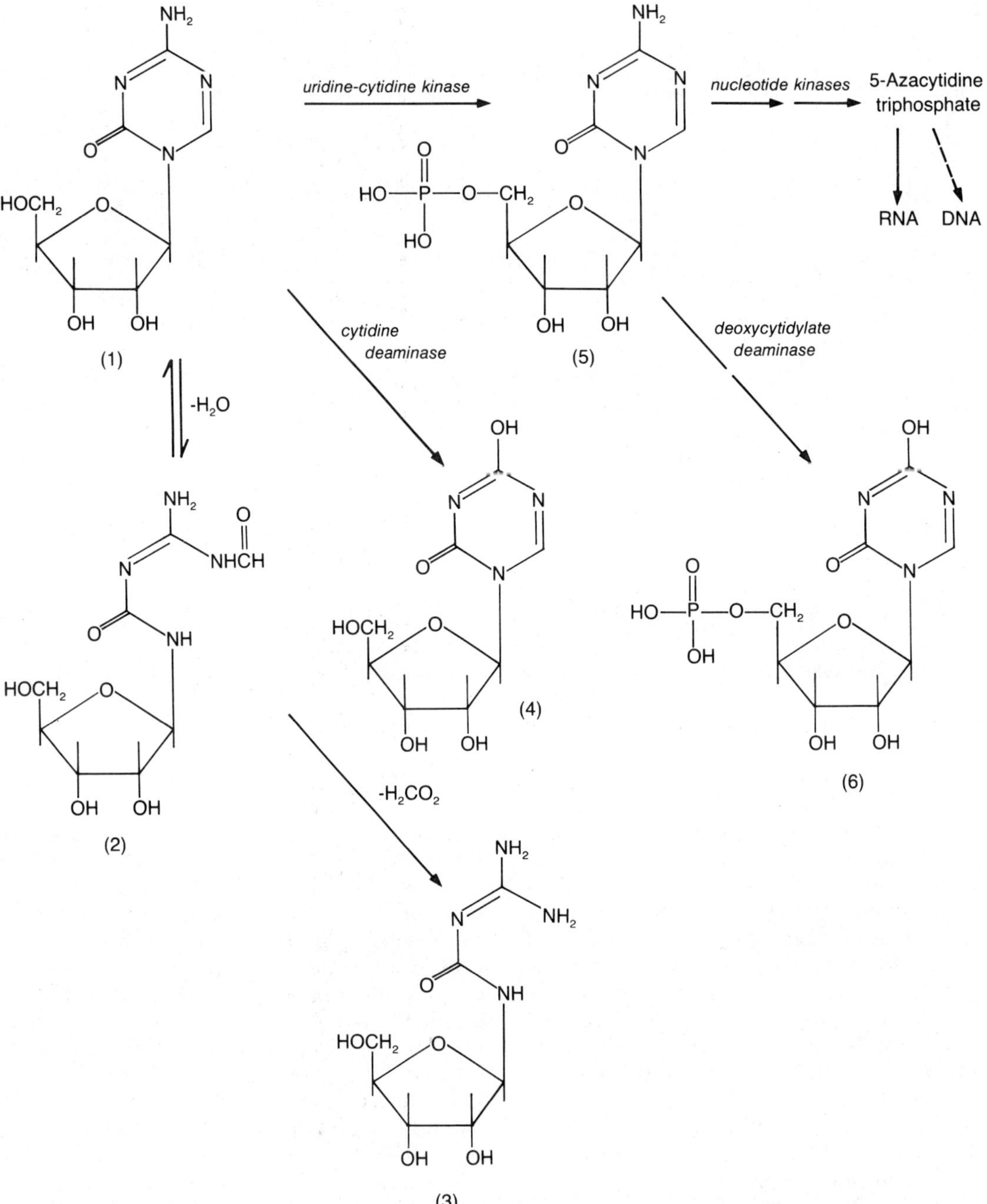

Figure 8–16. Transformation of 5-azacytidine (1), which undergoes reversible spontaneous decomposition to N-(formylamidino)-N′-β-D-ribofuranosylurea (2), which may further decompose to 1-β-D-ribofuranosyl-3-guanylurea (3). Enzymatic breakdown to 5-azauridine (4) also occurs, as well as activation to 5-azacytidine monophosphate (5) and higher nucleotides, with ultimate incorporation into RNA, and, to a lesser extent, DNA. Deamination of (5) to 5-azauridine monophosphate (6) is suspected but not proved.

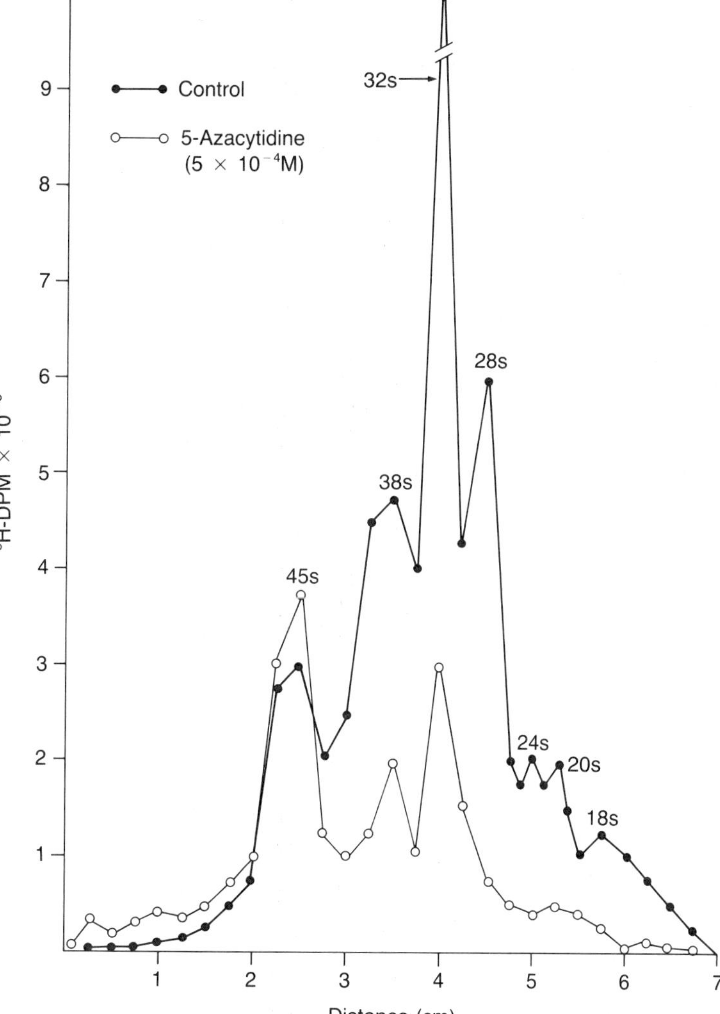

Figure 8–17. Electrophoresis of nucleolar RNA from control and 5-azacytidine–treated Novikoff hepatoma cells. 1.5 × 10^8 cells were incubated in media with or without 5-azacytidine, 5 × 10^{-4}M, for three hrs. ^{3}H-uridine was added to the medium for the final two hrs of incubation. RNA samples were electrophoresed on 2.1% acrylamide–0.6% agarose gels. Note the marked decrease in the lower molecular weight peaks (18s and 28s), and the relative increase in 45s RNA in the drug-treated cells. (After Weiss and Pitot.[122])

drug, 60 to 70 per cent of acid-soluble radioactivity was identified as 5-azaCTP.[128] The activation of 5-azacytidine to a triphosphate and its incorporation into nucleic acids are greatly augmented by preincubation of cells with pyrazofurin,[123, 142] an inhibitor of *de novo* pyrimidine synthesis, an effect probably mediated through decreased feedback inhibition of uridine-cytidine kinase.

Both drug concentration and duration of exposure are important determinants of 5-azacytidine cytotoxicity in tissue culture, a finding consistent with a preferential action on rapidly dividing cells. In tissue culture experiments, it has greatest lethality for cells in the S phase of the cell cycle, with relatively little effect against nondividing cells.[129, 143] However, dose-survival curves *in vivo* for L1210 and normal hematopoietic cells are both biphasic, indicating perhaps more than a single site or mechanism of cytotoxic action.[144]

In addition to its cytotoxic effects, 5-azacytidine has other biologic actions of possible importance in its clinical use. It stimulates the activity of various hepatic enzymes, including tyrosine aminotransferase[145] and uridine-cytidine kinase.[146] The latter enzyme increases four- to five-fold in activity 24 hours after a dose of 5-azacytidine, apparently owing to a decreased rate of degradation. It is not known whether a similar time-dependent increase in this enzyme's activity occurs in bone marrow or malignant cells, although such an increase could well affect the rate of activation of the drug. The "induced" hepatic uridine-cytidine kinase has greater thermal stability than the kinase found in untreated animals, indicating a selective stabilization of an isoenzyme.[146]

In addition, 5-azacytidine at minimally cytotoxic concentrations stimulates differentiation of the mouse embryo C3H 10T 1/2 C18 cells into striated muscle cells in culture.[147] Whether the drug has similar "differentiating" effects on malignant cells has not been examined. 5-Azacytidine given during the first six weeks of life markedly hastens the appearance of leukemia in AKR mice, a strain that harbors a leukemia virus. Leukemia is expressed in the first nine weeks of life in treated animals, as compared with four to nine months in control animals.[148]

The drug has mutagenic and teratogenic effects. Chromatid breaks have been noted in cultured hamster fibroblasts[149] and in L1210 cells,[129] but as yet no second malignancies related to 5-azacytidine treatment have been described in animals or humans. 5-Azacytidine has profound toxic effects on fertility in male mice,[150] but also causes teratogenic effects when administered during pregnancy.[151]

Schedule-dependent effects on immune function by 5-azacytidine have been reported. Simultaneous injection of the drug and sheep erythrocytes enhanced the formation of a primary antibody response in rats, and drug administration one to two days after antigen depressed the same response.[152]

ASSAY METHODS

At present no assay method specific for 5-azacytidine has been developed for clinical use. Future attempts to develop such methods will undoubtedly be complicated by the chemical instability of the drug, its very limited lipid solubility (which will complicate attempts at extraction and concentration from plasma), and the presence of cytidine deaminase in serum, an enzyme that will hydrolyze 5-azacytidine.

CLINICAL PHARMACOLOGY AND PHARMACOKINETICS

The limited information available on 5-azacytidine pharmacokinetics in animals and humans is based on studies employing ^{14}C-labeled drug,[119, 153-155] and provides an incomplete understanding of drug disposition because of the drug's extensive metabolism and chemical decomposition. ^{14}C-5-azacytidine is well absorbed after subcutaneous injection as judged by radioactivity levels in plasma.[155] Radioactivity distributes into a volume approximately equal to or greater than total body water (0.58 to 1.15 liters per kg) with little plasma protein binding. Peak plasma levels of 0.1 to 1.0 mM are reached by drug infusion at a rate of 2 to 6 mg per hour in adult patients. The primary half-life of radioactivity in plasma is approximately 3.5 hours after bolus intravenous injection, but after 30 minutes less than 2 per cent of radioactivity is associated with intact drug.[119] Isolated measurements of radioactivity in the cerebrospinal fluid (CSF) indicate poor penetration of drug, with a ratio of less than 0.1 for CSF as compared to plasma.

The identity of metabolites is unclear in humans. It is known that 5-azacytidine is susceptible to deamination by cytidine deaminase,[130] an enzyme found in high concentrations in liver, granulocytes, and intestinal epithelium, and in lower concentration in plasma. A variety of metabolic products have been identified in the urine of beagle dogs, including 5-azacytosine, 5-azauracil, and ring cleavage products.[153] The last-named may result from decomposition of the parent compound or of its deamination product, 5-azauridine.

TABLE 8–5. 5-Azacytidine in the Treatment of Acute Myelogenous Leukemia

Ref.	*Dose (mg/m²/day)*	*Bolus (B) or Infusion (I)*	*Toxicity**	*CR Rate*
114	150–200 × 5 day	B	N, V, D, M	5/14 (36%)
115	300–400 × 5 day	B	N, V, D, M	3/18 (17%)
116	150–200 × 5 day	I	M	11/45 (24%)
158	200–250 × 5 day	B	N, V, M, Neuro	5/18 (28%)

*N = nausea; V = vomiting; D = diarrhea; M = myelosuppression; Neuro = neuromuscular symptoms (see text).

Evidence for the importance of deamination in 5-azacytidine pharmacokinetics is provided by investigations of the effect of tetrahydrouridine, a cytidine deaminase inhibitor, on 5-azacytidine disposition in mice.[156] Tetrahydrouridine increases the toxicity and therapeutic activity of orally administered drug, and increases the drug concentration in plasma.

These initial observations, although incomplete, are compatible with a pharmacokinetic profile very similar to that of cytosine arabinoside, i.e., very rapid deamination, limited diffusion into cerebrospinal fluid and effusions, and rapid absorption into the intracellular space. However, a more precise identification of metabolic products is needed if alternative clinical schedules and drug combinations are to be developed on a rational basis.

TOXICITY

A variety of schedules of administration have been employed for 5-azacytidine,[114-117] including single weekly intravenous doses of up to 750 mg/m^2, daily doses of 150 to 200 mg/m^2 for five to ten consecutive days, and continuous infusion of similar daily doses for up to five days (Table 8–5). With each of these schedules, the primary toxicity has been leukopenia, although nausea and vomiting have been extremely bothersome for patients receiving the drug in bolus doses. Nausea and vomiting have not been readily controlled by antiemetics, leading some investigators to favor continuous intravenous infusion.[116] The latter schedule is also supported by cell kinetic considerations, in view of the drug's greater activity in the S phase of the cell cycle and its very rapid metabolism in man. The continuous infusion of 5-azacytidine requires fresh preparation of drug at frequent intervals, usually every three to four hours, because of the chemical instability of the agent. The response rate to 5-azacytidine in previously treated patients with acute myelogenous leukemia has varied from 17 to 36 per cent, and appears to be approximately equivalent for the bolus and continuous infusion schedules.

Maximal doses, as shown in Table 8–5, produce profound leukopenia and somewhat lesser thrombocytopenia. The nadir of WBC count occurs seven to 14 days after the last day of drug administration in most patients, but may be even more prolonged in some. Hepatotoxicity has also been observed, particularly in patients with preexisting hepatic dysfunction. Bellet and colleagues have described the development of fatal hepatic coma in four patients with extensive hepatic metastases, and have warned against the use of this agent in patients with hypoalbuminemia (less than 3 gm/dl) secondary to liver metastases.[157]

A syndrome of neuromuscular toxicity has been observed by Levi and co-workers in patients receiving 200 mg/m^2 per day by intravenous bolus injection.[158] Muscle tenderness and weakness developed after the second or third dose and were accompanied by progressive lethargy, confusion, and (in one patient) coma. It is unclear whether this peculiar reaction was related to the somewhat higher dose of drug used, but neurotoxicity has been reported only sporadically by other investigators using this agent.[117]

Several less worrisome acute toxicities have been associated with 5-azacytidine, including transient fever, a pruritic skin rash, and rarely hypotension during or immediately following bolus intravenous administration.[115]

DRUG INTERACTION AND COMBINATION THERAPY

Because of the single-agent activity of both 5-azacytidine and cytosine arabinoside against acute myelogenous leukemia, there has been interest in the use of these agents in combination. This interest is heightened by the fact that the most common mechanism of resistance to cytosine arabinoside in animal tumors is deletion of deoxycytidine kinase (see Chapter 18), a change that has no impact on 5-azacytidine metabolism. Experimental studies indicate a schedule-dependent interaction between these two agents. In treating L1210 leukemia,[159] maximal cell kill was achieved by a sequence of cytosine arabinoside followed six hours later by 5-azacytidine. Other workers[160, 161] found that simultaneous administration of these drugs gave inferior results to schedules employing the drugs separated by six to 48 hours in either possible sequence. A clinical study using cytosine arabinoside, daunomycin, and 5-azacytidine in combination against acute myelogenous leukemia had a complete remission rate of 53 per cent, a result that can be achieved by cytosine arabinoside and daunomycin alone.[162] Favorable interactions have been reported for oral 5-azacytidine and tetrahydrouridine (a cytidine deaminase inhibitor), and 5-azacytidine with pyrazofurin (an inhibitor of *de novo* pyrimidine synthesis), as mentioned previously in this chapter. Neither combination has received clinical trial.

References

Fluorinated Pyrimidines

1. Heidelberger C, Chaudhari NK, Danneberg P, et al.: Fluorinated pyrimidines. A new class of tumour-inhibitory compounds. Nature 179:663–666, 1957.
2. Rutman RJ, Cantarow A, and Paschkis KE: Studies on 2-acetylaminofluorene carcinogenesis. III. The utilization of uracil-2-C^{14} by pre-neoplastic rat liver. Cancer Res. 14:119–126, 1954.
3. Bosch L, Harbers E, and Heidelberger C: Studies on fluorinated pyrimidines. V. Effects on nucleic acid metabolism *in vitro*. Cancer Res. 18:335–343, 1958.
4. Santi DV, McHenry CS, and Sommer A: Mechanisms of interactions of thymidylate synthetase with 5-fluorodeoxyuridylate. Biochemistry 13:471–480, 1974.
5. Sommer A, and Santi DV: Purification and amino acid analysis of an active site peptide from thymidylate synthetase containing covalently bound 5-fluoro-2′-deoxyuridylate and methylene tetrachloride. Biochem. Biophys. Res. Commun. 57:689–696, 1974.
6. Fernandes DJ, and Bertino JR: 5-Fluorouracil-methotrexate synergy: enhancement of 5-fluorodeoxyuridylate binding to thymidylate synthetase by dihydropteroylpolyglutamates. Proc. Natl. Acad. Sci. USA 77:5663–5667, 1980.
7. Dolnick BJ, and Cheng Y-C: Human thymidylate synthetase derived from blast cells of patients with acute myelocytic leukemia. J. Biol. Chem. 252:7697–7703, 1977.
8. Ullman B, Lee M, Martin DW Jr, et al.: Cytotoxicity of 5-fluoro-2′-deoxyuridine: requirement for reduced folate cofactors and antagonism by methotrexate. Proc. Natl. Acad. Sci. USA 75:980–983, 1978.
9. Danenberg KD, and Danenberg PV: Evidence for sequential interaction of the subunits of thymidylate synthetase. J. Biol. Chem. 254:4345–4348, 1979.
10. Murinson DS, Anderson T, Schwartz HS, et al.: Competitive radioassay for 5-fluorodeoxyuridine 5′-monophosphate in tissues. Cancer Res. 39:2471–2479, 1979.
11. Washtein WL, and Santi DV: Assay of intracellular free and macromolecular-bound metabolites of 5-fluorodeoxyuridine and 5-fluorouracil. Cancer Res. 39:3397–3404, 1979.
12. Maybaum J, Ullman B, Mandel HG, et al.: Regulation of RNA- and DNA-directed actions of 5-fluoropyrimidines in mouse T-lymphoma (S-49) cells. Cancer Res. 40:4209–4215, 1980.
13. Evans RM, Laskin JD, and Hakala MT: Assessment of growth-limiting events caused by 5-fluorouracil in mouse cells and in human cells. Cancer Res. 40:4113–4122, 1980.
14. Madoc-Jones J, and Bruce WR: On the mechanism of the lethal action of 5-fluorouracil in mouse L-cells. Cancer Res. 28:1976–1981, 1968.
15. Spiegelman S, Nayak R, Sawyer R, et al.: Potentiation of the antitumor activity of 5-FU by thymidine and its correlation with the formation of (5-FU) RNA. Cancer 45:1129–1134, 1980.
16. Spiegelman S, Sawyer R, Nayak R, et al.: Improving the antitumor activity of 5-fluorouracil by increasing its incorporation into RNA via metabolic modulation. Proc. Natl. Acad. Sci. USA 77:4966–4970, 1980.
17. Santelli G, and Valeriote F: *In vivo* enhancement of 5-fluorouracil cytotoxicity to AKR leukemia cells by thymidine in mice. J. Natl. Cancer Inst. 61:843–847, 1978.
18. Carrico CK, and Glazer RI: Augmentation by thymidine of the incorporation and distribution of 5-fluorouracil into ribosomal RNA. Biochem. Biophys. Res. Commun. 87:664–670, 1979.
19. Kufe DW, and Egan EM: Enhancement of 5-fluorouracil incorporation into human lymphoblast ribonucleic acid. Biochem. Pharmacol. 30:129–133, 1981.
20. Murgo AJ, Fried J, Burchenal D, et al.: Effects of thymidine and thymidine plus 5-fluorouracil on the growth kinetics of a human lymphoid cell line. Cancer Res. 40:1543–1549, 1980.
21. Wilkinson DS, Tisty TD, and Hanas RJ: The inhibition of ribosomal RNA synthesis and maturation in Novikoff hepatoma cells by 5-fluorouridine. Cancer Res. 35:3014–3020, 1975.
22. Chaudhuri NK, Montag BJ, and Heidelberger C: Studies on fluorinated pyrimidines. III. The metabolism of 5-fluorouracil-2-^{14}C and 5-fluoroorotic-2-^{14}C acid *in vivo*. Cancer Res. 18:318–328, 1958.
23. Harbers E, Chaudhuri NK, and Heidelberger C: Studies on fluorinated pyrimidines. VIII. Further biochemical and metabolic investigations. J. Biol. Chem. 234:1255–1262, 1959.
24. Laskin JD, Evans RM, Slocum HK, et al.: Basis for natural variation in sensitivity to 5-fluorouracil in mouse and human cells in culture. Cancer Res. 39:383–390, 1979.
25. Carrico CK, and Glazer RI: The effect of 5-fluorouracil on the synthesis and translation of poly (A) RNA from regenerating liver. Cancer Res. 39:3694–3701, 1979.
26. Tseng W-C, Medina D, and Randerath K: Specific inhibition of transfer RNA methylation and modification in tissue of mice treated with 5-fluorouracil. Cancer Res. 38:1250–1257, 1978.
27. Glazer RI, and Legraverend M: The effect of 5-fluorouridine 5′-triphosphate on RNA transcribed in isolated nuclei *in vitro*. Mol. Pharmacol. 17:279–282, 1980.
28. Ingraham HA, Tseng BY, and Goulian M: Mechanism for exclusion of 5-fluorouracil from DNA. Cancer Res. 40:998–1001, 1980.
29. Walliser S, and Redmann K: Effect of 5-fluorouracil and thymidine on the transmembrane potential and potential of HeLa cells. Cancer Res. 38:3555–3559, 1978.
30. Kessel D: Cell surface alterations associated with exposure of leukemia L1210 cells to fluorouracil. Cancer Res. 40:322–324, 1980.

30A. Wohlhueter RM, McIvor RS, and Plagemann PGW: Facilitated transport of uracil and 5-fluorouracil, and permeation of orotic acid into cultured mammalian cells. J. Cell. Physiol. 104:209–319, 1980.

31. Bowen D, Diasio RB, and Goldman ID: Distinguishing between membrane transport and intracellular metabolism of fluorodeoxyuridine in Ehrlich ascites tumor cells by application of kinetic and high-performance liquid chromatographic techniques. J. Biol. Chem. 254:5333–5339, 1979.
32. Schwartz PM, and Handschmacher RE: Selective antagonism of 5-fluorouracil cytotoxicity by 4-hydroxypyrazolopyrimidine (allopurinol) *in vitro*. Cancer Res. 39: 3095–3101, 1979.
33. Reyes P, and Hall TC: Synthesis of 5-fluorouridine 5′-phosphate by a pyrimidine phosphoribosyltransferase

of mammalian origin. I. Some properties of the enzyme from P-1534J mouse leukemia cells. Biochemistry 8:2057–2062, 1969.

34. Houghton JA, and Houghton RJ: 5-Fluorouracil in combination with hypoxanthine and allopurinol: toxicity and metabolism in xenografts of human colonic carcinomas in mice. Biochem. Pharmacol. 29:2077–2080, 1980.
35. Kessel D, Deacon J, Coffey B, et al.: Some properties of a pyrimidine phosphoribosyltransferase from murine leukemia cells. Mol. Pharmacol. 8:731–739, 1972.
36. Benz C, and Cadman E: Modulation of 5-fluorouracil metabolism and cytotoxicity by antimetabolite pretreatment in human colorectal adenocarcinoma HCT-8. Cancer Res. 41:994–999, 1981.
37. Cory JG, Breland JB, and Carter GL: Effect of 5-fluorouracil on RNA metabolism in Novikoff hepatoma cells. Cancer Res. 39:4905–4913, 1979.
38. Cadman E, Davis L, and Heimer R: Enhanced 5-fluorouracil nucleotide formation following methotrexate: biochemical explanation for drug synergism. Science 205:1135–1137, 1979.
39. Moran RG, and Heidelberger C: Determinants of 5-fluorouracil sensitivity in human tumors. Bull. Cancer (Paris) 66:79–83, 1979.
40. Wahba AJ, and Friedkim M: The enzymatic synthesis of thymidylate. I. Early steps in the purification of thymidylate synthetase of *Escherichia coli*. J. Biol. Chem. 237:3794–3799, 1962.
41. Roberts D: An isotopic assay for thymidylate synthetase. Biochemistry 5:3546–3548, 1966.
42. Bresnick E, and Thompson UB: Properties of deoxythymidine kinase partially purified from animal tumors. J. Biol. Chem. 240:3967–3974, 1965.
43. Zaharko DS, Bolten BJ, Chiuten D, et al.: Pharmacokinetic studies during phase I trials of high-dose thymidine infusions. Cancer Res. 39:4777–4781, 1979.
44. Krenitsky TA: Pentosyl transfer mechanisms of the mammalian nucleoside phosphorylases. J. Biol. Chem. 243:2871–2875, 1968.
45. Nahas A, Savlov ED, and Hall TC: Phosphoribosyl transferase in colon tumor and normal mucosa as an aid in adjuvant chemotherapy with 5-fluorouracil (NSC-19893). Cancer Chemother. Rep. 58:909–912, 1974.
46. Reyes P, and Guganig M: A new and highly sensitive radiotracer assay for orotate phosphoribosyltransferase. Anal. Biochem. 46:276–286, 1972.
47. Reyes P, and Hall TC: Synthesis of 5-fluorouridine 5′-phosphate by a pyrimidine phosphoribosyltransferase of mammalian origin. II. Correlation between the tumor levels of the enzyme and 5-fluorouracil-promoted increase in survival of tumor-bearing mice. Biochem. Pharmacol. 18:2587–2590, 1969.
48. Kasbeker DK, and Greenberg DM: Studies on tumor resistance to 5-fluorouracil. Cancer Res. 23:818–825, 1963.
49. Reichard P, Sköld O, and Klein G: Possible enzymatic mechanisms for development of resistance against fluorouracil in ascites tumours. Nature 183:939–941, 1959.
50. Reichard P, Sköld O, Klein G, et al.: Studies on resistance against 5-fluorouracil. I. Enzymes of the uracil pathway during development of resistance. Cancer Res. 22:235–243, 1962.
51. Ardalan B, Cooney DA, Jayaram HN, et al.: Mechanisms of sensitivity and resistance of murine tumors to 5-fluorouracil. Cancer Res. 40:1431–1437, 1980.
52. Hande KR, and Chabner BA: Pyrimidine nucleoside monophosphate kinase from human leukemic blast cells. Cancer Res. 38:579–585, 1978.
53. Heidelberger C, Kaldor G, Mukherjee KL, et al.: Studies on fluorinated pyrimidines. XI. *In vitro* studies on tumor resistance. Cancer Res. 20:903–909, 1960.
54. Baskin F, Carlin SC, Kraus P, et al.: Experimental chemotherapy of neuroblastoma. II. Increased thymidylate synthetase activity in a 5-fluorodeoxyuridine-resistant variant of mouse neuroblastoma. Mol. Pharmacol. 11:105–117, 1975.
55. Priest DG, Ledford BE, and Doig MT: Increased thymidylate synthetase in 5-fluorodeoxyuridine-resistant cultured hepatoma cells. Biochem. Pharmacol. 29:1549–1553, 1980.
56. Kessel D, Hall TC, and Wodinsky I: Nucleotide formation as a determinant of 5-fluorouracil response in mouse leukemia. Science 154:911–913, 1966.
57. Myers CE, Young RC, and Chabner BA: Biochemical determinants of 5-fluorouracil response *in vivo*: the role of deoxyuridylate pool expansion. J. Clin. Invest. 56:1231–1238, 1975.
58. Klubes P, Connelly K, Cerna I, et al.: Effects of 5-fluorouracil on 5-fluorodeoxyuridine 5′-monophosphate and 2-deoxyuridine 5′-monophosphate pools and DNA synthesis in solid mouse L1210 and rat Walker 256 tumors. Cancer Res. 38:2325–2331, 1978.
59. Moran RG, Spears CP, and Heidelberger C: Biochemical determinants of tumor sensitivity to 5-fluorouracil: ultrasensitive methods for determination of 5-fluoro-2′-deoxyuridylate, 2′-deoxyuridylate, and thymidylate synthetase. Proc. Natl. Acad. Sci. USA 76:1456–1460, 1979.
60. Ardalan B, Buscaglia MD, and Schein PS: Tumor 5-fluorodeoxyuridylate concentrations as a determinant of 5-fluorouracil response. Biochem. Pharmacol. 27:2009–2013, 1978.
61. Sitar DS, Shaw DH, Thirwell MP, et al.: Disposition of 5-fluorouracil after intravenous bolus doses of a commercial formulation to cancer patients. Cancer Res. 37:3981–3984, 1977.
62. Buckpitt AR, and Boyd MR: A sensitive method for determination of 5-fluorouracil and 5-fluoro-2′-deoxyuridine in human plasma by high-pressure liquid chromatography. Anal. Biochem. 106:432–437, 1980.
63. Finn D, and Sadee W: Determination of 5-fluorouracil (NSC-19893) plasma levels in rats and man by isotope dilution-mass spectrography. Cancer Chemother. Resp. 59:279–285, 1975.
64. Cohen JL, and Brennan PB: GLC assay for 5-fluorouracil in biological fluids. J. Pharm. Sci. 62:572–575, 1973.
65. Ensminger WD, Rosowsky A, Raso VO, et al.: A clinical pharmacological evaluation of hepatic arterial infusion of 5-fluoro-2′-deoxyuridine and 5-fluorouracil. Cancer Res. 38:3784–3792, 1978.
66. Schreiber R, and Raso V: Radioimmunoassay for the detection and quantitation of 5-fluorodeoxyuridine. Cancer Res. 38:1889–1892, 1978.
67. Bruckner HW, and Creasey WA: The administration of 5-fluorouracil by mouth. Cancer 33:14–18, 1974.
68. Finch RE, Bending MR, and Lant AF: Plasma levels of 5-fluorouracil after oral and intravenous administration in cancer patients. Br. J. Clin. Pharmacol. 7:613–617, 1979.
69. Christophidis N, Vajda FJE, Lucas I, et al.: Fluorouracil therapy in patients with carcinoma of the large bowel: a pharmacokinetic comparison of various rates and routes of administration. Clin. Pharmacokinet. 3:330–336, 1978.
70. Cohen JL, Irwin LW, Marshall OJ, et al.: Clinical pharmacology of oral and intravenous 5-fluorouracil (NSC-19893). Cancer Chemother. Rep. 58:723–731, 1974.
71. Fraile RJ, Baker LH, Buroker TR, et al.: Pharmacokinetics of 5-fluorouracil administered orally by rapid intravenous and by slow infusion. Cancer Res. 40:2223–2228, 1980.
72. Almersjo OE, Gustavsson BG, Regardh CG, et al.: Pharmacokinetic studies of 5-fluorouracil after oral and intravenous administration in man. Acta Pharmacol. Toxicol. 46:329–336, 1980.
73. Hahn RG, Moertel CG, Schutt J, et al.: A controlled comparison of intensive courses of 5-FU by oral versus IV route in colorectal carcinoma. Proc. Am. Assoc. Cancer Res. 15:191, 1974.
74. Speyer JL, Collins JM, Dedrick RL, et al.: Phase I and pharmacologic studies of 5-fluorouracil administered intraperitoneally. Cancer Res. 40:567–572, 1980.

75. Clarkson B, O'Connor A, Winston L, et al.: The physiologic disposition of 5-fluorouracil and 5-fluoro-2'-deoxyuridine in man. Clin. Pharmacol. Ther. 5:581–610, 1964.
76. MacMillan WE, Wolberg WH, and Welling PG: Pharmacokinetics of fluorouracil in humans. Cancer Res. 38:3479–3482, 1978.
77. Jones RB, Buckpitt AR, Londer H, et al.: Potential clinical applications of a new method for quantitation of plasma levels of 5-fluorouracil and 5-fluorodeoxyuridine. Bull. Cancer (Paris) 66:75–78, 1979.
78. Cano JP, Rigault JP, Aubert C, et al.: Determination of 5-fluorouracil in plasma by GC/MS using an internal standard. Applications to pharmacokinetics. Bull. Cancer (Paris) 66:67–74, 1979.
79. Kirkwood JM, Ensminger W, Rosowsky A, et al.: Comparison of pharmacokinetics of 5-fluorouracil and 5-fluorouracil with concurrent thymidine infusions in a phase I trial. Cancer Res. 40:107–113, 1980.
80. Woodcock TM, Martin DS, Damin LEM, et al.: Clinical trials with thymidine and fluorouracil: a phase I and clinical pharmacologic evaluation. Cancer 45:1135–1143, 1980.
81. Collins JM, Dedrick RL, King FG, et al.: Nonlinear pharmacokinetic models for 5-fluorouracil in man: intravenous and intraperitoneal routes. Clin. Pharmacol. Ther. 28:235–246, 1980.
82. Mukherjee KL, Boohar J, Wentland D, et al.: Studies on fluorinated pyrimidines. XVI. Metabolism of 5-fluorouracil-2-C^{14} and 5-fluoro-2'-deoxyuridine-2-C^{14} in cancer patients. Cancer Res. 23:49–66, 1963.
83. Stolfi RL, Sawyer RC, Rabandranath N, et al.: Protection by testosterone from fluorouracil-induced toxicity without loss of anticancer activity against autochthonous murine breast tumors. Cancer Res. 40:2730–2735, 1980.
84. Seifert P, Baker L, Reed ML, et al.: Comparison of continuously infused 5-fluorouracil with bolus injection in treatment of patients with colorectal adenocarcinoma. Cancer 36:123–128, 1975.
85. Spiers ASD, Kasimis BS, and Janis MG: High-dose intravenous infusion of 5-fluorouracil for refractory solid tumors — the HI-FU regimen. Clin. Oncol. 6:63–69, 1980.
86. Ansfield F, Ramirez G, Skibba JL, et al.: Intrahepatic arterial infusion with 5-fluorouracil. Cancer 28:1147–1151, 1971.
87. Sullivan RD, Norcross JW, and Watkins E Jr: Chemotherapy of metastatic liver cancer by prolonged hepatic artery infusion. N. Engl J. Med. 270:321–327, 1964.
88. Burrows JH, Talley RW, Drake EH, et al.: Infusion of fluorinated pyrimidines into hepatic artery for treatment of metastatic carcinoma of liver. Cancer 20:1886–1892, 1967.
89. Narsete T, Ansfield F, Wirtanen G, et al.: Gastric ulceration in patients receiving intrahepatic infusion of 5-fluorouracil. Ann. Surg. 186:734–736, 1977.
90. Taylor I, Broman P, and Rowling JT: Adjuvant liver perfusion in colorectal cancer: initial results of clinical trial. Br. Med. J. 2:1320–1322, 1977.
91. Pottage A, Holt S, Ludgate S, et al.: Fluorouracil cardiotoxicity. Br. Med. J. 1:547, 1978.
92. Dent RG, and McColl I: 5-Fluorouracil and angina. Lancet 1:347–348, 1975.
93. Haidak DJ, Hurwitz BS, and Yeung KY: Tear-duct fibrosis (dacryostenosis) due to 5-fluorouracil. Ann. Intern. Med. 88:657, 1978.
94. Santelli J, and Valeriote F: *In vivo* potentiation of 5-fluorouracil cytotoxicity against AKR leukemia by purines, pyrimidines and their nucleosides and deoxynucleosides. J. Natl. Cancer Inst. 64:69–72, 1980.
95. Donehower R, Allegra J, Lippman M, et al.: Sequence-dependent effects of methotrexate and 5-fluoropyrimidine in serum-free cultures of human breast cancer. Proc. Am. Assoc. Cancer Res. 20:1024, 1979.
96. Tattersall MHN, Jackson RC, Connors TA, et al.: Combination chemotherapy: the interaction of methotrexate and 5-fluorouracil. Eur. J. Cancer 9:733–739, 1973.
97. Bertino JR, Sawicki WL, Linquist CA, et al.: Schedule-dependent antitumor effects of methotrexate and 5-fluorouracil. Cancer Res. 37:327–328, 1977.
98. Tattersall MHN, Jackson RC, Connors TA, et al.: Combination chemotherapy: the interaction of methotrexate and 5-fluorouracil. Eur. J. Cancer 9:733–739, 1973.
99. Donehower RC, Myers CE, and Chabner BA: Minireview. New developments on the mechanisms of action of antineoplastic drugs. Life Sci. 24:1–14, 1979.
100. Vogel SJ, Presant CA, Ratkin FA, et al.: Phase I study of thymidine plus 5-fluorouracil infusions in advanced colorectal carcinoma. Cancer treat. Rep. 63:1–5, 1979.
101. Hostege A, Herrmann B, and Leppler DOR: Increased formation of nucleotide derivatives of 5-fluorouridine in hepatoma cells treated with inhibitors of pyrimidine synthesis and D-galactosamine. FEBS Lett. 95:361–365, 1978.
101A. Erlichman C, Donehower RC, Speyer JL, et al.: A phase I–II trial of N-phosphonacetyl-L-aspartic acid and 5-fluorouracil given by bolus injection. J. Natl. Cancer Inst., in press.
102. Fox RM, Woods RL, and Tattersall MHN: Allopurinol modulation of high-dose fluorouracil toxicity. Cancer Treat. Rev. (Suppl.) 6:143–147, 1979.
103. Hall SW, Valdivieso M, and Benjamin RS: Intermittent high single dose ftorafur. A phase I clinical trial with pharmacologic-toxicity correlations. Cancer Treat. Rep. 61:1495–1498, 1977.
104. Benvenuto J, Lu K, Hall SW, et al.: Metabolism of 1-(tetrahydro-2-furanyl)-5-fluorouracil (ftorafur). Cancer Res. 38:3867–3870, 1978.
105. Au JL, Wu AT, Friedman MA, et al.: Pharmacokinetics and metabolism of ftorafur in man. Cancer Treat. Rep. 63:343–350, 1979.
106. Benvenuto JA, Liehr JG, Winkler T, et al.: Human urinary metabolites of 1-(tetrahydro-2-furanyl)-5-fluorouracil (ftorafur). Cancer Res. 39:3199–3201, 1979.
107. Au JL, and Sadee W: Activation of ftorafur (R,S-1-tetrahydro-2-furanyl)-5-fluorouracil to 5-fluorouracil and butyrolactone. Cancer Res. 40:2814–2819, 1980.
108. Valdivieso M, Bodey GP, Gottlieb JA, et al.: Clinical evaluation of ftorafur (pyrimidino-deoxyribose N_1-2'-furanidyl-5-fluorouracil). Cancer Res. 36:1821–1824, 1976.
109. Cook AF, Holman MJ, Kramer MJ, et al.: Fluorinated pyrimidine nucleosides. 3. Synthesis and antitumor activity of a series of 5'-deoxy-5-fluoropyrimidine nucleosides. J. Med. Chem. 22:1330–1335, 1979.
110. Bollag W, and Hartmann HR: Tumour inhibitory effects of a new fluorouracil derivative: 5'-deoxy-5-fluorouridine. Eur. J. Cancer 16:427–432, 1980.
111. Armstrong RD, and Diasio RB: Metabolism and biological activity of 5'-deoxy-5-fluorouridine, a novel fluoropyrimidine. Cancer Res. 40:3333–3338, 1980.

5-Azacytidine

112. Sorm F, Piskala A, Cihak A, et al.: 5-Azacytidine, a new highly effective cancerostatic. Experientia 20:202–203, 1964.
113. Hanka LJ, Evans JS, Mason DJ, et al.: Microbiological production of 5-azacytidine. 1. Production and biological activity. Antimicrob. Agents Chemother. 1966:619–624, 1966.
114. Karon M, Sieger L, Leimbrock S, et al.: 5-Azacytidine: a new active agent for the treatment of acute leukemia. Blood 42:359–365, 1973.
115. McCredie KB, Bodey GP, Burgess MA, et al.: Treatment of acute leukemia with 5-azacytidine (NSC-102816). Cancer Chemother. Rep. 57:319–323, 1973.
116. Vogler WR, Miller DS, and Keller JW: 5-Azacytidine (NSC-102816): a new drug for the treatment of myeloblastic leukemia. Blood 48:331–337, 1976.

117. Von Hoff DD, Slavik M, and Muggia FM: A new anticancer drug with effectiveness in acute myelogenous leukemia. Ann. Intern. Med. 85:237–245, 1976.
118. Beisler J: Isolation, characterization, and properties of a labile hydrolysis product of the antitumor nucleoside, 5-azacytidine. J. Med. Chem. 21:204–208, 1978.
119. Israili ZH, Vogler WR, Mingioli ES, et al.: The disposition and pharmacokinetics in humans of 5-azacytidine administered intravenously as a bolus or by continuous infusion. Cancer Res. 36:1453–1461, 1976.
120. Notari RE, and DeYoung JL: Kinetics and mechanisms of degradation of the antileukemic agent 5-azacytidine in aqueous solutions. J. Pharm. Sci. 64:1148–1157, 1975.
121. Vesely J, and Cihak A: 5-Azacytidine: mechanism of action and biological effects in mammalian cells. Pharmacol. Ther. 2:813–840, 1978.
122. Weiss JW, and Pitot HC: Inhibition of ribosomal precursor RNA maturation by 5-azacytidine and 8-azaguanine in Novikoff hepatoma cells. Arch. Biochem. Biophys. 165:588–596, 1974.
123. Lee T, and Karon MR: Inhibition of protein synthesis in 5-azacytidine-treated HeLa cells. Biochem. Pharmacol. 25:1737–1742, 1976.
124. Kalousek F, Raska K, Jurovik M, et al.: Effect of 5-azacytidine on the acceptor activity of sRNA. Colln. Czech. Chem. Commun. 31:1421–1424, 1966.
125. Cihak A, Vesela H, and Sorm F: Thymidine kinase and polyribosomal distribution in regenerating rat liver following 5-azacytidine. Biochim. Biophys. Acta 166:277–279, 1968.
126. Cihak A, and Vesely J: Prolongation of the lag period preceding the enhancement of thymidine and thymidylate kinase activity in regenerating rat liver by 5-azacytidine. Biochem. Pharmacol. 21:3257–3265, 1972.
127. Li LH, Olin EJ, Buskirk HH, et al.: Cytotoxicity and mode of action of 5-azacytidine on L1210 leukemia. Cancer Res. 30:2760–2769, 1970.
128. Plagemann PGW, Behrens M, and Abraham D: Metabolism and cytotoxicity of 5-azacytidine in cultured Novikoff rat hepatoma and P388 mouse leukemia cells and their enhancement by preincubation with pyrazofurin. Cancer Res. 38:2458–2466, 1978.
129. Li LH, Olin EJ, Fraser TJ, et al.: Phase specificity of 5-azacytidine against mammalian cells in tissue culture. Cancer Res. 30:2770–2775, 1970.
130. Chabner BA, Drake JC, and Johns DG: Deamination of 5-azacytidine by a human leukemia cell cytidine deaminase. Biochem. Pharmacol. 22:2763–2765, 1973.
131. Doskocil J, and Sorm F: The determination of 5-azapyrimidines and their derivatives in bacterial RNA. FEBS Lett. 2:30–32, 1974.
132. Cihak A: Modulation of orotate phosphoribosyltransferase and orotidine 5′-phosphate decarboxylase activities in regenerating rat liver by 5-azacytidine. Colln. Czech. Chem. Commun. 39:3782–3792, 1974.
133. Pliml J, and Sorm F: Synthesis of 2′-deoxy-D-furanosyl-5-azacytosine. Colln. Czech. Chem. Commun. 29:2576–2578, 1964.
134. Beisler JA, Abbasi MM, and Driscoll JS: Dihydro-5-azacytidine hydrochloride, a biologically active and chemically stable analog of 5-azacytidine. Cancer Treat. Rep. 60:1671–1674, 1976.
135. Futterman B, Derr J, Beisler JA, et al.: Studies on the cytostatic action, phosphorylation and deamination of 5-azacytidine and 5,6-dihydro-5-azacytidine in HeLa cells. Biochem. Pharmacol. 27:907–909, 1978.
136. Beisler JA, Abbasi MM, and Driscoll JS: The synthesis and antitumor activity of arabinosyl-5-azacytosine. Biochem. Pharmacol. 26:2469–2472, 1977.
137. Drake JC, Stoller RG, and Chabner BA: Characteristics of the enzyme uridine-cytidine kinase isolated from a cultured human cell line. Biochem. Pharmacol. 26:64–66, 1977.
138. Lee T, Karon M, and Momparler RL: Kinetic studies on phosphorylation of 5-azacytidine with the purified uridine-cytidine kinase from calf thymus. Cancer Res. 34:2481–2488, 1974.
139. Vadlamudi S, Padarathsingh M, Bonmassar E, et al.: Reduction of antileukemic and immunosuppressive activities of 5-azacytidine in mice by concurrent treatment with uridine. Proc. Soc. Exp. Biol. Med. 133:1232–1238, 1970.
140. Vadlamudi S, Choudry JN, Waravdekar VS, et al.: Effect of combination treatment with 5-azacytidine and cytidine on the life span and spleen and bone marrow cells of leukemic (L1210) and non-leukemic mice. Cancer Res. 30:362–369, 1970.
141. Vesely J, Cihak A, and Sorm F: Biochemical mechanisms of drug resistance. IV. Development of resistance to 5-azacytidine and simultaneous depression of pyrimidine metabolism in leukemic mice. Int. J. Cancer 2:639–646, 1967.
142. Cadman E, Eiferman F, Heimer R, et al.: Pyrazofurin enhancement of 5-azacytidine antitumor activity in L5178Y and human leukemia cells. Cancer Res. 38:4610–4617, 1978.
143. Lloyd HH, Dalmadge EA, and Wikoff LJ: Kinetics of the reduction in viability of cultured L1210 leukemic cells exposed to 5-azacytidine (NSC-102816). Cancer Chemother. Rep. 56:585–591, 1972.
144. Presant CA, Vietti TJ, and Valeriote F: Kinetics of both leukemic and normal cell population reduction following 5-azacytidine. Cancer Res. 35:1926–1930, 1975.
145. Cihak A, Lamar C, and Pitot HC: Studies on the mechanism of the stimulation of tyrosine aminotransferase activity *in vivo* by pyrimidine analogs: the role of enzyme synthesis and degradation. Arch. Biochem. Biophys. 156:176–187, 1973.
146. Cihak A, and Vesely J: Enhanced uridine kinase in rat liver following 5-azacytidine administration. J. Biol. Chem. 248:1307–1313, 1973.
147. Constantinides PG, Jones PA, and Gevers W: Functional striated muscle cells from non-myoblast precursors following 5-azacytidine treatment. Nature 267:364–366, 1977.
148. Vesely J, and Cihak A: High frequency induction *in vivo* of mouse leukemia in AKR strain by 5-azacytidine and 5-iodo-2′-deoxyuridine. Experientia 29:1132–1133, 1973.
149. Karon M, and Benedict W: Chromatid breakage: differential effect of inhibitors of DNA synthesis during G_2 phase. Science 178:62, 1972.
150. Seifertova M, Vesely J, and Cihak A: Enhanced mortality in offspring of male mice treated with 5-azacytidine prior to mating. Morphological changes in testes. Neoplasma 23:53–60, 1976.
151. Seifertova M, Vesely J, and Sorm F: Effect of 5-azacytidine on developing mouse embryo. Experientia 24:487–488, 1968.
152. Madar J, and Cihak A: Stimulatory effect of 5-azacytidine on 7s antibody production in rats. Proc. Soc. Exp. Biol. Med. 158:36–39, 1978.
153. Coles E, Thayer PS, Reinhold V, et al.: Pharmacokinetics and excretion of 5-azacytidine (NSC-102816) and its metabolites. Proc. Am. Assoc. Cancer Res. 16:91, 1974.
154. Chan KK, Staroscik JA, and Sadee W: Synthesis of 5-azacytidine-6-^{13}C and -6-^{14}C. J. Med. Chem. 20:598–600, 1977.
155. Troetel WM, Weiss AJ, Stambaugh JE, et al.: Absorption, distribution, and excretion of 5-azacytidine (NSC-102816) in man. Cancer Chemother. Rep. 56:405–411, 1972.
156. Neil GL, Moxley TE, Kuentzel SL, et al.: Enhancement by tetrahydrouridine (NSC-112907) of the oral activity of 5-azacytidine (NSC-102816) in L1210 leukemic mice. Cancer Chemother. Rep. 59:459–465, 1975.
157. Bellet RE, Mastrangelo MJ, Engstrom PF, et al.: Hepatotoxicity of 5-azacytidine (NSC-102816). A clinical and pathologic study. Neoplasma 20:303–309, 1973.
158. Levi J, and Wiernik P: A comparative clinical trial of 5-azacytidine and guanazole in previously treated adults with acute nonlymphocytic leukemia. Cancer 38:36–41, 1976.
159. Neil GL, Barger AE, Bhuyan BK, et al.: Combination

chemotherapy of L1210 leukemia with 1-β-D-arabinofuranosylcytosine and 5-azacytidine. Cancer Res. 36:1114–1120, 1976.
160. Momparler RL, Goodman J, and Karon M: *In vitro* biochemical and cytotoxicity studies with 1-β-D-arabinofuranosylcytosine and 5-azacytidine in combination. Cancer Res. 35:2853–2857, 1975.
161. Presant CA, Valeriote F, and Vietti TJ: Biological characterization of a prolonged antileukemic effect of 5-azacytidine. Cancer Res. 37:376–381, 1977.
162. Baehner RL, Bernstein ID, Higgins G, et al.: Improved induction remission response in children with acute nonlymphocytic leukemia treated with daunomycin, 5-azacytidine (D-ZAPO). Proc. Am. Assoc. Cancer Res. 18:349, 1977.

PURINE ANTIMETABOLITES

9

John J. McCormack

David G. Johns

6-MERCAPTOPURINE AND 6-THIOGUANINE

Hitchings and Elion, in a short introductory article for an early symposium[1] on 6-mercaptopurine (6-MP) (Fig. 9–1), commented that this compound and its 2-amino analogue, 6-thioguanine (6-TG), were first submitted for clinical evaluation as antitumor agents in 1951. Today, 30 years later, these purine derivatives, although they occupy an important role in the management of leukemia, are still the subjects of extensive biochemical, pharmacologic, and clinical investigation. At present, 6-TG is used primarily for remission induction in acute myelogenous leukemia, and 6-MP is used for maintenance therapy of acute lymphocytic and acute myelogenous leukemia. 6-Mercaptopurine (I) was synthesized by Elion et al.[2] and was the first purine analogue to achieve extensive clinical use in cancer chemotherapy. Burchenal and colleagues[3] initially established that 6-MP can induce remissions in patients with acute leukemia and chronic myelocytic leukemia, but noted that chronic lymphocytic leukemia, lymphomas, and various solid tumors generally show little or no response to treatment with this agent.

Thiation of the natural purine, guanine, yielded 6-thioguanine (II), which was found to exhibit antineoplastic activity in a variety of experimental systems[4] and which, at present, is the only other purine antimetabolite in clinical use as an anticancer agent in the United States. It is interesting to note that thioguanine has been isolated from the fermentation broth of a pseudomonad.[5]

In this chapter we emphasize the pharmacology of 6-MP and 6-TG because of their clinical significance. It should be noted, however, that a large number of purine derivatives have antineoplastic and immunosuppressant actions, and summaries of pertinent information on the chemistry and biology of such compounds are found in several chapters of a comprehensive collection of reviews published in 1975[6-11] and in an excellent article by Montgomery and Struck.[12]

Mechanism of Action

6-Mercaptopurine is converted to the ribonucleotide derivative, which is the form of the drug active in inhibiting important reactions at several metabolic loci.[13] Its metabolic transformations, and the responsible enzymes, are indicated in Figure 9–2. Despite many years of intensive investigation, there is still considerable controversy concerning the primary mechanism(s) by which 6-MP, in its activated form(s), exerts its antineoplastic effect, although it does seem clear that conversion to a nucleotide form is a prerequisite for drug activity. At present it is not possible to pinpoint any one of the several prominent effects observed in mammalian cells after treatment with 6-MP as the primary mechanism of cytotoxic action of this drug. Mammalian cells undoubtedly have the ability to convert 6-MP to 6-TG deoxyribonucleotide and to incorporate the latter residue into DNA.[14] However, the significance of incorporation has been questioned on the basis of observations[15] that some 6-MP–resistant cells incorporated more deoxythioguanosine residues into DNA than did sensitive cells. Mammalian cells are capable of incorporating 6-MP (as thioguanine residues) into RNA, and Melvin and Keir have described an efficient method to separate sulfur-containing RNA from RNA that does not contain sulfur.[16]

A prominent metabolic effect associated with administration of 6-MP is the inhibition of purine biosynthesis *de novo* (Fig. 9–3). Early investigations with 6-MP led to the conclusion that this drug is capable of producing substantial inhibition of the incorporation of simple precursors such as glycine or formate into purine derivatives.[17, 18]

X = O Hypoxanthine
X = S 6-Mercaptopurine

I

X = O Guanine
X = S 6-Thioguanine

II

Azathioprine

III

Figure 9–1. Chemical structures of purines and purine analogues.

The ribonucleotide derivative of 6-MP inhibits the enzyme glutamine-5-phosphoribosylpyrophosphate (PRPP) amidotransferase, which catalyzes the initial reaction in the purine biosynthetic pathway.[19] 6-Methylmercaptopurine ribotide also is capable of inhibiting this enzyme; the thiopurine nucleotides exert their inhibitory activity by producing a "negative feedback" effect on enzymatic activity, mimicking the effects of natural purine nucleotide modulators of purine biosynthesis. The ribonucleotide of 6-MP can also inhibit two purine nucleotide interconversion reactions that play an important role in the supply of purine precursors for nucleic acid synthesis. One such reaction is the conversion of inosinate (IMP) through adenylosuccinate to adenylate (AMP); the second reaction is the conversion of inosinate (IMP) to xanthylate (XMP), an obligatory process in the formation of guanylate (GMP).[13] Another interesting and potentially important action of 6-MP ribonucleotide is inhibition of the exonuclease repair activity of DNA polymerase.[20] Combined use of the adenosine analogue ara-A and 6-MP leads to increased incorporation of ara-A into DNA.

As in the case of 6-MP, it is difficult to identify a single locus of action for thioguanine.[21] One "active form" of 6-TG, 6-thioguanylic acid (thio-GMP), exerts biochemical effects similar to those described for the ribonucleotide derivative of 6-MP. 6-Thioguanylate is a good inhibitor of glutamine-PRPP amidotransferase (Fig. 9–3, step *a*), and of inosinic acid dehydrogenase (Fig. 9–3, step *b*), and therefore is capable of decreasing purine biosynthesis at two sites by suppressing both the rate of formation of the purine ring and the rate of conversion of inosinate to guanylate. It is important to emphasize, however, the considerable evidence indicating that a major mechanism of cytotoxicity produced by thioguanine administration involves incorporation of this compound (at the deoxynucleotide level) into DNA and the subsequent effects of such incorporation on DNA function.[22]

Relatively low levels of thioguanine are capable of inhibiting cell surface glycoprotein synthesis, presumably by reducing the levels of guanosine diphosphate sugar derivatives required for transfer reactions essen-

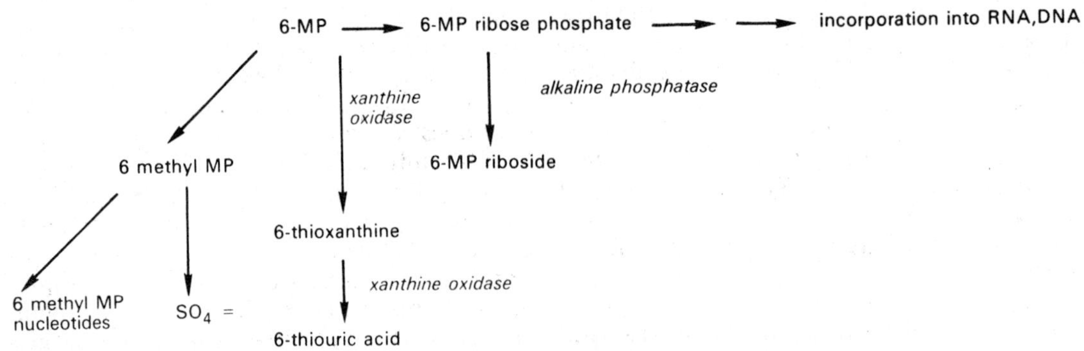

Figure 9–2. Metabolic transformations of 6-mercaptopurine.

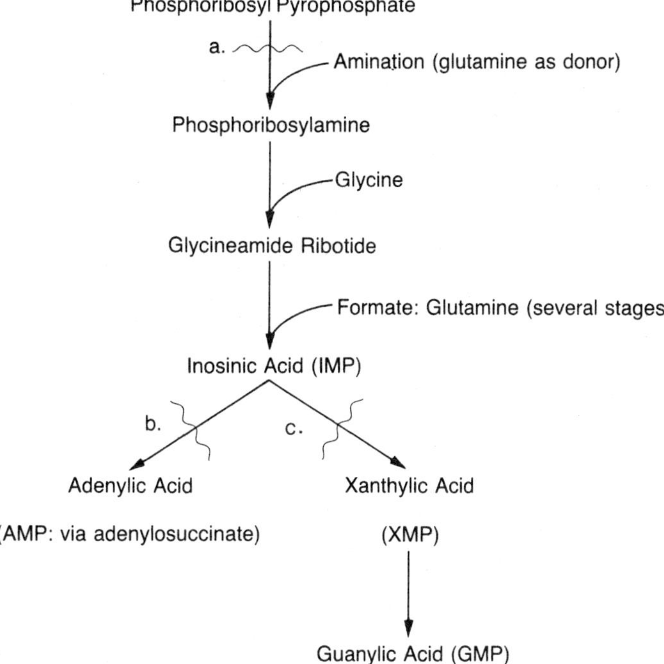

Figure 9–3. Sites of inhibition of purine biosynthesis by thioinosinic and thioguanylic acid. *a*, Glutamine-PRPP amidotransferase inhibited by both thioinosinic and thioguanylic acid. *b*, Adenylosuccinate synthetase inhibited by both thioinosinic and thioguanylic acid. *c*, Inosinic acid dehydrogenase inhibited by thioinosinic acid.

tial for glycoprotein synthesis.[23] The contribution of this effect to the cytotoxic action of thioguanine is not yet clear; a similar effect would be expected to occur with 6-MP under appropriate conditions.

Carrico and Sartorelli have provided evidence that thioguanine-induced inhibition of messenger-RNA synthesis may contribute to the cytotoxic action of this drug[24]; the mechanism(s) responsible for such inhibition have not been identified.

Resistance to Thiopurines

Clinical cross-resistance is generally observed between 6-MP and 6-TG. Several mechanisms of resistance to these agents have been described in experimental tumors. The most thoroughly studied mechanism of resistance is the diminished ability of resistant cells to "activate" 6-MP to 6-thioinosinic acid and 6-TG to 6-thioguanylic acid[25, 26] via the reaction catalyzed by hypoxanthine:guanine phosphoribosyltransferase (HGPRT). This mechanism appears to be relatively rare as a basis for resistance in human leukemic cells.[27] Another factor that possibly determines the sensitivity of a cell population to 6-MP and/or 6-TG is the capacity of the cells to degrade the drugs or their active metabolites. Wolpert and colleagues in 1971 reported that the resistance of sarcoma-180 cells to 6-MP is associated with an increase in the activity of membrane-bound alkaline phosphatase that converts the active mononucleotide to 6-thioinosine and inorganic phosphate.[28] A similar relationship between resistance to thiopurines and elevation of alkaline phosphatase has been reported in human leukemia patients.[29, 30] It is of considerable interest that the properties of alkaline phosphatases obtained from thiopurine-sensitive and -resistant cell lines differ significantly in their heat lability, pH maxima, and immunologic properties.[31, 32]

Assay Methods

Most current information about the pharmacokinetics of the thiopurines was obtained using assay techniques that depended on the use of radiolabeled drug, with separation of parent compound and metabolites by paper chromatography. The published pharmacokinetic data show considerable inconsistency and variability, and it is likely that a clearer understanding of this problem will be forthcoming from the application of newer assay techniques.

New assay methods have recently been described, but have not received detailed application. Tidd and Dedhar have utilized a preliminary oxidation of the thiopurines to sulfonate derivatives with alkaline permanganate,[33] followed by fluorometric detection. A somewhat different chemical method has been devised by Maddocks,[34] who separated 6-MP from interfering substances by converting the thiopurine to a phenyl mercury derivative, followed by extraction into toluene, back extraction with 0.1 N HCl, and fluorometric detection. This latter assay is sensitive to levels of 66 nM and can also be applied to the measurement of 6-MP generated as a metabolite of azathioprine in man. Other, less sensitive spectral methods have been applied to the study of 6-MP pharmacokinetics.[35, 36]

Bailey and co-workers have described a gas-chromatographic method for determination of 6-MP in serum; this method, however, was incapable of detecting levels of 6-MP in serum samples taken from 12 of 13 patients on oral maintenance doses of this drug.[37] Using their HPLC-fluorometric procedure, Tidd and Dedhar found levels of thioguanine in a patient with acute myelocytic leukemia to be approximately 2×10^{-7}M, on an oral dosage regimen of 180 mg per day. HPLC methods have also been developed for studies of 6-MP and its metabolites in cellular materials.[38] The paired-ion assay of Day et al. has a sensitivity of 1 μM and separates the parent compound from two metabolites, 6-thiouric acid and 6-methylmercaptopurine.[39]

6-Mercaptopurine and 6-TG require metabolic "activation" in order to exert their characteristic biologic effects. HGPRT is the enzyme responsible for conversion of these agents to their respective active ribonucleotide metabolites, 6-thioinosinic acid (6-MP ribose phosphate) (Fig. 9–2) and 6-thioguanylic acid.[40] It is pertinent to stress that, because the active form(s) of 6-MP and related compounds are intracellular nucleotides, measurements of plasma levels of parent drug (such as 6-MP) may be of relatively limited value, a point that applies to many purine and pyrimidine antimetabolites, and which was well made by Elion and Hitchings in a review of the 6-MP derivative, azathioprine.[8]

Pharmacokinetics

The major elimination mechanism for both 6-MP and 6-TG involves metabolic alteration; renal excretion of unchanged drug is a minor route of elimination with conventional clinical dosage schedules. With high doses of intravenous 6-MP, the renal excretion of unchanged drug becomes quantitatively very significant (20 to 40 per cent of administered dose)[41]; excretion of unmetabolized 6-MP in children receiving high doses (1000 mg/m^2) of 6-MP has resulted in hematuria and crystalluria.[42] 6-MP ordinarily is administered orally. Absorption is somewhat erratic from the intestine after oral administration; approximately 50 per cent of an oral dose reaches the systemic circulation. Distribution into most peripheral compartments is rather uniform, but the drug is not transported efficiently across the blood–brain barrier. 6-MP is bound to plasma proteins to the extent of about 30 per cent; however, the binding is not tight since the drug-protein complex can be dissociated readily by dialysis. Estimates of the plasma half-life for 6-MP range from 20 to 60 minutes (average 50 min) after intravenous administration to adults[43]; the estimated serum half-life was significantly lower (20 min) in children. Loo and colleagues[43] have stressed the importance of specificity of analytical methods used for pharmacokinetic studies of this type, as exemplified by differences in half-lives observed in studies using colorimetric rather than radioisotopic methods. The metabolic alteration of 6-MP is a relatively rapid process; one important pathway for metabolism of 6-MP involves initial oxidation of the drug in position 8 of the imidazole portion of the molecule, mediated by xanthine oxidase, and subsequent oxidation in the pyrimidine portion of the molecule to a product, 6-thiouric acid, devoid of antitumor activity (Fig. 9–2).

It is essential to recognize the importance of the xanthine oxidase pathway in modulating the biologic effect of 6-MP in clinical situations, particularly since patients who receive both 6-MP and the xanthine oxidase inhibitor allopurinol may be at considerable risk of severe toxicity.[44] For example, severe bleeding associated with leukopenia and thrombocytopenia were observed in a young patient on a regimen that included full doses of allopurinol and 6-MP.[45] Because of the increased toxicity that can occur if a standard dose of 6-MP is administered to a patient receiving allopurinol, it is recommended that the dosage of 6-MP be reduced to approximately 25 per cent of the standard dose when allopurinol is included in the drug regimen. In the presence of allopurinol, thioxanthine (and not thiouric acid) becomes the major oxidation product of 6-MP.[46, 47] The enzyme(s) responsible for the partial oxidation to thioxanthine during allopurinol administration have not been identified, but it is extremely unlikely that the conversion is attributable to xanthine oxidase, in view of the blockade of catalytic activity of this enzyme under these conditions.

It is possible that thioxanthine arises from oxidation of 6-MP mediated by human liver aldehyde oxidase; no information on this point appears to be available, although Krenitsky and colleagues[48] have reported that rabbit liver aldehyde oxidase oxidizes 6-MP to 8-hydroxy-6-mercaptopurine and not to thioxanthine. Incubation of 6-MP with rat liver microsomes, in the presence of NADPH, results in drug binding to microsomal protein[49]; thus, it is possible that the occurrence of a cytochrome P-450–dependent metabolic activation of 6-MP to a toxic metabolite plays a role in liver damage associated with 6-MP administration. Other metabolic processes also influence the levels of 6-MP in patients; for example, several methylated purine sulfonic acid derivatives are formed from 6-MP in man,[13] and these purine sulfonic acid derivatives appear to undergo conversion to oxypurines with liberation of inorganic sulfate. Methylation of the sulfur function of 6-MP is probably mediated by an S-adenosylmethionine–dependent methyltransferase[50]; it is important to note that 6-methylmercaptopurine riboside, as well as 6-MP, can be converted to potentially active methylmercaptopurine ribonucleotides.[51, 52]

6-Thioguanine, like 6-MP, is absorbed incompletely after oral administration; the plasma half-life after intravenous injection is reported to be approximately 90 minutes (median value:range 25 to 240 min). Methylation of the sulfur function in position 6, yielding 2-amino-6-methylthiopurine, is an important reaction in the metabolism of this drug; as with 6-MP, subsequent oxidation of the methylthio group results ultimately in the release of inorganic sulfate.[53] 6-TG is also converted to 6-thioxanthine in a reaction presumably mediated by hepatic guanine deaminase ("guanase"), and the 6-thioxanthine thus formed is oxidized to 6-thiouric acid by xanthine oxidase. There is some controversy about the quantitative significance of the deamination-oxidation pathway in man. Earlier clinicopharmacologic studies of thioguanine are incomplete, unfortunately, with no quantitative data given on percentages of various metabolites. Studies of the interaction of 6-TG with rat liver guanine deaminase have demonstrated that the former has an affinity for this enzyme approximately 1000 times lower than that of the natural substrate guanine.[54] A recent clinicopharmacologic study[55] of oral thioguanine in patients with acute myelogenous leukemia indicates that peak plasma levels occur two to four hours after drug administration and that these levels can vary widely (from 3×10^{-8}M to 5×10^{-7}M). Absorption appeared to be slowed and plasma levels reduced by food intake, and also in patients with nausea. 6-TG is not a substrate for xanthine oxidase, and therefore dosage reduction for this agent is not required during concomitant administration of allopurinol.

Clinical Use

6-Mercaptopurine, in combination with other agents, has found application in both the induction and maintenance phases of chemotherapeutic regimens for patients with acute lymphoblastic leukemia.[56] Although 6-MP does have activity in acute myelocytic leukemia, thioguanine is used more frequently as a component of both induction and maintenance regimens.[57]

In addition, 6-MP is used as a second-line drug in the treatment of chronic myelocytic leukemia, and may be employed in the acute blastic phase. Recent reports suggest a possible role for 6-MP in maintenance of remissions induced by other drugs in patients with diffuse histiocytic and diffuse undifferentiated lymphomas.[58] Bryan and colleagues have suggested "cautious use" of 6-TG in combination with cytosine arabinoside for treatment of patients with acute lymphocytic leukemia who do not respond to conventional modes of therapy.[59]

Toxicology

Early animal studies revealed three major types of toxic manifestations after administration of 6-MP:myelosuppression, damage to the intestinal epithelium, and hepatic dysfunction.[60] Thioguanine was found to produce myelosuppression (agranulocytosis, thrombocytopenia) in experimental animals to a degree similar to that observed with 6-MP, but intestinal and hepatic damage were less common. In man the toxicity observed during therapeutic use of thiopurines resembles that noted in animal studies. 6-MP produces significant gastrointestinal toxicity, with anorexia, nausea, and vomiting occurring in approximately 30 per cent of adult patients; gastrointestinal toxicity is reported to occur less commonly in children.[61]

Diarrhea and stomatitis are also observed in patients receiving 6-MP. Hematologic disturbances produced by 6-MP in man include leukopenia, thrombocytopenia and anemia; these disturbances may increase in severity after drug treatment is discontinued, indicating persistent disruption of the hematopoietic system. Both hematologic and gastrointestinal toxicities are dose-related, as evidenced by reports of adverse effects in patients on an experimental high-dose 6-MP protocol.[62] Liver dysfunction has been reported in a number of patients receiving 6-MP, and generally is manifested as a reversible cholestatic jaundice,[63] although high doses of 6-MP appear capable of producing frank hepatic necrosis.[64]

Since 6-MP itself may produce liver damage, administration of this drug along with other potentially hepatotoxic agents should be avoided if possible. Should concomitant use of 6-MP and another hepatotoxic drug be required, it is obvious that close attention must be paid to indices of liver function. A surprisingly high incidence of hepatic toxicity (10 of 19 patients) was reported by Rodriguez and colleagues in an experimental regimen of 6-MP and doxorubicin (Adriamycin).[65] Thioguanine produces gastrointestinal toxicity less frequently than does 6-MP, but the qualitative aspects of gastrointestinal toxicity are similar for the two drugs. Jaundice has been reported in patients receiving thioguanine. Thioguanine also produces significant bone marrow depression in man, and leukopenia and thrombocytopenia are common indications of drug toxicity. The interesting observation has been made that the toxicity to experimental animals of 6-MP at high dosage is enhanced considerably by bacterial endotoxin, but the clinical significance of this phenomenon remains to be established.[66] In patients receiving 6-MP or 6-TG, periodic (weekly) determinations of leukocyte and platelet counts and of hemoglobin levels are recommended; either drug should be discontinued if abnormal depression of hematologic values occurs.

6-Mercaptopurine and 6-TG are drugs with definite teratogenic potential; their use in pregnant patients, especially during the first trimester, requires exceedingly careful assessment of the risk-benefit ratio. Fetal group C trisomy has been reported as a possible consequence of intensive chemotherapy with 6-TG and cytosine arabinoside in a pregnant woman with acute myelocytic leukemia[67]; on the other hand, the same drug combination, begun during the 26th week of pregnancy, resulted in complete remission of acute myelocytic leukemia and delivery of a normal infant at term.[68]

Dosage Scheduling and Drug Interactions in Man

6-Mercaptopurine is usually given by the oral route at a dose of 75 to 100 mg per m^2 (2.0 to 2.5 mg/kg) per day. Dose reduction in patients with impaired renal or hepatic function has been recommended,[69] but the bases

TABLE 9–1.

Drug	*Usual Dose*	*t½**	*Major Elimination Route*	*Drug Interactions*
6-Mercaptopurine	75–100 mg/m^2	1 hr	Metabolism	Allopurinol; other hepatotoxic drugs; warfarin (?)
6-Thioguanine	75 mg/m^2	1–5 hrs	Metabolism	Other hepatotoxic drugs
Azathioprine	120 mg/m^2 (initial)	5 hrs	Metabolism	Allopurinol; neuromuscular blockers; hepatotoxic drugs

*These values are based on disappearance of isotopically labeled drug and are included as rough estimates, *not* as definitive values.

for guidelines for dosage reduction in renal impairment appear to be obscure.[70] 6-MP has been reported to inhibit the anticoagulant action of warfarin in a patient with acute myelocytic leukemia, but a mechanism for this interaction has not been convincingly established.[71] The important interaction between 6-MP and allopurinol has been described earlier in this chapter. Thioguanine is given at an oral dose of approximately 75 mg per m^2 (2 mg/kg); after about four weeks of treatment with no discernible clinical response and no significant toxicity, the dose may be increased cautiously to 90 to 100 mg per m^2 (up to 3 mg/kg). A similar increase in "standard" dosage may be made with 6-MP under appropriate circumstances.

Attempts have been made to increase 6-MP dosage.[72] In a trial of bolus doses of 1000 mg per m^2 per day for five days, no responses were observed in a test group of 20 patients with various solid tumors. Six patients experienced severe myelosuppression, and one died of drug-related toxicity. No pharmacologic studies were conducted in conjunction with this trial.

AZATHIOPRINE

Azathioprine (6-[(1-methyl-4-nitro-5-imidazolyl)thio]purine (Fig. 1, compound III)) was originally synthesized as a "protected" form of 6-MP that would resist rapid systemic oxidation and methylation and release 6-MP at various sites in the body. The generation of 6-MP from azathioprine can be mediated non-enzymatically by sulfhydryl compounds such as glutathione,[73] or by other nucleophilic agents. Recent communications also have described enzymatic conversions of azathioprine to 6-MP.[74, 75] Elion and Hitchings[8] have identified several other processes that can modulate the actions of azathioprine, and have cautioned against oversimplification of the chemical and biochemical mechanisms by which this drug exerts its characteristic biologic effects. Azathioprine is employed primarily as an immunosuppressant agent, a use exemplified by its role in management of patients receiving renal transplants and of patients with severe rheumatoid arthritis unresponsive to more conventional therapy. Azathioprine has produced remissions in patients with leukemia,[76] but has not received widespread use as an antineoplastic agent in clinical settings. The preference of azathioprine to 6-MP for clinical use as an immunosuppressant agent is attributed to an improvement in the therapeutic index for azathioprine compared with 6-MP.[77] The complex interactions of azathioprine and 6-MP on aspects of immunologic function have been reviewed by Elion.[77] Interesting differential effects of azathioprine on human lymphocytes *in vitro* have been described; for example, B cells were found to be highly susceptible to suppressant effects of low concentrations of azathioprine, whereas "helper" T cells were quite resistant to this drug.[78]

Azathioprine can be administered either orally or intravenously to prevent homograft rejection; the drug is given intravenously during the first one to four days after surgery, and orally before surgery and as maintenance therapy after IV administration has been discontinued. Dosage of azathioprine, as with other drugs of comparably high toxic potential, must be adjusted to an individual basis. The usual initial dose ranges from 3 to 5 mg per kg and, under appropriate circumstances, 30 to 40 per cent of this dose level will suffice for maintenance. Extensive conversion of azathioprine to 6-MP occurs in man. One method described for 6-MP analysis can also be applied to analysis of azathioprine in biologic fluids.[29] When conventional doses of azathioprine are administered orally, relatively small amounts of unchanged azathioprine are detected in the urine of patients.[46, 79] It has been suggested that the small degree of excretion of unchanged azathioprine in man reflects almost complete metabolism of lower doses of the drug in clinical situations, as compared with doses used in experimental animals.[80] Azathioprine absorption from the gastrointestinal tract is adequate but not complete in man; approximately 50 per cent of a given dose of radiolabeled drug appears in the urine over a period of 24 hours following oral administration. In one patient, peak plasma levels (1 to 2 μg/ml) appeared at two hours following azathioprine administration, and serum radioactivity declined with a half-life of about five hours.

The above pharmacokinetic data, as Elion has emphasized clearly, must be interpreted in light of the fact that the analytical studies carried out measured azathioprine in conjunction with several metabolites, and not azathioprine alone.[81] Indeed, as recently stated by Trounce,[81a] considerable refinement of classical pharmacokinetic approaches appears necessary to optimize clinical use of cytotoxic drugs in general. Thiouric acid, derived from 6-MP by the action of xanthine oxidase, is a prominent urinary metabolite of azathioprine. Although Chalmers and colleagues[82] have found that mammalian aldehyde oxidase is capable of oxidizing azathioprine to the 8-hydroxy derivative, the significance of this reaction appears extremely limited in man.[77] Because xanthine oxidase plays a critical role in controlling levels of 6-MP formed from azathioprine *in vivo*, dosage of azathioprine must be reduced to approximately one fourth of a "full" dose in patients medicated concomitantly with allopurinol. There is a possible danger of hepatotoxicity associated with azathioprine (and/or its active metabolite, 6-MP); for this reason, and also because hepatic metabolism plays a role in the inactivation of 6-MP, Kaplan and Calabresi[83] have recommended reduction of azathioprine dosage in patients with compromised liver function. However, these authors do not advocate dosage reduction in renal insufficiency, a practice that is considered prudent by others.[84,85] As would be anticipated from its extensive conversion to 6-MP, the toxicity of azathioprine is qualitatively similar to that of 6-MP.

Myelosuppression, manifested in leukopenia and less commonly in thrombocytopenia and anemia, is the principal adverse effect associated with azathioprine therapy. Liver dysfunction and gastrointestinal toxicity also have occurred in patients receiving azathioprine. Acute pancreatitis has been reported to be produced by azathioprine; one communication describes an episode of pancreatitis in a patient receiving azathioprine and prednisone for systemic lupus erythematosus.[86] Azathioprine is able to antagonize neuromuscular blockade produced by nondepolarizing neuromuscular blocking agents (curariform drugs) and to potentiate blockade produced by succinylcholine; it is proposed that these neuromuscular effects are attributable to inhibition of cyclic AMP phosphodiesterase.[87] An unusual dermatologic complication, manifested as a sensation of ants crawling in the skin (formication), has been described in a patient receiving azathioprine.[88] Reduced immunologic competence produced by azathioprine (and concurrently administered agents such as corticosteroids) renders patients susceptible to opportunistic pathogens such as fungi, protozoa (e.g., *Pneumocystis*), and viruses. The increased susceptibility to infection observed in patients given azathioprine also may occur in those receiving 6-MP or 6-TG as part of antineoplastic drug regimens. The observation of a relatively high incidence of neoplasms in renal homograft patients treated with azathioprine and corticosteroids may reflect the carcinogenic potential of azathioprine (and/or its metabolic products), reduction of immunologic surveillance mechanisms, or a combination of these and other factors.[89-91] Chromosome damage by azathioprine has been reported in a number of experimental systems, and such results were confirmed by studies of lymphocytes from children on long-term azathioprine therapy.[92]

9-β-D-ARABINOFURANOSYLADENINE (ara-A)

Over the past two decades, many analogues of adenosine and 2′-deoxyadenosine have received extensive preclinical study as potential antitumor and/or antiviral agents. Among these are 9-β-D-arabinofuranosyladenine (ara-A), 9-β-D-xylofuranosyladenine (xylosyl-A), formycin A, cordycepin, and tubercidin. In addition, both parent purine nucleosides for this series (i.e., adenosine and 2′-deoxyadenosine) show a variety of pharmacologic effects, including antitumor activity,[93] when administered at supraphysiologic dose levels. Among purine antimetabolites, however, only ara-A and a "slow-release" form of the latter, ara-A-5′-P, have received extensive clinical study. The former compound, which exhibits a wide spectrum of antiviral activity, is now marketed for use in the treatment of ocular herpes infections and has also received clinical trial as an antitumor agent,[94] while its monophosphorylated derivative, ara-A-5′-P, is presently undergoing clinical trial both as an antiviral and as an antitumor agent.[95] Detailed reviews of the biochemistry and pharmacology of the adenosine analogues have appeared[96-98]; this discussion will be confined primarily to ara-A and ara-A-5′-P, the two compounds in the series that have received clinical study.

The major obstacle to the development of this class of agents has been their rapid deamination by the widely distributed enzyme adenosine deaminase to inactive metabolites; among the compounds listed above, only tubercidin (7-deaza-adenosine) is not a substrate for this enzyme.[99] In early studies with a variety of animal model tumor systems, LePage and co-workers showed that tumors with low deaminase and high adenosine kinase levels were responsive to ara-A, whereas tumors with unfavorable deaminase-kinase ratios were not.[100] In addition, the aqueous solubility of ara-A is low, rendering it impractical to compensate for a rapid deamination rate merely by administering a larger dose of the drug. Thus, despite unequivocal evidence of the antitumor activity of the drug in early clinical trial,[94] this promising line of investigation was temporarily abandoned because of the combined disadvantages of administering high doses of the agent in a large volume of solvent.

These disadvantages appear to have been overcome in the case of ara-A with the development of the phosphomonoester ara-A-5′-P. This agent is much more water-soluble than ara-A, and although rapidly cleaved enzymically to ara-A in many mammalian species, it undergoes only relatively slow cleavage in man, so that in human subjects ara-A-5′-P can be regarded as a "slow-release" form of the drug.[101]

Chemistry, Metabolism, and Analytical Methodology

The synthesis of ara-A (Fig. 9–4) was described in 1960 by Lee and co-workers[102]; a more convenient source of the drug, however, is its isolation from fermentation broths of *Streptomyces antibioticus*.[103] Ara-A-5′-P is prepared by chemical phosphorylation of the nucleoside. *In vivo*, the major conversion products of ara-A are the mono-, di-, and triphosphates, and the product of deamination, arahypoxanthine. Quantitation of these compounds in body fluids and cell supernatants is largely dependent on the use of chromatographic methodology generally applicable to purine nucleosides and nucleotides; many of these methods have been adapted successfully for high-performance liquid chromatography (HPLC), with significant increase in speed and convenience of assay.[104] The use of ^3H-labeled ara-A has facilitated the localization and identification of drug metabolites after chromatography in the presence of naturally occurring purine nucleosides and nucleotides.

Mode of Action

Ara-A exerts its pharmacologic activity after intracellular conversion to the triphosphate ara-ATP; the latter compound is an inhibitor of both mammalian and viral DNA polymerases.[105-107] Ara-AMP, administered parenterally, is thought to be cleaved by plasma and cell membrane phosphomonoesterases to the nucleoside ara-A, prior to its intracellular anabolic conversion to mono-, di-, and triphosphates; the possibility exists, however, that a significant fraction of the parenterally administered drug can enter cells as the monophosphate.[108]

Since its site of action is inhibition of DNA polymerases, it would appear that ara-A resembles in its pharmacologic activity the more widely used antitumor agent ara-C (1-β-D-arabinofuranosylcytosine), which is also thought to act by this mechanism after anabolic conversion to the triphosphate.[109] The similarity of ara-A and ara-C effects on DNA synthesis have been emphasized by Bell and Fridland,[110] who examined the action of these compounds on DNA synthesis in CEM cells. They found that both analogues inhibit the formation of new replicating segments of DNA (replicons) at drug concentrations that inhibit overall DNA synthesis by only 50 to 70 per cent. These authors concluded that the arabinose nu-

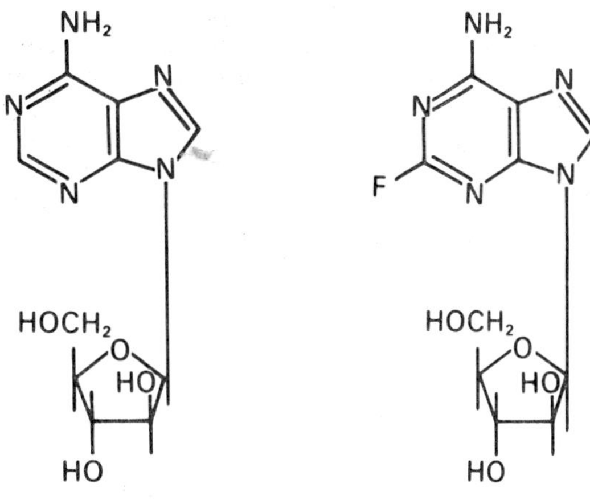

Figure 9–4. Chemical structures of 9-β-D-arabinofuranosyladenine (ara-A) and 2-fluoro-ara-A.

cleosides had greater effects on chain initiation than on elongation. Ara-CTP was 10- to 15-fold more potent than ara-ATP in this inhibitory action.

The ara nucleotides have other biochemical actions that may contribute to their antitumor effects. Both ara triphosphates inhibit the reduction of CDP to dCDP by ribonucleotide reductase.[111] Ara-ATP is more potent in this regard than ara-CTP. Although these effects are unlikely to account for cytotoxicity, they might influence deoxynucleotide pools, which in turn determine antimetabolite effectiveness and influence drug interactions. Deoxyadenosine (AdR) and ara-A also bind tightly to adenosylhomocysteine hydrolase, an enzyme that mediates the breakdown of adenosylhomocysteine. The latter acts as an inhibitor of the formation of S-adenosylmethionine (SAM),[112] a methyl donor in many important biologic reactions, including methylation of RNA and DNA. There is evidence that inhibition of SAM formation has little role in cytotoxicity. Ara-A nucleotide formation is not required for the SAM-depletion mechanism described above, but is required for ara-A toxicity, since mutants lacking adenosine kinase are resistant to ara-A.

Ara-A action is attenuated in some cells, particulary T lymphocytes and tumors derived from these cells, by adenosine deaminase (Fig. 9–5). Ho and colleagues[113] have examined the adenosine deaminase concentrations in various human tissues and found the highest levels in the following organs: spleen > intestine > lung > colon > brain > liver > bone marrow > kidney. The highest deaminase activity was found in acute lymphocytic leukemia cells, followed closely by acute myeloblastic leukemia, and chronic myeloblastic leukemia in blastic crisis. Chronic lymphocytic leukemia cells had little adenosine deaminase by comparison (Table 9–2). The latter findings indicate that the effectiveness of ara-A or ara-AMP would likely be enhanced to a significant degree by deaminase inhibitors such as deoxycoformycin (2′-dCF). Indeed, significant increases in the therapeutic potency and therapeutic index of ara-A are achieved as a consequence of treatment of lymphoblastic leukemias with a combination of ara-A and an adenosine deaminase inhibitor.[114-116]

Although *de novo* resistance to the ara-A type of analogues may result from high concentrations of adenosine deaminase, sensitive cells cultured with ara-A develop resistance on the basis of deletion of adenosine kinase, the initial activating enzyme in the salvage pathway.[117] These cells are resistant to both ara-A and ara-AMP, an indication that the latter compound undergoes hydrolysis to ara-A before entering the cell. A 5′ ecto-nucleotidase that hydrolyzes ara-AMP is present on the cell membrane of both sensitive and resistant cell lines. Alteration in the properties of DNA polymerases, associated with a decrease in sensitivity to inhibition by ara-ATP, has also been implicated as a factor in ara-A resistance.[118]

Clinical Studies

The most extensive clinical studies with ara-A have been carried out in trials prior to its use as an antiviral agent.[119] As an antitumor agent, ara-A was examined by Bodey et al.[94, 120] Twenty-eight patients were studied; clinical responses were seen in two of four patients with blastic transformation of chronic myelogenous leukemia and in four of ten patients with acute lymphocytic leu-

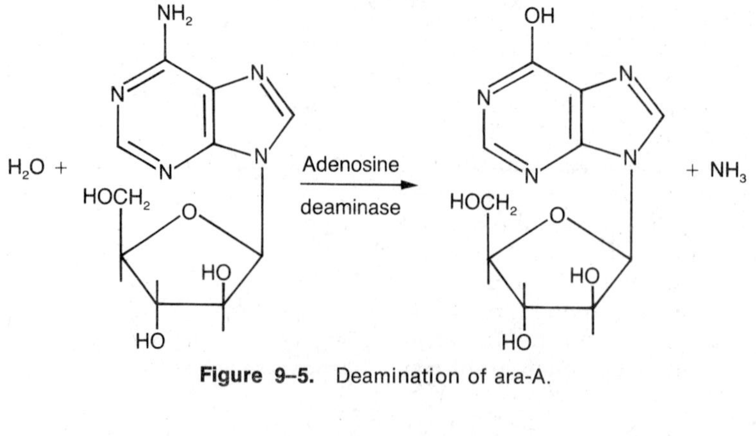

H_2O + [ara-A: NH₂ purine, HOCH₂ sugar, HO, HO] —Adenosine deaminase→ [OH purine, HOCH₂ sugar, HO, HO] + NH_3

Figure 9–5. Deamination of ara-A.

kemia. Because of the low solubility and rapid deamination of the drug, however, this approach was later abandoned in favor of studies with the monophosphorylated derivative, ara-A-5′-P.[121] Twenty-four patients were treated with one to four courses of ara-A-5′-P at 750 to 1500 mg per m^2 per day ara-A equivalent; objective responses were noted in one patient with chronic myelogenous leukemia in blast crisis, one with non-Hodgkin's lymphoma, one with ovarian carcinoma, two with myelomas, and one with malignant melanoma. Hematologic improvement was seen in four other cases of leukemia.

Deaminase-resistant Adenosine Analogues

2-Fluoro-ara-A (F-ara-A), an analogue synthesized by Montgomery and Hewson[121a] more than 10 years ago, has significant biochemical advantages as compared with ara-A (Fig. 9–4). It is not hydrolyzed by adenosine deaminase, and thus is active as a single agent against tumors containing high concentrations of the degradative enzyme. Second, F-ara-A is activated by a different pathway from that of ara-A. The former is converted to a monophosphate by deoxycytidine kinase (the same enzyme responsible for ara-C activation), whereas the latter is phosphorylated by adenosine kinase.[122] Thus, ara-A–resistant cells (which lack adenosine kinase) may not be cross-resistant to F-ara-A. Third, F-ara-A is more potent than the combination of ara-A and dCF versus the T-lymphocyte cell line CEM, and F-ara-ATP is a more potent inhibitor of DNA synthesis on a molar basis.[123] Whether it will have selective toxicity for tumor cells as opposed to normal tissues is not known.

Additional, newer adenosine analogues have been synthesized. 2′-Azido-2′-deoxy-ara-A (Fig. 9–6) is approximately equally inhibitory for L1210 cells in culture, but is 25 times more soluble than ara-A.[124] Its activity, like that of ara-A, is enhanced by inhibition of adenosine deaminase. De Clercq and colleagues[125] have synthesized a number of 2′- and 3′-NH_2 or -azido derivatives of the purines. The most interesting is 2′-NH_2-2′-deoxyguanosine (Fig. 9–6), which was selectively toxic for L1210 cells but not for normal kidney cells. Its ID_{50} (50 per cent inhibitory concentration) for the tumor cells was 3.9 μg/ml, compared with an ID_{50} of 26 μg/ml for ara-A and 0.007 μg/ml for ara-C. A more potent compound is 9-deaza-adenosine (Fig. 9–6), which has an ID_{50} of 0.0008 μg/ml versus L1210 cells in culture.[126]

TABLE 9–2. Adenosine Deaminase Activity in Human Leukemic Cells

	Deaminase (μmol product/min/mg × 10^{-2}) MEAN ± SE	RANGE
Acute myelocytic leukemia	683 ± 170	157–2570
Chronic myelocytic leukemia	195 ± 15	90–270
Chronic myelocytic leukemia (blast crisis)	618 ± 105	508–828
Acute lymphocytic leukemia	805	668–940
Chronic lymphocytic leukemia	112	107–118

ADENOSINE DEAMINASE INHIBITORS

A new approach to the clinical use of adenosine analogues as antitumor and antiviral agents has been suggested by the development of the potent adenosine deaminase inhibitors 2′-deoxycoformycin (2′-dCF) and erythro-9-(2-hydroxy-3-nonyl)-adenine (EHNA) (Fig. 9–7). As discussed above, adenosine deaminase is widely distributed at high levels in mammalian tissues, its role presumably being to provide a protective effect against accumulation of the physiologic nucleosides adenosine and 2′-deoxyadenosine. The adenine nucleosides and their respective nucleotides can be shown to exert a variety of toxic effects, but the initial and dose-limiting toxicity in man appears to be severe lymphocytopenia and a consequent impairment in lymphocyte-mediated immunity. These results present an interesting parallel to the severe impairment in lymphocyte function observed in patients who lack adenosine deaminase as a consequence of an inherited genetic defect (severe combined immunodeficiency disease), and who usually succumb to infections in infancy. The accumulation of nucleotides of 2′-deoxyadenosine, with consequent feedback inhibition of ribonucleoside diphosphate reductase and a general inhibition of DNA synthesis, may be responsible for the defective replication of lymphocytes in this condition, and also after the administration of adenosine deaminase inhibitors such as 2′-dCF. T lymphocytes appear to be particularly susceptible to the toxic effects of adenosine nucleotides because of their lack of 5′-nucleotidase to cleave the accumulated toxic products.[127]

2′-NH$_2$-2′-deoxy-ara-adenine 2′-NH$_2$-2′-deoxyguanosine

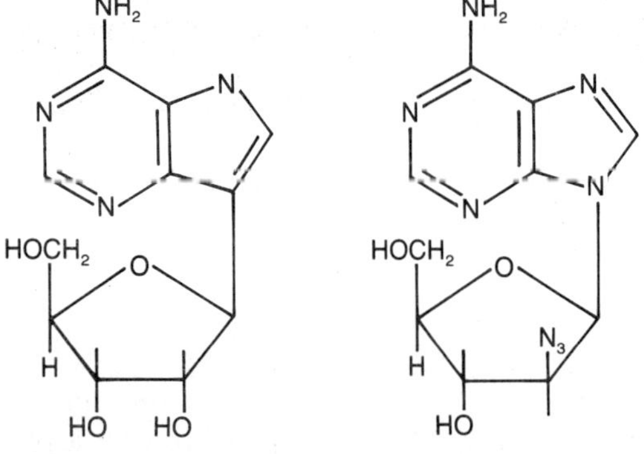

9-deaza-adenosine 2′-azido-2′-deoxy-ara-adenine

Figure 9–6. New adenosine and guanosine analogues.

The following dual observations are of immediate practical importance from the point of view of cancer chemotherapy, however:

1. 2′-Deoxycoformycin (and other potent adenosine deaminase inhibitors) can be shown to result in a significant increase not only in intracellular ara-ATP and in antitumor potency, but also in the therapeutic index of a number of adenosine analogues, including ara-A, xylosyl-A (Table 9–3), and cordycepin.[114-116, 128] The effect is most marked in tumors with high adenosine deaminase levels.

2. 2′-Deoxycoformycin, when administered as a single agent, exerts a specific antilymphocytic effect of possible therapeutic value in the treatment of lymphocytic malignancies. This effect is likely to be greatest in tumors derived from T lymphocytes or in the blastic phase of chronic granulocytic leukemia.[129]

Chemistry and Assay Methodology

2′-Deoxycoformycin (and its ribose analogue coformycin) are obtained from broths of *Streptomyces antibioticus.* The trivial names of these agents are derived from the original isolation procedures, where these compounds were detected by their ability to potentiate the cytotoxic activity of formycin A. Subsequent studies revealed that this activity was due to inhibition of the conversion of formycin A to formycin B by adenosine deaminase. These compounds are the most potent inhibitors of adenosine deaminase yet described, with K_i values of 2.5×10^{-12}M for 2′-dCF and 1.0×10^{-12}M for coformycin.[130] Structurally, these compounds are diazepine derivatives (Fig. 9–7), and they are chemically unstable in aqueous solution below pH 7. Because of their potency as adenosine deaminase inhibitors, the compounds can easily be quantitated by enzyme inhibition titration assay.[131] A microbiologic assay for 2′-dCF has also been described,[132] and the compound has been prepared in radiolabeled form for metabolic studies *in vivo.*[133]

EHNA (Fig. 9–7) was synthesized by Schaeffer and Schwender as the result of a systematic search for potent transition-state adenosine deaminase inhibitors.[134] A feature of considerable practical interest is that, although considerably higher doses are required, EHNA is as effective as 2′-dCF in potentiating the antitumor activity of adenosine analogues *in vivo.*[135]

2′-DCF EHNA

Figure 9–7. Chemical structures of adenosine deaminase inhibitors. *Left,* 2′-deoxycoformycin (pentostatin or 2′-dCF). *Right, erythro*-9-(2-hydroxy-3-nonyl)-adenine hydrochloride (EHNA).

TABLE 9–3. Effect of 2′-dCF and EHNA on Antitumor Activity of 9-β-D-Xylofuranosyladenine (Xylosyladenine) in Mice with P388 Ascites Leukemia*

Drug	*Optimal Daily Dose (mg/kg)*	*Median Survival Time (Days)*	*% Long-term Survivors*
Controls, saline		12	0
2′-dCF	0.25	12	0
EHNA	6.2–12.5	12	0
Xylosyladenine	50	17	0
Xylosyladenine + 2′-dCF (0.25 mg/kg)	3.1	30	20
Xylosyladenine + EHNA (12.5 mg/kg)	12.5	38	30

*Mice received 10^6 tumor cells intraperitoneally. Drug treatment began 24 hrs later by the intraperitoneal route and was continued for 9 days. In combination experiments, 2′-dCF and EHNA were administered 10 min prior to xylosyladenine. (Reproduced from Adamson et al.[135]).

Clinical Activity

Several clinical pharmacology/Phase I trials of single-agent 2′-dCF have been carried out, and at least four such studies have been published.[136-139] In the initial study,[136] partial responses were seen in three of seven patients with acute lymphocytic leukemia. In subsequent studies, responses have also been reported in mycosis fungoides[137, 138] and in chronic lymphocytic leukemia (CLL).[137] Severe, dose-limiting toxicities have been noted at higher dose levels of 2′-dCF (> 10 mg m^2 daily for three days); these include CNS effects (somnolence and coma) and impairment in renal function. Conjunctivitis has also been encountered frequently, but is not dose-limiting. In view of the toxicity of therapeutically effective doses of the compound in man, the future of 2′-dCF appears uncertain. One of the most promising applications appears to be the maintenance therapy of otherwise refractory cases of CLL;[137] patients with refractory CLL have been maintained in remission with low weekly doses (4 mg/m^2) of 2′-dCF for periods of up to seven months.

Although extensive studies of 2′-dCF (and other adenosine deaminase inhibitors) in combination with ara-A, xylosyl A, formycin A, and other adenosine analogues have been carried out in animal test systems, clinical trials of such combinations in either antiviral or antitumor therapy have not yet been conducted. It appears likely that these agents, in view of their potency as adenosine deaminase inhibitors, together with their ability to potentiate a variety of adenosine analogues with known pharmacologic activity, will prove applicable to clinical medicine. Their eventual clinical role, however, remains to be established.

References

1. Hitchings GH, and Elion GB: The chemistry and biology of purine analogs. Ann. N.Y. Acad. Sci. 60:195, 1954.
2. Elion GB, Burgi E, and Hitchings GH: Studies on condensed pyrimidine systems IX. The synthesis of some 6-substituted purines. J. Am. Chem. Soc. 74:411, 1952.
3. Burchenal JH, Murphy ML, Ellison RR, et al.: Clinical evaluation of a new antimetabolite, 6-mercaptopurine, in the treatment of acute leukemia and allied diseases. Blood 8:965, 1953.
4. Elion GB, and Hitchings GH: The synthesis of 6-thioguanine. J. Am. Chem. Soc. 77:1676, 1955.
5. Scannell JP, Preuss DL, Kellett M, et al.: Antimetabolites produced by microorganisms III. 2-Aminopurine-6-thiol (Thioguanine). J. Antibiot. 24:328, 1971.
6. Montgomery JA: Rational design of purine nucleoside analogs. *In* Sartorelli AC, and Johns DG (eds.): Handbook of Experimental Pharmacology 38, Part 1. Springer-Verlag, Berlin, 1975, p. 76.
7. Patterson ARP, and Tidd DM: 6-Thiopurines. *In* Sartorelli AC, and Johns DG (eds.): Handbook of Experimental Pharmacology 38, Part 2. Springer-Verlag, Berlin, 1975, p. 384.
8. Elion GB, and Hitchings GH: Azathioprine. *In* Sartorelli AC, and Johns DG (eds.): Handbook of Experimental Pharmacology 38, Part 2. Springer-Verlag, Berlin, 1975, p. 404.
9. LePage GA: Purine arabinosides, xylosides and lyxosides. *In* Sartorelli AC, and Johns DG (eds.): Handbook of Experimental Pharmacology 38, Part 2. Springer-Verlag, Berlin, 1975, p. 426.
10. Nichol CA: Antibiotics resembling adenosine. *In* Sartorelli AC, and Johns DG (eds.): Handbook of Experimental Pharmacology 38, Part 2. Springer-Verlag, Berlin, 1975, p. 434.
11. Parks RE Jr, and Agarwal KC: 8-Azaguanine. *In* Sartorelli AC, and Johns DG (eds.): Handbook of Experimental Pharmacology 38, Part 2. Springer-Verlag, Berlin, 1975, p. 458.
12. Montgomery JA, and Struck RF: The relationship of the metabolism of anticancer agents to their activity. Prog. Drug Res. 17:320, 1973.
13. Elion GB: Biochemistry and pharmacology of purine analogs. Fed. Proc. 26:898, 1967.
14. Tidd DM, and Patterson ARP: A biochemical mechanism for the delayed cytotoxic reaction of 6-mercaptopurine. Cancer Res. 34:738, 1974.
15. Scannell JP, and Hitchings GH: Thioguanine in deoxyribonucleic acid from tumors of 6-mercaptopurine treated mice. Proc. Soc. Exp. Biol. Med. 122:627, 1966.
16. Melvin WT, and Keir HM: Interaction of 6-thiopurines and thiol containing RNA with a cellulose mercurial. Anal. Biochem. 92:324, 1979.
17. Skipper HE. On the mechanism of action of 6-mercaptopurine. Ann. N.Y. Acad. Sci. 60:315, 1954.
18. Fernandes JF, LePage GA, and Lindner A: The influence of

azaserine and 6-mercaptopurine on the *in vivo* metabolism of ascites tumor cells. Cancer Res. 16:154, 1956.

19. Hill DL, and Bennett LL Jr.: Purification and properties of 5-phosphoribosyl pyrophosphate amidotransferase from adenocarcinoma 758 cells. Biochemistry 8:122, 1969.
20. Lee MYWT, Byrnes JJ, Downey KM, et al.: Mechanism of inhibition of deoxyribonucleic acid synthesis by 1-β-D-arabinofuranosyl adenosine triphosphate and its potentiation by 6-mercaptopurine ribonucleoside 5′-monophosphate. Biochemistry 19:215, 1980.
21. Crabtree GW: Pyrimidine and purine analogs. *In* Brodsky I, Kahn SB, and Conroy JF (eds.): Cancer Chemotherapy III. Grune & Stratton, New York, 1978.
22. Nelson JA, Carpenter JW, Rose LM, et al.: Mechanisms of action of 6-thioguanine, 6-mercaptopurine and 8-azaguanine. Cancer Res. 35:2872, 1975.
23. Lazo JS, Hwang KM, and Sartorelli AC: Inhibition of L-fucose incorporation into glycoprotein of sarcoma 180 ascites cells by 6-thioguanine. Cancer Res. 37:4250, 1977.
24. Carrico CK, and Sartorelli AC: Effects of 6-thioguanine on macromolecular events in regenerating rat liver. Cancer Res. 37:1868, 1977.
25. Brockman RW: Mechanism of resistance to anticancer agents. Adv. Cancer Res. 7:129, 1963.
26. Van Diggelen OP, Donahue TF, and Shin SI: Basis for differential cellular sensitivity to 8-azaguanine and 6-thioguanine. J. Cell. Physiol. 98:59, 1979.
27. Rosman M, and Williams HE: Leukocyte purine phosphoribosyl transferases in human leukemia sensitive and resistant to 6-thiopurines. Cancer Res. 33:1202, 1973.
28. Wolpert MK, Damle SP, Brown JE, et al.: The role of phosphohydrolases in the mechanism of resistance to 6-thiopurines. Cancer Res. 31:1620, 1971.
29. Rosman M, Lee ML, Creasey WA, et al.: Mechanisms of resistance to 6-thiopurines in human leukemia. Cancer Res. 34:1952, 1974.
30. Scholar EM, and Calabresi P: Increased activity of alkaline phosphatases in leukemic cells from patients resistant to thiopurines. Biochem. Pharmacol. 28:445, 1979.
31. Lee MH, Huang YM, and Sartorelli AC: Alkaline phosphatase activities of 6-thiopurine–sensitive and –resistant sublines of sarcoma 180. Cancer Res. 38:2413, 1978.
32. Lee MH, Huang YM, and Sartorelli AC: Immunological studies on alkaline phosphatases of 6-thiopurine–sensitive and –resistant sublines of sarcoma 180. Cancer Res. 38:2419, 1978.
33. Tidd DM, and Dedhar S: Specific and sensitive combined HPLC flow fluorimetric assay for intracellular 6-thioguanine metabolites of 6-mercaptopurine and 6-thioguanine. J. Chromatogr. 145:237, 1978.
34. Maddocks JL: Assay of azathioprine, 6-mercaptopurine and a novel thiopurine metabolite in human plasma. Br. J. Clin. Pharmacol. 8:273, 1979.
35. Finkel JM: A fluorimetric method for the estimation of 6-mercaptopurine in serum. Anal. Biochem. 21:362, 1967.
36. Tterlikkis L, Ortega E, Solomon R, et al.: Pharmacokinetics of 6-mercaptopurine. J. Pharm. Sci. 66:1454, 1977.
37. Bailey DG, Wilson TW, and Johnson EG: A gas chromatographic method for measuring 6-mercaptopurine in serum. J. Chromatogr. 111:305, 1975.
38. Breter HJ, Maidof A, and Zahn RK: The quantitative determination of metabolites of 6-mercaptopurine in biological materials. III. The determination of ^{14}C-labeled 6-thiopurines in L5178Y cell extracts using high-pressure liquid cation-exchange chromatography. Biochim. Biophys. Acta 518:205, 1978.
39. Day JL, Tterlikkis L, Neimann R, et al.: Assay of mercaptopurine in plasma using paired-ion high-performance liquid chromatography. J. Pharm. Sci. 67:1027, 1978.
40. Brockman RW, and Anderson EP: Biochemistry of cancer. Annu. Rev. Biochem. 32:463, 1963.
41. Coffey JJ, White CA, Lesk AB, et al.: Effect of allopurinol on the pharmacokinetics of 6-mercaptopurine (NSC 755) in cancer patients. Cancer Res. 32:1283, 1972.
42. Duttera MJ, Carolla RL, Gallelli JF, et al.: Hematuria and crystalluria after high-dose 6-mercaptopurine administration. N. Engl. J. Med. 287:292, 1972.
43. Loo TL, Luce JK, Sullivan MP, et al.: Clinical pharmacologic observations on 6-mercaptopurine and 6-methylpurine riboside. Clin. Pharmacol. Ther. 9:180, 1968.
44. Ascione FJ: Allopurinol with mercaptopurine. Drug Ther. 7(12):69, 1977.
45. Berns A, Rubenfeld S, and Rymzo WT: Hazard of combining allopurinol and thiopurine. N. Engl. J. Med. 286:730, 1972.
46. Elion GB, Callahan S, Rundles RW, et al.: Relationship between metabolic fates and anticancer activities of thiopurines. Cancer Res. 23:1207, 1963.
47. Elion GB, Callahan S, Nathan H, et al.: Potentiation by inhibition of drug degradation: 6-substituted thiopurines and xanthine oxidase. Biochem. Pharmacol. 12:85, 1963.
48. Krenitsky TA, Neil SM, Elion GB, et al.: A comparison of the specificities of xanthine oxidase and aldehyde oxidase. Arch. Biochem. Biophys. 150:585, 1972.
49. Hyslop RM, and Jardine I: Cytochrome P-450 dependent irreversible binding of 6-thiopurine to rat liver microsomal protein *in vitro* and protection by glutathione. Res. Commun. Chem. Pathol. Pharmacol. 22:163, 1978.
50. Romy CN: Metabolism of thiopyrimidines and thiopurines. S-Methylation with S-adenosylmethionine transmethylase and catabolism in mammalian tissues. J. Biol. Chem. 238:1078, 1963.
51. Zimmerman TP, Chu L-C, Rugge CJL, et al.: Identification of 6-methylmercaptopurine ribonucleoside-5′-diphosphate and 5′-triphosphate as metabolites of 6-mercaptopurine in man. Cancer Res. 34:221, 1974.
52. Zimmerman TP, Chu L-C, Rugge CJL, et al.: Formation of 5′-nucleotides of 6-methylmercaptopurine ribonucleoside in human tissues *in vitro*. Biochem. Pharmacol. 23:2737, 1974.
53. LePage GA, and Whitecar JP Jr: Pharmacology of 6-thioguanine in man. Cancer Res. 31:1627, 1971.
54. Lin H-L, Kwang KM, and Loo TL: Metabolism of 6-thioguanine by rat liver guanine deaminase. Proc. Am. Assoc. Cancer Res. 20:137, 1979.
55. Belch A, Birkett L, and Brox L: Clinical pharmacology of oral thioguanine in acute myelogenous leukemia. Proc. Am. Assoc. Cancer Res. 20:280, 1979.
56. Henderson ES: Acute lymphoblastic leukemia. *In* Holland JF, and Frei E III (eds.): Cancer Medicine. Lea & Febiger, Philadelphia, 1973, p. 1173.
57. Gale RP: Advances in the treatment of acute myelogenous leukemia. N. Engl. J. Med. 300:1189, 1979.
58. Lister TA, Cullen MH, Brearley RB, et al.: Combination chemotherapy for advanced non-Hodgkin's lymphoma of unfavourable histology. Cancer Chemother. Pharmacol. 1:107, 1978.
59. Bryan JH, Henderson ES, and Leventhal BG: Cytosine arabinoside and 6-thioguanine in refractory acute lymphocytic leukemia. Cancer 33:539, 1974.
60. Philips FS, Sternberg SS, Hamilton L, et al.: The toxic effects of 6-mercaptopurine and related compounds. Ann. N.Y. Acad. Sci. 60:283, 1954.
61. Burchenal JH, and Ellison RR: Pyrimidine and purine antagonists. Clin. Pharmacol. Ther. 2:523, 1961.
62. Esterhay RJ Jr, Aisner J, Levi JA, et al.: High-dose 6-mercaptopurine in advanced refractory cancer. Cancer Treat. Rep. 62:1229, 1978.
63. Einhorn M, and Davidsohn I: Hepatotoxicity of 6-mercaptopurine. J.A.M.A. 188:802, 1964.
64. Clark PA, Hsia YE, and Huntsman RG: Toxic complications of treatment with 6-mercaptopurine: two cases with hepatic necrosis and intestinal ulceration. Br. Med. J. 1:393, 1960.
65. Rodriguez V, Bodey GP, McCredie KB, et al.: Combination 6-mercaptopurine–Adriamycin in refractory adult acute leukemia. Clin. Pharmacol. Ther. 18:462, 1975.

66. Higuchi T, Nakamura T, and Uchino H: Mechanisms of enhanced toxicity of 6-mercaptopurine with endotoxin. Biochem. Pharmacol. 27:2507, 1978.
67. Mauer LH, Forcier RJ, McIntyre OR, et al.: Fetal group C trisomy after cytosine arabinoside and thioguanine. Ann. Intern. Med. 75:809, 1971.
68. Raich PC, and Curet LB: Treatment of acute leukemia during pregnancy. Cancer 36:861, 1975.
69. LePage GA, and Loo TL: Purine antagonists. *In* Holland JF, and Frei E III (eds.): Cancer Medicine. Lea and Febiger, Philadelphia, 1973, p. 754.
70. Shinn AF, Rutkowski D, Wilner FM, et al.: Dosage modifications of cancer chemotherapeutic agents in renal failure. Drug Intell. Clin. Pharmacy 11:140, 1977.
71. Spiers ASD, and Mibashan RS: Increased warfarin requirement during mercaptopurine therapy. Lancet 2:221, 1974.
72. Esterhay RJ, Aisner J, and Levi JA, et al.: High-dose 6-mercaptopurine in advanced refractory cancer. Cancer Treat. Rep. 62:1229, 1978.
73. Elion GB, Callahan S, Bieber S, et al.: A summary of investigations with 6-[1-methyl-4-nitro-5-midazolyl] thiopurine. Cancer Chemother. Rep. 14:93, 1961.
74. Kaplowitz N, and Kuhlenkamp J: Inhibition of hepatic metabolism of azathioprine *in vivo*. Gastroenterology 74:90, 1978.
75. Watanabe A, Hubara N, and Nagashima H: Demonstration of enzymatic activity converting azathioprine to 6-mercaptopurine. Acta Med. Okayama 32:173, 1978.
76. Rundles RW, Laszlo J, Ituga T, et al.: Clinical and hematological study of 6-[(1-methyl-4-nitro-5-imidazolyl)-thio]purine and related compounds. Cancer Chemother. Rep. 14:99, 1961.
77. Elion GB: Immunosuppressive agents. Transplant. Proc. 9:975, 1975.
78. Dimitriu A, and Fauci AS: Activation of human B lymphocytes. XI. Differential effects of azathioprine on B lymphocytes and lymphocyte subpopulations regulating B cell function. J. Immunol. 121:2335, 1978.
79. Chalmers AH: A spectrophotometric method for the estimation of urinary azathioprine, 6-mercaptopurine and 6-thiouric acid. Biochem. Med. 12:234, 1975.
80. DeMiranda P, Beacham LM III, Creagh TH, et al.: The metabolic disposition of ^{14}C-azathioprine in the dog. J. Pharmacol. Exp. Ther. 195:50, 1975.
81. Elion GB: Significance of azathioprine metabolites. Proc. R. Soc. Med. 65:257, 1972.
81a. Trounce JR: Dosage and pharmacokinetics of cytotoxic drugs. Br. J. Clin. Pharmacol. 8:205, 1979.
82. Chalmers AH, Knight PR, and Atkinson MR: 6-Thiopurines as substrates and inhibitors of purine oxidases: a pathway for conversion of azathioprine into 6-thiouric acid without release of 6-mercaptopurine. Aust. J. Exp. Biol. Med. Sci. 47:263, 1969.
83. Kaplan SR, and Calabresi P: Immunosuppressive agents. N. Engl. J. Med. 289:1234, 1973.
84. American Medical Association Department of Drugs. Azathioprine. AMA Drug Eval., 3rd ed., 1978, p. 1207.
85. Gamelli RL, and Foster RS: Increased azathioprine toxicity after ureteral ligation and nephrectomy. Surg. Forum 29:358, 1978.
86. Herskowitz LJ, Olansky S, and Lang PG: Acute pancreatitis associated with long-term azathioprine therapy. Arch. Dermatol. 115:179, 1979.
87. Dretchen KL, Morgenroth VH III, Standaert FG, et al.: Azathioprine: effects on neuromuscular transmission. Anesthesiology 45:604, 1976.
88. Brandt LJ: Formication and azathioprine therapy. Ann. Intern. Med. 87:458, 1977.
89. Sieber SM, and Adamson RH: Toxicity of antineoplastic agents in man: chromosomal aberrations, antifertility effects, congenital malformations and carcinogenic potential. Adv. Cancer Res. 22:57, 1975.
90. Scharf J, Nahir M, Eidelman S, et al.: Carcinoma of the bladder with azathioprine therapy. J.A.M.A. 237:152, 1977.
91. Gilmore IT, Holden G, and Roden KS: Acute leukemia during azathioprine therapy. Postgrad Med. J. 53:173, 1977.
92. VanWent GF: Investigations into the mutagenic activity of azathioprine (Imuran) in different test systems. Mutat. Res. 68:153, 1979.
93. Harrap KR, and Paine RM: Use of a regulatory effector as a potential antitumour agent. *In* Davis W, and Harrap KR (eds.): Advances in Tumour Prevention, Detection and Characterization, Vol. 4. Characterization and Treatment of Human Tumours. Proceedings of the Seventh International Symposium on the Biological Characterization of Human Tumours. Excerpta Medica, Amsterdam, 1978, pp. 239–246.
94. Bodey GP, Gottlieb J, McCredie KB, et al.: Arabinosyl adenine (ara-A) as an antitumor agent. Proc. Am. Assoc. Cancer Res. 15:129, 1974.
95. LePage GA, and Khaliq A: Responses of patients to arabinosyladenine-5′-phosphate correlated with an *in vitro* test. Adv. Enzyme Regul. 17:437, 1978.
96. Pavan-Langston D, Buchanan RA, and Alford CA Jr (eds.): Adenine Arabinoside: An Antiviral Agent. Raven Press, New York, 1975.
97. LePage GA: Purine arabinosides, xylosides and lyxosides. *In* Sartorelli AC, and Johns DG (eds.): Antineoplastic and Immunosuppressive Agents, Vol. II. Springer-Verlag, New York–Heidelberg, 1975, pp. 426–433.
98. Suhadolnik RJ: Naturally occurring nucleoside and nucleotide antibiotics. Prog. Nucleic Acid Res. Mol. Biol. 22:193, 1979.
99. Agarwal RP, Sagar SM, and Parks RE Jr.: Adenosine deaminase from human erythrocytes. Biochem. Pharmacol. 24:693, 1975.
100. LePage GA: Alterations in enzyme activity in tumors and the implications for chemotherapy. Adv. Enzyme Regul. 8:323, 1969.
101. LePage GA, Naik SR, Katakkar SB, et al.: 9-β-D-Arabinofuranosyladenine 5′-phosphate metabolism and excretion in humans. Cancer Res. 35:3036, 1975.
102. Lee WW, Benitez A, Goodman L, et al.: Potential anticancer agents. XL. Synthesis of the β-anomer of 9-(D-arabinofuranosyl) adenine J. Am. Chem. Soc. 82:2648, 1960.
103. Shannon WM: Adenine arabinoside: antiviral activity *in vitro*. *In* Pavan-Langston D, Buchanan RA, and Alford CA Jr (eds.): Adenine Arabinoside: An Antiviral Agent. Raven Press, New York, 1975, pp. 1–43.
104. Plunkett W, and Cohen SS: Increased toxicity of 9-β-D-arabinofuranosyladenine in the presence of an inhibitor of adenosine deaminase. Ann. N.Y. Acad. Sci. 284:91, 1977.
105. York JL, and LePage GA: A proposed mechanism for the action of 9-β-D-arabinofuranosyladenine as an inhibitor of the growth of some ascites cells. Can. J. Biochem. 44:19, 1966.
106. Furth JJ, and Cohen SS: Inhibition of mammalian DNA polymerase by the 5′-triphosphate of 9-β-D-arabinofuranosyladenine. Cancer Res. 27:1528, 1967.
107. Müller WEG, Zahn RK, Bittlingmaier K, et al.: Inhibition of herpesvirus DNA synthesis by 9-β-D-arabinofuranosyladenine in cellular and cell-free systems. Ann. N.Y. Acad. Sci. 284:34, 1977.
108. Plunkett W, Lapi L, Ortiz PJ, et al.: Penetration of mouse fibroblasts by the 5′-phosphate of 9-β-D-arabinofuranosyladenine and incorporation of the nucleoside into DNA. Proc. Natl. Acad. Sci. USA 71:73, 1974.
109. Furth JJ, and Cohen SS: Inhibition of mammalian DNA polymerase by the 5′-triphosphate of 1-β-D-arabinofuranosylcytosine and the 5′-triphosphate of 9-β-D-arabinofuranosyladenine. Cancer Res. 28:2061, 1968.
110. Bell DE, and Fridland A: Mode of action of 9-β-D-arabinosyladenine on DNA synthesis in human lymphoblasts. Biochim. Biophys. Acta 606:57, 1980.
111. Chang CH, and Cheng YC: Effects of deoxyadenosine triphosphate and 9-β-D-arabinofuranosyladenine 5′-triphosphate on human ribonucleotide reductase from molt-4F cells and the concept of "self-potentiation." Cancer Res. 40:3555, 1980.

112. Hersfield MS: Apparent suicide inactivation of human lymphoblast S-adenosylhomocysteine hydrolase by 2′-deoxyadenosine and adenine arabinoside. J. Biol. Chem. 254:22, 1979.
113. Ho DHW, ,Pincus C, Carter CJ, et al.: Distribution and inhibition of adenosine deaminase in tissues of man, rat, and mouse. Cancer Treat. Rep. 64:629, 1980.
114. LePage GA, Worth LS, and Kimball AP: Enhancement of the antitumor activity of arabinofuranosyladenine by 2′-deoxycoformycin. Cancer Res. 36:1481, 1976.
115. Johns DG, and Adamson RH: Enhancement of the biological activity of cordycepin (3′-deoxyadenosine) by the adenosine deaminase inhibitor 2′-deoxycoformycin. Biochem. Pharmacol. 25:1441, 1976.
116. Adamson RH, Zaharevitz DW, and Johns DG: Enhancement of the biological activity of adenosine analogs by the adenosine deaminase inhibitor 2′-deoxycoformycin. Pharmacology 15:84, 1977.
117. Juranka P, and Chan VL: Relative cytotoxicity of 9-β-D-arabinofuranosyladenine and 9-β-D-arabinofuranosyladenine 5′-monophosphate. Cancer Res. 40:4123, 1980.
118. LePage GA: Resistance to 9-β-D-arabinofuranosyladenine in murine tumor cells. Cancer Res. 38:2314, 1978.
119. Alford CA Jr: Summary of parenteral use of adenine arabinoside. *In* Pavan-Langston D, Buchanan RA, and Alford CA Jr (eds.): Adenine Arabinoside: An Antiviral Agent. Raven Press, New York, 1975, pp. 287–291.
120. Bodey GP, Gottlieb J, McCredie KB, et al.: Adenine arabinoside in cancer chemotherapy. *In* Pavan-Langston D, Buchanan RA, and Alford CA Jr (eds.): Adenine Arabinoside: An Antiviral Agent. Raven Press, New York, 1975, pp. 281–285.
121. LePage GA, and Khaliq A: Responses of patients to arabinosyladenine-5′-phosphate correlated with an *in vitro* test. Adv. Enzyme Regul. 17:437, 1979.
121a. Montgomery JA, and Hewson K: Nucleosides of 2-fluoroadenosine. J. Med. Chem. 12:498, 1969.
122. Brockman RW, Cheng YC, Schabel FM, et al.: Metabolism and chemotherapeutic activity of 9-β-D-arabinofuranosyl-2-fluoradenine against murine leukemia L1210 and evidence for its phosphorylation by deoxycytidine kinase. Cancer Res. 40:3610, 1980.
123. Plunkett W, Chubb S, Alexander L, et al.: Comparison of the toxicity and metabolism of 9-β-D-arabinofuranosyl-2-fluoroadenine and 9-β-D-arabinofuranosyladenine in human lymphoblastoid cells. Cancer Res. 40:2349, 1980.
124. Lee SH, Unger FM, Christian R, et al.: Cytotoxic activity of the adenine arabinoside analogs, 2′-azido- and 2′-amino-2′-deoxy-β-D-arabinofuranosyladenine. Biochem. Pharmacol. 28:1267, 1979.
125. De Clercq E, Balzrini J, Descamps J, et al.: Antiviral, antimetabolic and antineoplastic activities of 2′- or 3′-amino or -azido-substituted deoxyribonucleosides. Biochem. Pharmacol. 29:1849, 1980.
126. Lim MI, and Klein RS: Synthesis of "9-deazaadenosine"; a new cytotoxic C-nucleoside isostere of adenosine. Tetra. Lett. 22:25, 1981.
127. Wortmann RL, Mitchell BS, Edwards NL, et al.: Biochemical basis for differential deoxyadenosine toxicity to T and B lymphoblasts: role for 5′-nucleotidase. Proc. Natl. Acad. Sci. USA 76:2434, 1979.
128. Plunkett W, Alexander L, Chubb S, et al.: Biochemical basis of the increased activity of 9-β-D-arabinofuranosyladenine in the presence of inhibitors of adenosine deaminase. Cancer Res. 39:3655, 1979.
129. Smyth JF, Poplack DG, Holiman BJ, et al.: Correlation of adenosine deaminase activity with cell surface markers in acute lymphoblastic leukemia. J. Clin. Invest. 62:710, 1978.
130. Agarwal RP, Spector T, and Parks RE Jr: Tight-binding inhibitors. IV. Inhibition of adenosine deaminase by various inhibitors. Biochem. Pharmacol. 26:359, 1977.
131. Chassin MM, Adamson RH, Zaharevitz DW, et al.: Enzyme inhibition titration assay for 2′-deoxycoformycin and its application to the study of the relationship between drug concentration and tissue adenosine deaminase in dogs and rats. Biochem. Pharmacol. 28:1849, 1979.
132. McConnell WR, Suling WJ, Rice LS, et al.: Use of microbiologic and enzymatic assays in studies on the disposition of 2′-deoxycoformycin in the mouse. Cancer Treat. Rep. 62:1153, 1978.
133. Borondy PE, Chang T, Maschewske E, et al.: Inhibition of adenosine deaminase by co-vidarabine and its effect on the metabolic disposition of adenine arabinoside (vidarabine). Ann. N.Y. Acad. Sci. 284:9, 1977.
134. Schaeffer HJ, and Schwender CF: Enzyme inhibitors. 26. Bridging hydrophobic and hydrophilic regions on adenosine deaminase with some 9-(2-hydroxy-3-alkyl)-adenines. J. Med. Chem. 17:6, 1974.
135. Adamson RH, Chassin MM, Chirigos MA, et al.: Some aspects of the pharmacology of the adenosine deaminase inhibitors 2′-deoxycoformycin and erthro-9-(2′-hydroxy-3-nonyl)-adenine. *In* Siegenthaler W, and Lüthy R (eds.): Current Chemotherapy: Proceedings of the 10th International Congress of Chemotherapy, Vol. II. American Society for Microbiology, Washington, 1978, pp. 1116–1118.
136. Smyth JF, Paine RM, Jackman AL, et al.: The clinical pharmacology of the adenosine deaminase inhibitor 2′-deoxycoformycin. Cancer Chemother. Pharmacol. 5:93, 1980.
137. Grever MR, Siaw MFE, Jacob WF, et al.: The biochemical and clinical consequences of 2′-deoxycoformycin in refractory lymphoproliferative malignancy. Blood 57:406, 1981.
138. Poplack DG, Sallan SE, Rivera G, et al.: Phase I study of 2′-deoxycoformycin in acute lymphoblastic leukemia. Cancer Res. 41:3343, 1981.
139. Major PP, Agarwal RP, and Kufe DW: Clinical pharmacology of deoxycoformycin. Blood 58:91, 1981.

METHOTREXATE

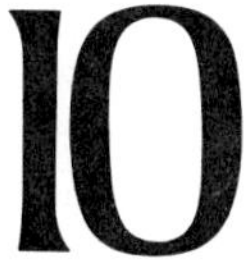

Bruce A. Chabner

INTRODUCTION

The folic acid vitamins present a particularly attractive target for the design of antitumor chemotherapy because of their role in the synthesis of DNA precursors. Reduced forms of folic acid (called tetrahydrofolates) are required for synthesis of both purines and pyrimidine, as shown in Figure 10–1. N^{10}-formyl-tetrahydrofolate and $N^{5\text{-}10}$-methenyltetrahydrofolate contribute their labile one-carbon groups to the synthesis of inosinic acid, the precursor of adenylate (AMP) and guanylate (GMP). In a second important synthetic pathway, $N^{5\text{-}10}$-methylenetetrahydrofolate provides a methyl group and two hydrogens for the synthesis of thymidylate (dTMP) from deoxyuridylate (dUMP). Farber and associates reasoned that analogues of folic acid might have inhibitory effects on the proliferation of malignant cells, a hypothesis confirmed by the initial trials of aminopterin (2,4-diamino,4-deoxy-folic acid) (Fig. 10–2) in 1948.[1] This compound has since been supplanted in clinical usage by its N^{10}-methyl derivative, methotrexate (MTX). The pharmacologic properties of this latter agent have been extensively studied and it is probably the best understood of the cancer chemotherapeutic drugs.

MECHANISM OF ACTION

The critical structural change that leads to antitumor activity of folate analogues is the substitution of an amino group for the hydroxyl at the 4 position of the pteridine ring. This single change transforms the folate molecule from substrate to a tight-binding inhibitor of the key enzyme in intracellular folate metabolism, dihydrofolate reductase (Fig. 10–1).

In order to understand the action of methotrexate and other antifolates, it is necessary to appreciate the critical role of this enzyme in folate metabolism. Folic acid compounds are active as coenzymes only in their fully reduced form as tetrahydrofolates. In the thymidylate synthesis reaction, shown in Figure 10–1, $N^{5\text{-}10}$-methylenetetrahydrofolic acid is converted to dihydrofolic acid. This inactive cofactor then becomes a substrate for dihydrofolate reductase, which transfers two hydrogen atoms from the cofactor NADPH to dihydrofolic acid to form tetrahydrofolic acid. In cells with rapidly ongoing thymidylate synthesis, inhibition of dihydrofolate reductase by MTX or similar analogues leads to accumulation of folate cofactors in the inactive form of dihydrofolic acid, with resultant inhibition of the synthesis of both purines and thymidylate.

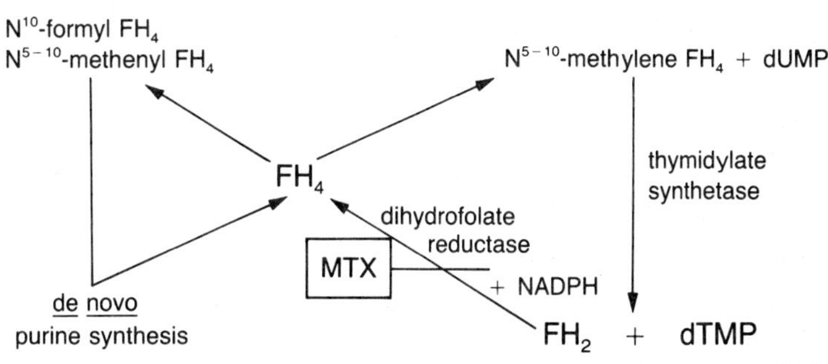

Figure 10–1. Central role of dihydrofolate reductase in maintaining intracellular pool of tetrahydrofolic acid (FH_4). FH_4 serves as a source for the active folate cofactors required for synthesis of purines and pyrimidines. Methotrexate (MTX) inhibits the reductase reaction, leading to accumulation of intracellular folates as FH_2.

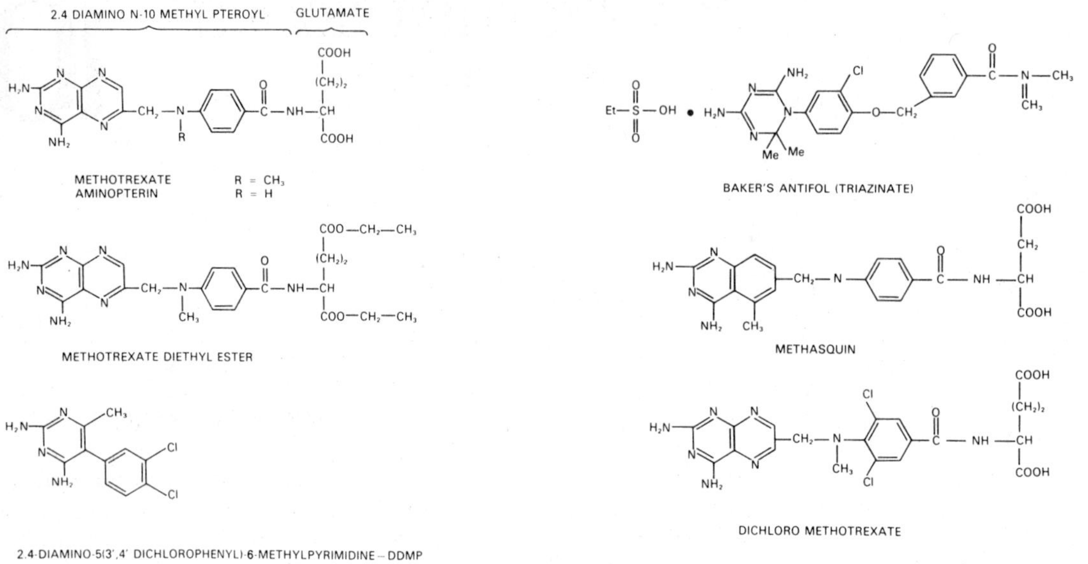

Figure 10–2. Folate analogues of clinical interest. Addition of glutamate groups in peptide linkage to the γ-carboxyl group of methotrexate creates polyglutamate derivatives, which are also potent inhibitors of dihydrofolate reductase.

Chemical Structure

A variety of heterocyclic ring structures with the 2,4-diamino configuration (Fig. 10–2) have antifolate activity, including diaminopyrimidines such as pyrimethamine (Daraprim), trimethoprim, DDMP, and DAMP[2, 2A, 3]; triazinates[4]; quinazolines such as methasquin*[5]; esters of MTX[6]; and halogenated derivatives of MTX such as dichloromethotrexate.[7] Many of these compounds inhibit dihydrofolate reductase with a potency equal to or greater than MTX, but none has replaced MTX, primarily because of clinical familiarity with the older agent and the lack of evidence that the newer compounds are capable of circumventing antifolate resistance.

Commercially available MTX contains at least seven impurities, including 4-amino-N^{10}-methyl pteroic acid and N^{10}-methylfolic acid.[8, 9] These impurities constitute 10 to 15 per cent of the administered material and are thought to arise from contaminants present in the bulk products used to synthesize the drug, rather than from degradation of MTX during storage. The possible role of these impurities in the toxicities or therapeutic activity of the clinical formulation is unproved. None have strong reductase inhibiting activity. Improved methods for drug manufacture are now available and it is expected that a purer commercial product will be available in the near future.

CELLULAR PHARMACOLOGY AND MECHANISMS OF RESISTANCE

In this section the sequence of events that lead to the cytotoxic action of MTX will be considered, beginning with drug movement across the cell membrane, followed by its transformation to polyglutamate derivatives, binding to dihydrofolate reductase, depletion of intracellular reduced folates, and inhibition of DNA synthesis. Each of these steps has importance in determining response to treatment and toxicity.

Transmembrane Transport

The movement of MTX and other antifolates across cell membranes has received much attention because of the potential relevance of transport abnormalities to resistance. The general characteristics of mech-

*The quinazoline antifolates also inhibit thymidylate synthetase directly; the 2,4-diamino-5-methyl derivative described by Calvert el al. (Eur. J. Cancer 16:713, 1980) has a K_i of 0.47 μM for this enzyme and a K_i of 0.6 pM for dihydrofolate reductase, and requires both folinic acid and thymidine for rescue, in contrast to the sufficiency of folinic acid alone for rescue of classical antifolates.

anisms for transmembrane movement of drugs and the specific features of antifolate transport are discussed in greater detail in Chapter 2. The classic studies of Goldman et al.[10] established that MTX enters cells by means of an energy-dependent, temperature-sensitive, and concentrative process that likely depends on a specific intramembrane protein. The influx process can be observed in isolated membrane vesicles.[11] Macromolecules that bind folates have been isolated from membranes of mammalian cells,[12] but have no proved role in transport.

The carrier mechanism that transports MTX in murine and human leukemia cells is also utilized by the naturally occurring reduced folates, including the rescue agent 5-formyltetrahydrofolate (leucovorin). Thus, MTX and the reduced folates compete for entry into cells. In addition, through a process known as heteroexchange, free intracellular MTX is forced to efflux from cells when high concentrations of extracellular reduced folate enter the cells.[13]

The affinity of the influx carrier for MTX lies between 1 and 6 μM for various tumor cell lines (both murine and human),[10, 14-16] whereas that of isolated intestinal epithelial cells is somewhat less (Km = 87 μM).[17] This greater affinity of the tumor cell carrier is believed to account for the longer intracellular persistence of unbound drug in tumor as compared with normal epithelial cells, and may contribute to the selectivity of antifolate action against tumor as opposed to normal tissue.

The accumulation of MTX in tumor cells can be influenced by other antitumor agents, including drugs commonly used with the antifolate in combination therapy. Vincristine increases intracellular MTX by inhibiting drug efflux.[18] The concentration of vincristine required to produce this effect (10 μM) is not readily achieved during clinical chemotherapy, which produces peak vincristine blood levels of less than 0.1 μM. MTX influx is inhibited by ouabain, glucocorticoids, and cephalothin,[19] although none of these interactions has been shown to affect clinical chemotherapy.

The proliferative, or kinetic, state of cells strongly influences the transport process.[20] Rapidly proliferating murine leukemia cells have a threefold greater rate of MTX uptake and a decreased rate of drug efflux as compared with cells in the stationary phase of growth. The growth rate dependency of transport may contribute to greater cytotoxicity of MTX for rapidly dividing cells, although increased requirements for reduced folate in phases of rapid growth may also contribute to the relatively greater cytotoxicity.

In addition to the high-affinity active transport process described above, a second entry mechanism comes into play at high drug concentrations (in excess of 20 μM).[15, 21] It is not clear at present whether the second process is merely passive diffusion or a saturable and specific carrier process. Additional features of this second transport process are a lack of competition between MTX and reduced folates for entry, and an absence of heteroexchange of MTX and reduced folates. This second entry mechanism would account for the ability of transport-resistant cells to take up drug at high extracellular concentrations, and provides a rationale for the use of high-dose MTX clinically.

The accumulation and persistence of drug may determine the duration of drug action in specific tissues. Greater peak levels of intracellular drug and much longer persistence of drug were observed in MTX-sensitive murine leukemic cells than in intestinal epithelium (Fig. 10–3), while the resistant sarcoma 180 cell line accumulated lower concentrations of drug, had briefer periods of inhibition of DNA synthesis, and was unaffected by drug in chemotherapy experiments.[22] Specific *in vitro* analysis of drug uptake rates by murine leukemia cells has provided a similar positive correlation between drug response and transport.[23]

Significant differences in drug transport characteristics exist for the various antifolates. The quinazoline antifolates (Fig. 10–2) have a lower rate of efflux and a higher rate of influx than MTX; these differences correlate with the greater intracellular accumulation of the quinazolines, as compared with MTX, after equimolar doses *in vivo*.[24]

The importance of MTX transport in determining clinical response is uncertain. Other resistance mechanisms, particularly an increase in dihydrofolate reductase concentration as the result of gene amplification (see below), have been documented in both human and murine tumors exposed to low concentrations of drug *in vitro*, and may be an equally important mechanism of resistance in clinical practice, but the necessary

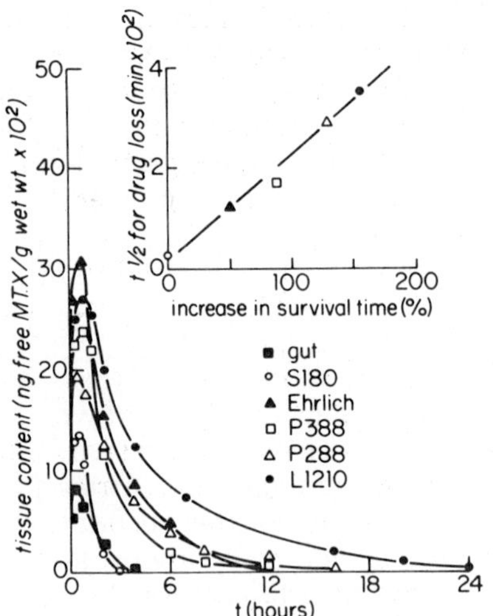

Figure 10–3. Uptake and loss of methotrexate in murine tumor cells and intestinal epithelium after 3 mg/kg dose IP. Each data point represents free intracellular drug concentration. The insert demonstrates correlation of therapeutic result and half-time of drug retention by various tumors. (Reproduced with permission from Sirotnam FM, and Donsbach RC: Further evidence for a basis of selective activity and relative responsiveness during antifolate therapy of murine tumors. Cancer Res. 35:1737–1744, 1975.)

clinical studies of antifolate resistance have not been performed.

New approaches aimed at circumventing resistance due to transport deficiency have been proposed and await clinical testing. Lipid-soluble antifolates such as MTX esters, diaminopyrimidines, and triazinates have excellent antitumor activity in cell culture and in the experimental treatment of rodent tumors, and should penetrate transport-deficient cells. The dibutyl ester of MTX also has the unusual property of inhibiting thymidine incorporation into DNA, apparently owing to an inhibition of nucleoside transport.[25] The diesters of MTX are rapidly hydrolyzed to the parent compound in mouse plasma,[6] but are more stable in the plasma of monkey, dog, and man; when incubated in the latter plasmas, the dibutyl ester is converted to an alpha- or gamma-monobutyl derivative, which is a stable and effective inhibitor of dihydrofolate reductase.[26] The transport properties of the monobutyl ester have not been defined.

Conjugates of MTX and polylysine, which are toxic to transport-deficient hamster ovary cells in culture,[27] also offer promise of overcoming transport resistance. Since the polylysine-MTX conjugate does not itself inhibit dihydrofolate reductase, it is likely that the compound undergoes intracellular cleavage to liberate the antifolate.

Intracellular Transformation

Although most MTX is eliminated unchanged after administration to animals or man, a small fraction undergoes polyglutamation in normal and malignant cells. The addition of glutamate groups to the terminal glutamic acid of naturally occurring folic acid cofactors is known to occur in many mammalian tissues; this reaction appears to serve as a mechanism for retaining these cofactors within the cell in a less readily transported form and increases cofactor affinity for important enzymes such as thymidylate synthetase. MTX may also undergo polyglutamation (Fig. 10–2), with addition of one to four additional glutamate groups.[27A] This transformation occurs in various tissues, including normal human liver[28, 28A] cultured human fibroblasts,[29] human breast cancer cells,[30] and murine leukemia cells.[31] In human breast cancer cells continuously incubated with MTX, the percentage of intracellular drug found in the polyglutamate form increases with time, reaching approximately 80 per cent at 24 hours.[30] Much of the drug bound to reductase at this time is in the form of polyglutamate rather than the parent compound. The mono- and di-glutamyl derivatives have at least equal inhibitory potency for dihydrofolate reductase,[32] although their binding kinetics have not been carefully evaluated.

The monoglutamate of MTX (methotrexate plus one glutamate or MTX-G_1) penetrates cells by active transport, but in L1210 cells has a maximal uptake velocity only 1/15th that of methotrexate.[33] Once inside the cell, it slowly undergoes deglutamation. The Km for MTX-G_1 influx is 50 μM in L1210 cells or 16-fold higher than MTX. The ability of polyglutamates to leave cells is controversial. Mono- and diglutamates are detected in the culture medium after preloading of L1210 cells with MTX but it is uncertain that the higher polyglutamates are able to leave the cell.[33A]

Polyglutamation has potential importance as a determinant of response to antifolate chemotherapy. Formation of polyglutamates in cultured human fibroblasts leads to a prolonged inhibition of ^{3}H-UdR incorporation into DNA when cells are resuspended in drug-free medium.[31] It remains to be established whether this prolonged inhibition by polyglutamates results from their greater affinity for dihydrofolate reductase,[32] or from their selective retention within tumor cells in the absence of free extracellular drug,[28A, 29] as has been suggested by preliminary work. Mono- and diglutamates of MTX can be detected in the culture medium of cells during an efflux period following exposure to MTX, but the rate of exit of these compounds has not been characterized.[33A]

The enzyme that converts folate and folate analogues to polyglutamates (folyl polyglutamate synthetase) has been partially purified from liver,[34] which forms MTX polyglutamates rapidly[35] and retains these compounds for months after drug administration.[28] The hepatic enzyme has higher affinity for MTX as substrate than for folic acid, apparently owing to the 4-NH_2 substituent. The enzyme adds glutamates to other folic acid analogues as well, including aminopterin and 5-methyltetrahydro-homofolate. The accumulation of MTX polyglutamates reduces polyglutamation of naturally occurring folates in rat liver,[36] an effect of possible importance in chronic hepatic toxicity of MTX.

Binding to Dihydrofolate Reductase

The physical characteristics of binding of NADPH and MTX to dihydrofolate reductase have been established by x-ray crystallographic studies and amino acid sequencing of native and chemically modified enzyme. Enzymes from both bacterial and mammalian sources have been studied[35-42]; the amino acid sequences, as shown in Figure 10–4, have striking similarities in positions implicated in cofactor and inhibitor binding.[43] In general, a long hydrophobic pocket binds MTX and is formed in part by the isoleucine-(or leucine)-7, alanine-9, leucine-31, phenylalanine-34, and other residues. Two particularly important interactions contribute to the binding potency of the 4-amino antifolates: (1) the carbonyl oxygen of isoleucine-7 is hydrogen bonded to the 4-amino group of the inhibitor; and (2) the carboxyl group of aspartate- (or glutamate)-30 protonates the N-1 position of MTX, but does not bind to the physiologic substrates. In addition, the physiologic substrates seem to be bound to the enzyme in an inverted, or

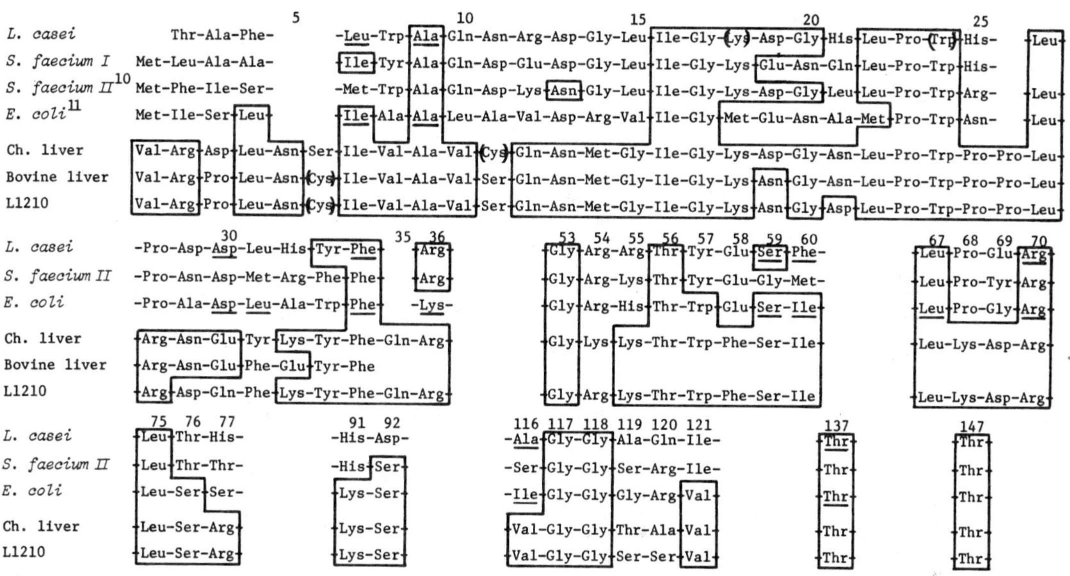

Figure 10–4. Amino acid sequence of dihydrofolate reductase from various bacterial and animal sources. Amino acids are numbered according to chicken liver sequence and gaps are inserted to maximize homology. Residues implicated in binding to methotrexate are underlined. Homologous regions are enclosed in solid line. (Reproduced with permission from Freisheim et al.: Structure-function relationships of dihydrofolate reductases: sequence homology considerations and active center residues. *In* Kisliuk RL, and Brown GM (eds.): Chemistry and Biology of Pteridines. Elsevier, North Holland, New York, 1979, pp. 419–424.

"upside down," configuration as compared with the inhibitor.[41] The reader is referred to more detailed reviews of this subject for consideration of substrate and cofactor binding characteristics.[40, 41, 43]

In the presence of excess NADPH, the binding affinity of MTX for reductase has been estimated to lie between 1 nM and 1 pM,[44] although this affinity is significantly affected by pH, salt concentration, and the status of enzyme sulfhydryl groups. Under conditions of low pH and with a low ratio of inhibitor to enzyme, binding is essentially stoichiometric[45]; i.e., each molecule of MTX will be bound to one molecule of enzyme. The enzyme–NADPH–inhibitor complex is extremely stable, surviving gel electrophoresis and gel filtration.

Binding of MTX to the reductase from S. *faecium* generates a slowly formed complex with an inhibitor K_i of 5.8×10^{-11}M.[41] The overall process has been termed slow, tight-binding inhibition.[46, 47] Other folate analogues, including the diaminopyrimidines trimethoprim and aminopterin, follow the same "slow, tight-binding" kinetic process, whereas pteridines lacking the aminobenzoic acid group behave as classic competitive inhibitors of the enzyme.

In the therapeutic setting, MTX acts as a tight-binding but reversible inhibitor. Under conditions of high concentrations of competitive substrate (dihydrofolate) and at normal intracellular pH, a considerable excess of free drug is required to inhibit the enzyme fully. In cell culture and in cell-free systems, ^{3}H-MTX bound to intracellular enzyme can be displaced by exposure of cells to unlabeled drug, indicating a slow but definite "off-rate" or dissociation of MTX from the enzyme.[48, 49] This off-rate is tenfold faster than calculated in experiments utilizing purified enzyme in the presence of excess NADPH. The reason is unclear, but this difference may be the result of differences in the ionic environment or may be due to involvement of drug in lower-affinity complexes with enzyme and $NADP^+$ or with enzyme alone. Thus, an excess of "free," or unbound, drug is required to maintain total inhibition of dihydrofolate reductase and to halt thymidylate synthesis.[30] For example, if one incubates tumor cells with high concentrations of the drug to allow total titration of the enzyme, and then removes the unbound drug from solution, thymidylate synthesis will resume immediately despite the persistence of intracellular drug bound to the enzyme.

These observations indicate that, in the

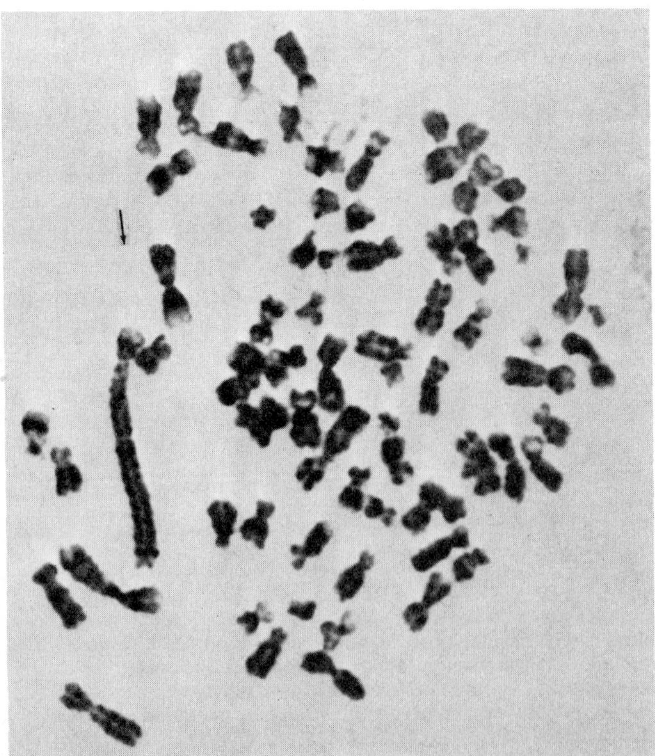

Figure 10–5. Marker chromosomes found in methotrexate-resistant breast cancer cells. A human breast cancer cell line, MCF-7, resistant to methotrexate was isolated by growing cells in gradually increasing drug concentrations. These cells are resistant to drug concentrations greater than 200-fold those that kill wild type cells, and contain more than 30-fold increases in dihydrofolate reductase. The arrow indicates a marker chromosome with a greatly expanded homogeneously staining region. (Photograph courtesy of Cowan K, Lippman M, and Douglas P, National Cancer Institute, Bethesda, MD 20205.)

absence of free drug, a small fraction of intracellular reductase, either through new synthesis or perhaps through dissociation from the inhibitor, becomes available for catalytic activity and is adequate to restore tetrahydrofolate pools in the cell. The requirement for excess free drug to inhibit enzyme activity completely is extremely important in understanding the clinical effects and toxicity of this agent, and will be the foundation for our understanding of the relationship between pharmacokinetics and toxicity.

Jackson et al. have reported a close correlation between initial drug sensitivity and the affinity of drug binding to reductase for a series of murine leukemias of varying responsiveness to MTX.[44] However, resistance induced by treatment with MTX is not clearly related to changes in enzyme binding affinity. A more common finding in resistant cells is an increase in total enzyme activity with no change in affinity.[51] Elevated enzyme concentrations may be detected by assay of a homogenate of tumor cells or by labeling of the enzyme with a fluorescent MTX derivative. The latter procedure allows separation of high-reductase mutants by a fluorescence-activated cell sorter.[52] This elevation in enzyme activity may be partially explained by a decreased rate of catabolism of enzyme bound to drug,[53] but these elevated enzyme levels persist for many generations of cell renewal in tumor cells from resistant patients.[54] In resistant murine leukemic cells the increased reductase activity results from reduplication of the dihydrofolate reductase gene (Fig. 10–5), a process that can be reproduced by exposing cells in culture to stepwise increases in drug concentration.[52,55,55A] Gene reduplication is a stable property in some cell lines and is associated with the presence of new pieces of chromosomal material called double minutes, which may become integrated into larger chromosomes and appear as new, homogeneously staining regions[56] (Fig. 10–5). In other cell lines, double minutes do not become integrated into larger chromosomes, and a reversion to the original low-reductase genotype occurs in the absence of drug. The occurrence of this unique mode of resistance, called "gene amplification," suggests that gene reduplication may be going on continuously in normal and malignant cells, but only becomes apparent in the presence of selective pressures, such as cytotoxic drug exposure. Gene amplification has also been detected as a mechanism of resistance to the new pyrimidine antagonist and aspartate transcarbamylase inhibitor, PALA (phosphonoacetyl-L-aspartic acid.)[57]

Although increased reductase levels account for resistance to MTX in cell lines exposed to graded increases in drug concentration *in vitro,* this mechanism is only one of several changes observed in resistant cells. Some resistant cell lines contain a second species of enzyme of somewhat lower molecular weight (20,000 daltons versus 21,000 for the native enzyme)[58]; this lower-molecular-weight enzyme is amplified in the resistant cells.[58A,58B] Other cell lines have a deficient transport system in addition to elevated enzyme levels, and this transport deficiency appears to be responsible for resistance, since hybridization of the resistant cells with a sensitive line resulted in a drug-sensitive hybrid with an intact transport capability and elevated enzyme concentrations.[59] Flintoff and Essani have described MTX-resistant cells that contain amplified levels of a reductase that has lower binding affinity for MTX.[59A]

Cline and associates have made novel use of the amplified dihydrofolate reductase gene.[60] They have transferred calcium phosphate precipitates of genetic material from MTX-resistant tumor cells to normal mouse bone marrow cells, thus creating a drug-resistant normal hematopoietic cell line that can then be selected out in recipient mice by exposure to the drug. After infusion of transfected marrow, recipient mice become tolerant to drug doses that produce marrow hypoplasia in control animals. These experiments have far-reaching implications for cancer chemotherapy as well as genetic engineering. They suggest the possibility of transferring dihydrofolate reductase genes to the hematopoietic stem cells of cancer patients in order to increase their tolerance to chemotherapy, and, second, insertion of "drug-resistance" genes coupled to genes coding for proteins that might correct inborn errors of metabolism such as immunodeficiency or hemoglobinopathy. These experiments will require the use of MTX for the *in vivo* selection of transformed cells.

Consequences of Reductase Inhibition

The critical result produced by MTX inhibition of dihydrofolate reductase is the depletion of intracellular-reduced folate pools;

owing to ongoing thymidylate synthesis (Fig. 10–1), $N^{5\text{-}10}$-methylenetetrahydrofolate is converted to dihydrofolate, but cannot be recycled to the reduced tetrahydrofolate form, and intracellular folates accumulate as inactive dihydrofolate. The biosynthesis of both thymidylate and purines requires reduced folate cofactors, although thymidylate synthesis is more sensitive to a drop in the intracellular-reduced folate pool. Zaharko and colleagues have shown that in mouse bone marrow a block in thymidylate synthesis was established by MTX concentrations of 10^{-8}M or greater, whereas inhibition of purine synthesis occurred only at drug levels of 10^{-7}M or higher.[61] These findings imply that purine synthesis may be conserved at the expense of thymidylate synthesis, under conditions of minimal folate depletion. Further work with human breast cancer cells in culture has confirmed this difference in sensitivity of the two folate-dependent pathways.[62]

The antipurine effect of MTX appears to be a function of the growth rate of cells. In an examination of four hepatoma cell lines of differing growth rate, the most rapidly proliferating cells were most sensitive to the combination of MTX and thymidine, a combination that should allow isolated inhibition of purine synthesis. The slowest growing cells were least sensitive to this combination.[63] In addition, differences in sensitivity to antipurine effects are found among rapidly growing tumor cells. Tattersall et al. noted that the antipurine effect correlated with the relative cellular activities of $N^{5\text{-}10}$-methylenetetrahydrofolate dehydrogenase and thymidylate synthetase.[64] Cells with higher dehydrogenase activity, and presumably greater purine synthesis, showed greater sensitivity to the antipurine effects of MTX. The former enzyme converts 5,10-methylenetetrahydrofolate to $N^{5\text{-}10}$-methenyltetrahydrofolate, one of two folates required for purine biosynthesis. The relative activities of these enzymes may determine the distribution of intracellular-reduced folates and, ultimately, the relative vulnerability of the purine versus pyrimidine pathways to folate depletion.

On the basis of the multiple effects of antifolates on nucleotide biosynthesis, several ultimate mechanisms of cell death have been proposed. Thymidine triphosphate (dTTP) and deoxypurine nucleotides are required for both the synthesis of DNA and its repair. Inhibition of thymidylate and purine synthesis leads to a cessation of DNA synthesis, but it is unclear that this inhibition by itself kills cells. It is doubtful whether MTX inhibition of DNA repair synthesis is sufficient to explain cytotoxicity since the drug has little effect on nondividing cells.

Another hypothesis that seeks to explain MTX cytotoxicity concerns the increase in intracellular dUMP that occurs as a consequence of inhibition of thymidylate synthesis. It is clear that the high concentrations of dUMP may lead to substitution of uracil for thymine in DNA; in the presence of 10 μM MTX, human lymphoblasts incorporate about 1 pmole of dUMP per μmole DNA.[65, 66] A specific enzyme, uracil-DNA-glycosylase, excises uracil bases from DNA, a process that may be responsible for the fragments of DNA observed in cells with high levels of uracil incorporation.[67] Although this theory has afforded new insight into the potential and consequences of uracil incorporation into DNA, it does not explain the marked toxicity of MTX-thymidine combinations, which must act through an antipurine effect.

Pharmacokinetic and Cytokinetic Determinants of Cytotoxicity

At least two pharmacokinetic factors — drug concentration and duration of cell exposure — are critical determinants of cytotoxicity. In tissue culture and in intact animals, extracellular drug concentrations of 1 $\times$ 10^{-8}M are required to inhibit thymidylate synthesis in normal bone marrow. This same drug concentration is associated with depletion of bone marrow cellularity if maintained for 24 hours or longer. The rate of cell loss from murine bone marrow increases with increasing drug concentrations up to 1 $\times$ 10^{-5}M (Fig. 10–6). Similar findings have been reported in studies of murine tumor cells. In addition to drug concentration, the duration of tissue exposure is a critical factor in determining cell death. For a given dose of drug, cell loss is approximately proportional to the time period of exposure. This relationship is likely the result of the S-phase specificity of MTX. With longer durations of exposure, more cells are allowed to enter the vulnerable DNA synthetic phase of the cell cycle.

The cytotoxic effects of MTX on murine bone marrow are mitigated at drug concen-

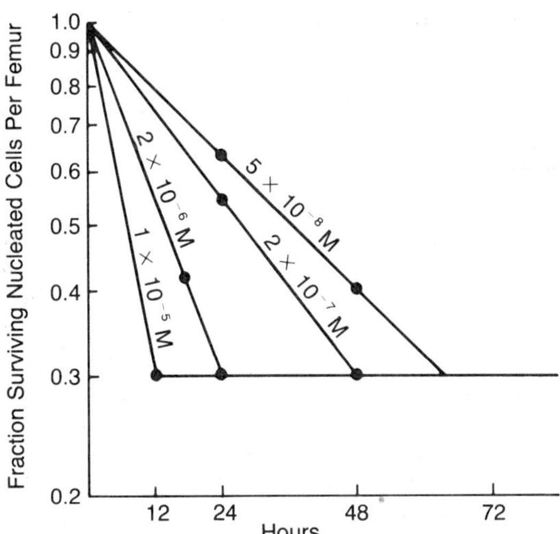

Figure 10–6. Nucleated cells per femur remaining after constant infusion of methotrexate into mice to achieve indicated drug concentration for various periods of time. (Reproduced with permission from Pinedo et al.: The relative contribution of drug concentration and duration of exposure to mouse bone marrow toxicity during continuous methotrexate infusion. Cancer Res. 37:445–450, 1977.)

trations above 1 μM by recruitment of uncommitted precursor cells (CFU-S) into myeloid colony formation.[69] It is not known whether similar recruitment occurs in malignant cell populations in response to MTX.

The time and concentration correlates of cytotoxicity for human tumor cells are poorly understood. Hryniuk and Bertino found variable inhibition of thymidylate synthetase by human leukemic cells in short-term culture when these cells were exposed to 1 μM MTX for one hour or less.[70] More extensive investigation of these parameters is now possible with the improvement in technology for growth of human tumors *in vitro*.

In addition to pharmacokinetic and cytokinetic factors, physiologic compounds in the cellular environment may profoundly affect the cytotoxicity of MTX. Most prominent among these factors are the naturally occurring purine bases and nucleosides, and thymidine. As discussed previously, in bone marrow and intestinal epithleium both thymidylate and *de novo* purine synthesis are blocked by concentrations of MTX above 0.1 μM, but cells can survive this block if bone marrow is supplied with 10 μM thymidine and a purine source (adenosine, inosine, or hypoxanthine) in similar concentrations. Thymidine alone was not capable of reversing the MTX effect.[71] Thymidine levels in plasma of man have been reported to be approximately 0.2 μM,[72] while the concentration of the purine bases and nucleosides was somewhat higher (0.5 μM).[73] Thus, under basal conditions, neither the purines nor the thymidine concentration would be adequate to rescue cells. However, pharmacologic intervention, such as allopurinol (which elevates circulating hypoxanthine concentrations), and chemotherapy, with attendant tumor lysis, might well raise levels of these compounds and ameliorate toxicity to tumor or host tissues. These possibilities have not been adequately investigated at present.

In an effort to improve MTX antitumor activity and reduce its toxicity to normal tissue, investigators have tested combinations of MTX and thymidine in animals and man. This combination is based on the rationale that normal tissues might be less sensitive to the antipurine effects of MTX and might have greater ability to utilize thymidine than do tumor cells.* In non–tumor-bearing animals, thymidine is ineffective in reversing or preventing toxicity to normal tissues, probably owing to the low concentrations of circulating purines.[74] In tumor-bearing animals, thymidine rescue does ameliorate host toxicity, and the combination produces results superior to those of MTX alone in selected test systems.[75, 76] The toxic and therapeutic results of clinical trials of this combination clearly indicate that antifolate toxicity is lessened in man by thymidine, but the therapeutic value of the combination remains in doubt. These results are discussed in greater detail in a subsequent section of this chapter.

A third factor of importance in determining antifolate effect is the concentration of reduced folate in the circulation. 5-Methyltetrahydrofolate (the predominant circulating folate cofactor), if present in sufficient concentration, can readily reverse MTX toxicity,[77] as can 5-formyltetrahydro-

*Jackson has shown that if cells are exposed to thymidine prior to MTX, the high levels of intracellular dTTP formed inhibit ribonucleotide reductase, lower the intracellular pool of dUMP, and inhibit the consumption of reduced folates in the thymidylate synthetase reaction.[73A] The antipurine effect of MTX is negated in this sequence. If, however, MTX is administered first, the reduced folate pool is depleted and the antipurine effect is established. Subsequent exposure to thymidine only reverses the antithymidylate action of MTX.

folate, also known as leucovorin.[78] Circulating levels of 5-methyltetrahydrofolate are approximately 0.01 μM and are inadequate to reverse the effect of higher concentrations of MTX achieved by most clinical regimens. Exogenously administered reduced folates are able to reverse MTX toxicity in a competitive manner. Leucovorin is commonly used after MTX administration to reduce or prevent toxicity, and is effective if the duration of MTX treatment has been less than 48 hours. The concentration of 5-formyltetrahydrofolate required to prevent MTX toxicity increases as the drug concentration increases.[71] This competitive relationship is illustrated in Figure 10–7. The reasons for this competition are not clear, although it is known that MTX and leucovorin share a common transport mechanism across cell membranes. A second reason for the competitive relationship may be that leucovorin is rapidly converted to dihydrofolate in the process of thymidylate synthesis, and as the dihydrofolate pool builds, the binding of methotrexate gradually is reversed.[133] At high concentrations of MTX (greater than 10 μM), the competitive rescue relationship no longer holds true. Leucovorin in 100-fold greater concentrations (1 mM) is unable to protect bone marrow cells, a finding that bears on the failure of leucovorin rescue in the occasional patient with exceedingly high concentrations of circulating drug.

METHOTREXATE ASSAY

Two methods exist for assay of MTX: those based on its tight binding to dihydrofolate reductase, and those that depend on antibody-drug interactions. Both procedures provide extremely sensitive measurement at levels of 10^{-8}M or less in biologic fluids, but there are significant differences in the time required for their performance and their specificity for parent compound as opposed to metabolites. The first widely used method,[79] the enzyme inhibition assay, measures MTX concentration by determining the ability of a clinical sample to inhibit dihydrofolate reductase enzyme activity. This method requires the availability of the enzyme and a recording spectrophotometer; samples are assayed in sequence, and serial dilutions of the sample must be tested in order to find a dilution that inhibits enzyme in a readable range of 25 to 75 per cent inhibition. Thus, the enzyme inhibition assay is time-consuming and impractical if results must be reported on the same day.

A competitive binding assay that utilizes dihydrofolate reductase as the binding protein has since been developed, and preserves the advantages of specificity for parent compound found in the enzyme inhibition assay. In the binding assay, MTX in a biologic sample competes for reductase binding sites with a known quantity of radiolabeled drug.

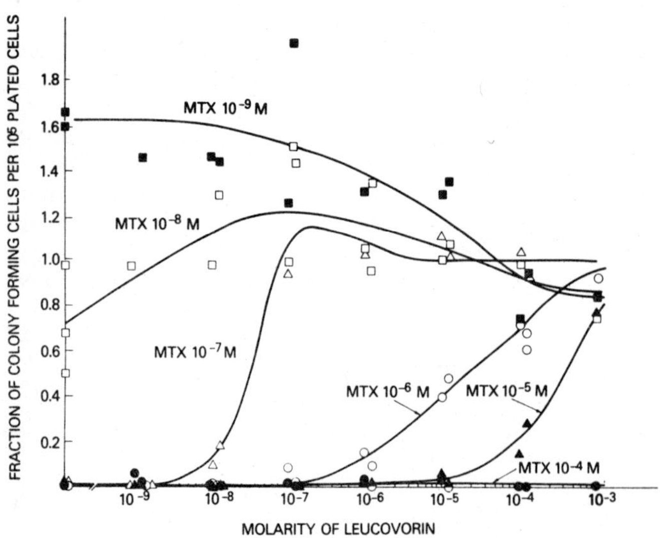

Figure 10–7. Effect of various combinations of leucovorin and methotrexate on formation of granulocyte colonies *in vitro* by mouse bone marrow. Values are normalized to control value for marrow incubated without either drug. Methotrexate concentrations: ■ — 10^{-9}M; □ — 10^{-8}M; △ — 10^{-7}M; ○ — 10^{-6}M; ▲ — 10^{-5}M; ● — 10^{-4}M. (Reproduced with permission from Pinedo et al.: The reversal of methotrexate cytotoxicity to mouse bone marrow cells by leucovorin and nucleosides. Cancer Res. 36:4418–4424, 1976.)

Enzyme-bound ^{3}H-MTX is separated from free drug by albumin-coated charcoal adsorption of the unbound material, and the bound fraction remaining in the supernatant is counted (Fig. 10–8). Multiple samples can be run simultaneously and results can be reported on the same day.[80]

Radioimmunoassays for MTX are also available for routine clinical use, and employ antibodies generated by a MTX:bovine serum albumin complex.[81] These assays have the same sensitivity and speed as the competitive reductase binding procedure, but have somewhat different specificity. The immunoassay antibodies cross-react with one MTX metabolite, 2,4-diamino-N^{10}-methyl pteroic acid (DAMPA), but not with 7-OH-MTX (Fig. 10–9). At later time points after drug administration, DAMPA is found in plasma in relatively high concentrations (equal to or greater than MTX). Thus MTX levels in plasma, as measured by RIA, are an average two- to fourfold higher than by the reductase binding method.[82] A variant of the radioimmunoassay, based on antibody inhibition of an enzyme:MTX complex, has equal sensitivity and is the most rapid assay available, but also cross-reacts with DAMPA.[83]

High-pressure liquid chromatography can be used to separate MTX and metabolites and to quantitate these individual products (Fig. 10–10), but this technique is not practical for routine clinical monitoring.[82]

PHARMACOKINETICS

Although the pharmacologic properties of MTX are well understood on a biochemical level, clinical utilization of this knowledge depends on a detailed understanding of the moment-to-moment changes in drug concentration in extracellular fluid and, further, the complicated relationship of drug levels to effects on specific tissues. Great strides have been made in the past decade in defining antifolate pharmacokinetics, but the important second step — the definition of relationships between drug concentration and effect — has not been completed.

The first attempts to define the distribution and disposition of MTX in a comprehensive manner were reported by Zaharko et al.[84] in their study of ^{3}H-MTX in mice. These authors developed a detailed model for MTX pharmacokinetics that accurately predicted drug-derived radioactivity in various tissue compartments for a four-hour period follow-

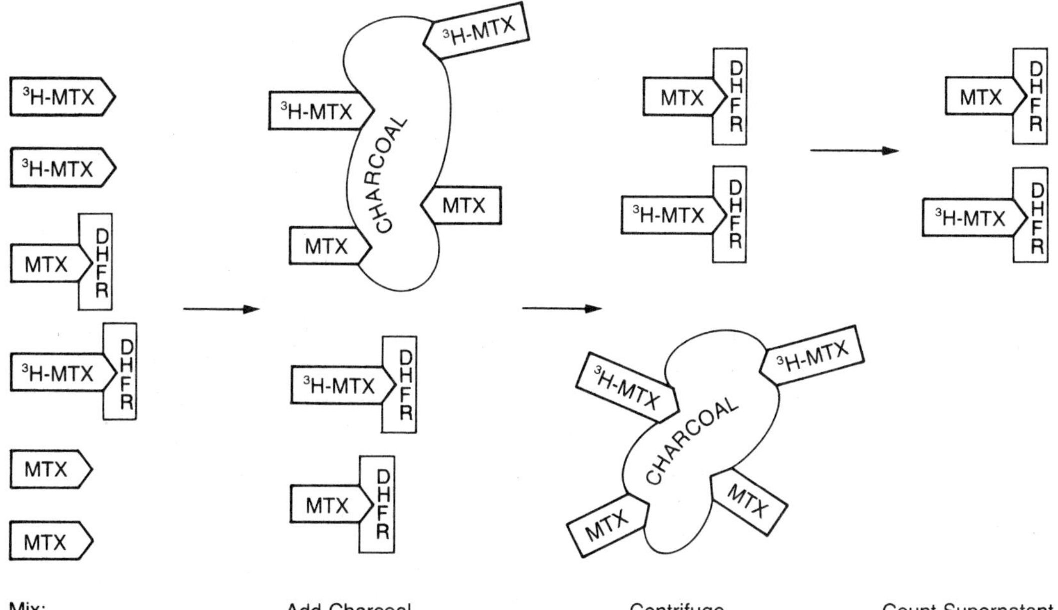

Figure 10–8. Competitive protein binding assay for methotrexate (MTX) using dihydrofolate reductase (DHFR) as binding protein. The MTX content of the sample determines the fraction of ^{3}H-MTX bound to DHFR.

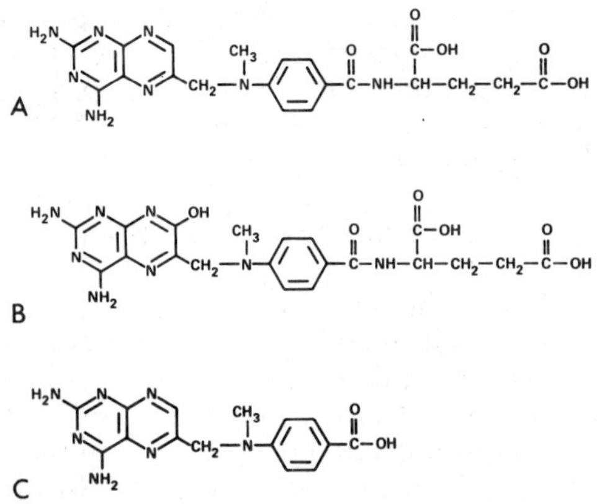

Figure 10–9. Methotrexate metabolites in man. A is the parent compound, B is 7-OH-methotrexate, and C is 2,4-diamino-N^{10}-methyl pteroic acid (DAMPA).

ing drug administration. The primary elements of that model were: (1) elimination of MTX by renal excretion; (2) an active enterohepatic circulation; (3) metabolism of at least a small fraction of drug within the gastrointestinal tract by intestinal flora; and (4) multiple drug half-lives in plasma, the longest of which was found to be approximately three hours. Each of these elements has been observed in man, although we now appreciate a longer terminal half-life variously estimated at eight to 27 hours, depending on the specificity of the assay method employed.[85] High-pressure liquid chromatography has also disclosed extensive metabolism of MTX in both mouse and man. Thus, studies employing specific assay procedures have extensively modified earlier conceptions of MTX pharmacokinetics, while confirming in a qualitative sense most of the conclusions drawn from the earlier work.

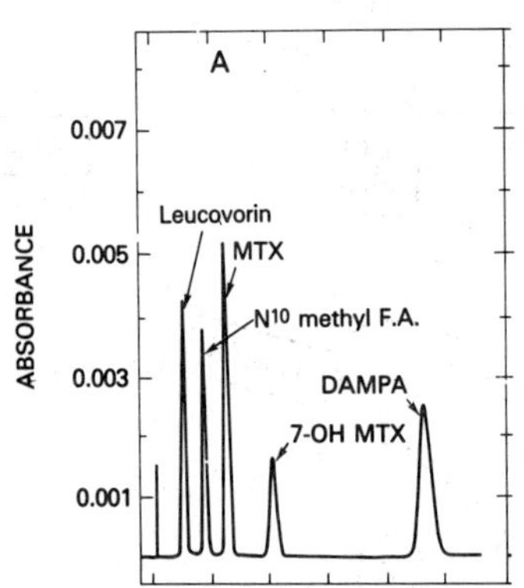

Figure 10–10. Separation of methotrexate and two primary metabolites, 7-OH-methotrexate and DAMPA, and a frequent pharmaceutical contaminant, N^{10}-methyl folic acid, by high-pressure liquid chromatography, using a reversed phase system. (Reproduced with permission from Donehower et al.: Presence of 2,4-diamino-N^{10}-methyl pteroic acid after high-dose methotrexate. Clin. Pharmacol. Ther. 26:63–72, 1979.)

Absorption

Methotrexate is well absorbed from the gastrointestinal tract by active transport[86] at doses below approximately 30 mg per m^2.[87] At higher doses, absorption is incomplete; bioavailability for total doses of 50 mg per m^2 or greater may be enhanced by subdivision of the dose as opposed to a single large dose.[88]

It should be remembered that drug absorbed in the intestine enters the portal circulation and thus must pass through the liver, where hepatocellular uptake, polyglutamation, and storage all occur; orally administered drug is further subject to degradation by intestinal flora to DAMPA (see above), a metabolite that is inactive pharmacologically[82] but which cross-reacts in the commonly used radioimmunoassay system for MTX. Drugs taken orally are also subject to the variability of intestinal absorption created by drug-induced epithelial denudation, motility changes, and alterations in flora. One or all of these factors may be responsible for the variability in peak plasma concentration observed in children receiving small doses of MTX (20 mg/m^2) by mouth.[89] For these reasons, MTX is usually given by systemic routes, primarily by intravenous infusion.

Distribution

The volume of distribution of MTX is approximately that of total body water. The drug is loosely bound to serum albumin, with approximately 60 per cent binding at or above 1 μM concentrations in plasma.[90] It can be displaced from this binding by weak organic acids such as aspirin,[91] but this displacement has no proved clinical significance.

The drug penetrates slowly into third-space collections of fluid, such as pleural effusions[92] or ascitic fluid,[93] reaching equilibrium with plasma concentrations in approximately six hours. It also exits slowly from these compartments, producing a concentration gradient of several-fold in favor of the loculated fluid (Fig. 10–11) at later time points. For example, the clearance of MTX from peritoneal fluid is about 5 ml per minute, or substantially less than the clearance from the plasma compartment, which equals or exceeds glomerular filtration (120 ml/min). The reason for accumulation of drug in closed spaces has been discussed by Chabner et al.,[93] and forms the basis for current trials of intraperitoneal chemotherapy with MTX and other agents. To summarize briefly, the limited permeability of the peritoneal surface to ionized compounds and to high-molecular-weight compounds[94] allows only small amounts of drug to pass across the peritoneal membrane into the portal circulation. Drug not retained or metabolized in the liver passes into the systemic circulation and is excreted rapidly in the urine.

Third-space retention of intravenously administered drug is associated with a prolongation of the terminal drug half half-life in plasma, owing apparently to the slow reentry of sequestered drug into the blood stream.[93] This effect should be kept in mind when treating patients with ascites or pleural fluid. No strict guidelines for dose adjustment have been provided by the few studies of MTX pharmacokinetics in patients with third-space accumulations; however, it is advisable to evacuate this fluid before treatment, to monitor plasma drug concentrations in such patients, and to reduce dosage in proportion to the terminal half-life of the drug.

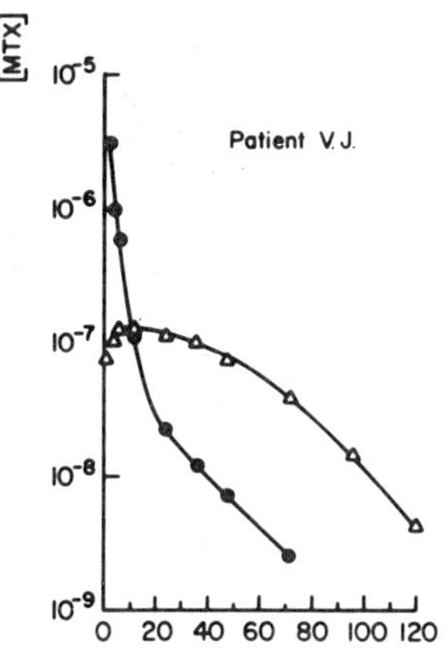

Figure 10–11. Intraperitoneal (△—△) and plasma (●—●) methotrexate concentration after intravenous administration of 25 mg/m^2 in a patient with ovarian cancer. (Reproduced with permission from Chabner et el.: Methotrexate disposition in humans: case studies in ovarian cancer and following high-dose infusion. Drug Metab. Rev. 8:107–117, 1978.)

Plasma Pharmacokinetics

Following the initial distribution phase, which lasts a relatively few minutes, at least two phases of drug disappearance from plasma are observed in man and in laboratory animals. Conventional doses of 25 to 100 mg per m^2 produce peak plasma concentrations of 1 to 10 μM, while high-dose infusion regimens using 1.5 gm per m^2 or greater yield peak levels of 0.1 to 1 mM.[95] It is unclear whether plasma concentrations are strictly proportional to dose. Lawrence et al. found a 50 per cent decrease in MTX clearance and disproportionately higher plasma levels after 100 mg intravenous MTX as compared with 25 mg doses in the same patient. This nonlinearity was ascribed to saturation of the tubular secretory mechanism for MTX, although no direct evidence for this hypothesis was presented.[96] The initial phase of drug disappearance from plasma has a half-life of two to three hours, with no apparent variation as doses are increased to the "high-dose" range. This phase extends for the first 12 to 24 hours after drug administration and is largely determined by the rate of renal excretion of MTX. Prolongation of this phase, as well as the terminal phase of drug disappearance from plasma, is observed in patients with renal dysfunction, with a half-life that is approximately proportional to the serum creatinine.[97] In patients with normal creatinine clearance, the half-life of the initial phase of drug disappearance increases with advancing age of the patient, lending additional variability to plasma levels, disappearance kinetics, and toxicity.

The final phase of drug disappearance has a considerably longer half-life of eight to ten hours[93, 95, 98, 99]; this half-life may further lengthen in patients with renal dysfunction or third-space fluid such as ascites. Following conventional doses of 25 to 100 mg per m^2, this terminal phase begins at drug concentrations above the threshold for toxicity to bone marrow and gastrointestinal epithelium. Thus, any prolongation of the terminal half-life is likely to be associated with significant and unexpected toxicity.

The use of MTX by constant infusion has

received increasing consideration, since it offers the advantage of providing predictable blood and cerebrospinal fluid concentrations for a specific period. Bleyer[100] has used the following formulae for achieving a desired plasma concentration in a patient with normal renal function:

[a] Priming dose (in mg/m^2) = $(1.5 \times 10^7) \cdot (MTX)_{plasma}$
[b] Infusion dose (in $mg/m^2/hr$) = $(3 \times 10^6) \cdot MTX)_{plasma}$

An approximate correction for renal function may be made by reducing the infusion doses in proportion to the reduction in creatinine clearance, based on a normal creatinine clearance of 60 ml per min per m^2.

Renal Excretion

The bulk of drug is excreted in the urine in the first 12 hours after administration. Estimates of the percentage renal excretion vary form 44 to virtually 100 per cent of the administered dose,[95, 98, 99, 101] and the higher figure is likely to be correct in patients with normal renal function. MTX clearance by the kidney has exceeded creatinine clearance in some patients studied; Hande et al. calculated MTX renal clearance to be 194 ml per minute in a patient recovering from drug-induced renal failure,[102] and Monjanel consistently found MTX clearance to exceed creatinine clearance.[103] However, other studies have placed MTX clearance at a level somewhat lower than creatinine clearance.[101]

During high-dose infusion, rapid drug excretion may lead to high MTX concentrations in the urine. These concentrations, approaching 10 mM, exceed the solubility of the drug below pH 7.0 (Table 10–1) and are believed to be responsible for intrarenal precipitation of drug, leading to renal failure. Thus, in high-dose regimens, hydration and alkalinization of the urine are recommended in order to avoid renal toxicity (Table 10–2); this is discussed in greater detail later in this chapter. Intensive hydration does not affect the clearance of MTX or the plasma pharmacokinetics, aside from its effects that are related to prevention of renal damage.[104]

The actual excretion mechanism of MTX in the human kidney has not been elucidated. In the dog and monkey, active secretion of MTX takes place in the proximal renal tubule, with reabsorption in the distal tubule.[105] As noted above, the high clearance values in excess of creatinine clearance suggest that active tubular secretion of MTX occurs in man. In addition, MTX excretion is inhibited by the weak organic acid, aspirin,[66] and by probenecid, an inhibitor of organic acid secretion.[106] Simultaneous folic acid administration blocks MTX reabsorption, suggesting that leucovorin might accelerate MTX excretion in high-dose rescue regimens.

Methotrexate pharmacokinetics are not entirely predictable on the basis of knowledge of renal function in the individual

TABLE 10–1. Aqueous Solubility of Methotrexate and Metabolites

	pH 5.0	*pH 6.0* MG/ML	*pH 7.0*
MTX	0.39	1.55	9.04
7-OH-MTX	0.13	0.37	1.55
DAMPA	0.05	0.10	0.85

TABLE 10–2. High-Dose Methotrexate Therapy

Prehydration
In 12 hrs prior to treatment, establish diuresis with 1.5 liters/m^2 with 100 mEq HCO_3^- and 20 mEq KCl per liter. Test urine pH to ensure neutrality (pH 7.0 or >) at time of drug infusion.

Drug Infusion
1. Jaffe regimen: 50–250 mg/kg MTX over 6-hr infusion. Continue hydration for 24 hrs. Begin leucovorin 2 hrs after end of infusion, 15 mg/m^2 IM q6h × 7 doses.
2. Alternative: Bolus administration of 50 mg/m^2 MTX IV followed by infusion of MTX over 36-hr period at dose of 1.5 gm/m^2. At 36 hrs, begin leucovorin infusion 200 mg/m^2 for 12 hrs. At 48 hrs, give leucovorin 25 mg/m^2 IM q6h × 6 doses.

Monitor Points
For Jaffe regimen and for 36-hr infusion, drug levels above 5×10^{-7}M at 48 hrs require additional leucovorin rescue.

DRUG LEVEL	DOSE LEUCOVORIN
5×10^{-7}M	15 mg/m^2 q6h × 8 doses
1×10^{-6}M	100 mg/m^2 q6h × 8 doses
2×10^{-6}M	200 mg/m^2 q6h × 8 doses

Drug levels should be repeated every 48 hrs and leucovorin dose adjusted until drug concentration is less than 5×10^{-8}M.

patient.[103] In one study of 20 patients with normal serum creatinine, the total body clearance of MTX varied from 40 to 400 ml per minute. Decreased renal tubular function, not reflected in creatinine clearance, may be responsible for this variability.

In high-dose MTX therapy, despite interindividual variability in pharmacokinetics, blood levels of drug may be accurately predicted by a preliminary determination of drug clearance using a small (50 mg/m^2) test dose. Pharmacokinetic measurements made during the trial dose provide a basis for calculating high-dose infusion rates according to the formula:

$$\text{Clearance (ml/min)} = \frac{\text{Dose (50 mg/m}^2\text{)}}{\text{Area under C} \times \text{T curve}}$$

$$\text{Infusion rate} = (\text{MTX})_{\text{plasma}} \cdot (\text{Clearance}_{\text{MTX}})$$

Thus, the desired infusion rate is the product of the target steady-state concentration multiplied by the MTX clearance rate, as determined during the test dose period.[103] The extrapolation from the test dose of 50 mg per m^2 to the high-dose infusion has proved reliable as long as renal function remains normal during the infusion period.

Hepatic Uptake and Biliary Excretion

Methotrexate undergoes uptake, storage, and metabolism in the liver, but the specific contribution of these processes to human pharmacokinetics is unclear at this time.

Methotrexate is transported into hepatocytes by an active uptake system that appears to have several components; these include a high-affinity, low-capacity carrier[107] and a low-affinity, high-capacity mechanism.[108] The low-affinity system is believed to be distinct from that used by the naturally occurring reduced folates. In the hepatocyte, MTX is converted to polyglutamate forms that persist for several months after drug administration.[28] The parent drug also undergoes excretion into the biliary tract and is reabsorbed into the systemic circulation from the small intestine. Strum et al.[109] have found that other chemotherapeutic agents affect hepatic uptake and biliary secretion of MTX. Vincristine and cyclophosphamide inhibit both hepatic uptake and biliary excretion, but the net effect of these actions is to produce a fall in intrahepatic drug concentration. Actinomycin D strongly inhibits biliary secretion of MTX, with little effect on hepatic uptake, and causes a marked increase in intrahepatic levels of the drug. The pharmacokinetic effects of these drug interactions have not been examined in detail in man; the possibility exists that the combination of MTX and actinomycin D may increase MTX levels in liver and enhance its hepatic toxicity.

There are widely divergent estimates of the quantitative importance of biliary excretion of MTX in man. Leme et al.,[110] using ^{3}H-MTX, found only 0.41 per cent of an administered dose in the bile of a patient with a biliary fistula. Subsequent studies have variously estimated that 6.7 to 9 per cent[111] or 20 per cent[101] of an administered dose enters the biliary tract. Calvert and co-workers used the highly specific reductase inhibition assay to measure biliary concentrations of MTX, and found that biliary levels were 2500- to 10,000-fold higher than simultaneous concentrations in the plasma.[101] Despite these high concentrations in bile, less than 10 per cent of an intravenous dose of MTX is eliminated in the feces. Most MTX excreted in bile is reabsorbed as intact drug, while an undefined fraction is metabolized by intestinal flora to the inactive derivative DAMPA (Fig. 10–9).[112] The intraluminal metabolism of MTX by intestinal flora can be reduced by nonabsorbable antibiotics. Shen and Azarnoff[111] have observed that patients pretreated with kanamycin have higher levels of intact MTX and lower concentrations of metabolites in their plasma, presumably owing to decreased metabolism in the gastrointestinal tract.

METHOTREXATE METABOLISM

The introduction of high-dose MTX regimens has led to recognition of at least two MTX metabolites in man, both of which have been discussed previously in connection with drug assay. Jacobs et al. employed ion exchange chromatography to identify 7-hydroxymethotrexate (7-OH-MTX) in the urine of patients receiving high-dose infusions (Fig. 10–9)[113]; 7-OH-MTX constituted 20 to 46 per cent of material excreted in the urine in the time interval between 12 and 24 hours after the start of the infusion. The fraction of drug in the form of metabolite was estimated to be as high as 86 per cent in the time period from 24 to 48 hours. A second metabolite, DAMPA, has also been identified by high-pressure liquid chromatography in plasma and urine, and becomes an important fraction of drug-derived material at later time points, comprising a mean of 25 per cent of material excreted in the time interval from 24 to 48 hours.[82] Neither of these metabolites contributes a majority fraction of total material excreted in the urine, but both are known to accumulate in plasma in increasingly high percentage at later time points; at 24 to 48 hours after high-dose MTX administration, they account for most of the MTX-derived material found in plasma.

Both metabolites can be separated and quantified by high-pressure liquid chromatography; in the reverse-phase system described by Donehower et al.[82] the metabolites have longer retention times than the parent compound, and constitute prominent peaks in both plasma and urine samples (Fig. 10–10). As previously discussed, DAMPA cross-reacts strongly with antibodies to MTX prepared by conjugating the glutamate end of the MTX molecule to serum albumin.

The pharmacokinetics of 7-OH-MTX have been studied after bolus or infusion doses of MTX, and it has been found to reach equivalent plasma levels with MTX 10 hours after bolus administration. At 24 hours, the ratio of 7-OH to MTX was between 1:1 and 30:1 in eight patients studied.[114]

The sites of MTX metabolism have not been definitively identified. The 7-OH metabolite is probably formed by aldehyde oxidase in the liver. This reaction has been clearly demonstrated in rabbits but not in man. At this time, no dosage adjustment appears to be necessary for persons with hepatic dysfunction or a history of previous methotrexate treatment. The pteroic acid metabolite DAMPA is probably formed by the action of bacterial carboxypeptidases in the gastrointestinal tract; enzymes specific for glutamate terminal peptide bonds have been characterized from bacterial sources,[115] but not from mammalian tissues. DAMPA is also produced by the enzymatic cleavage of MTX in a novel rescue regimen for treating brain tumors[116]; in this protocol, high-dose systemic MTX is followed by the infusion of the bacterial enzyme carboxypeptidase G_1, which degrades MTX in the systemic circulation but leaves drug intact in the brain and cerebrospinal fluid.

The role of these metabolites in producing MTX toxicity or therapeutic activity is uncertain. Both 7-OH-MTX and the pteroic acid metabolite have lesser solubility than the parent drug (Table 10–1). Jacobs demonstrated that 7-OH-MTX constituted more than 50 per cent of precipitated intrarenal material in his study of MTX-induced renal failure in monkeys,[113] but the role of either metabolite in the clinical syndrome of renal toxicity secondary to MTX is unproved.

Neither metabolite retains significant ability to inhibit dihydrofolate reductase. The 7-OH metabolite has 1/10th the activity of MTX, and the pteroic acid metabolite has less than 1/100th the inhibitory activity. The ability of either metabolite to cross cell membranes has not been established.

As mentioned previously, MTX may also be converted to polyglutamate forms in the liver, and probably in other tissues as well. These derivatives have not been found in the blood stream as yet, and the process of polyglutamation has no proved quantitative importance in MTX pharmacokinetics at present.

TOXICITY

The primary toxic effects of folate antagonists are myelosuppression and gastrointestinal mucositis. The intestinal and oral epithelium is somewhat more sensitive than granulocyte and platelet precursors, in that drug schedules that produce intense mucositis (particularly those with prolonged, low drug concentrations) may cause little marrow suppression. The threshold plasma concentration of MTX required to inhibit DNA synthesis in bone marrow has been estimated to be 1×10^{-8}M, whereas gastrointestinal epithelium is inhibited at 5×10^{-9}M plasma concentrations.[117] This greater sensitivity of gastrointestinal epithelium is believed to result from greater accumulation and persistence of MTX in intestinal epithelium, as opposed to bone marrow.[118] Mucositis usually appears three to seven days after drug administration, and precedes the onset of a fall in white blood count or platelet count by several days. The duration and intensity of these acute toxicities are generally determined by drug dose and individual pharmacokinetics. In patients with compromised renal function, small doses on the order of 25 mg may provide cytotoxic blood levels for three to five days and may result in serious bone marrow toxicity. Myelosuppression and mucositis usually are completely reversed within two weeks, unless drug excretion mechanisms are severely impaired.

The introduction of high-dose MTX regimens,[119] with leucovorin rescue, has led to the appreciation of a new spectrum of clinical toxicities and has required a more careful monitoring of drug pharmacokinetics in individual patients. These regimens employ otherwise lethal doses in a six- to 42-hour infusion, followed by a 24- to 48-hour period of multiple leucovorin injections to terminate the toxic effect of MTX. Several of the more common high-dose regimens and their related pharmacokinetics are presented in Table 10–2. In each regimen, successful rescue by leucovorin depends on the rapid elimination of MTX by the kidneys. However, early experience with high-dose regimens indicated that MTX itself may have acute toxic effects on renal function during the period of drug infusion,[119] leading to delayed drug clearance, ineffective rescue by leucovorin, and a host of secondary toxicities, including severe myelosuppression, mucositis, and epithelial desquamation.[95, 98] At least 30 fatalities have occurred as a direct result of high-dose MTX infusions.[120]

The etiology of drug-induced renal dysfunction, which is usually detected as an abrupt rise in serum creatinine and BUN and a fall in urine output, is thought to be the precipitation of MTX and possibly its less soluble metabolites, 7-OH-MTX and DAMPA, in acidic urine.[113, 114] However, a direct toxic effect of antifolates on the renal tubule is suggested by the finding that aminopterin, an equally soluble compound that is used in one tenth the dose of MTX, also causes renal toxicity.[121] Jacobs et al.[113] have reproduced the syndrome of MTX-induced renal failure in monkeys and have demonstrated precipitation of 7-OH-MTX and the parent compound in renal tubules, both of which have limited solubility at acid pH. In order to prevent precipitation, most centers now use vigorous hydration (3 liters of fluid per m^2 per 24 hours, beginning 12 hours prior to infusion and continuing for 36 hours), and alkalinize the urine (1 ampule of $NaHCO_3$ per liter of intravenous fluid). The MTX infusion should not begin until urine flow exceeds 100 ml per hour and urine pH is 7.0 or higher, and these parameters should be monitored during the course of the infusion.

With this regimen, the incidence of renal failure and myelosuppression at the National Cancer Institute has been reduced from approximately 10 per cent to less than 1 per cent, and other institutions have reported similar favorable results. No change in the rate of MTX excretion or alteration of plasma pharmacokinetics results from the intense hydration used in the preparatory regimen described above[104]; thus, these "safety" measures should have no deleterious effect on the therapeutic efficacy of the regimen.

Despite careful attention to the details of hydration and alkalinization, occasional patients develop serious or even fatal toxicity.[120] In almost all cases, these toxic episodes are associated with delayed MTX clearance from plasma and can be predicted by routine monitoring of drug concentration in plasma at appropriate times after drug infusion.[122] The specific time for monitoring, and the guidelines for distinguishing between normal and dangerously elevated levels, must be determined for each regimen and for each assay procedure. Examples are given in Table 10–2, but in general a time point well into the final phase of drug disappearance, such as 24 to 36 hours after the start of infusion, should be chosen. The value of monitoring has been established by numerous studies. The experience of the National Cancer Institute group in administering adjuvant therapy for osteosarcoma is typical. These investigators used a regimen described in Table 10–2: a six-hour infusion of 50 to 250 mg per kg MTX, followed two hours after infusion by 15 mg per m^2 leucovorin repeated every six hours for seven doses.[119] Their experience, summarized in Figure 10–12, was that, in each of seven patients with moderate-to-severe myelosuppression, plasma MTX concentration at 48 hours after drug administration was 9×10^{-7}M or higher; this finding alerted physicians to the high risk of toxicity. In three of these seven patients, renal function remained normal; this finding confirmed the unreliability of serum creatinine determinations as a predictor of toxicity.[98] Earlier time points may be used for monitoring drug disappearance and for guiding patient management. After a six-hour high-dose infusion regimen, plasma concentrations of less than 5×10^{-6}M at 24 hours are associated with a low incidence of toxicity.[123]

Early detection of elevated concentrations of MTX allows institution of specific clinical measures; continuous medical supervision

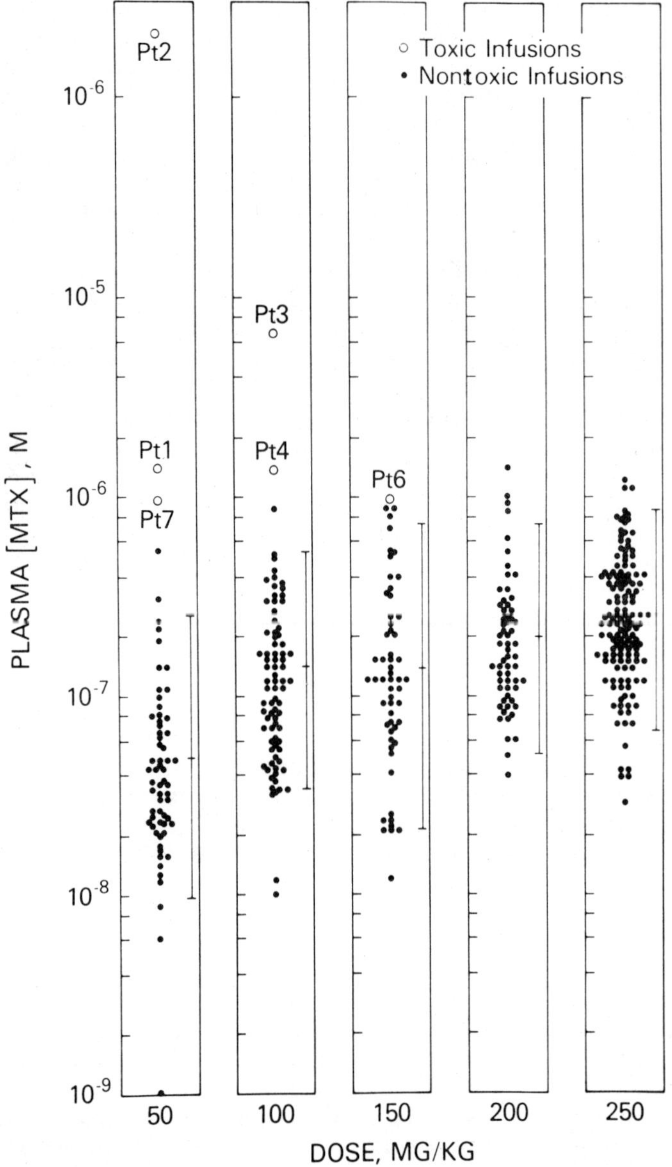

Figure 10–12. Relationship between 48-hour plasma methotrexate concentration and toxicity in patients treated with 6-hour infusion of methotrexate at indicated doses. All toxic patients had plasma concentrations above 9×10^{-7}M, and patients with lower levels of methotrexate had no signs of toxicity. (Reproduced with permission from Stoller et al.: Use of plasma pharmacokinetics to predict and prevent methotrexate toxicity. N. Engl. J. Med. 297:630–634, 1977.)

is warranted until the severity and duration of myelosuppression can be determined. Leucovorin in increased doses is required and must be continued until plasma MTX concentration falls below 5×10^{-8}M. Because of the competitive relationship between MTX and leucovorin, the leucovorin dose must be increased in proportion to the plasma concentration of MTX. Small doses of leucovorin are not able to prevent toxicity in patients with elevated drug levels, even if leucovorin is continued beyond 48 hours.[98,122] In the osteosarcoma study of the National Cancer Institute,[122] leucovorin doses of 50 to 100 mg per m^2 every six hours successfully rescued four of four patients with MTX levels above 9×10^{-7}M at 48 hours, whereas five of five patients with similarly high levels who received 12 to 30 mg per m^2 of leucovorin experienced severe myelosuppression. It seems reasonable to use 100 mg per m^2 leucovorin every six hours for patients with MTX levels of 1 μM and to increase this dose in proportion to the methotrexate level up to a maximum of 500 mg per m^2 leucovorin, with leucovorin dose adjustments based on repeated assays of plasma MTX at 24-hour intervals. The results of *in vitro* studies of leucovorin rescue and of limited, unpublished personal experience indicate that leucovorin may not be able to rescue patients who have plasma MTX concentrations above 1×10^{-5}M; in these patients, supportive care, including antibiotics, platelet transfusion, and hydration, must be relied on to carry them through the prolonged period of myelosuppression.

Leucovorin is usually adminstered intravenously to ensure its absorption; oral leucovorin is also well absorbed, but is not available commercially.

The persistence of high concentrations of MTX in plasma presents a serious danger to patients who have received high-dose MTX. Because of the variable effectiveness of leucovorin in preventing toxicity in patients with levels of 1×10^{-5}M or greater at 48 hours, alternative methods of rescue have been proposed. Both hemodialysis and peritoneal dialysis are ineffective in removing significant quantities of MTX; clearance by the former was estimated to be 40 ml per minute,[102] but only 5 ml per minute for the latter. In one carefully studied patient, despite the presence of moderate renal failure, renal clearance of MTX exceeded hemodialysis clearance by greater than twofold.[102] Although hemodialysis produced a momentary decrease in plasma concentration of MTX, a rapid rebound to pre-dialysis levels was observed upon cessation of the procedure. This rebound was likely the result of re-entry of drug into the plasma space from deeper compartments. The use of charcoal hemoperfusion columns is capable of removing MTX and other antineoplastic drugs from whole blood, but again encounters the problem of re-entry from deeper compartments[124]; in addition, platelets adhere to these columns, leading to thrombocytopenia. Abelson and co-workers have used a bacterial enzyme, carboxypeptidase G_1,[116] which inactivates MTX by removal of its terminal glutamate, to destroy circulating MTX. The regimen of high-dose MTX followed by intravenous carboxypeptidase was well tolerated, but this form of enzymatic rescue carries a risk of hypersensitivity to the bacterial enzyme. Bertino et al. have demonstrated the feasibility of attaching the enzyme to hollow fiber tubing, which can then be used in an extracorporeal shunt for drug removal,[125] and thus might avoid immune sensitization. A disadvantage of carboxypeptidase G_1 is its high affinity for natural folates as well as MTX. An alternative enzyme that cleaves MTX but not reduced folates has been isolated by Albrecht and co-workers,[126] but has not been extensively purified or characterized.

The rationale for rescue of MTX with thymidine has been discussed previously. Preliminary reports have described the successful prevention of MTX toxicity in man using six- to 40-hour infusions of the antifolate followed by a 72-hour infusion of thymidine at a rate of 8 gm per m^2 per day.[72, 127, 128] Patients receiving a bolus dose of MTX, 3 gm per m^2, were successfully rescued by thymidine infusion (1 gm/m^2/day); the infusion was begun 24 hours after MTX and continued until plasma MTX concentration in the plasma reached 5×10^{-8}M.[129]* Few antitumor responses were noted in these initial trials, but the number of treated patients was small and the therapeutic value of this approach remains unproved.

In the experimental setting, MTX toxicity can also be blocked by drugs that prevent cell progression into the DNA synthetic phase of the cell cycle. The best example of this effect is the antagonistic effect of L-asparaginase on MTX toxicity; through depletion of the amino acid, asparagine, the enzyme inhibits protein synthesis and prevents entry of cells into DNA synthesis.[130] Rescue regimens[131] that employ high doses of MTX (up to 400 mg/m^2), followed within 24 hours by 20,000 to 40,000 units per m^2 L-asparaginase, produce minimal bone marrow toxicity and mucositis, and appear to have some effectiveness in patients refractory to low-dose MTX alone. Yap et al.[131] reported a complete remission rate of 62 per cent (13/21) in adult patients with acute lymphoblastic leukemia who had failed initial therapy with conventional induction regimens (vincristine, prednisone, daunomycin). The regimen is less effective in previously treated patients with acute myeloblastic leukemia, producing a remission rate of only 18 per cent. Capizzi has concluded[132] that continued responsiveness to L-asparaginase is a requirement for achievement of complete remission with this regimen.

---

*Thymidine infusions of 1 gm/m^2/day produced only a twofold rise in serum thymidine concentration, indicating a very steep dose-response relationship for thymidine rescue. The serum concentration of thymidine is proportional to thymidine dose up to infusion rates of 3 gm/m^2/day. Above that rate, there is little further increase in serum thymidine concentration.[129]

Methotrexate toxicity is also blocked by drugs that block the thymidylate synthetase reaction, thereby preventing consumption of the reduced folate pool and negating the effect of dihydrofolate reductase inhibition. This effect has been studied in detail and seems to explain the antagonism of pretreatment with fluoropyrimidines followed by MTX.[133] The interaction of MTX and fluoropyrimidine is discussed more fully in Chapter 8. It should be remembered that this antagonism has not been carefully studied or, in fact, demonstrated in clinical practice.

Other Toxicities

In addition to its inhibitory effects on replicating tissues, MTX has toxic effects on nondividing tissues not easily explained by its primary action on DNA synthesis. Chronic MTX therapy is associated with portal fibrosis and, in occasional cases, cirrhosis. Chronic liver disease has occurred most frequently in patients with psoriasis or in children with acute leukemia who have been receiving maintenance therapy over a period of several years. The incidence of frank cirrhosis has been estimated to be 10 per cent in MTX-treated psoriatic patients, but reaches 25 per cent in those treated for five years or longer.[134] A high underlying incidence of chronic hepatic disease related to alcohol or to arsenicals used for psoriasis treatment is found in this patient population.[135] Cirrhosis does not always progress with continued antifolate treatment. Of 11 psoriatic patients with cirrhotic changes on liver biopsy who received continued treatment, only three showed progression on subsequent biopsy, and three had no pathologic findings on a subsequent biopsy.[134]

Acute elevations of liver enzymes (SGOT, SGPT, LDH) are commonly found in the blood following high-dose MTX administration, and usually return to normal within ten days. Liver biopsy in such patients has revealed fatty infiltration, but no evidence of hepatocellular necrosis or periportal fibrosis. The late occurrence of cirrhosis in patients treated with high-dose MTX in the adjuvant situation has not been reported.

The biochemical basis for liver toxicity is not known. MTX causes increased lipid deposition in liver, possibly through interference with synthesis of choline (which requires a one-carbon transfer).[136] Acute MTX hepatotoxicity in rats can be reversed by choline administration.

Methotrexate also causes a poorly characterized, self-limited pneumonitis, with fever, cough, and an interstitial pulmonary infiltrate.[137, 138] Eosinophilia has not been a consistent finding, either in the peripheral blood or in open lung biopsy specimens. Lung biopsies have revealed a variety of findings, from simple interstitial edema and a mononuclear infiltrate to noncaseating granulomas. The possibility that MTX pneumonitis represents a hypersensitivity phenomenon has been questioned because of the failure of patients to react to a reinstitution of MTX therapy. It is possible that many earlier case reports of "MTX lung" in fact represented unrecognized viral infections or allergic reactions to unsuspected allergens. No specific therapy for this entity is recommended except that of withholding MTX treatment during the acute reaction. Careful diagnostic work-up is indicated to exclude the possibility of tumor or an opportunistic infection.

True anaphylactic reactions to MTX are rare. Two cases of acute hypersensitivity reaction to MTX have been described[139]; the first patient experienced acute cardiovascular collapse, which was reproduced on rechallenge of the patient. In the second case the acute reaction consisted of facial edema, rash, and generalized pruritus, and again was elicited on repeated rechallenges. Both patients were receiving bacillus Calmette-Guérin (BCG) in conjunction with MTX at the time of these reactions, and thus may have developed heightened sensitivity to the drug on this basis.

PHARMACOKINETICS AND TOXICITY OF METHOTREXATE IN THE CENTRAL NERVOUS SYSTEM

Because of its high degree of ionization at physiologic pH, MTX crosses the blood-brain barrier and penetrates into the cerebrospinal fluid (CSF) with difficulty. The ratio of venous MTX concentration to CSF concentration is approximately 30:1 at equilibrium during a constant intravenous infusion of drug.[140] Thus, plasma levels in excess of 100 μM would be required to achieve the 1 μM concentration thought to be necessary for killing of leukemic cells. The blood-brain barrier can be reversibly disrupted by intracarotid arterial infusion of 25 per cent mannitol, a procedure that allows a tenfold increase in brain uptake of MTX.[140A] It is not known whether a similar degree of enhanced uptake occurs in brain tumors or brain metastases, which probably do not have an intact blood-brain barrier. Protocols for prophylaxis against meningeal leukemia and lymphoma employing systemic high-dose infusions of MTX are currently being pursued to answer the question of the relative efficacy of systemic versus intrathecal drug.

Direct intrathecal injection of MTX has been used for more than two decades in the treatment and prophylaxis of meningeal malignancy. Drug injected into the intrathecal space distributes in a total volume of approximately 120 ml for persons over three years of age. Thus, a maximal total dose of 12 mg is advised for all persons over three years, lower doses being indicated for younger children. Bleyer[100] has suggested 6 mg for age one year or younger, 8 mg for ages one to two, and 10 mg for ages two to three. The peak CSF concentration achieved by this schedule is approximately 100 μM. The lumbar CSF concentration of drug declines in a biphasic pattern, with half-lives of 1.7 and 6.6 hours.[140B] This terminal phase of disappearance may be considerably prolonged in patients with active meningeal disease, with increased intracranial pressure,[140B] in those of older age,[141] or by administration of probenecid. MTX is cleared from spinal fluid by the bulk resorption of spinal fluid (so-called "bulk flow"); a second component of resorption is the active transport of this organic anion by the choroid plexus. This active transport process is inhibited by probenecid.[140B] A prolongation of the terminal half-life is also found in patients who develop drug-related neurotoxicity, although a causal relationship between abnormal pharmacokinetics and neurotoxicity has not been established.[141]

Methotrexate administered into the lumbar space distributes poorly over the cerebral convexities and into the ventricular spaces.[140] The concentration gradient between lumbar and ventricular CSF may exceed 10:1. Although this maldistribution has no proved importance in the relapse of patients treated for meningeal leukemia, awareness of this problem had led to trials of direct intraventricular injection of MTX via a permanent intracerebral Ommaya reservoir. Bleyer[142] had demonstrated that a "C × T" (concentration × time) regimen, employing 1 mg MTX injected into the Ommaya reservoir every 12 hours for three days, yielded continuous CSF levels above 5×10^{-7}M and gave equivalent therapeutic results as compared with the conventional intralumbar injection of 12 mg per m^2 every four days. However, the "C × T" regimen was associated with a considerable reduction in neurotoxic side effects, presumably owing to the avoidance of the high peak levels of drug associated with the larger dose.

Three types of neurotoxic reactions to intrathecal MTX have been observed in children with acute leukemia.[100] The most common, and most immediate, neurotoxic side effect is an acute chemical arachnoiditis manifested as severe headache, nuchal rigidity, vomiting, fever, and inflammatory cell pleocytosis of the spinal fluid. This constellation of symptoms appears to be a function of the frequency and dose of drug administered, and may be ameliorated by dosage reduction or a change in therapy to intrathecal cytosine arabinoside. A less acute but more serious neurotoxic syndrome has been observed in approximately 10 per cent of patients treated with 12 to 15 mg per m^2 of intrathecal MTX; this subacute toxicity appears during the second or third week of treatment, usually in adult patients with active meningeal leukemia, and is manifested as motor paralysis of the extremities, cranial nerve palsy, seizures, or coma. Because of the associated abnormal drug pharmacokinetics found in these patients, it is suspected that this toxicity may be the result of toxic drug concentrations present for an extended time period.[141]

Finally, a more chronic demyelinating encephalopathy has been observed in children months or years after they have received intrathecal MTX. The primary symptoms of this toxicity are dementia, limb spasticity, and, in more advanced cases, coma. Computerized axial tomography has revealed ventricular enlargement, cortical thinning, and diffuse intracerebral calcification in children who have received prophylactic intrathecal methotrexate.[143] Most of these patients had also received cranial irradiation (greater than 2000 rads) and all had received systemic chemotherapy. A few patients treated only with repeated courses of high-dose intravenous MTX also developed encephalopathy[144]; in these patients, dementia and paret-

TABLE 10-3. Methotrexate Interactions with Other Antineoplastic Agents

Sequence					
Drug 1	*Drug 2*	*Interval Between*	*Biochemical Basis of Interaction*	*Chemotherapy Effect*	*Ref.*
WITH FLUOROPYRIMIDINES					
MTX	5-FU	3–24 hrs	MTX increases PRPP and enhances nucleotide formation	Increased cell kill in culture	145
5-FU or 5-FUdR	MTX	0–24 hrs	MTX effect negated by inhibition of thymidylate synthetase	Decreased MTX cytotoxicity	146
WITH L-ASPARAGINASE					
MTX	L-Asp	24 hrs	MTX toxicity attenuated by block in protein synthesis	Decreased MTX toxicity to normal tissue	130–132
L-Asp	MTX	0–?	MTX toxicity attenuated by block in protein synthesis	Decreased MTX cell kill	130–132
WITH CYTOSINE ARABINOSIDE					
MTX	ara-C	1–72 hrs	Increased ara-C nucleotide formation, mechanism unknown	Enhanced kill in tissue culture	147
WITH VINCRISTINE					
VCR	MTX	0–1 hr	Blocks MTX efflux	None *in vivo*	19
MTX	VCR	8–48 hrs	Unknown	Enhanced survival of mice with L1210	148

ic symptoms developed in the second or third month after treatment was begun and were associated with diffuse cortical hypodensity on CAT scan. Thus, the contribution of each of these additional treatment modalities is not clear. There is no evidence to support the use of leucovorin, either acutely following intrathecal MTX or chronically in patients who develop neurotoxic symptoms.

The etiology of CNS toxicity of MTX is unknown. Dihydrofolate reductase is found in brain tissue, but is probably of little biochemical importance in the function of the cerebral cortex, the primary site of MTX neurotoxicity.

CLINICAL DOSAGE SCHEDULES

A variety of possible dosage schedules and routes of administration are used clinically. These range from weekly intravenous or intramuscular injections of 25 to 50 mg per m^2, oral administration of 10 mg per m^2 twice weekly, or single intermittent parenteral doses of 50 to 100 mg per m^2. Other variations are possible with the addition of leucovorin rescue, which allows administration of high-dose infusion up to 42 hours in length with minimal toxicity in most patients. The selection of the appropriate schedule largely depends on the physician's analysis of the disease, the other drugs or irradiation to be employed, the patient's likely tolerance for toxicity, and factors that might alter pharmacokinetics and lead to serious toxicity. For example, maintenance schedules in acute leukemia generally employ small oral doses given regularly over long periods. The chances of acute toxicity are low in these schedules, although long-term side effects such as hepatic fibrosis and chronic immunosuppression present definite risks. Higher-dose parenteral schedules are preferred for induction therapy regimens in which maximal concentrations and durations of exposure are desirable in the effort to achieve complete remission. Regimens employing rescue with leucovorin offer the additional advantage of minimal bone marrow toxicity, a particularly attractive feature in combination chemotherapy. However, this regimen can safely be employed only in patients with normal renal and cardiac function and with no large extracellular accumulations of fluid. As emphasized earlier, high-dose regimens should be instituted only if plasma monitoring is available to help determine the adequacy of drug clearance and the risk of serious toxicity.

DRUG INTERACTIONS

In experimental tumor systems, MTX has significant synergistic or antagonistic interactions with other antineoplastic drugs. These are briefly summarized in Table 10–3. Most of these interactions are highly dependent on the specific sequence and timing of administration of MTX and the second agent. For example, MTX dramatically enhances the formation of 5-fluorouracil nucleotides in L1210 leukemia cells if the antifolate exposure precedes 5-fluorouracil addition by three hours.[145] If the sequence of administration is reversed, antagonism of 5-fluorouracil nucleotide formation results. The biochemical basis for these results is more fully discussed in Chapter 8.

As previously mentioned, vincristine given 30 minutes to one hour prior to MTX enhances the uptake of the antifolate by blocking its efflux from the cell.[19] However, in experimental chemotherapy of L1210 leukemia, this sequence of administration does not improve survival of tumor-bearing animals. For unexplained reasons, vincristine given eight to 48 hours after MTX does produce synergistic therapeutic effects.[148]

The reader is referred to the comprehensive review of Warren et al.[149] for further discussion of MTX-related drug interactions. It should be remembered that these interactions have no proved importance in the clinical use of MTX, although, in the absence of evidence to the contrary, they should logically be taken into consideration in the design of clinical protocols.

References

1. Farber S, Diamond LK, Mercer RD, et al.: Temporary remissions in acute leukemia in children produced by folic antagonist 4-amethopteroylglutamic acid (aminopterin). N. Engl. J. Med. 238:787–793, 1948.
2. Price LA, Hill BT, and Goldie JH: DDMP and selective folinic acid protection in the treatment of malignant disease: a further report. Clin. Oncol. 3:281–286, 1977.
2A. Hill BT, and Price LA: DDMP (2,4-diamino-5-(3′,4′-dichlorophenyl)-methyl pyrimidine. Cancer Treat. Rev. 7:95, 1980.
3. Zakrezewski SF, Dave C, Mead LH, et al.: Studies with a new antifolate 2,4-diamino-5-adamantyl-6-methyl pyrimidine (DAMP). Tissue distribution and disposition of 2,4-diamino-5-ademantyl-6-methyl pyrimidine (DAMP) and its metabolites. J. Pharmacol. Exp. Ther. 205:19–26, 1978.
4. Skeel RT, Cushmore AR, Sawicki WL, et al.: Clinical and pharmacological evaluation of triazinate in humans. Cancer Res. 36:48–54, 1976.
5. Hutchison, DJ: Quinazoline antifolates: biologic activities. Cancer Chemother. Rep. 52:697–705, 1968.
6. Johns DG, Farquhar D, Chabner BA, et al.: Antineoplastic activity of lipid-soluble dialkyl esters of methotrexate. Experientia 29:1104–1105, 1973.
7. Goldin A, Humphreys SR, Venditti JM, et al.: Prolongation of the lifespan of mice with advanced leukemia (L1210) by treatment with halogenated derivatives of amethopterin. J. Natl. Cancer Inst. 22:811–823, 1959.
8. Hignite CE, Shen DD, and Azarnoff DL: Separation and identification of impurities of parenteral methotrexate dosage forms. Cancer Treat. Rep. 62:13–18, 1978.
9. Chatterji DC, Frazier AG, and Galelli JF: Identification and quantitation of impurities in methotrexate. J. Pharm. Sci. 67:622–624, 1978.
10. Goldman ID, Lichtenstein NS, and Oliverio VT: Carrier-mediated transport of the folic acid analogue, methotrexate, in the L1210 leukemia cell. J. Biol. Chem. 243:5007–5017, 1968.
11. Yang CH, Peterson RH, Sirotnak FM, et al.: Folate analog transport by plasma membrane vesicles isolated from L1210 leukemia cells. J. Biol. Chem. 254:1402–1407, 1979.
12. McHugh M, and Cheng Y-C: Demonstration of a high affinity folate binder in human cell membranes and its characterization in cultured human KB cells. J. Biol. Chem. 254:11312, 1979.
13. Goldman ID: A model system for the study of heteroexchange diffusion: methotrexate-folate interactions in L1210 leukemia and Ehrlich ascites tumor cells. Biochim. Biophys. Acta 233:624–634, 1971.
14. Sirotnak FM, and Donsbach RC: Kinetic correlates of methotrexate transport and therapeutic responsiveness in murine tumors. Cancer Res. 36:1151–1158, 1976.
15. Warren RD, Nichols AP, and Bender RA: Membrane transport of methotrexate in human lymphoblastoid cells. Cancer Res. 38:668–671, 1978.
16. Fyfe MJ, and Goldman ID: Characteristics of the vincristine-induced augmentation of methotrexate uptake in Ehrlich ascites tumor cells. J. Biol. Chem. 248:5067–5073, 1973.
17. Chello PL, Sirotnak FM, Dorck DM, et al.: Therapeutic relevance of differences in the structural specificity of the transport systems for folate analogs in L1210 tumor cells and in isolated murine intestinal epithelial cells. Cancer Res. 37:4297–4303, 1977.
18. Warren RD, Nichols AP, and Bender RA: The effect of vincristine on methotrexate uptake and inhibition of DNA synthesis by human lymphoblastoid cells. Cancer Res. 37:2993–2997, 1977.
19. Zager RF, Frisby SA, and Oliverio VT: The effects of antibiotics and cancer chemotherapeutic agents on cellular transport and antitumor activity of methotrexate in L1210 murine leukemia. Cancer Res. 33:1670–1676, 1973.
20. Chello PL, Sirotnak FM, and Dorick DM: Alterations in the kinetics of methotrexate transport during growth of L-1210 murine leukemia cells in culture. Mol. Pharmacol. 18:274, 1980.
21. Hill BT, Bailey BD, White JC, et al.: Characteristics of transport of 4-amino antifolates and folate compounds by two lines of L5178Y lymphoblasts, one with impaired transport of methotrexate. Cancer Res. 39:2440–2446, 1979.
22. Sirotnak FM, and Donsbach RC: Further evidence for a basis of selective activity and relative responsiveness during antifolate therapy of murine tumors. Cancer Res. 35:1737–1744, 1975.
23. Kessel D, Hall TC, Roberts D, et al.: Uptake as a determinant of methotrexate response in mouse leukemias. Science 150:752–754, 1965.
24. Sirotnak FM, and Donsbach RC: Comparative studies on the transport of aminopterin, methotrexate, and methasquin by the L1210 leukemia cell. Cancer Res. 32:2120–2126, 1972.

25. Rosowsky A, and Yu C-S: New methods of neutral esterification of methotrexate and related compounds. *In* Kisliuk RL, and Brown GM (eds.): Chemistry and Biology of Pteridines. Elsevier/North Holland, New York, 1979, pp. 273–277.
26. Rosowsky A, Beardsley GP, Ensminger WD, et al.: Methotrexate analogues. II. Unambiguous chemical synthesis and *in vitro* biological evaluation of α- and γ-monoesters as potential prodrugs. J. Med. Chem. 21:380–386, 1978.
27. Ryser HJP, and Shen WC: Conjugation of methotrexate to poly (L-lysine) increases drug transport and overcomes resistance in cultured cells. Proc. Natl. Acad. Sci. USA 75:3867–3870, 1978.
27A. Jolivet J, and Schilsky, RL: High pressure liquid chromatography analysis of MTX polyglutamates in cultured human breast cancer cells. Biochem Pharmacol. 30: 1387–1390, 1981.
28. Jacobs SA, Derr CJ, and Johns DG: Accumulation of methotrexate diglutamate in human liver during methotrexate therapy. Biochem. Pharmacol. 26:2310–2313, 1977.
28A. Gewirtz DA, White JC, Randolph JK, et al.: Transport, binding, and polyglutamation of methotrexate in freshly isolated rat hepatocytes. Cancer Res. 40:573, 1980.
29. Rosenblatt DS, Whitehead VM, Dupont MM, et al.: Synthesis of methotrexate polyglutamates in cultured human cells. Mol. Pharmacol. 14:210–214, 1978.
30. Schilsky RL, Bailey BD, and Chabner BA: Methotrexate polyglutamate synthesis by cultured human breast cancer cells. Proc. Natl. Acad. Sci. USA 77:2919, 1980.
31. Whitehead VM: Synthesis of methotrexate polyglutamates in L1210 murine leukemia cells. Cancer Res. 37:408–412, 1977.
32. Jacobs SA, Adamson RH, Chabner BA, et al.: Stoichiometric inhibition of mammalian dihydrofolate reductase by the γ-glutamyl metabolite of methotrexate, 4-amino-4-deoxy-N^{10}-methylpteroylglutamyl-γ-glutamate. Biochem. Biophys. Res. Commun. 63:692–698, 1975.
33. Sirotnak FM, Chello PL, Piper JR, et al.: Growth inhibitory, transport and biochemical properties of the γ-glutamyl and γ-aspartyl peptides of methotrexate in L1210 leukaemia cells *in vitro*. Biochem. Pharmacol. 27:1821–1825, 1978.
33A. Poser RG, Sirotnak FM, and Chello PL: Extracellular recovery of methotrexate polyglutamates following efflux from L1210 leukemia cells. Biochem. Pharmacol. 29: 2701, 1980.
34. McGuire JJ, Kitamoto Y, Hsieh P, et al.: Characterization of mammalian folyl polyglutamate synthetase. *In* Kisliuk RK., and Brown GM (eds.): Chemistry and Biology of Pteridines. Elsevier/North Holland, New York, 1979, pp. 471–476.
35. Gewirtz DA, White JC, Randolph JK, et al.: Rapid polyglutamation of methotrexate in rat hepatocytes. Cancer Res. 39:2914–2918, 1979.
36. Shin YS, Buehring KU, and Stokstad ELR: The metabolism of methotrexate in *Lactobacillus casei* and rat liver and the influence of methotrexate on metabolism of folic acid. J. Biol. Chem. 249:5772–5777, 1974.
37. Gupta SV, Greenfield NJ, Poe M, et al.: Dihydrofolate reductase from a resistant subline of the L1210 lymphoma: purification by affinity chromatography, ultraviolet difference spectrophotometric and circular dichroic studies. Biochemistry 16:3073–3079, 1977.
38. Nakamura H, and Littlefield J: Purification, properties, and synthesis of dihydrofolate reductase from wild type and methotrexate-resistant hamster cells. J. Biol. Chem. 247:179–187, 1972.
39. Gready JE: Dihydrofolate reductase: the current story. Nature 282:674, 1979.
40. Matthews DA, Alden RA, Bolin JT, et al.: X-ray structural studies of dihydrofolate reductase. *In* Kisliuk RL, and Brown GM (eds.): Chemistry and Biology of Pteridines. Elsevier/North Holland, New York, 1979, pp. 465–470.
41. Charlton PA, Young DW, Birdsall B, et al.: Stereochemistry of reduction of folic acid using dihydrofolate reductase. Chem. Commun. 20:922–924, 1979.
42. Matthews DA, Alden RA, Bolin JT, et al.: Dihydrofolate reductase x-ray structure of the binary complex with methotrexate. Science 197:452–455, 1977.
43. Freisheim JH, Kumar AA, and Blankenship DT: Structure-function relationships of dihydrofolate reductases: sequence homology considerations and active center residues. *In* Kisliuk RL, and Brown GM (eds.): Chemistry and Biology of Pteridines. Elsevier/North Holland, New York, 1979, pp. 419–424.
44. Jackson RC, Hart LI, and Harrap KR: Intrinsic resistance to methotrexate of cultured mammalian cells in relation to the inhibition kinetics of their dihydrofolate reductase. Cancer Res. 36:1991–1997, 1980.
45. Werkheiser WC: The biochemical, cellular, and pharmacological action and effects of the folic acid antagonists. Cancer Res. 23:1277–1285, 1963.
46. Cha S: Tight-binding inhibitors. III. A new approach for the determination of competition between tight-binding inhibitors and substrates — inhibition of adenosine deaminase by coformycin. Biochem. Pharmacol. 25:2695–2702, 1976.
47. Williams JW, Duggleby RG, Cutler R, et al.: The inhibition of dihydrofolate reductase by folate analogues: structural requirements for slow- and tight-binding inhibitors. Biochem. Pharmacol. 29:589–595, 1980.
48. Cohen M, Bender RA, Donehower RC, et al.: Reversibility of high affinity binding of methotrexate in L1210 murine leukemia cells. Cancer Res. 38:2866–2870, 1978.
49. Jackson RC, Niethammer D, and Hart LI: Reactivation of dihydrofolate reductase inhibited by methotrexate or aminopterin. Arch. Biochem. Biophys. 182:646–656, 1977.
50. White CJ, Loftfield S, and Goldman ID: The mechanism of action of methotrexate. III. Requirement of free intracellular methotrexate for maximal suppression of (^{14}C) formate incorporation into nucleic acids and protein. Mol. Pharmacol. 11:287–297, 1975.
51. Friedkin M, Crawford E, Humphreys SR, et al.: The association of increased dihydrofolate reductase with Amethopterin resistance in mouse leukemia. Cancer Res. 22:600–606, 1962.
52. Kaufman RJ, Bertino JR, and Schimke RT: Quantitation of dihydrofolate reductase in individual parental and methotrexate-resistant murine cells: use of a fluorescence activated cell sorter. J. Biol. Chem. 253:5852–5860, 1978.
53. Hillcoat BL, Swett V, and Bertino JF: Increase in dihydrofolate reductase activity in cultured mammalian cells after exposure to methotrexate. Proc. Natl. Acad. Sci. USA 58:1632–1637, 1967.
54. Bertino JR, Donohue DR, Simmons B, et al.: Induction of dihydrofolate reductase activity in leukocytes and erythrocytes of patients treated with Amethopterin. J. Clin. Invest. 42:466–475, 1963.
55. Alt FW, Kellems RE, and Schimke RT: Synthesis and degradation of folate reductase in sensitive and methotrexate-resistant lines of S180 cells. J. Biol. Chem. 251:3063–3074, 1976.
55A. Alt FW, Kellems RE, Bertino JR, et al.: Selective multiplication of dihydrofolate reductase genes in methotrexate-resistant variants of cultured murine cells. J. Biol. Chem. 253:1357, 1978.
56. Kaufman RJ, Brown PC, and Schimke RT: Amplified dihydrofolate reductase genes in unstably methotrexate-resistant cells are associated with double minute chromosomes. Proc. Natl. Acad. Sci. USA 76:5669–5673, 1979.
57. Wahl GM, Padgett RA, and Stark GR: Gene amplification causes overproduction of the first three enzymes of UMP synthesis in N-(phosphonacetyl)-L-aspartate–resistant hamster cells. J. Biol. Chem. 254:8679, 1979.
58. Malera PW, Wolgemuth D, Hession C, et al.: Evidence for the overproduction of two dihydrofolate reductases encoded by separate mRNAs in antifolate-resistant Chinese hamster cells. J. Cell Biol. 83:407, 1979.
58A. Melera PW, Wolgemuth D, Biedler JL, et al.: Antifolate-

resistant Chinese hamster cells. J. Biol. Chem. 255:319, 1980.

58B. Melera PW, Lewis JA, Biedler JL, et al.: Antifolate-resistant Chinese hamster cells. J. Biol. Chem. 255:7024, 1980.

59. Fenwick RG: Sensitivity to aminopterin in the face of dihydrofolate reductase overproduction. J. Cell Biol. 79:390, 1978.

59A. Flintoff WF, and Essani K: Methotrexate-resistant Chinese hamster ovary cells contain a dihydrofolate reductase with an altered affinity for methotrexate. Biochemistry 19:4321, 1980.

60. Cline MJ, Stang H, Mercola K, et al: Gene transfer in intact animals. Nature 284:422–425, 1980.

61. Zaharko DS, Fung W-P, and Yang K-H: Relative biochemical aspects of low and high doses of methotrexate in mice. Cancer Res. 37:1602–1607, 1977.

62. Donehower RC, Allegra JC, Lippman ME, et al.: Combined effects of methotrexate and 5-fluoropyrimidine on human breast cancer cells in serum-free cultures. Eur. J. Cancer 16:655–661, 1980.

63. Jackson RC, and Weber G: Enzyme pattern directed chemotherapy: the effects of combinations of methotrexate, 5-fluorodeoxyuridine and thymidine on rat hepatoma cells *in vitro.* Biochem. Pharmacol. 25:2613–2618, 1976.

64. Tattersall MH, Jackson RC, Jackson ST, et al.: Factors determining cell sensitivity to methotrexate: studies of folate and deoxyribonucleotide triphosphate pools in five mammalian cell lines. Eur. J. Cancer 10:819–826, 1974.

65. Fridland A: Effect of methotrexate on deoxynucleotide pools and DNA synthesis in human lymphocyte cells. Cancer Res. 34:1883–1888, 1974.

66. Goulian M, Bleile B, and Tseng BY: Methotrexate-induced misincorporation of uracil into DNA. Proc. Natl. Acad. Sci. USA 77:1956–1960, 1980.

67. Grafstrom RH, Tseng BY, and Goulian M: The incorporation of uracil into animal cell DNA *in vitro.* Cell 15:131–140, 1978.

68. Pinedo HM, Zaharko DS, Bull JM, et al.: The relative contribution of drug concentration and duration of exposure to mouse bone marrow toxicity during continuous methotrexate infusion. Cancer Res. 37:445–450, 1977.

69. Pinedo HM, Chabner BA, Zaharko DS, et al.: Evidence for early recruitment of granulocyte precursors during high-dose methotrexate infusion in mice. Blood 48:301–307, 1976.

70. Hryniuk WM, and Bertino JR: Treatment of leukemia with large doses of methotrexate and folinic acid: clinical-biochemical correlates. J. Clin. Invest. 48:2140–2155, 1969.

71. Pinedo HM, Zaharko DS, Bull JM, et al.: The reversal of methotrexate cytotoxicity to mouse bone marrow cells by leucovorin and nucleosides. Cancer Res. 36:4418–4424, 1976.

72. Howell SB, Ensminger WD, Krishan A, et al.: Thymidine rescue of high-dose methotrexate in humans. Cancer Res. 38:325–330, 1978.

73. Rustum Y: High-pressure liquid chromatography quantitative separation of purine and pyrimidine nucleosides and bases. Anal. Biochem. 90:289–299, 1978.

73A. Jackson RC: Modulation of methotrexate toxicity by thymidine: sequence-dependent biochemical effects. Mol. Pharmacol. 18:281, 1980.

74. Straw JA, Talbot DC, Taylor GA, et al.: Some observations on the reversibility of methotrexate toxicity in normal proliferating tissues. J. Natl. Cancer Inst. 58:91–97, 1977.

75. Tattersall MHN, Brown B, and Frei E III: The reversal of methotrexate toxicity by thymidine with maintenance of antitumour effects. Nature 253:198–200, 1975.

76. Semon JH, and Grindey GB: Potentiation of the antitumor activity of methotrexate by concurrent infusion of thymidine. Cancer Res. 38:2905–2911, 1978.

77. Novelli A, Mini E, Liuffi M, et al.: Clinical data on rescue of high-dose methotrexate with N^5-methyltetrahydrofolate in human solid tumors. *In* Periti P (ed.): High-Dose Methotrexate Pharmacology, Toxicology and Chemotherapy. Giuntina, Firenze, 1978, pp. 299–309.

78. Goldin A, Mantel N, Greenhouse SW, et al.: Effect of delayed administration of citrovorum factor on antileukemic effectiveness of Amethopterin in mice. Cancer Res. 14:43–48, 1954.

79. Bertino JR, and Fischer GA: Techniques for study of resistance to folic acid antagonists. Methods Med. Res. 10:297, 1964.

80. Myers CE, Lippman ME, Eliot HM, et al.: Competitive protein binding assay for methotrexate. Proc. Natl. Acad. Sci. USA 72:3683–3686, 1975.

81. Bertino JR, and Isacoff WH: Methods of measuring methotrexate in body fluids. *In* Pinedo HM (ed.): Clinical Pharmacology of Antineoplastic Drugs. Elsevier/North Holland, Amsterdam, 1978, pp. 3–11.

82. Donehower RC, Hande KR, Drake JC, et al.: Presence of 2,4-diamino-N^{10}-methyl pteroic acid after high-dose methotrexate. Clin. Pharmacol. Ther. 26:63–72, 1979.

83. Oellerich M, Engelhardt P, Schaadt M, et al.: Determination of methotrexate in serum by a rapid, fully mechanized enzyme in immunoassay (EMIT). J. Clin. Chem. Clin. Biochem. 18:169–174, 1980.

84. Zaharko DS, Dedrick RL., and Bischoff KB: Methotrexate tissue distribution: prediction by a mathematical model. J. Natl. Cancer Inst. 46:775–784, 1971.

85. Huffman DH, Wan SH, Azaranoff DL, et al.: Pharmacokinetics of methotrexate. Clin. Pharmacol. Ther. 14:572–579, 1973.

86. Chungi VS, Bourne DWA, and Dittert LW: Drug absorption. VIII. Kinetics of GI absorption of methotrexate. J. Pharm. Sci. 67:560–561, 1978.

87. Henderson ES, Adamson RH, and Oliverio VT: The metabolic fate of tritiated methotrexate. II. Absorption and excretion in man. Cancer Res. 25:1018–1024, 1965.

88. Stuart JFB, Calman KC, Watters J, et al.: Bioavailability of methotrexate: implications for clinical use. Cancer Chemother. Pharmacol. 3:239–241, 1979.

89. Kearney PJ, Light PA, Preece A, et al.: Unpredictable serum levels after oral methotrexate in children with acute lymphoblastic leukemia. Cancer Chemother. Pharmacol. 3:117–120, 1979.

90. Steele WH, Stuart JB, Lawrence JR, et al.: Methotrexate protein binding. Br. J. Cancer 40:316, 1979.

91. Liegler DG, Henderson ES, Hahn MA, et al.: The effect of organic acids on renal clearance of methotrexate in man. Clin. Pharmacol. Ther. 10:849–857, 1969.

92. Wan SH, Huffman DH, Azarnoff DL, et al.: Effect of route of administration and effusion on methotrexate pharmacokinetics. Cancer Res. 34:3487–3491, 1974.

93. Chabner BA, Stoller RG, Hande KR, et al.: Methotrexate disposition in humans: case studies in ovarian cancer and following high-dose infusion. Drug Metab. Rev. 8:107–117, 1978.

94. Torres IJ, Litterst CL, and Guarino AM: Transport of model compounds across the peritoneal membrane in the rat. Pharmacology 17:330–340, 1978.

95. Stoller RG, Jacobs SA, Drake JC, et al.: Pharmacokinetics of high-dose methotrexate. Cancer Chemother. Rep. 6:19–24, 1975.

96. Lawrence JR, Steele WH, Stuart JFB, et al.: Dose-dependent methotrexate elimination following bolus intravenous injection. Eur. J. Clin. Pharmacol. 17:371–374, 1980.

97. Kristenson L, Weismann K, and Hutters L: Renal function and the rate of disappearance of methotrexate from serum. Eur. J. Clin. Pharmacol. 8:439–444, 1975.

98. Nirenberg A, Mosende C, Mehte B, et al.: High-dose methotrexate with citrovorum factor rescue: predictive value of serum methotrexate concentrations and corrective measures to avert toxicity. Cancer Treat. Rep. 61:779–783, 1977.

99. Isacoff WH, Morrison PF, Aroesty J, et al.: Pharmacokinetics of high-dose methotrexate with citrovorum factor rescue. Cancer Treat. Rep. 61:1665–1674, 1977.

100. Bleyer WA: The clinical pharmacology of methotrexate. Cancer 41:36–51, 1978.
101. Calvert AH, Bondy PK, and Harrap KR: Some observations on the human pharmacology of methotrexate. Cancer Treat. Rep. 61:1647–1656, 1977.
102. Hande KR, Balow JE, Drake JC, et al.: Methotrexate and hemodialysis. Ann. Intern. Med. 87:495–596, 1977.
103. Monjanel S, Rigault JP, Cano JP, et al.: High-dose methotrexate: preliminary evaluation of a pharmacokinetic approach. Cancer Chemother. Pharmacol. 3:189–196, 1979.
104. Romolo JL, Goldberg NH, Hande KR, et al.: The effect of hydration on plasma methotrexate levels. Cancer Treat. Rep. 61:1393–1395, 1977.
105. Huang KC, Wenczak BA, and Liu YK: Renal tubular transport of methotrexate in the rhesus monkey and dog. Cancer Res. 39:4843–4848, 1979.
106. Aherne GW, Prall E, Marks V, et al.: Prolongation and enhancement of serum methotrexate concentrations by probenecid. Br. Med. J. 1:1097–1099, 1978.
107. Gewirtz DA, White JC, and Goldman ID: Transport, binding, and polyglutamation of methotrexate (MTX) in freshly isolated hepatocytes. Proc. Am. Assoc. Cancer Res. 20:147, 1979.
108. Strum WB, and Liem HH: Hepatic uptake, intracellular protein binding and biliary excretion of Amethopterin. Biochem. Pharmacol. 26:1235–1240, 1977.
109. Strum WB, Liem HH, and Muller-Eberhard U: Effect of chemotherapeutic agents on the uptake and excretion of Amethopterin by the isolated perfused rat liver. Cancer Res. 38:4734–4736, 1978.
110. Leme PR, Creaven PJ, Allen LM, et al.: Kinetic model for the disposition and metabolism of moderate and high-dose methotrexate in man. Cancer Chemother. Rep. 59:811–817, 1975.
111. Shen DD, and Azarnoff DL: Clinical pharmacokinetics of methotrexate. Clin. Pharmacokinet. 3:1–13, 1978.
112. Valerino DM, Johns DG, Zaharko DS, et al.: Studies of the metabolism of methotrexate by intestinal flora. Biochem. Pharmacol. 21:821–831, 1972.
113. Jacobs SA, Stoller RG, Chabner BA, et al.: 7-Hydroxy methotrexate as a urinary metabolite in human subjects and rhesus monkeys receiving high-dose methotrexate. J. Clin. Invest. 57:534–538, 1976.
114. Lankelma, J, and van der Klein E: The role of 7-hydroxy methotrexate during methotrexate anticancer chemotherapy. Cancer Lett. 9:133–142, 1980.
115. McCullough JL, Chabner BA, and Bertino JR: Purification and properties of carboxypeptidase G_1. J. Biol. Chem. 246:7203–7213, 1971.
116. Abelson HT, Ensminger W, Rosowsky A, et al.: Comparative effects of citrovorum factor and carboxypeptidase G_1 on cerebrospinal fluid methotrexate pharmacokinetics. Cancer Treat. Rep. 62:1549–1552, 1978.
117. Chabner BA, and Young RC: Threshold methotrexate concentration for *in vivo* inhibition of DNA synthesis in normal and tumorous target tissues. J. Clin. Invest. 52:1804–1811, 1973.
118. Sirotnak F, and Moccio DM: Pharmacokinetic basis for differences in methotrexate sensitivity of normal proliferative tissues in the mouse. Cancer Res. 40:1230–1234, 1980.
119. Jaffe N: Recent advances in the chemotherapy of metastatic osteogenic sarcoma. Cancer 30:1627–1631, 1972.
120. Von Hoff DD, Penta JS, Helman LJ, et al.: Incidence of drug-related deaths secondary to high-dose methotrexate and citrovorum factor administration. Cancer Treat. Rep. 61:745–748, 1977.
121. Glode LM, Pitman SW, Ensminger WD, et al.: A phase I study of high doses of aminopterin with leucovorin rescue in patients with advanced metastatic tumor. Cancer Res. 39:3707, 1979.
122. Stoller RG, Hande KR, Jacobs SA, et al.: Use of plasma pharmacokinetics to predict and prevent methotrexate toxicity. N. Engl. J. Med. 297:630–634, 1977.
123. Evans WE, Pratt CB, Taylor H, et al.: Pharmacokinetic monitoring of high-dose methotrexate. Cancer Chemother. Pharmacol. 3:161–166, 1979.
124. Djerassi I, Ciesielka W, and Kim JS: Removal of methotrexate by filtration-adsorption using charcoal filters or by hemodialysis. Cancer Treat. Rep. 61:751–752, 1977.
125. Bertino JR, Condos S, Horvath C, et al.: Immobilized carboxypeptidase G_1 in methotrexate removal. Cancer Res. 38:1936–1941, 1978.
126. Albrecht AM, Boldizsar E, and Hutchison DJ: Carboxypeptidase displaying differential velocity in hydrolysis of methotrexate, 5-methyltetrahydrofolic acid, and leucovorin. J. Bacteriol. 134:506–513, 1978.
127. Ensminger WD, and Frei E III: The prevention of methotrexate toxicity by thymidine infusions in humans. Cancer Res. 37:1857–1863, 1977.
128. Schornagel JH, Leyva A, Bucsa JM, et al.: Thymidine prevention of methotrexate toxicity in head-and-neck cancer. *In* Pinedo HM (ed.): Clinical Pharmacology of Antineoplastic Drugs. Elsevier/North Holland, Amsterdam, 1978, pp. 83–95.
129. Howell SB, Herbst K, Boss GR, et al.: Thymidine requirements for the rescue of patients treated with high-dose methotrexate. Cancer Res. 40:1824–1829, 1980.
130. Capizzi RL: Schedule-dependent synergism and antagonism between methotrexate and L-asparaginase. Biochem. Pharmacol. 23:151–161, 1974.
131. Yap BS, McCredie KB, Benjamin RS, et al.: Refractory acute leukaemia in adults treated with sequential colaspase and high-dose methotrexate. Br. Med. J. 2:791–793, 1978.
132. Lobel JS, O'Brien RT, McIntosh S, et al.: Methotrexate and asparaginase combination chemotherapy in refractory acute lymphoblastic leukemia of childhood. Cancer 43:1089–1094, 1979.
133. Moran RG, Mulkins M, and Heidelberger C: Role of thymidylate synthetase activity in development of methotrexate cytotoxicity. Proc. Natl. Acad. Sci. USA 76:5924–5928, 1979.
134. Zachariae H, Kragballe K, and Søgaard H: Methotrexate-induced cirrhosis. Br. J. Dermatol. 102:407–412, 1980.
135. Dahl MGC, Gregory MM, and Scheuer PJ: Liver damage due to methotrexate in patients with psoriasis. Br. Med. J. 1:625–630, 1971.
136. Tuma DJ, Barak AJ, and Sorrell MF: Interaction of methotrexate with lipotropic factors in rat liver. Biochem. Pharmacol. 24:1327–1331, 1975.
137. Clarysse AM, Catney WJ, Cartwright GE, et al.: Pulmonary disease complicating intermittent therapy with methotrexate. J.A.M.A. 209:1861–1864, 1969.
138. Sostman HD, Matthay RA, Putman C, et al.: Methotrexate-induced pneumonitis. Medicine 55:371–388, 1976.
139. Goldberg NH, Romolo JL, Austin EH, et al.: Anaphylactoid type reactions in two patients receiving high-dose intravenous methotrexate. Cancer 41:52–55, 1978.
140. Shapiro WR, Young DG, and Mehta BM: Methotrexate distribution in cerebrospinal fluid after intravenous, ventricular, and lumbar injections. N. Engl. J. Med. 293:161–166, 1975.
140A. Neuwelt EA, Frenkel EP, Rapoport S, et al.: Effect of osmotic blood-brain barrier disruption on methotrexate pharmacokinetics in the dog. Neurosurgery 7:36, 1980.
140B. Bode U, Magrath IT, Bleyer WA, et al.: Active transport of methotrexate from cerebrospinal fluid in humans. Cancer Res. 40:2184, 1980.
141. Bleyer WA, Drake JC, and Chabner BA: Neurotoxicity and elevated cerebrospinal-fluid methotrexate concentration in meningeal leukemia. N. Engl. J. Med. 289:770–773, 1973.
142. Bleyer WA, Poplack DG, and Simon RM: "Concentration × time" methotrexate via a subcutaneous reservoir: a less toxic regimen for intraventricular chemotherapy of central nervous system neoplasms. Blood 51:835–842, 1978.
143. Peylan-Ramu N, Poplack DG, Blei CL, et al.: Computer-assisted tomography in methotrexate encephalopathy. J. Comput. Assist. Tomogr. 1:216–221, 1977.
144. Shapiro WR, Allen JC, and Horten BC: Chronic methotrexate toxicity to the central nervous system. Clin. Bull. Memorial-Sloan Kettering 10:49–52, 1980.
145. Cadman E, Heimer R, and Davis L: Enhanced 5-

fluorouracil nucleotide formation after methotrexate administration: explanation for drug synergism. Science 205:1135–1137, 1979.

146. Bowen D, White JC, and Goldman ID: Basis for fluoropyrimidine-induced antagonism to methotrexate in Ehrlich ascites tumor cells *in vitro*. Cancer Res. 38:219–222, 1978.

147. Cadman E, and Eiferman P: Mechanism of synergistic cell killing when methotrexate precedes cytosine arabinoside. Study of L1210 and human leukemic cells. J. Clin. Invest. 64:788–797, 1979.

148. Chello PL, Sirotnak FM, and Dorick DM: Different effects of vincristine on methotrexate uptake by L1210 cells and mouse internal epithelia *in vitro* and *in vivo*. Cancer Res. 39:2106–2112, 1979.

149. Warren RD, and Bender RA: Drug interactions with antineoplastic drugs. Cancer Treat. Rep. 61:1231–1241, 1977.

150. Pinedo HM, and Chabner BA: Role of drug concentration, duration of exposure, and endogenous metabolites in determining methotrexate cytotoxicity. Cancer Treat. Rep. 61:709–715, 1977.

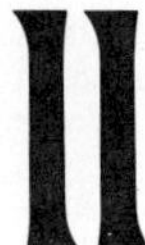

TUBULIN BINDING AGENTS

Richard A. Bender

Bruce A. Chabner

VINCA ALKALOIDS

INTRODUCTION

Although plant derivatives have been a traditional source of folk medicine, and remain important agents in cardiovascular therapeutics and for pain relief, the search for antineoplastic principals of plant origin has been minimally successful. The only effective plant products used in cancer treatment at present are semisynthetic derivatives of the mandrake plant (the epipodophyllotoxins) and alkaloids of the periwinkle plant *(Vinca rosea)*.[1,2] The epipodophyllotoxins, which have gained increasing significance in the treatment of testicular carcinoma, lymphomas, and small cell carcinoma of the lung, are discussed later in this chapter. We will first consider the vinca family, which includes vincristine (VCR), vinblastine (VB), and vindesine (VDS); VCR and VB have gained a prominent role in the curative treatment of Hodgkin's disease and the non-Hodgkin's lymphomas, childhood acute lymphoblastic leukemia, and various pediatric solid tumors. Vindesine, which has received only preliminary clinical evaluation, appears to have a broad range of activity, but has not displaced the original vinca alkaloids in primary treatment regimens at this time.

STRUCTURE

Vincristine and vinblastine are formed of two structurally similar, multiringed units, vindoline and catharanthine, which are linked by a carbon-carbon bridge; the two derivatives differ only in the single substitution on the catharanthine group (Fig. 11–1). Vindesine, or desacetyl vinblastine carboxyamide, was originally isolated as a VB metabolite, but has antitumor activity of its own and a somewhat different spectrum of clinical toxicity from that found with either VCR or VB. All three derivatives are believed to share a common mechanism of action, the inhibition of tubulin formation, but differ

A

VINBLASTINE R—CH_3
VINCRISTINE R—CHO

B

Figure 11–1. Molecular structures of vinblastine and vincristine *(A)* and vindesine *(B)*.

significantly in their pharmacologic properties and spectra of clinical activity.

CELLULAR PHARMACOLOGY

The vinca alkaloids appear to cross the cell membrane by an energy-dependent transport system.[3] The affinity constant for VCR transport is approximately 10 μM in murine and human leukemic cells, and this transport is competitively inhibited by VB, suggesting a common carrier for these closely related compounds. Glutamate also competitively inhibits VB uptake.[4] Recent work with P388 murine leukemia cells suggests an alternative mechanism. These investigators found VCR transport to be nonsaturable and energy-independent at substrate concentrations in excess of 100 μM, and suggest diffusion as the mechanism for transmembrane movement.[5]

Evidence from the study of cross-resistance patterns in animal tumors suggests that VCR may share its transport system with other high-molecular-weight antitumor agents. For example, Ehrlich ascites tumor cells resistant to daunomycin are also resistant to VCR,[6] and Chinese hamster ovary cells resistant to actinomycin D are similarly resistant to VB and VCR, as well as to mithramycin, daunomycin, and mitomycin C.[7] P388 murine leukemia cells resistant to VCR are also resistant to actinomycin D and the anthracyclines,[8] although they retain sensitivity to the closely related plant alkaloid VP-16.[9] Since the vinca alkaloids, anthracyclines, and antibiotics are believed to have quite different mechanisms of action, cross-resistance in these cell lines might be due to deletion of a common transport carrier. This possibility is supported by the observation that resistant P388 murine leukemia cells exhibit increased efflux of the anthracyclines and actinomycin D.[10,11] Alterations in cell surface glycoproteins have been found in cultured human leukemia lymphoblasts resistant to vinca alkaloids, lending further support to the importance of membrane transport in vinca alkaloid resistance.[11A,11B]

Interaction with Tubulin

The vinca alkaloids exert their biologic effects through their binding to tubulin, a protein of dimeric structure that polymerizes to form microtubules,[12] as shown in Figure 11–2. A number of cellular functions, including mitosis, transport of solutes, cell movement, and structural integrity, depend on the microtubular system. These tubules are cylindric organelles 250Å wide and several microns long.[13] In eukaryotic cells, microtubules form the mitotic spindle that appears and then regresses during mitosis. Microtubules perform specialized functions in nerve cell axons[14] (neurotransmitter movement along axons) and in secretory cells (conducting proteins and hormones from ribosomes to the cell membrane). The microtubular apparatus exists in a dynamic equilibrium with the soluble pool of cytoplasmic tubulin, undergoing continuous formation at a growing end and dissolution at the opposite pole.

Vincristine and vinblastine share a common pair of binding sites on each tubulin dimer, sites distinct from the binding locus for two other tubulin-binding alkaloids, colchicine and podophyllotoxin.[15] The binding affinity (K_D) of VCR and VB for soluble tubulin is about 0.1 μM; the K_D for tubulin crystals is somewhat weaker, 4 μM.[16] Binding leads to an inhibition of the assembly of tubulin into microtubules[17] and the formation of tubulin-rich intracellular crystals.[18] Vinca binding ultimately leads to disappearance of the microtubular structures and a dissolution of the mitotic spindle structure.[19]

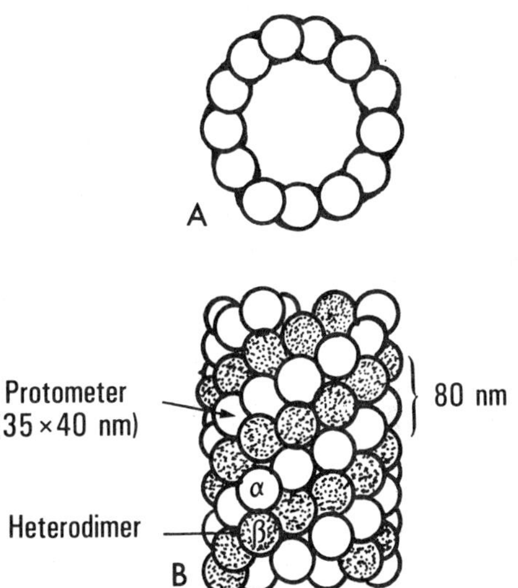

Figure 11–2. Model of a microtubule, cross-sectional *(A)* and longitudinal *(B)* views. There are 13 protofilaments in each microtubule. The protofilaments are made up of heterodimers consisting of α and β tubulin subunits.

Only minute concentrations of vinca alkaloids (less than 0.1 μM in cell culture) are required to inhibit microtubule formation,[17] possibly because inhibition of the assembly process results from the incorporation of a single drug-tubulin complex into the growing end of the microtubule.*

Consistent with an inhibitory effect on mitotic spindle formation, the tubulin-binding agents arrest cells in metaphase of mitosis. Exposure to colchicine provides a convenient method for synchronizing cells, since washout of the drug reverses this block and leads to a resumption of mitosis. The mitotic arrest produced by VCR and VB is incompletely reversed by drug washout, depending on experimental conditions and the specific cell lines studied.[20-23] For example, Chinese hamster ovary cells exposed briefly to VB undergo spindle dissolution, but retain viability after drug removal, as judged by colony formation.[24]

*An interesting new antitumor plant alkaloid, taxol, enhances polymerization of tubulin and blocks its depolymerization by colchicine. (See Schiff PB, and Horowitz SB: Proc. Natl. Acad. Sci. USA 77:1561, 1980.)

Despite the preponderance of evidence that cytotoxicity is intimately related to metaphase arrest, cultured cells are killed by exposure to drug during all phases of the cell cycle and are most sensitive to the vinca alkaloids if exposed during the late S phase of the cell cycle.[20, 25] In addition, flow microfluorometric studies have indicated that these drugs also produce a progression delay in G_2.[25] These characteristics of drug actions are not readily explained on the basis of interaction with tubulin.

The concentrations of vinca alkaloid required to produce cytotoxicity in cell culture are extremely low.[26] VCR concentrations of 4×10^{-8}M produced 50 per cent cell kill (Fig. 11–3). Proliferation of a human T-lymphoblastoid cell line (CEM) is completely inhibited by 1×10^{-8}M VCR. The possibility that normal cells and tumor cells have different sensitivity to VCR was suggested by the finding that morphologic changes indicative of drug effects were produced in normal lymphocytes by 1.2×10^{-5}M VCR, but tenfold lower doses produced the same effect in chronic lymphocytic leukemia cells.[27] This observation might explain the

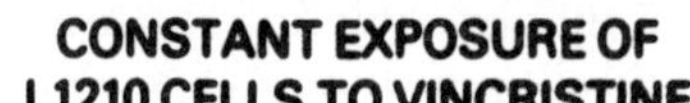

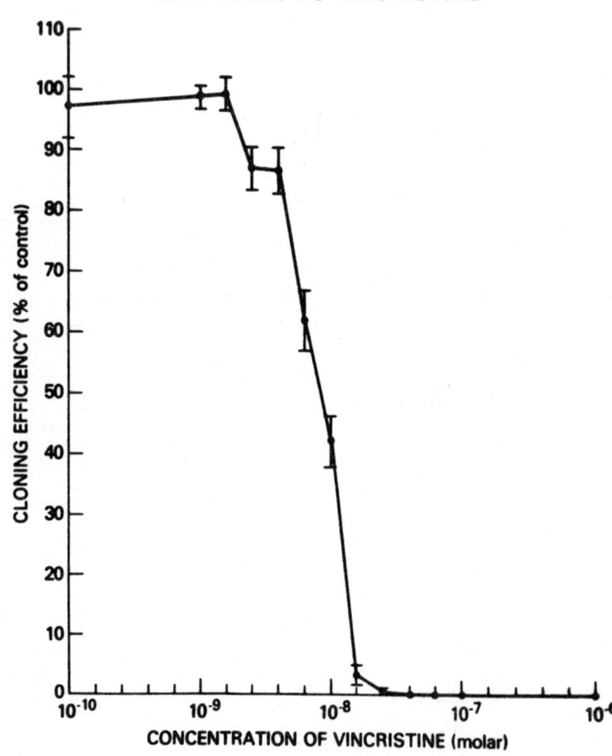

Figure 11–3. Cytotoxicity of vincristine for L1210 murine leukemia cells as measured by cloning efficiency. Cells were placed in soft agar containing vincristine at the specified concentration, and colonies were counted 14 days later and expressed as a percentage of colonies that developed from unexposed (control) cells. (Reproduced with permission from Jackson DV, and Bender RA: Cytotoxic thresholds of vincristine in L1210 murine leukemia and a human lymphoblastic cell line *in vitro.* Cancer Res. 39:4346–4349, 1979.)

exquisite sensitivity of some human lymphocytic malignancies at doses that produce no measurable effect on peripheral lymphocyte count.

Although most experimental evidence supports the hypothesis that vinca alkaloids kill cells through their inhibition of tubulin synthesis, this class of compounds has other toxic effects. High concentrations of VB (1000-fold greater than achieved *in vivo*) inhibit the incorporation of uridine into RNA and incorporation of thymidine into DNA of cells in culture.[28, 29] Vinca alkaloids also inhibit lipid and protein synthesis.[30] Both VCR and VB block the entry of glutamic acid into tumor cells and into rat brain synaptosomes.[31] However, none of these actions has been directly implicated in vinca cytotoxicity. They may well be secondary effects of the inhibition of tubulin assembly and, because of this likelihood, have not attracted much research interest.

Mechanisms of Resistance

No detailed investigations of mechanisms of tumor cell resistance to VCR or VB have been conducted, but several possible mechanisms have been inferred from observations regarding transport and tubulin binding in resistant cells. As mentioned previously, the vinca alkaloids are cross-resistant with other antibiotic antitumor agents in various murine leukemia cell lines, despite the fact that these drugs have widely divergent mechanisms of action. A possible explanation, still unproved, is that these drugs share a common transport mechanism. The decreased uptake of vinca alkaloids, actinomycin D, and the phthalanilide antibiotics in murine tumor cells appears to result from an accelerated exit of these drugs[32] owing to an amplified membrane glycoprotein.[32A] Second, decreased intracellular binding of VCR correlates with sensitivity of murine tumor cell lines to this agent.[32B] Both the transport and tubulin binding theories of drug resistance require verification by more careful examination of these processes at the molecular level.

CLINICAL PHARMACOLOGY

Clinical assessment of the pharmacokinetics and metabolism of the vinca alkaloids has been greatly hampered by the very small doses used in clinical chemotherapy and the lack of suitably sensitive drug assays. Thus, radiolabeled drug has been the mainstay for most clinical studies to date. The recent development of a radioimmunoassay for VCR should lead to a better understanding of the pharmacokinetics of this drug.[33, 33A] A summary of pharmacokinetic information is given in Table 11–1.

Bender and colleagues separated ^{3}H-VCR from metabolites by high-pressure liquid chromatography[34] (Fig. 11–4) and found peak plasma levels of approximately 0.4 μM. They defined a triphasic disappearance of drug from plasma thereafter, with half-lives of 0.85, 7.4, and 164 minutes. The earliest half-life very likely represents drug distribution into the extracellular compartment. VCR is extensively concentrated in platelets, with lesser amounts in white blood cells and erythrocytes. The extensive uptake by platelets has led to the use of vinca-loaded platelets for treatment of idiopathic thrombocytopenic purpura and other disorders of platelet consumption.

TABLE 11–1. Pharmacokinetics of Vinca and Epipodophyllotoxin Derivatives

	Peak Plasma Level (μM)	*Plasma $t^{1/2}$ (min)* α	β	γ	*Primary Route of Excretion*
VINCA					
Vincristine	0.4	0.8	7	164	Hepatic metabolism, biliary excretion
Vinblastine	0.4	3.9	53	1200	"
Vindesine	0.4	3.9	99	1200	"
EPIPODOPHYLLOTOXINS					
VP–16	20	30	230	1600	Hepatic metabolism, biliary and renal excretion
VM–26	40	–	168	900	Hepatic metabolism, and renal excretion of parent compound

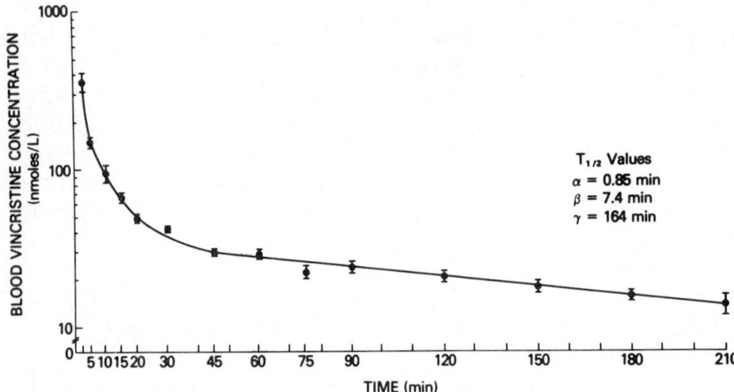

Figure 11–4. The blood disappearance curve of tritiated vincristine in man. The t½ values are derived by linear regression analysis. Correction for metabolism and/or decomposition is not included in the concentration measurements. (Reproduced with permission from Bender et al.: The pharmacokinetics of [^{3}H] vincristine in man. Clin. Pharmacol. Ther. 22:430–438, 1977.)

Hepatic metabolism plays a primary role in the elimination of VCR.[35, 36] In man, less than 15 per cent of an administered dose is excreted in the urine, whereas 70 per cent or more appears in the feces in the form of metabolites or possibly decomposition products.[33] The large quantity of VCR-derived material in the feces results from biliary excretion of metabolites, a process confirmed by studies of a patient with an indwelling choledochal T tube.[37] Bile concentrations of VCR-derived material are 100-fold higher than simultaneous levels in plasma two to four hours after administration, and remain 20-fold higher than plasma at 72 hours after injection. Cumulative biliary excretion in the single patient studied accounted for at least 50 per cent of injected drug (Fig. 11–5).

Although hepatic metabolism is undoubtedly responsible for most degradation of VCR observed in these experiments, the radioactive material itself is unstable in buffered solution at 37° C; in addition, exchange of the tritium label could account for some of the apparent metabolism.[37]

Vincristine enters the central nervous system rapidly after intravenous injection into primates. Concentrations above 1 nM are maintained in spinal fluid for longer than 72 hours after a single dose.[38] However, in the limited clinical pharmacokinetics studies to date, drug penetration into the CSF, as monitored from an indwelling CSF reservoir, was 20- to 30-fold lower than corresponding plasma drug concentrations, and never exceeded 1.1×10^{-9}M[38A] in the two carefully studied patients.

Vinblastine displays similar pharmacokinetics to those of VCR in man, as determined by studies employing ^{3}H-labeled drug.[39] A biphasic disappearance from plasma has been observed, with half-lives of 4.5 and 190

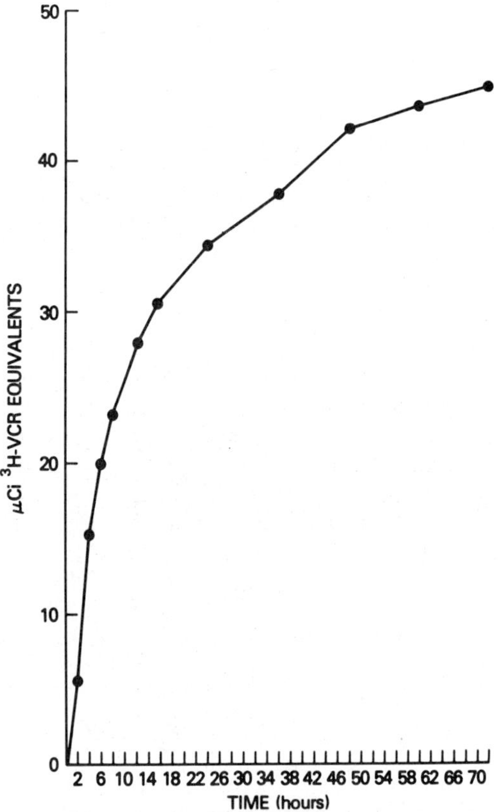

Figure 11–5. Cumulative biliary excretion of tritiated vincristine in man. Total radioactivity excreted has been measured and correction for metabolism and/or decomposition has not been carried out. Samples were collected from an indwelling T tube located in the common bile duct following intravenous injection of 158 μCi of tritiated drug. (Reproduced with permission from Jackson et al.: Biliary excretion of vincristine. Clin. Pharmacol. Ther. 24:101–107, 1978.)

minutes. Somewhat different results have been forthcoming from the use of radioimmunoassay, which detected half-lives of 3.9 and 53 minutes, and a terminal phase with a half-life of 20 hours.[40] Peak plasma concentration is 0.4 μM at usual clinical doses and, as in the case of VCR, platelets avidly concentrate the drug, with lesser uptake by white and red blood cells.

Less than 15 per cent of administered VB is excreted in the urine, but fecal excretion of the parent compound is low also (less than 10 per cent of dose in one study) as determined by radioimmunoassay.[40] A much larger fraction of ^3H labeled drug appears in the feces, probably representing metabolites that do not cross-react in the radioimmunoassay. One of the metabolites of VB is VDS, a more potent cytotoxic compound than the parent drug in experimental systems and a clinical antitumor agent in its own right.

Only preliminary information is available regarding VDS pharmacokinetics, but again the pattern of excretion and plasma disappearance is similar to that of the other vinca alkaloids. Radioimmunoassay results indicate a triphasic disappearance from plasma with half-lives of 3.2 and 99 minutes, and a final phase of 20 hours.[33] These results have been confirmed by a second pharmacokinetic study that reported half-lives of 2 minutes, 50 minutes, and 24 hours.[40A] Less than 15 per cent of a dose is excreted in the urine in 24 hours. Fecal and biliary excretion have not been measured in man, but appear to be the primary route of drug elimination in the rat.[41]

Drug Dosage and Schedules

Vincristine is administered intravenously in doses of 1 to 1.4 mg per m^2. Total doses in excess of 2 mg frequently lead to a progressive and disabling neurotoxicity, particularly if given on a weekly basis.[42, 43] Thus, many protocols specify a single-dose limitation of 2 mg. Vinblastine is administered as a single agent in doses of 0.1 to 0.3 mg per kg, and repeat doses are given at weekly intervals with escalation according to patient tolerance.[42] The lower range of doses is used in combination therapy with other myelosuppressive drugs. VB may also be administered by a prolonged, continuous intravenous infusion, a schedule that takes advantage of the dependence of cell kill on duration of exposure.[44] Response rates of 30 per cent have been reported in advanced, previously treated breast cancer cases, using a five-day continuous-infusion regimen with doses of 1.5 to 2.0 mg per m^2 per day. Because of erratic absorption and unpredictable toxicity, VB is not administered orally. It should be noted that patients resistant to VCR, such as those who have Hodgkin's disease previously treated with MOPP (nitrogen mustard, Oncovin[vincristine], procarbazine, and prednisone), may remain responsive to VB. Thus, the two agents do not demonstrate cross-resistance in clinical use.

Vindesine has been used in various schedules, such as slow infusion,[45] single weekly injections, or multiple weekly injections. The total weekly dose for each of these schedules is 3 to 7 mg per m^2.[45, 45A, 45B] The most common schedules employ single weekly doses of 3 to 4 mg per m^2.[46] The drug appears to be most effective in lymphocytic malignancies, in the blastic phases of chronic granulocytic leukemia, and in systemic mastocytosis, and does not exhibit cross-resistance with VCR.[47, 48]

Toxicity

Although the vinca alkaloids are very similar in structure and mechanism of action, they exhibit very different patterns of clinical toxicity. Neuropathy is the most frequent and dose-limiting toxicity of VCR.[49] Neurotoxicity occurs also in a small percentage of patients treated with VDS, but rarely arises at usual clinical doses of VB. VCR neurotoxicity is most frequent in patients above 40 years of age and is related to total cumulative dose. Its primary manifestations are a symmetric neuropathy affecting both sensory and motor functions. Initial manifestations are usually a loss of the deep tendon reflexes of the lower extremities, followed by paresthesias of the fingers and toes, and ultimately a loss of strength in the dorsiflexors of the lower extremities and in the small musculature of the hand and wrist. "Footdrop" and "wristdrop" are observed in patients with advanced VCR motor neuropathy and are often irreversible after drug discontinuation. Cranial motor nerves may also be affected, causing hoarseness, diplopia, or facial palsies. Autonomic neuropathies are unusual and occur primarily as a consequence of high-dose VCR therapy (single dose > 2 mg/m^2) or in patients with altered hepatic function; these patients may develop paralytic ileus, with bloating, abdominal cramps, and obstipation, as well as urinary retention or (rarely) arterial hypotension. Rarely, alterations in mental status may also result from VCR treatment, with symptoms such as depression, confusion, or insomnia. Direct intrathecal injection of VCR, an inadvertent clinical mishap, has been reported to cause ascending sensory and motor neuropathy, encephalopathy, and death.[49A] Thus, it is probably fortunate that VCR penetrates poorly into the cerebrospinal fluid. Many of these side effects also occur during VDS therapy; a loss of reflexes is reported in most patients treated with VDS, but dose-limiting neurotoxicity is observed in less than 10 per cent of patients.

Neuropathic side effects are not usually accompanied by slowed nerve conduction on clinical testing,[49] but abnormal nerve conduction has been reported in patients with advanced motor neuropathy.[50] In such cases, electromyography may disclose evidence of denervation. Pathologic examination of affected nerves reveals axonal degeneration and demyelination. In experimental studies, the motor end-plate may also be disrupted.[50] Unmyelinated fibers may be the most sensitive to the toxic effects of VCR, thus explaining the early onset of loss of deep tendon reflexes.[51, 52]

Vincristine has been implicated as a cause of inappropriate antidiuretic hormone (IADH) secretion, and may cause symptomatic hyponatremia with seizures in patients receiving intensive hydration as part of their treatment.[53] The IADH syndrome, which is accompanied by an actual increase in serum ADH concentration, usually remits within two to three days of onset. Other side effects associated with VCR therapy include dysphagia,[54] possibly Raynaud's phenomenon,[55] and (infrequently) myelosuppression in patients with severely compromised marrow function. At low doses (1 mg/m^2 or less), VCR may cause an actual increase in circulating platelets as the result of endoreduplication of megakaryocytes.[56]

In contrast, the dose-limiting toxicity of VB is myelosuppression. Both thrombocytopenia and leukopenia reach their nadir seven to ten days after treatment. Mucositis is also a frequent and bothersome side effect. VB rarely causes neurotoxic symptoms or inappropriate antidiuretic effects, and then only at high doses.[56A] VDS causes a moderate, reversible leukopenia without thrombocytopenia and mild VCR-like neurotoxicity as its primary side effects. The neurotoxicity is primarily sensory, its manifestations being paresthesias, diminished deep tendon reflexes, and a flu-like syndrome of muscle aching and weakness.[45, 45A, 45B]

Because of the lack of precise pharmacokinetic information, only general guidelines can be offered for dosage modification in patients with hepatic dysfunction. A 50 per cent reduction of dose seems logical in patients with bilirubin above 3 mg per dl. No change in dosage is necessary for patients with abnormal renal function.

Drug Interactions

Both VCR and VB are frequently used in drug combinations because they have a unique mechanism of action and a broad spectrum of antitumor activity, and because VCR has no significant myelosuppressive effects. However, there have been few studies of the pharmacologic interaction of these agents with other antitumor drugs.

The only interaction well documented experimentally is the enhancement of methotrexate (MTX) accumulation by tumor cells in the presence of VCR[57] and VB.[58] This effect is mediated by VCR blockade of MTX exit from cells and is more fully described in Chapter 10. MTX reaches higher steady-state levels in humans in both acute myeloblastic and lymphoblastic leukemia cells in the presence of VCR,[58, 59] but the minimal VCR concentration required to achieve this effect, 0.1 μM, in myeloblasts is realized only momentarily in clinical treatment, and even higher VCR concentrations are needed to produce enhancement of MTX uptake in lymphoblasts. Schedules of experimental chemotherapy that employ VCR followed by MTX have not demonstrated therapeutic synergism in the L1210 murine leukemia model.[60] Synergy between these two agents has been reported in the opposite sequence when VCR follows MTX, but the latter schedule is less likely to reflect enhancement of MTX uptake. Thus, there appears to be little justification for routine use of VCR pretreatment in high-dose MTX protocols.

Low concentrations of glutamic acid, aspartic acid, ornithine, citrulline, and arginine completely reverse the cytotoxic effect of VB in tissue culture,[2] probably through inhibition of VB transport. Thus, caution should be exercised in the use of intravenous hyperalimentation with amino acids in conjunction with VB therapy.

EPIPODOPHYLLOTOXINS

INTRODUCTION

The roots and rhizomes of the May apple or mandrake plant, *Podophyllum peltatum*, have long been used as a source of folk medicines because of their cathartic, emetic, and anthelmintic properties.[61, 62] The active principle in these preparations, podophyllotoxin, is an antimitotic agent that binds to a site on tubulin distinct from that occupied by the vinca alkaloids. A number of semi-synthetic derivatives have been made and tested clinically.[63] Two glycosidic derivatives of podophyllotoxin,[64] VM-26 and VP-16, have highly significant clinical acitivity against Hodgkin's disease, diffuse histiocytic lymphoma, small cell carcinoma of the lung, and testicular tumors, and are undergoing extensive clinical trials to establish the range of their activity.

These drugs share a common multiringed structure, epipodophyllotoxin, linked to a glucopyranose sugar, and differ only in the single substitution on the 4,6-acetal carbon (Fig. 11–6). Both drugs concentrate in the cell at levels that exceed those in extracellular fluid, and bind to high- and low-affinity intracellular sites.[65] VM-26 concentrations intracellularly exceed those of VP-16 by seven- to tenfold. It is not clear whether transport of either is "active" or energy-dependent.

Despite their structural similarity to podophyllotoxin, a potent inhibitor of tubulin polymerization,[66, 67] the synthetic congeners have no effect on microtubule assembly at concentrations as high as 100 μM, nor do they promote dissolution of microtubules.[68] These agents do not arrest cells in mitosis, but rather exert their maximal effects late in S or G_2 phase and prevent cells from entering mitosis.[69, 70] Cells are arrested in G_2, and this effect is not reversed by washout of the drug, in contrast to the reversibility of mitotic arrest by the vincas or by podophyllotoxin. The epipodophyllotoxins inhibit nucleoside transport into HeLa cells in tissue culture[66] and inhibit nucleoside incorporation into RNA and DNA,[71] but it is uncertain whether these actions are primary mechanisms of toxicity. Other *in vitro* actions include the induction of single-stranded DNA breaks[68] and chromosomal aberrations[72] in cultured cells.

A comparison of the properties of the epipodophyllotoxins and their nonglycosidic bases is instructive. The nonglycosidic analogue of VP-16 also inhibits nucleoside transport but, in contrast to the parent compound, blocks assembly of microtubules *in vitro*. It is not known whether the clinically useful epipodophyllotoxins, VP-16 and VM-26, are converted to their base compounds *in vivo*; obviously this conversion would drastically alter the properties of these compounds.

CLINICAL PHARMACOLOGY

Most current pharmacokinetic information about the podophyllotoxin derivatives has come from studies of the disposition of radio-labeled drug,[73, 74] although specific ana-

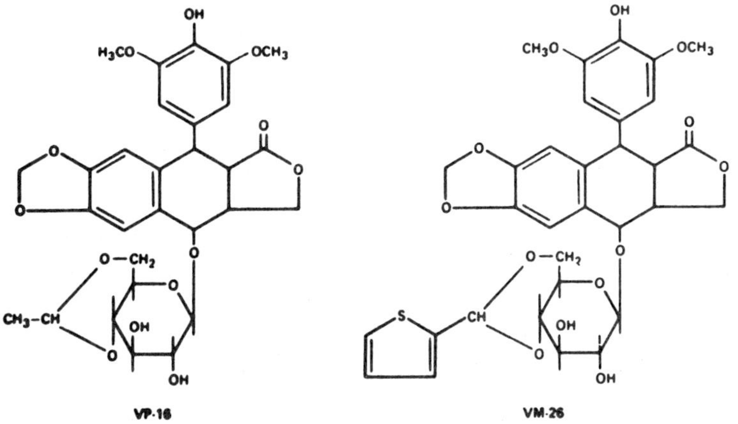

Figure 11–6. Molecular structures of VP-16 and VM-26.

lytic techniques employing high-pressure liquid chromatography have been developed more recently.[74A, 74B] Considerable uncertainty still exists as to the nature and extent of metabolism of these agents in man.

The assay described by Sinkule et al.[74B] begins with methanol extraction of plasma, followed by reverse-phase chromatography on a μBondapak phenyl column, with isocratic elution using a water/acetonitrile/acetic acid buffer [74/25/1]. This system allows identification of either VM-26 or VP-16, their known hydroxy acid metabolites, picro-lactone isomers, and potential metabolites (aglycones). The only metabolites identified thus far in man are the hydroxy acids,[74A] which are the primary metabolites found in the urine in adult patients.

The primary pharmacokinetic characteristics of VP-16 and VM-26 are given in Table 11–1.[73, 74]

Following an intravenous bolus injection of VP-16, 290 mg per m^2, peak plasma concentrations reach 30 μg/ml, and decline thereafter in a biphasic pattern with half-lives of 2.8 and 15.1 hours. The mechanism of elimination has not been completely defined. Approximately 45 per cent of the administered dose is excreted in the urine, of which two thirds is unchanged drug, and 15 per cent is excreted in the feces. The remainder of administered drug has not been accounted for in these initial studies. Cerebrospinal fluid concentrations of VP-16 are less than 10 per cent of simultaneous plasma levels during the initial 26 hours after dosage.

The agent VM-26 has somewhat different pharmacokinetic characteristics: (1) slower renal clearance of 2.2 ml per min, versus 13.6 ml per min for VP-16; (2) more extensive metabolism of material recovered in the urine (80 per cent metabolite, versus 20 per cent for VP-16); and (3) a longer terminal half-life of 26 hours. As with VP-16, a significant fraction of administered VM-26 has not been accounted for in initial studies of its elimination in man. Cerebrospinal fluid concentrations are less than 1 per cent of those found in simultaneous blood samples.

A drinking ampule has been formulated for oral administration of VP-16.[76, 77] Oral absorption of drug given in this way is approximately 50 per cent, and initial clinical reports suggest that the oral and intravenous routes provide equivalent therapeutic results in patients with small cell carcinoma of the lung.[78]

Schedules of Administration

The agent VP-16 has been used in various schedules and by both oral and intravenous routes of administration. Single daily doses give superior results in comparison with schedules of intermittent administration, according to both preclinical and clinical trials. The maximal-tolerated intravenous doses are 45 mg per m^2 per day for seven days, 86 mg per m^2 per day twice weekly, or a single dose of 290 mg per m^2 per week.[79] When given orally in the form of a drinking ampule (a soft gelatin capsule), VP-16 dosage is increased two- to fivefold to compensate for incomplete absorption and/or first-pass elimination in the liver.

Fewer schedules have been used for VM-26. The most common protocol employs weekly doses of 67 mg per m^2 intravenously.[80]

The dose-limiting toxicity of VP-16 and VM-26 is leukopenia.[78, 81] Thrombocytopenia (less than 100,000 platelets per mm^3) occurs in less than 25 per cent of patients. Large intravenous doses of VP-16, 170 mg per m^2, cause a higher incidence of leukopenia than smaller daily doses of 50 mg per m^2.

The epipodophyllotoxins cause nausea and vomiting in approximately 15 per cent of patients treated by the intravenous route; the incidence of these complaints rises to 55 per cent in patients receiving oral VP-16.[78] Alopecia is common with both drugs. Other less frequent toxicities include phlebitis, fever, mild abnormalities of liver function tests, and peripheral neuropathy. The neuropathy is usually of minor significance, except in patients receiving concurrent VCR.

Acute arterial hypotension results from rapid intravenous infusion of these agents, and is believed to be caused by the vehicle Tween 80 (polysorbate 80) plus polyethylene glycol for formulation of these highly water-insoluble compounds. This bothersome side effect can be avoided by administering the drugs over a 30-minute period of infusion.[82]

Precise guidelines for dose modification in patients with renal or hepatic compromise have not been established. However, since the renal clearance of VP-16 is sixfold greater than that of VM-26, it is likely that renal impairment would have a greater effect on VP-16 pharmacokinetics. The low fecal excretion of both drugs suggests that biliary excretion has a limited role in elimination of these agents.

MAYTANSINE

INTRODUCTION

Of the more than 180,000 plant extracts screened by the National Cancer Institute between 1950 and 1980, only 4 per cent have had antitumor activity in experimental test systems, and 19 of these compounds have reached the state of actual clinical trial. One of these compounds, maytansine, an alkaloid derived from the African shrub *Maytenus serrata,* has attracted considerable research interest because of its potent antimitotic activity. However, it has not shown sufficient clinical activity to warrant combination therapy trials or marketing.

The structure of maytansine is shown in Figure 11–7.[83] It belongs to the general chemical class called ansa macrolides, a class that includes the streptovaricins and rifamycins. Four additional maytansine-like compounds lacking the C-3 ester have been isolated from related plants,[84] but lack antitumor activity,[85] indicating that the ester group may be an important determinant of biologic activity. Further analogue development in this class will likely rely on large-scale fermentation of plant cells, as described for production of ansamycin antibiotics.[86]

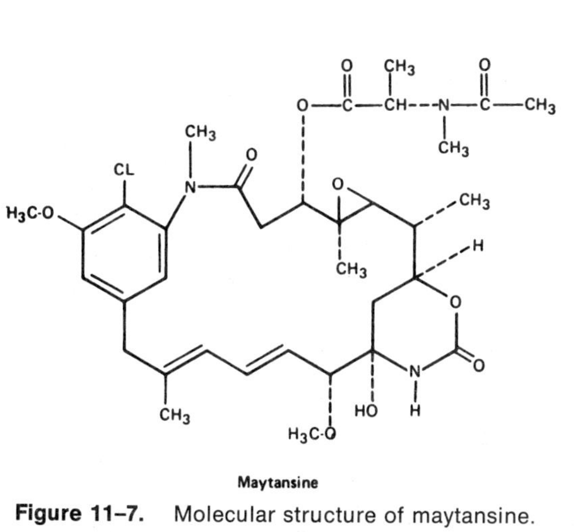

Maytansine

Figure 11–7. Molecular structure of maytansine.

CELLULAR PHARMACOLOGY

The mode of entry of maytansine into cells has not been investigated. Inside the cell, maytansine binds to tubulin and inhibits the progression of cells through mitosis. In the initial screening of maytansine against murine tumors, it was noted that concentrations of 0.01 μM produced a tenfold increase in the number of L1210 cells in mitosis.[87] Maytansine was observed to be 100-fold more potent than vincristine in inhibiting mitosis in sea urchin eggs,[88] although these two agents were equipotent in blocking tubulin polymerization in cell-free systems.

Maytansine binds reversibly to tubulin with a K_D of 6.7×10^{-7}M.[87] The dissociation constant for VCR is quite similar (2×10^{-6}M). Maytansine competitively inhibits the binding of both VB and VCR,[89, 90] but is incompletely displaced from its own tubulin binding sites by VCR. Twenty-five per cent of bound maytansine remains bound to tubulin in the presence of excess VCR, indicating that maytansine may bind to a unique site. Colchicine, which binds to a site distinct from the vinca alkaloids,[15] does not compete with maytansine for binding to tubulin.[90]

Tubulin binding is the most likely mechanism of maytansine cytotoxicity and antitumor activity. Flow microfluorometric examination of treated leukemic cells has disclosed a progressive increase in the fraction of cells in the intermitotic (G_2) and mitotic (M) phases of the cell cycle,[91, 92] and a multiplicity of changes characteristic of tubulin-binding agents: endoreduplication of cellular DNA beyond the tetraploid state, chromosomal aberrations, and dissolution of microtubules in the axonal processes of nerves.[93] Maytansine cytotoxicity is cell cycle phase–specific. Mitotic and G_2 cells are most sensitive, G_1 cells are resistant, and S-phase cells are intermediate in sensitivity.[94]

Maytansine produces cell death in tissue culture at concentrations in the range of 1 nM, and is thus one of the most potent antineoplastic compounds yet discovered. The 50 per cent cytotoxic drug concentration for sensitive murine leukemia cell lines in culture, including the P388, L1210, and L5178Y tumors, lies in the range of 0.6 to 2.0 nM.[87] This cytotoxic effect can be reversed by resuspending cells in drug-free medium after 24 hours of exposure; longer durations of exposure produce irreversible damage.

Maytansine has no primary effect on nucleic acid or protein synthesis.[94] High drug concentrations depress thymidine incorporation into DNA,[87] probably as a secondary effect of accumulation of cells in G_2 and M. Maytansine has no inhibitory effect on RNA polymerase, in contrast to other ansa macrolides such as rifamycin.

Little is known concerning the mechanism of resistance to maytansine. Murine cell lines resistant to VCR, such as P388/VCR and L1210, are also resistant to maytansine;[87] the P388/VCR line is sensitive to VP-16, an indication that the epipodophyllotoxins do not mediate their antitumor effect by binding to tubulin.[9]

CLINICAL PHARMACOLOGY

There are no established methods for measuring maytansine in biologic specimens, and thus there is no pharmacokinetic information regarding the use of this agent in man. Two basic dose schedules have been employed in initial clinical trials, the first a daily intravenous schedule of 0.4 mg per m^2 per day for three to five days,[95, 96] and the second a single intravenous dose of 1.6 to 2.0 mg per m^2 given once every three weeks.[97]

The primary clinical side effects are gastrointestinal and neurologic.[95-97] Nausea, vomiting, and diarrhea are consistent complaints arising from the schedules described above. At higher doses, diarrhea may become intractible and life-threatening. Patients who receive a single injection of maytansine every three weeks experience a syndrome of profound weakness, nausea, and vomiting that lasts three to five days. A similar syndrome of lesser severity may occur in patients receiving maytansine on a schedule of daily doses for three days. Neurologic complaints may include transient paresthesias, which increase in severity with doses above 0.6 mg per m^2.[95]

Maytansine administration has been associated with mild elevations of serum transaminases[95, 97] in patients with normal hepatic function prior to treatment, but in one report three patients with pre-existing liver function impairment developed clinical jaundice following doses of 0.6 to 0.9 mg per m^2 daily for three days.[96] Myelosuppression, rarely seen as a side effect of maytansine, has been reported in patients with abnormal liver function,[96] indicating that this drug, like the vinca alkaloids, probably undergoes hepatic uptake and biliary excretion.

References

1. Johnson IS, Armstrong JG, Gorman M, et al.: The vinca alkaloids: a new class of oncolytic agents. Cancer Res. 23:1390–1427, 1963.
2. Johnson IS, Wright HF, Svoboda GH, et al.: Antitumor principles derived from *Vinca rosea* Linn. I. Vincaleukoblastine and leurosine. Cancer Res. 20:1016–1022, 1960.
3. Bleyer WA, Frisby SA, and Oliverio VT: Uptake and binding of vincristine by murine leukemia cells. Biochem. Pharmacol. 24:633–639, 1975.
4. Creasey WA, Bensch KG, and Malawista SE: Colchicine, vinblastine, and griseofulvin: pharmacological studies with human leukocytes. Biochem. Pharmacol. 20:1579, 1971.
5. Bender, RA, and Kornreich WD: Cellular entry of vincristine in murine leukemia cells. Proc. Am. Assoc. Cancer Res. 22:227, 1981.
6. Dano K: Development of resistance to daunomycin (NSC-83151) in Ehrlich ascites tumor. Cancer Chemother. Rep. 55:133–141, 1971.
7. Biedler JL, and Riehm H: Cellular resistance to actinomycin D in Chinese hamster cells *in vitro*: cross-resistance, radioautographic, and cytogenetic studies. Cancer Res. 30:1174–1184, 1970.
8. Wilkoff LJ, and Dulmadge EA: Resistance and cross-resistance of cultured leukemia P388 cells to vincristine, Adriamycin, Adriamycin analogs, and actinomycin D. J. Natl. Cancer Inst. 61:1521–1524, 1978.
9. Wilkoff LJ, and Dulmadge EA: Sensitivity and resistance of cultured leukemia P388 cells to vincristine (VCR) and 4′-dimethyl podophyllotoxin (VP-16-213). Proc. Am. Assoc. Cancer Res. 18:37, 1978.
10. Inaba, M, and Johnson RK: Uptake and retention of Adriamycin and daunorubicin by sensitive and anthracycline-resistant sublines of P388 leukemia. Biochem. Pharmacol. 27:2123–2130, 1978.
11. Inaba M, Kobayashi H, Sakurai Y, et al.: Active efflux of daunorubicin and Adriamycin in sensitive and resistant sublines of P388 leukemia. Cancer Res. 39:2200–2203, 1979.

11A. Beck WT, Mueller TJ, and Tanzer LR: Altered cell surface membrane glycoproteins in vinca-alkaloid–resistant human leukemic lymphoblasts. Cancer Res. 39:2070, 1979.

11B. Baskin F, Rosenberg RN, and Dev V: Correlation of double-minute chromosomes with unstable multidrug cross-resistance in uptake mutants of neuroblastoma cells. Proc. Natl. Acad. Sci. USA 78:3654–3658, 1981.

12. Luduena RF, Shooter EM, and Wilson L: Structure of the tubulin dimer. J. Biol. Chem. 252:7006–7014, 1977.
13. Olmstead JB, and Borisy GG: Microtubules. Annu. Rev. Biochem. 43:507–540, 1973.
14. Wilson L: Action of drugs on microtubules. Life Sci. 17:303, 1975.
15. Owellen RJ, Owens AH, and Donigan DW: The binding of vincristine, vinblastine and colchicine to tubulin. Biochem. Biophys. Res. Commun. 47:685–691, 1972.
16. Wilson L, Morse NC, and Bryan J: Characterization of acetyl-^{3}H-labelled vinblastine binding to vinblastine-tubulin crystals. J. Mol. Biol. 121:255–268, 1978.

17. Owellen RJ, Hartke CA, Dickerson RM, et al.: Inhibition of tubulin-microtubule polymerization by drugs of the vinca alkaloid class. Cancer Res. 36:1499–1502, 1976.
18. Bryan J: Vinblastine and microtubules. II. Characterization of two protein subunits from the isolated crystals. J. Mol. Biol. 66:157–168, 1972.
19. Bensch KG, and Malawista SE: Microtubule crystals in mammalian cells. J. Cell Biol. 40:95–107, 1969.
20. Madoc-Jones H, and Mauro F: Interphase action of vinblastine and vincristine: differences in their lethal action through the mitotic cycle of cultured mammalian cells. J. Cell Physiol. 72:185–196, 1968.
21. Bruchovsky N, Owen AA, Becker AJ, et al.: Effects of vinblastine on the proliferative capacity of Earle's L-cells and their progress through the division cycle. Cancer Res. 25:1232–1237, 1965.
22. Krishan A: Time-lapse ultrastructure studies on the reversal of mitotic arrest induced by vinblastine sulfate in Earle's L-cells. J. Natl. Cancer Inst. 51:581–595, 1968.
23. Tucker RW, Owellen RJ, and Harris SB: Correlation of cytotoxicity and mitotic spindle dissolution by vinblastine in mammalian cells. Cancer Res. 37:4346–4351, 1977.
24. Jellinghaus W, Schultze B, and Maurer W: The effect of vincristine on mouse jejunal crypt cells of differing cell age: double labeling autoradiographic studies using ^{3}H and ^{14}C TdR. Cell Tissue Kinet. 10:147–156, 1977.
25. Stoehr M, and Fischinger W: Microfluorometric investigations on the cell cycle progression of experimental ascites tumors treated with alkaloidic drugs. Drug Res. 28:977–981, 1978.
26. Jackson DV, and Bender RA: Cytotoxic thresholds of vincristine in L1210 murine leukemia and a human lymphoblastic cell line *in vitro*. Cancer Res. 39:4346–4349, 1979.
27. Schrek R: Cytotoxicity of vincristine to normal and leukemic cells. Am. J. Clin. Pathol. 62:1–7, 1974.
28. Creasey WA, and Markiw ME: Biochemical effects of the vinca alkaloids. I. Effect of vinblastine on nucleic acid synthesis in mouse tumor cells. Biochem. Pharmacol. 12:135–142, 1964.
29. Creasey WA, and Markow ME: Biochemical effects of the vinca alkaloids. III. The synthesis of ribonucleic acid and the incorporation of amino acids in Ehrlich ascites cells *in vitro*. Biochim. Biophys. Acta 103:635–645, 1965.
30. Creasey WA: Modifications in biochemical pathways produced by the vinca alkaloids. Cancer Chemother. Rep. 52:501–507, 1968.
31. Peterson NA, Raghupathy E, and Estey SJ: Effects of vinca alkaloids on uptakes of amino acids by rat brain synaptosomes. Biochem. Pharmacol. 25:1389–1395, 1976.
32. Burchenal JH, Coley V, Purple JR, et al.: Studies on the mechanisms of action of various phthalanilide derivatives by cross-resistance and tissue culture. Cancer Res. 23:1364–1374, 1963.
32A. Riordan JR, and Ling V.: Purification of a P-glycoprotein from plasma membrane vesicles of Chinese hamster ovary cell mutants with reduced colchicine permeability. J. Biol. Chem. 254:1270, 1979.
32B. Ling, V, Aubin JE, Chase A, et al.: Mutants of Chinese hamster ovary (CHO) cells with altered colcemid-binding activity. Cell 18:423, 1979.
33. Owellen RJ, Root MA, and Hains FO: Pharmocokinetics of vindesine and vincristine in humans. Cancer Res. 37:2603–2607, 1977.
33A. Sethi VS, Burton SS, and Jackson DV: A sensitive radioimmunoassay for vincristine and vinblastine. Cancer Chemother. Pharmacol. 4:183, 1980.
34. Bender RA, Castle MC, Margileth DA, et al.: The pharmacokinetics of [^{3}H] vincristine in man. Clin. Pharmacol. Ther. 22:430–438, 1977.
35. Castle, MC, Margileth DA, and Oliverio VT: Distribution and excretion of [^{3}H]vincristine in the rat and the dog. Cancer Res. 36:3684–3689, 1976.
36. El Dareer SM, White VM, Chen FP, et al.: Distribution and metabolism of vincristine in mice, rats, dogs and monkeys. Cancer Treat. Rep. 61:1269–1277, 1977.
37. Jackson DV, Castle MC, and Bender RA: Biliary excretion of vincristine. Clin. Pharmacol. Ther. 24:101–107, 1978.
38. Jackson DV, Castle MC, Poplack DG, et al.: Pharmacokinetics of vincristine in the cerebrospinal fluid of sub-human primates. Cancer Res. 40:722–724, 1980.
38A. Jackson DV, Sethi VS, Spurr CL, et al.: Pharmacokinetics of vincristine in the cerebrospinal fluid of humans. Cancer Res. 41:1466, 1981.
39. Owellen RJ, and Hartke CA: The pharmacokinetics of 4-acetyl tritium vinblastine in two patients. Cancer Res. 35:975–980, 1975.
40. Owellen RJ, Hartke CA, and Hains FO: Pharmacokinetics and metabolism of vinblastine in humans. Cancer Res. 37:2597–2602, 1977.
40A. Nelson RL, Dyke RW, and Root MA: Clinical pharmacokinetics of vindesine. Cancer Chemother. Pharmacol. 2:243, 1979.
41. Culp HW, Daniels WD, and McMahon RE: Disposition and tissue levels of [^{3}H]vindesine in rats. Cancer Res. 37:3053–3056, 1977.
42. Livingston RB, and Carter SK: Single Agents in Cancer Chemotherapy. Plenum Press, New York, 1970.
43. Sandler SG, Tobin W, and Henderson ES: Vincristine-induced neuropathy: a clinical study of fifty leukemic patients. Neurology 19:367, 1969.
44. Yap H-Y, Blumenschein GR, Hortobagyi GN, et al.: Continuous 5-day infusion vinblastine in the treatment of refractory advanced breast cancer. Proc. Am. Assoc. Cancer Res. 20:334, 1979.
45. Dyke RW, and Nelson RL: Phase I anticancer agents. Vindesine (desacetyl vinblastine amide sulfate). Cancer Treat. Rev. 4:135–142, 1977.
45A. Bayssas M, Gouveia J, deVassal F, et al.: Vindesine: a new alkaloid. Recent Results Cancer Res. 74:91, 1980.
45B. Ohnuma T, Greenspan EM, and Holland JF: Initial clinical study with vindesine: tolerance to weekly IV bolus and 24-hour infusion. Cancer Treat. Rep. 64:25, 1980.
46. Sklaroff RB, Straus D, and Young C: Phase II trial of vindesine in patients with malignant lymphoma. Cancer Treat. Rep. 63:793–794, 1979.
47. Mathe G, Misset JL, de Vassal F, et al.: Phase II clinical trial with vindesine for remission induction in acute leukemia, blastic crisis of chronic myeloid leukemia, lymphosarcoma, and Hodgkin's disease; absence of cross-resistance with vincristine. Cancer Treat. Rep. 62:805, 1978.
48. Gralla RJ, Raphael BC, Golbey RB, et al.: Phase II evaluation of vindesine in patients with non-small cell sarcoma of the lung. Cancer Treat. Rep. 63:1343, 1979.
49. Weiss HD, Walker MD, and Wiernik PH: Neurotoxicity of commonly used antineoplastic agents. N. Engl. J. Med. 291:127–133, 1974.
49A. Slyter H, Liwnicz B, Herrick MK, et al.: Fatal myeloencephalopathy caused by intrathecal vincristine. Neurology 30:867, 1980.
50. Bradley WG, Lassman LP, Pearce GW, et al.: The neuropathy of vincristine in man. Clinical, electrophysiological, and pathological studies. J. Neurol. Sci. 10:107, 1970.
51. Donoso JA, Green LS, Heller-Bettinger E, et al.: Action of the vinca alkaloids vincristine, vinblastine, and desacetyl vinblastine amide on axonal fibrillar organelles *in vitro*. Cancer Res. 37:1401–1407, 1977.
52. Goldstein BD, and Lowndes HE: Motor nerve function in vincristine neuropathy — lack of evidence of a dying-back neuropathy. Pharmacologist 20:162, 1978.
53. Robertson GL, Bhoopalam N, and Zelkowitz LJ: Vincristine neurotoxicity and abnormal secretion of antidiuretic hormone. Arch. Intern. Med. 132:717, 1973.
54. Chrisholm RC, and Curry SB: Vincristine-induced dysphagia. South. Med. J. 71:1364–1365, 1978.
55. Rothberg H: Raynaud's phenomenon after vinblastine-bleomycin chemotherapy. Cancer Treat. Rep. 62:569–570, 1978.
56. Bunn PA, Ford SS, and Shackney SE: The effects of Colcemid on hematopoiesis in the mouse. J. Clin. Invest. 58:1280–1285, 1976.
56A. Antony A, Robinson WA, Roy C, et al.: Inappropriate

antidiuretic hormone secretion after high-dose vinblastine. J. Urol. 123:783, 1980.

57. Bender RA, Bleyer WA, Frisby SA, et al.: Alteration of methotrexate uptake in human leukemia cells by other agents. Cancer Res. 35:1305–1308, 1975.
58. Zagar RF, Frisby SA, and Oiverio VT: The effects of antibiotics and cancer chemotherapeutic agents on the cellular transport and antitumor activity of methotrexate in L1210 murine leukemia. Cancer Res. 33:1670–1676, 1973.
59. Warren RD, Nichols AP, and Bender RA: The effect of vincristine on methotrexate uptake and inhibition of DNA synthesis by human lymphoblastoid cells. Cancer Res. 37:2993–2997, 1977.
60. Bender RA, Nichols AP, Norton L, et al.: Lack of therapeutic synergism of vincristine and methotrexate in L1210 murine leukemia *in vivo*. Cancer Treat. Rep. 62:997–1003, 1978.
61. Kelly MG, and Hartwell JL: The biological effects and the chemical composition of podophyllin. A review. J. Natl. Cancer Inst. 14:967–1010, 1954.
62. Bentley R: New American remedies. 1. *Podophyllum peltatum*. Pharm. J. Trans. 3:456–464, 1961.
63. Vaitkevicius VK, and Reed ML: Clinical studies with podophyllum compounds SPI-77 (NSC-72274) and SPG-827 (42076). Cancer Chemother. Rep. 50:565–571, 1966.
64. Keller-Juslen C, Kuhn M, Stahelin H, et al.: Synthesis and antimitotic activity of glycosidic lignan derivatives related to podophyllotoxin. J. Med. Chem. 14:936–940, 1971.
65. Allen L: The role of drug disposition kinetics on cellular transport of the antineoplastic agent VM-26. Drug Metab. Rev. 8:119–135, 1978.
66. Loike JD, and Horwitz SB: Effects of podophyllotoxin and VP-16-213 on microtubule assembly *in vitro* and nucleoside transport in HeLa cells. Biochemistry 15:5435–5442, 1976.
67. Cortese F, Bhattacharyya B, and Wolff J: Podophyllotoxin as a probe for the colchicine binding site of tubulin. J. Biol. Chem. 252:1134–1140, 1977.
68. Loike JD, and Horwitz SB: Effect of VP-16-213 on the intracellular degradation of DNA in HeLa cells. Biochem. 15:5443–5448, 1976.
69. Krishan A, Paika K, and Frei E: Photofluorometric studies on the action of podophyllotoxin and epipodophyllotoxins (VM-26, VP-16-213) on the cell cycle traverse of human lymphoblasts. J. Cell Biol. 66:521–530, 1975.
70. Drewinko B, and Barlogie B: Survival and cycle-progression delay of human lymphoma cells *in vitro* exposed to VP-16-213. Cancer Treat. Rep. 60:1295–1306, 1976.
71. Grieder A, Maurer R, and Staehelin H: Effect of an epipodophyllotoxin derivative (VP-16-213) on macromolecular synthesis and mitosis in mastocytoma cells *in vitro*. Cancer Res. 34:1788–1794, 1974.
72. Haung CC, Hou Y, and Wang JJ: Effects of a new antitumor agent epipodophyllotoxin on growth and chromosomes in human hematopoietic cell lines. Cancer Res. 33:3123–3129, 1973.
73. Creaven PJ, and Allen LM: EPEG, a new antineoplastic epipodophyllotoxin. Clin. Pharmacol Ther. 18:221–226, 1975.
74. Creaven PJ, and Allen LM: PTG, a new antineoplastic epipodophyllotoxin. Clin. Pharmacol. Ther. 18:227–233, 1975.
74A. Strife RJ, Jarrdine I, and Colvin M: Analysis of the anticancer drugs VP16-213 and VM-26 and their metabolites by high-performance liquid chromatography. J. Chromatogr. 182:211, 1980.
74B. Sinkule JA, Rivera G, and Evans WE: Clinical pharmacokinetics of VM 26 (Teniposide) in children with acute lymphocyte leukemia. Proc. Am. Soc. Clin. Pharmacol., May, 1981.
75. Allen LM, and Creaven PJ: Comparison of the human pharmacokinetics of VM-26 and VP-16, two antineoplastic epipodophyllotoxin glucopyranoside derivatives. Eur. J. Cancer 11:697–707, 1975.
76. Nissen NI, Dombernowsky P, Hansen HH, et al.: Phase I clinical trial of an oral solution of VP-16-213. Cancer Treat. Rep. 60:943–945, 1976.
77. Falkson G, van Dyk JJ, van Eden EB, et al.: A clinical trial of the oral form of 4′-demethylepipodophyllotoxin-β-D ethylidene gludoside (NSC-141540) VP-16-213. Cancer 35:1141–1144, 1975.
78. Radice PA, Bunn PA, and Ihde DC: Therapeutic trials with VP-16-213 and VM-26: active single agents in small cell lung cancer, non-Hodgkin's lymphoma, and other malignancies. Cancer Treat. Rep. 63:1231–1239, 1979.
79. Creaven PJ, Newman SJ, Selawry OS, et al.: Phase I clinical trials of weekly administration of 4′-demethylepipodophyllotoxin-9-(4,6,0-ethylidene-β-D-glucopyranoside) (NSC-141540; VP-16-213). Cancer Chemother. Rep. 58: 901–907, 1974.
80. Muggia FM, Selawry OS, and Hansen HH: Clinical studies with a new podophyllotoxin derivative, epipodophyllotoxxin, 4′-demethyl-9-(4,6-0-2-thenylidine-β-D-glucopyranoside) (NSC-122819). Cancer Chemother. Rep. 55: 575–581, 1971.
81. Rozencweig, M, Von Hoff DD, Henney JE, et al.: VM-26 and VP-16-213: a comparative analysis. Cancer 40:334–342, 1977.
82. Cavalli F, Sonntag RW, Ryssel HJ, et al.: Lack of severe hypotension with VP-16-213 administered directly IV. Cancer Treat. Rep. 61:1411, 1977.
83. Kupchan SM, Komoda Y, Court WA, et al.: Maytansine, a novel antileukemic ansa macrolide from *Maytenus ovatus*. J. Am. Chem. Soc. 94:1354–1356, 1972.
84. Kupchan SM, Komoda Y, Brantman AR, et al.: Novel maytansinoids. Structural interrelations and requirements for antileukemic activity. J. Am. Chem. Soc. 96:3706–3708, 1974.
85. Kupchan SM, Sneden AT, Brantman AR, et al.: Structural requirements for antileukemic activity among the naturally occurring and semisynthetic maytansinoids. J. Med. Chem. 21:31–37, 1978.
86. Higashide E, Asai M, Ootsu K, et al.: Ansamitocin, a group of novel maytansinoid antibiotics with antitumour properties from Nocardia. Nature 270:721–722, 1977.
87. Wolpert-DeFilippes MK, Adamson RH, Cysyk RL, et al.: Initial studies on the cytotoxic action of maytansine, a novel ansa macrolide. Biochem. Pharmacol. 24:751–754, 1975.
88. Remillard S, Rebhun LI, Howie GA, et al.: Antimitotic activity of the potent tumor inhibitor maytansine. Science 189:1002–1005, 1975.
89. Bhattacharyya B, and Wolff J: Maytansine binding to the vinblastine site of tubulin. Fed. Eur. Biochem. Soc. Lett. 75:159–162, 1977.
90. Mandelbaum-Shavit F, Wolpert-DeFilippes MK, and Johns DG: Binding of maytansine to rat brain tubulin. Biochem. Biophys. Res. Commun. 72:47–54, 1976.
91. Sieber SM, Wolpert DK, Adamson RM, et al.: Experimental studies with maytansine — a new antitumour agent. Bibl. Haematol. 43:495–500, 1976.
92. Alabaster O, and Cassidy M: Flow microfluorometric analysis of P388 murine leukemia after administration of vincristine and maytansine *in vivo*. J. Natl. Cancer Inst. 60:649–652, 1978.
93. Donoso JA, Watson DF, Heller-Bettinger IE, et al: Maytansine action on fast axoplasmic transport and the ultrastructure of vagal axons. Cancer Res. 38:1633–1637, 1978.
94. Rao PN, Freireich EJ, Smith ML, et al: Cell cycle phase–specific cytotoxicity of the antitumor agent maytansine. Cancer Res. 39:3152–3155, 1979.
95. Blum RH, and Kahert T: Maytansine. A phase I study of an ansa macrolide with antitumor activity. Cancer Treat. Rep. 62:435–438, 1978.
96. Cabanillas F, Rodriguez V, Hall SW, et al: Phase I study of maytansine using a 3-day schedule. Cancer Treat. Rep. 62:425–428, 1978.
97. Chabner BA, Levine AS, Johnson BL, et al: Initial clinical trials of maytansine, an antitumor plant alkaloid. Cancer Treat. Rep. 62:429–433, 1978.

HYDROXYUREA

Ross C. Donehower

12

INTRODUCTION

Hydroxyurea (HU) is a simple structural analogue of urea that was first synthesized more than 100 years ago.[1] Its potential biologic significance was recognized in 1928 by Rosenthal and co-workers, who noted leukopenia and anemia with megaloblastosis in animals treated with this compound.[2] After antitumor activity was observed in several mammalian tumor systems,[3, 4] the drug entered clinical trials in the early 1960s. Although responses were noted in a variety of human neoplasms,[5-9] the routine clinical use of HU is limited to chronic myelogenous leukemia (CML).[7, 9-11] Although HU is as effective as busulfan in the initial therapy of CML,[11] it is most commonly used in patients whose disease is no longer responsive to busulfan. HU is also of modest benefit in the accelerated phase and blastic transformation of CML.[12, 13] Responses have been noted in the hypereosinophilic syndrome (eosinophilic leukemia), and HU is currently the drug of choice in corticosteroid-resistant cases of this unusual disease.[14, 15] HU is also effective in preventing complications of intracerebral leukostasis in patients with acute myelogenous leukemia who present with markedly elevated peripheral blood blast counts.[13, 16]

The initial promising results in the treatment of malignant melanoma with HU[6, 8] have not been confirmed in subsequent studies using the drug as a single agent[17, 18] or in combination with dacarbazine (DTIC) and carmustine (BCNU).[19] In small series of patients, HU has had modest activity in the therapy of squamous cell carcinoma of the head and neck,[8, 20] renal cell carcinoma,[21, 22] transitional cell carcinoma of the bladder,[22, 23] and carcinoma of the prostate.[24] Whether HU can be effectively incorporated into combination regimens for these refractory diseases has not been established. It has also been used successfully in the treatment of psoriasis,[25] but indications for this use are declining.

Based on *in vitro* studies demonstrating that HU was able to synchronize cells in a radiation-sensitive phase of the cell cycle,[26] the drug has been studied in combination with radiation therapy. Select groups of patients with advanced cervical cancer have had modest increases in survival when treated with radiation and HU as compared with radiation alone.[27-29] Similar studies of primary intracranial neoplasms have shown minimal differences in favor of the combined treatment group.[30, 31] Therapeutic results of the HU-radiation combination in head and neck cancer have been conflicting,[32-36] and the results in lung cancer have shown no evidence of improved response rates.[37-39] The proposed mechanism of this interaction is discussed below, but these results have done little to encourage further clinical study.

STRUCTURE

The enzymic conversion of ribonucleotides to deoxyribonucleotides by ribonucleotide reductase is a potentially important target site for antineoplastic agents because of the critical role of this reaction in the regulation of DNA synthesis. HU is the only generally available agent that inhibits this reaction as its primary mechanism of action. Its structure is shown in Figure 12–1.

Early studies of the structure-activity relationship of HU and its analogues by Young et al.[40] suggested that the –NOH group was essential for activity, whereas the carbonyl group was not. This information led to the synthesis of HU analogues, including a series of aliphatic and aromatic hydroxamic

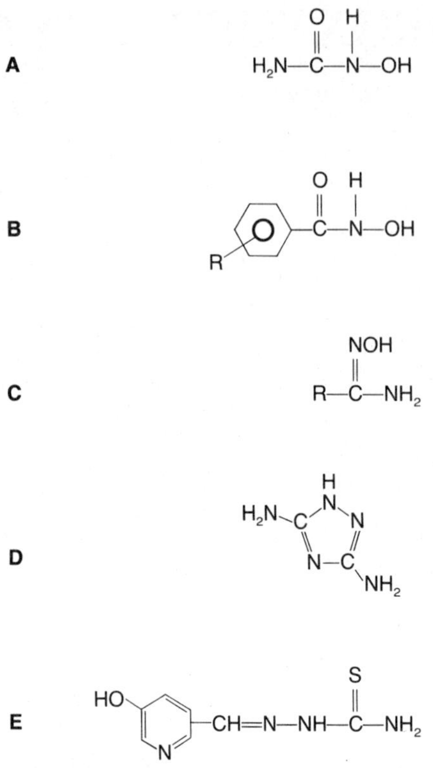

Figure 12–1. Shown here are the structures of: *A*, Hydroxyurea; *B*, the unsubstituted benzohydroxamic acid; *C*, the general amidoxime structure; *D*, guanazole; and *E*, 5-hydroxy-2-formylpyridine thiosemicarbazone, a representative of this class of compounds that entered clinical trial.

acids,[41-44] amidoximes,[45] and cyclic molecules of varying ring size, all containing the $-\overset{O}{\overset{\|}{C}}-\overset{OH}{\overset{|}{N}}-$ group.[46] Many of these compounds have demonstrated antitumor activity in animal tumor systems and the ability to inhibit ribonucleotide reductase *in vitro.* Although several of the benzohydroxamic acids (Fig. 12–1) are more potent inhibitors than HU *in vitro* and are capable of prolonging the life span of L1210 leukemic mice at lower doses than HU, there is no significant improvement in survival when maximal nonlethal doses of these drugs are compared with HU.[44] These analogues have not yet been evaluated clinically.

Guanazole and the α-(N)-heterocyclic carboxaldehyde thiosemicarbazones (Fig. 12–1) represent other structural classes of compounds that are inhibitors of ribonucleotide reductase and which have antitumor activity in animal tumors.[47, 48] Both have undergone brief clinical trial but are no longer actively under study.[49, 50]

MECHANISM OF ACTION

The major cytotoxic action of HU is inhibition of the ribonucleotide reductase system. Early experimental studies demonstrated a rapid and apparently specific inhibition of DNA synthesis *in vivo,*[51, 52] in cultured mammalian cells,[53, 54] and in bacteria[55, 56] with little or no effect on other macromolecular synthesis. This effect is thought to result from ribonucleotide reductase inhibition because of the ability of HU and other hydroxamic acids to inhibit the bacterial and mammalian enzyme *in vitro*[57, 58]; the view that ribonucleotide reductase is the target is further supported by the correlation of inhibition of DNA synthesis with decreased deoxyribonucleotide pools in intact HU-treated cells.[59-61]

Although the effects of HU on some cell lines are completely reversed by the addition of exogenous deoxyribonucleosides,[61-63] other cell lines are not rescued.[64, 65] This fact has been used in support of an additional mechanism of action, although a lack of deoxyribonucleoside kinase activity could explain this failure of nucleoside rescue.

The ribonucleoside diphosphate reductase reaction, as characterized for the *E. coli* enzyme,[66-68] with cytidine diphosphate (CDP) as substrate, can be depicted as follows:

[1] NADPH + H^+ thioredoxin-S_2 → thioredoxin-$(SH)_2$ + $NADP^+$
[2] thioredoxin-$(SH)_2$ + CDP → thioredoxin-S_2 + dCDP

In reaction [1], thioredoxin reductase catalyzes the reduction of disulfide bonds of thioredoxin, a small molecular weight protein, in the presence of NADPH. The product serves as the physiologic reducing agent in the formation of dCDP in a reaction catalyzed by ribonucleotide reductase (reaction[2]). The catalytically active ribonucleotide reductase complex contains two nonidentical protein subfractions, referred to as proteins B1 and B2 in the *E. coli* enzyme.[69, 70] Mammalian ribonucleotide reductase is also composed of two different subunits.[71, 72] Enzymatic reduction of ribonucleotide diphosphates is regulated in a complex manner by multiple nucleotide effectors at allosteric sites, presumably on protein B1 or its equivalent.[73, 74] Although some variability exists among enzymes from various tissue sources, the regulatory effects of various nucleoside triphosphates on the reduction of substrates by ribonucleotide reductase can be summarized as shown in Table 12–1.[73, 75, 76] The reduction of all substrates is inhibited, and the enzyme complex dissociates, in the presence of dATP.[72] The reduction of any nucleoside diphosphate is also inhibited noncompetitively by the presence of other diphosphates.[77] Which of these regulatory interactions are of the greatest importance in the intact cell has not been established.

Protein B2, a non-heme iron-containing protein,[78] is the catalytic subunit of the enzyme and the site of HU inhibition. This subunit is irreversibly inactivated by HU in cell-free enzyme preparations.[79] The partial reversibility of enzyme inhibition *in vitro* by the addition of ferrous iron,[80] its augmentation by an iron chelating agent,[81] and the fact that HU and other inhibitory hydroxamic acids are capable of complex formation with metal ions[40] all suggest that the inhibitory action of HU is the result of an interaction with the tightly bound non-heme iron cofactor.

Other proposed mechanisms of HU action are concerned principally with direct chemical damage to DNA by HU or by products of its degradation. HU and hydroxylamine cause fragmentations, translocations, and rearrangements of metaphase chromosomes of mouse embryo and Chinese hamster cells.[82] HU also induces breaks in template strands of replicating cellular DNA.[83] Such effects increase in the presence of drug-metabolizing systems, such as liver microsomes and NADPH,[84] or when HU has been in solution for a prolonged period,[85] suggesting that metabolic or degradative products are involved.

The determinants of the lethal effects of HU have been studied extensively in mammalian cell systems. HU selectively kills cells in S phase both *in vivo* and *in vitro*.[86-88] Within a population of cells in S phase, those that are most rapidly synthesizing DNA are most sensitive to HU.[89, 90] The lethal effects are dose- or concentration-related[86, 88-90] and correlate with the duration of drug exposure.[88, 91] Drug effects may be reversed completely or partially by the addition of exogenous deoxyribonucleosides or ferrous iron, as noted above. After brief periods of drug exposure, DNA synthesis returns rapidly to control levels when the drug is removed.[54, 86, 88] The fact that cellular DNA synthesis recovers rapidly following removal of HU, in contrast to the irreversible inactivation of the partially purified enzyme, suggests either that cells rapidly regenerate the enzyme or that proper conditions have not been found for regenerating the inactivated enzyme in the cell-free system.

In addition to its biochemical effects, HU causes kinetic changes, including partial synchronization in the G_1 or S phase. HU exerts its maximal lethal effect during S phase; cells in other phases progress normally through the cell cycle until they reach the G_1-S interface, at which point they are prevented from entering S phase.[80] Similar results have been observed in both *in vivo*[86, 92, 93] and *in vitro* systems.[94, 95] Other investigators have found that the G_1 to S progression is not totally prevented, but DNA synthesis proceeds slowly, resulting in abnormally short chains of DNA.[96, 97] Bulk DNA synthesis does not resume until the drug is removed.

The ability of HU to synchronize cells at the G_1-S interface forms the basis for the combined clinical use of radiation and HU described earlier. Increased lethality was noted in irradiated Chinese hamster cells in the presence of HU.[26] These cells are least sensitive to the effects of irradiation in S phase[98]; it was proposed that HU killed the fraction of cells in S phase and synchronized the remainder in G_1, a more radiosensitive phase of the cell cycle. The effects of irradiation are also increased when HU is added after irradiation,[26, 99] possibly as a result of impaired DNA repair in the postirradiation period.[100, 101]

Several possible mechanisms of resistance to HU have been suggested by experimental findings, including (1) a ribonucleotide reductase with decreased sensitivity to HU inhibition,[102, 103] and (2) markedly elevated

TABLE 12–1. Regulatory Effects of Nucleotide Triphosphate on Ribonucleotide Reductase

Substrate	*Activators*	*Inhibitors*
CDP UDP	ATP	dATP, dGTP, dUTP, dTTP, dATP
ADP	dGTP, GTP	dATP dTTP
GDP	dTTP	dATP, dGTP

levels of enzyme with normal sensitivity to HU inhibition.[104] Whether these elevated enzyme levels are the result of gene reduplication, as is the case with some instances of methotrexate resistance, has not been established.[105] The resistance of human cells *in vivo* has not been characterized.

CLINICAL PHARMACOLOGY AND PHARMACOKINETICS

The pharmacokinetic behavior of HU in man has been studied in a preliminary way, using colorimetric assays that measure the reaction product of the drug with either picryl chloride[106] or diacetylmonoxime and sodium *p*-diphenylaminesulfonate.[107] These assays have a practical limit of sensitivity of 5 μg/ml (65 μM).

Following the oral administration of HU, plasma levels peak in approximately one hour.[106-110] Peak levels attained after clinically relevant doses range from 30 to 150 μg/ml (0.3 to 2.0 mM).[106-109] The drug is apparently well absorbed, as indicated by studies demonstrating equivalent plasma levels following oral or intravenous administration[106] and peak plasma levels proportional to the administered dose,[108] although these findings have not been uniform.[110, 110A] The primary half-life after the end of intravenous drug infusions varied from 220 to 267 minutes.[110A]

Drug distribution occurs rapidly, as indicated by studies in mice and rats that show that, 30 to 60 minutes following an intraperitoneal injection of HU, the drug is found in body tissues in quantities proportional to organ weight.[111] HU readily enters cerebrospinal fluid (CSF) and ascites. Ratios for simultaneous plasma and CSF determinations of 4:1 to 9:1 and for plasma:ascites of 2:1 to 7.5:1 have been observed in small groups of patients.[108] The time course of drug disappearance from these extravascular sites has not been studied.

Following attainment of its peak levels, HU disappears rapidly from the plasma. Levels are undetectable after 24 hours, using the insensitive assays described above. The major route of elimination is renal excretion. However, there is wide variation in the amount of unchanged drug recovered in the urine. In one series, cumulative renal excretion in the first 24 hours ranged from 9.5 to 95 per cent.[106] In this study, a few patients excreted an additional 5 to 10 per cent in the second 24 hours. Other investigators report a more consistent 50 to 80 per cent recovery in the first 24 hours.[107] This variability in urinary excretion could be accounted for by incomplete gastrointestinal absorption, excretion by another route, or metabolism.

Animal studies strongly suggest that HU may undergo several types of metabolic transformation, but none of these reactions has been conclusively demonstrated in man. HU is degraded by urease, an enzyme found in intestinal bacteria.[112] Hydroxylamine (NH_2OH), a product of this reaction, has not been identified in man. However, acetohydroxamic acid is found in the plasma of patients receiving HU therapy,[112] and may represent the product of a reaction between hydroxylamine and acetylcoenzyme A, a major thioester in mammalian tissue. The conversion of HU to urea in mice has also been reported.[111] An enzyme system capable of this conversion is found in mouse liver, with the greatest activity localized in the mitochondrial subcellular fraction.[113] In this reduction, either NADPH or NADH may serve as the electron donor and the reaction is stimulated by the addition of flavin adenine dinucleotide. However, the full extent and significance of HU metabolism in man has not been established.

TOXICITY

The principal toxicity of HU is related to inhibition of DNA synthesis in bone marrow. Megaloblastic changes are detectable in marrow granulocyte and erythrocyte precursors within 48 hours of the first dose,[10, 114] and the peripheral leukocyte count begins to fall in two to five days. A more rapid fall in white cell count is seen in patients with CML or acute leukemia. Leukopenia is usually the dose-limiting toxicity of HU, but anemia and thrombocytopenia also occur. The primary advantage of HU in the leukemias lies in the rapidity of its effect on the circulating leukemic cell pool, and the equally brief duration of its action. Thus, the clinician has more immediate and predictable control over an elevated white cell count, in comparison with the more delayed and prolonged action of busulfan.

Although the effects on granulocyte precursor proliferation are rapidly reversible, the nadir in platelet count may lag seven to ten days behind the nadir of the granulocyte count.[5, 10] Early studies demonstrated that all patients receiving 80 mg per kg per day developed leukopenia in 14 days or less, and 70 per cent of those treated with 40 mg per kg per day developed leukopenia requiring discontinuation of therapy in a similar period.[5] These findings prompted the trial of alternative dosage schedules. A dose of 80 mg per kg given every third day results in less hematologic toxicity,[115] but no difference in tumor response has been noted.[116]

Gastrointestinal disturbances, although widely reported, rarely necessitate discontinuation of therapy. These side effects may include anorexia, nausea and vomiting, diarrhea, constipation, and (less frequently) ulcers of the oral mucosa or gastrointestinal tract.

Dermatologic side effects are occasionally seen and include a pruritic, maculopapular rash; hyperpigmentation; dry skin with cutaneous and subcutaneous atrophy; brittle and atrophic nails; and erythema, principally of the face and hands.[11, 117] Biopsies of involved skin have demonstrated histologic changes that resemble lichen planus.[117] Affected individuals have generally been receiving HU for at least several months. Alopecia is an infrequent side effect. Patients receiving HU have an increased tissue reaction to irradiation,[32, 33] and may have a recurrence of cutaneous erythema and hyperpigmentation in areas of previous radiation.[118]

Other side effects less frequently documented include transient abnormalities of renal function manifested by elevated serum urea nitrogen and creatinine, albuminuria, and granular casts; neurologic symptoms such as drowsiness, dizziness, and headache; abnormal liver function tests; and an increased incidence of chromosomal abnormalities.[5, 119-121]

References

1. Dresler WFC, and Stein R: Uber den Hydroxylharnstoff. Justus Liebigs Ann. Chemie 150:242–252, 1869.
2. Rosenthal F, Wislicki L, and Koller L: Uber die Beziehungen von schwersten Blutgiften zu Abbauprodukten des Eiweisses. Ein Beitrag zum Entstehungmechanismus der perniziosen Anemie. Klin. Wochenschr. 7:972–977, 1928.
3. Stearns B, Losee KA, and Bernstein J: Hydroxyurea. A new type of potential antitumor agent. J. Med. Chem. 6:201, 1963.
4. Tarnowski GS, and Stock CC: Chemotherapy studies on the RC and S790 mouse mammary carcinomas. Cancer Res. 18:1–45, 1958.
5. Thurman WG, Bloedow C, Howe CD, et al.: A phase I study of hydroxyurea. Cancer Chemother. Rep. 29:103–107, 1963.
6. Bloedow CE: A phase II study of hydroxyurea in adults: miscellaneous tumors. Cancer Chemother. Rep. 40:39–41, 1964.
7. Fishbein WN, Carbone PP, Freireich EJ, et al.: Clinical trials of hydroxyurea in patients with cancer and leukemia. Clin. Pharmacol. Ther. 5:574–580, 1964.
8. Ariel IM: Therapeutic effects of hydroxyurea: experience with 118 patients with inoperable tumors. Cancer 25:705–714, 1970.
9. Krakoff IH, Savel H, and Murphy ML: Phase II studies of hydroxyurea in adults: clinical evaluation. Cancer Chemother. Rep. 40:53–55, 1964.
10. Kennedy BJ, and Yarbro JW: Metabolic and therapeutic effects of hydroxyurea in chronic myelogenous leukemia. J.A.M.A. 195:1038–1043, 1966.
11. Kennedy BJ: Hydroxyurea therapy in chronic myelogenous leukemia. Cancer 29:1052–1056, 1972.
12. Schwartz JH, and Canellos GP: Hydroxyurea in the management of the hematologic complications of chronic granulocytic leukemia. Blood 46:11–16, 1975.
13. Hoaglund HC, and Perry MC: Blast cell crisis in acute or chronic leukemia. J.A.M.A. 235:1888–1889, 1976.
14. Chusid MJ, and Dale DC: Eosinophilic leukemia remission with vincristine and hydroxyurea. Am. J. Med. 59:297–300, 1975.
15. Parrillo JE, Fauci AS, and Wolff SM: The hypereosinophilic syndrome: dramatic response to therapeutic intervention. Trans. Assoc. Am. Physicians 90:135–144, 1977.
16. Grund FM, Armitage JO, and Burns CP: Hydroxyurea in the prevention of the effects of leukostasis in acute leukemia. Arch. Intern. Med. 137:1246–1247, 1977.
17. Luce JK: The chemotherapy of malignant melanoma. Cancer 30:1604–1615, 1972.
18. Gottlieb JA, Frei E III, and Luce JK: Dose-schedule studies with hydroxyurea in malignant melanoma. Cancer Chemother. Rep. 55:277–280, 1971.
19. Costanzi JJ, Vaitkevicius VK, Quagliana JM, et al.: Combination chemotherapy for disseminated malignant melanoma. Cancer 35:342–346, 1975.
20. Lerner HJ, Beckloff GL, and Godwin MC: Hydroxyurea intermittent therapy in malignant disease. Cancer Chemother. Rep. 53:385–395, 1969.
21. Nevinny H, and Hall TC: Chemotherapy with hydroxuyrea in renal cell carcinoma. J. Clin. Pharmacol. 88:352–359, 1968.
22. Carter SK, and Wasserman TH: The chemotherapy of urologic cancer. Cancer 36:729–747, 1975.
23. Beckloff GL, Lerner HJ, Cole DR, et al.: Hydroxyurea in bladder carcinoma. Invest. Urol. 6:530–534, 1976.
24. Lerner HJ, and Malloy TR: Hydroxyurea in stage D carcinoma of the prostate. Urology 10:35–38, 1977.
25. Leavell UW, and Yarbro JW: Hydroxyurea: a new treatment for psoriasis. Arch. Dermatol. 102:144–150, 1970.
26. Sinclair WK: The combined effect of hydroxyurea and x-rays on Chinese hamster cells *in vitro*. Cancer Res. 28:198–206, 1968.
27. Piver MS, Barlow JJ, Vongtama V, et al.: Hydroxyurea and radiation therapy in advanced cervical cancer. Am. J. Obstet. Gynecol. 120:969–972, 1974.
28. Piver MS, Barlow JJ, Vongtama V, et al.: Hydroxyurea as a radiation sensitizer in women with carcinoma of the uterine cervix. Am. J. Obstet. Gynecol. 129:379–383, 1977.
29. Hreshchyshyn MM, Aron BS, Boronow RC, et al.: Hydroxyurea or placebo combined with radiation to treat stages IIIB and IV cervical cancer confined to the pelvis. Int. J. Radiat. Oncol. Biol. Phys. 5:317–322, 1979.
30. Lerner HJ, Beckloff GL, and Godwin MC: Treatment of astrocytoma with hydroxyurea and irradiation. Am. Surg. 36:401–402, 1970.
31. Lerner HJ: Hydroxyurea and radiation therapy in primary intracranial malignant glial tumors. Proc. Am. Assoc. Cancer Res. 16:243, 1975 (abstr.).
32. Rominger CJ: Hydroxyurea and radiation therapy in advanced neoplasms of the head and neck. Am. J. Roentgenol. 111:103–108, 1971.
33. Richards GJ, and Chambers RG: Hydroxyurea in the treat-

ment of neoplasms of the head and neck. Am. J. Surg. 126:513–518, 1973.

34. Lipschutz H, and Lerner HJ: Six year survival in the combined treatment of far advanced head and neck cancer under a combined therapy program. Am. J. Surg. 126:519–522, 1973.
35. Stefani S, Eells RW, and Abbate J: Hydroxyurea and radiation therapy in head and neck cancer. Radiology 101:391–396, 1971.
36. Hussey DH, and Abrams JP: Combined therapy in head and neck cancer: hydroxyurea and radiotherapy. Prog. Clin. Cancer 6:79–86, 1975.
37. LePar E, Faust DS, Brady LW, et al.: Clinical evaluation of the adjunctive use of hydroxyurea in radiation therapy of carcinoma of the lung. Radiol. Clin. Biol. 36:32–40, 1967.
38. Landgren RC, Hussey DH, Barkley HT, et al.: Split-course irradiation compared to split-course irradiation plus hydroxyurea in the operable bronchogenic carcinoma. Cancer 34:1598–1601, 1974.
39. Petrovich Z, Ohanian M, and Cox J: Clinical research on the treatment of locally advanced lung cancer. Cancer 42:1129–1134, 1978.
40. Young CW, Schochetman G, Hodas S, et al.: Inhibition of DNA synthesis by hydroxyurea: structure-activity relationships. Cancer Res. 27:535–540, 1967.
41. Gale GR, and Hynes JB: Effects of certain arylhydroxamic acids on deoxyribonucleic acid synthesis by Ehrlich ascites tumor cells *in vitro*. J. Med. Chem. 11:191–194, 1968.
42. Gale GR, Hynes JB, and Smith AB: Synthesis of additional arylhydroxamic acids which inhibit nucleic acid biosynthesis *in vitro*. J. Med. Chem. 13:571–574, 1970.
43. van't Riet B, Wampler GL, and Elford HL: Synthesis of hydroxy- and amino-substituted benzohydroxamic acids: inhibition of ribonucleotide reductase and antitumor activity. J. Med. Chem. 22:589–592, 1979.
44. Elford HL, Wampler GL, and van't Riet B: New ribonucleotide reductase inhibitors with antineoplastic activity. Cancer Res. 39:844–851, 1979.
45. Flora KP, van't Riet B, and Wampler GL: Antitumor activity of amidoximes (hydroxyurea analogs) in murine tumor systems. Cancer Res. 38:1291–1295, 1978.
46. Chou JT, Beck WT, Khwaja T, et al.: Synthesis and anticancer activity of novel cyclic N-hydroxyureas. J. Pharm. Sci. 66:1556–1561, 1977.
47. Brockman RW, Shaddix S, Laster WR Jr, et al.: Inhibition of ribonucleotide reductase, DNA synthesis, and L1210 leukemia by guanazole. Cancer Res. 30:2358–2368, 1970.
48. Agrawal KC, and Sartorelli AC: α-(N)-Heterocyclic carboxaldehyde thiosemicarbazones. *In* Sartorelli AC, and Johns, DG (eds.): Handbook of Experimental Pharmacology, Vol. 38. Springer-Verlag, New York, 1975, pp. 793–807.
49. Yakar D, Holland JF, Ellison RR, et al.: Clinical pharmacological trial of guanazole. Cancer Res. 33:972–975, 1973.
50. DeConti RC, Toftness BR, Agrawal KC, et al.: Clinical and pharmacologic studies with 5-hydroxy-2-formylpyridine thiosemicarbazone. Cancer Res. 32:1455–1462, 1972.
51. Yarbro JW, Niehaus WG, and Barnum CP: Effect of hydroxyurea on regenerating rat liver. Biochem. Biophys. Res. Commun. 19:592–597, 1965.
52. Schwartz HS, Garofalo M, Sternberg SS, et al.: Inhibition of deoxyribonucleic acid synthesis in regenerating rat liver. Cancer Res. 25:1867–1870, 1965.
53. Young CW, and Hodas S: Hydroxyurea: inhibitory effect on DNA metabolism. Science 146:1172–1174, 1964.
54. Yarbro JW, Kennedy BJ, and Barnum CP: Hydroxyurea inhibition of DNA synthesis in ascites tumor. Proc. Natl. Acad. Sci. USA 53:1033–1035, 1965.
55. Rosenkranz HS, Garro AJ, Levy JA, et al.: Studies with hydroxyurea. I. The reversible inhibition of bacterial DNA synthesis and the effect of hydroxyurea on bactericidal action of streptomycin. Biochim. Biophys. Acta 114:501–505, 1966.
56. Gale GR, Kendall SM, McLain HH, et al.: Effect of hydroxyurea on *Pseudomonas aeruginosa*. Cancer Res. 24:1012–1019, 1964.
57. Elford HL: Effect of hydroxyurea on ribonucleotide reductase. Biochem. Biophys. Res. Commun. 33:129–135, 1968.
58. Turner MK, Abrams R, and Lieberman I: Meso-α,β,-diphenylsuccinate and hydroxyurea as inhibitors of deoxycytidylate synthesis in extracts of Ehrlich ascites and L cells. J. Biol. Chem. 241:5777–5780, 1966.
59. Neuhard J: Studies on the acid-soluble nucleotide pool in *Escherichia coli*. IV. Effects of hydroxyurea. Biochim. Biophys. Acta 145:1–6, 1967.
60. Skoog L, and Nordenskjold B: Effects of hydroxyurea and 1-β-D-arabinofuranosyl cytosine on deoxynucleoside triphosphate pools in mouse embryo cells. Eur. J. Biochem. 19:81–89, 1971.
61. Plagemann PGW, and Erbe J: Intracellular conversions of deoxyribonucleotides by Novikoff rat hepatoma cells and effects of hydroxyurea. J. Cell Physiol. 83:321–326, 1924.
62. Young CW, Schochetman G, and Karnofsky DA: Hydroxyurea-induced inhibition of deoxyribonucleotide synthesis: studies in intact cells. Cancer Res. 27:526–534, 1967.
63. Adams RLP, and Lindsay JG: Hydroxyurea. Reversal of inhibition and use as a cell synchronizing agent. J. Biol. Chem. 242:1314–1317, 1967.
64. Yarbro JW: Further studies on the mechanism of action of hydroxyurea. Cancer Res. 28:1082–1087, 1968.
65. Pollak RD, and Rosenkranz HS: Metabolic effects of hydroxyurea on BHK-21 cells transformed with polyoma virus. Cancer Res. 27:1214–1224, 1967.
66. Holmgren A, Reichard P, and Thelander L: Enzymatic synthesis of deoxyribonucleotides. VIII. The effects of ATP and dATP in the CDP reductase from *E. coli*. Proc. Natl. Acad. Sci. USA 54:830–836, 1965.
67. Laurent TC, Moore EC, and Reichard P: Enzymatic synthesis of deoxyribonucleotides. IV. Isolation and characterization of thioredoxin, the hydrogen donor from *E. coli*. J. Biol. Chem. 239:3436–3444, 1964.
68. Moore EC, Reichard P, and Thelander L: Enzymatic synthesis of deoxyribonucleotides. V. Purification and properties of thioredoxin reductase for *E. coli*. J. Biol. Chem. 239:3445–3452, 1964.
69. Brown NC, Larsson A, and Reichard P: On the subunit structure of ribonucleoside diphosphate reductase. J. Biol. Chem. 242:4272–4273, 1967.
70. Brown NC, and Reichard P: Ribonucleotide diphosphate reductase formation of active and inactive complexes of proteins B1 and B2. J. Mol. Biol. 46:25–38, 1969.
71. Chang C-H, and Cheng Y-C: Demonstration of two components and association of adenosine diphosphate-cytidine diphosphate reductase from cultured human lymphoblast cells (Molt-4F). Cancer Res. 39:436–442, 1979.
72. Cory JG, Fleischer AE, and Munro JB III: Reconstitution of the ribonucleotide reductase in mammalian cells. J. Biol. Chem. 253:2898–2901, 1978.
73. Moore EC, and Hurlbert RB: Regulation of mammalian deoxyribonucleotide biosynthesis by nucleotides as activators and inhibitors. J. Biol. Chem. 241:4802–4809, 1966.
74. Reichard P: Control of deoxyribonucleotide synthesis *in vitro* and *in vivo*. Adv. Enzyme Reg. 10:3–16, 1972.
75. Eriksson S, Thelander L, and Akerman M: Allosteric regulation of calf thymus ribonucleotide diphosphate reductase. Biochemistry 18:2948–2952, 1979.
76. Chang C-H, and Cheng Y-C: Effects of nucleoside triphosphates on human ribonucleotide reductase from Molt-4F cells. Cancer Res. 39:5087–5092, 1979.
77. Chang C-H, and Cheng Y-C: Substrate specificity of human ribonucleotide reductase from Molt-4F cells. Cancer Res. 39:5081–5086, 1979.
78. Brown NC, Eliasson R, Reichard P, et al.: Non-heme iron as a cofactor in ribonucleotide reductase from *E. coli*. Biochem. Biophys. Res. Commun. 30:522–527, 1968.

79. Krakoff I, Brown NC, and Reichard P: Inhibition of ribonucleoside diphosphate reductase by hydroxyurea. Cancer Res. 28:1559–1565, 1968.
80. Moore EC: The effects of ferrous iron and dithioerythritol on inhibition by hydroxyurea of ribonucleotide reductase. Cancer Res. 29:291–295, 1969.
81. Brockman RW, Shaddix S, Stringer V, et al.: Enhancement by desferoxamine of inhibition of DNA synthesis by ribonucleotide reductase inhibitors. Proc. Am. Assoc. Cancer Res. 13:88, 1972 (abstr.).
82. Borenfreund E, Krim M, and Bendich A: Chromosomal aberrations induced by hyponitrite and hydroxylamine derivatives. J. Natl. Cancer Inst. 32:667–680, 1969.
83. Walker IG, Yatscoff RW, and Sridhar R: Hydroxyurea: induction of breaks in template strands of replicating DNA. Biochem. Biophys. Res. Commun. 77:403–408, 1977.
84. Andrae U, and Greim H: Induction of DNA repair replication by hydroxyurea in human lymphoblastoid cells mediated by liver microsomes and NADPH. Biochem. Biophys. Res. Commun. 87:50–58, 1979.
85. Rosenkranz HS, and Rosenkranz S: Degradation of DNA by carbamoyloxyurea — an oxidation product of hydroxyurea. Biochim. Biophys. Acta 114:501–505, 1966.
86. Philips FS, Sternberg SS, Schwartz HS, et al.: Hydroxyurea. I. Acute cell death in proliferating tissues in rats. Cancer Res. 27:61–74, 1967.
87. Farber E, and Baserga R: Differential effects of hydroxyurea on survival of proliferating cells *in vivo*. Cancer Res. 29:136–139, 1969.
88. Sinclair WK: Hydroxyurea: differential lethal effects on cultured mammalian cells during the cell cycle. Science 150:1729–1731, 1965.
89. Ford SS, and Shackney SE: Lethal and sublethal effects of hydroxyurea in relation to drug concentration and duration of drug exposure in sarcoma 180 *in vitro*. Cancer Res. 37:2628–2637, 1977.
90. Kim JH, Gelbard AS, and Perez AG: Action of hydroxyurea on the nucleic acid metabolism and viability of HeLa cells. Cancer Res. 27:1301–1305, 1967.
91. Moran RE, and Straus MJ: Cytokinetic analysis of L1210 leukemia after continuous infusion of hydroxyurea *in vivo*. Cancer Res. 39:1616–1622, 1979.
92. Rajewsky MF: Synchronization *in vivo*: kinetics of a malignant cell system following temporary inhibition of DNA synthesis with hydroxyurea. Exp. Cell Res. 60:269–276, 1970.
93. Rabes HM, Iseler G, Czichos S, et al.: Synchronization of hepatocellular DNA synthesis in regenerating rat liver by continuous infusion of hydroxyurea. Cancer Res. 37:1105–1111, 1977.
94. Bacchetti S, and Whitmore GF: The action of hydroxyurea on mouse L-cells. Cell Tissue Kinet. 2:193–211, 1969.
95. Bhuyan BK, Fraser TJ, Gray LG, et al.: Cell-kill kinetics of several S-phase specific drugs. Cancer Res. 32:398–407, 1972.
96. Walters RA, Tobey RA, and Hildebrand CE: Hydroxyurea does not prevent synchronized G_1 Chinese hamster cells from entering DNA synthetic period. Biochem. Biophys. Res. Commun. 69:212–217, 1976.
97. Cress AE, and Gerner EW: Hydroxyurea inhibits ODC induction, but not the G_1 to S-phase transition. Biochem. Biophys. Res. Commun. 87:773–780, 1979.
98. Sinclair WK, and Morton RA: X-ray sensitivity during the cell generation cycle of cultured Chinese hamster cells. Radiat. Res. 29:450–474, 1966.
99. Phillips RA, and Tolmach LJ: Repair of potentially lethal damage in X-irradiated HeLa cells. Radiat. Res. 29:413–432, 1966.
100. Collins ARS, Schor SL, and Johnson RT: The inhibition of repair in UV-irradiated human cells. Mutat. Res. 42:413–422, 1977.
101. Francis AA, Blevins RD, Carrier WL, et al.: Inhibition of DNA repair in ultraviolet-irradiated human cells by hydroxyurea. Biochim. Biophys. Acta 563:385–392, 1979.
102. Lewis WH, and Wright JA: Altered ribonucleotide reductase activity in mammalian tissue culture cells resistant to hydroxyurea. Biochem. Biophys. Res. Commun. 60:926–933, 1974.
103. Lewis WH, and Wright JA: Ribonucleotide reductase from wild type and hydroxyurea-resistant Chinese hamster ovary cells. J. Cell. Physiol. 97:87–98, 1978.
104. Lewis WH, and Wright JA: Isolation of hydroxyurea Chinese hamster cells with altered levels of ribonucleotide reductase. Somat. Cell Genet. 5:83–96, 1979.
105. Alt FW, Kellems RE, Bertino JR, et al.: Selective multiple of dihydrofolate reductase genes in methotrexate-resistant variants of cultured murine cells. J. Biol. Chem. 253:1357–1370, 1978.
106. Bolton BH, Woods LA, Kaung DT, et al.: A simple method of colorimetric analysis for hydroxyurea. Cancer Chemother. Rep. 46:1–5, 1965.
107. Davidson JD, and Winter TS: A method of analyzing for hydroxyurea in biological fluids. Cancer Chemother. Rep. 27:97–110, 1963.
108. Beckloff GL, Lerner HJ, Frost D, et al.: Hydroxyurea in biologic fluids: dose-concentration relationship. Cancer Chemother. Rep. 48:57–58, 1963.
109. Creasey WA, Capizzi RL, and DeConti RC: Clinical and biochemical studies of high-dose intermittent therapy of solid tumors with hydroxyurea. Cancer Chemother. Rep. 54:191–194, 1970.
110. Rosner F, Rubin H, and Parise F: Studies on the absorption, distribution and excretion of hydroxyurea. Cancer Chemother. Rep. 55:167–173, 1971.
110A. Belt RJ, Haas CD, Kennedy J, et al.: Studies of hydroxyurea administered by continuous infusion. Cancer 46: 455, 1980.
111. Adamson RH, Ague SL, Hess SM, et al.: The distribution, excretion, and metabolism of hydroxyurea-^{14}C. J. Pharmacol. Exp. Ther. 150:322–327, 1965.
112. Fishbein WN, and Carbone PP: Hydroxyurea: mechanism of action. Science 142:1069–1070, 1963.
113. Colvin M, and Bono VH Jr: The enzymatic reduction of hydroxyurea to urea by mouse liver. Cancer Res. 30:1516–1519, 1970.
114. Bergsagel DE, Frenkel EP, Alfrey CP Jr, et al.: Megaloblastic erythropoiesis induced by hydroxyurea. Cancer Chemother. Rep. 40:15–17, 1964.
115. Lerner HJ, and Beckloff GL: Hydroxyurea administered intermittently. J.A.M.A. 192:1168–1170, 1965.
116. Ariel IM: Anticancer therapy with hydrea: comparative study of daily versus intermittent oral dosage. J. Surg. Oncol. 6:73–78, 1974.
117. Kennedy BJ, Smith LR, and Goltz RW: Skin changes secondary to hydroxyurea. Arch. Dermatol. 111:183–187, 1975.
118. Sears ME: Erythema in areas of previous irradiation in patients treated with hydroxyurea. Cancer Chemother. Rep. 40:31–32, 1965.
119. Kaung DT, and Swartzendruber AA: Effect of chemotherapeutic agents in chromosomes of patients with lung cancer. Dis. Chest 55:98–100, 1969.
120. Samuels ML, and Howe CD: Renal abnormalities induced by hydroxyurea. Cancer Chemother. Rep. 40:9–13, 1965.
121. Heddle R, and Calvert AF: Hydroxyurea-induced hepatitis. Med. J. Aust. 1:121, 1980.

13 THE ALKYLATING AGENTS

Michael Colvin

The alkylating agents are those antitumor drugs whose cytotoxic activity is mediated through the covalent bonding of alkyl groups (one or more saturated carbon atoms) to cellular molecules. Historically, the alkylating agents have played an important role in the development of cancer chemotherapy. The nitrogen mustards, mechlorethamine (HN2, "nitrogen mustard") and tris (β-chloroethyl)amine (HN3), were the first nonhormonal agents to show significant antitumor activity in man.[1-3] The clinical trials of nitrogen mustards in patients with lymphomas evolved from clinical observations of the victims of sulfur mustard gas used in World War I (Fig. 13–1). This compound was found to produce lymphoid aplasia in addition to the expected irritation of the lungs and mucous membranes, and was evaluated as an antitumor agent.[4] The related, but less reactive, bischloroethylamines (nitrogen mustards, Fig. 13–2) were found to be less toxic and to cause regressions of lymphoid tumors in mice. The first clinical studies produced some dramatic tumor regressions in lymphoma patients, and the antitumor effects were confirmed by an organized multi-institution study.[1-3] The demonstration of the clinical utility of the nitrogen mustards encouraged further efforts to find chemical agents with antitumor activity, leading to the wide variety of antitumor agents in use today.

CHEMISTRY

Mechanisms of Alkylating Reactions

Traditionally, alkylating reactions have been classified as S_N1 (nucleophilic substitution, first-order, Fig. 13–3) or S_N2 (nucleophilic substitution, second-order, Fig. 13–4). In the S_N1 reaction there is an initial formation of a highly reactive intermediate, followed by the rapid reaction of this intermediate with a nucleophile to produce the alkylated product. In this reaction the rate-limiting step is the initial formation of the reactive intermediate. Thus, the reaction exhibits first-order kinetics with regard to the concentration of the original alkylating agent and the rate is essentially independent of the concentration of the substrate, hence the designation S_N1.

The S_N2 alkylation reaction represents a bimolecular nucleophilic displacement. The rate of this reaction is dependent on the concentration of both the alkylating agent and the target nucleophile. Therefore, the reaction follows second-order kinetics. The terms S_N1 and S_N2 are defined kinetically, but normally are used in reference to the mechanism of action.

It would be expected that those compounds that alkylate via a highly reactive intermediate, such as the aliphatic nitrogen mustard mechlorethamine, would be less

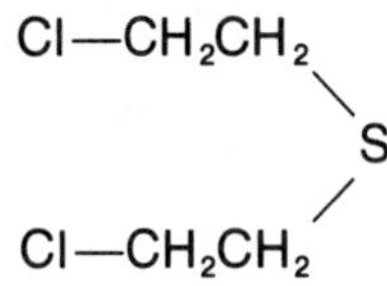

Figure 13–1. Bischloroethylsulfide (sulfur mustard).

Cl—CH$_2$CH$_2$
N—R
Cl—CH$_2$CH$_2$

Figure 13–2. Bischloroethylamine (nitrogen mustard general structure). —R = —CH_3 in mechlorethamine. —R = —CH_2CH_2Cl in tris(β-chloroethyl)amine.

$$RX \longrightarrow R^+ + X^- \xrightarrow{+Y^-} RY + X^-$$

Figure 13–3. S_N1 reaction.

selective in their alkylation targets than the less reactive S_N2 reagents, such as the alkyl alkane sulfonate busulfan. However, there is no simple relationship between the therapeutic effects of an alkylating agent and its chemical reactivity. The clinically useful agents include drugs that alkylate through an S_N1 mechanism, agents that alkylate through an S_N2 mechanism, and some compounds that alkylate through reactions with characteristics of both an S_N1 and an S_N2 mechanism.[5-7] Thus, the selectivity of a given alkylating agent obviously depends on a number of factors, including the reactivity, charge, and membrane permeability of the alkylating agent. If the agent is an S_N1 type reacting through an alkylating intermediate with a brief existence, the biologic half-life and membrane-penetrating properties of this intermediate may determine the selectivity. In the complex environment of the cell, especially the nucleus, chemical half-lives of nanoseconds and nanometer distances may be important in determining sites of alkylation. Application of techniques such as nuclear magnetic resonance and mass spectrometry to the study of the alkylation mechanism and the chemical nature of the intermediates involved are making possible a detailed understanding of these alkylation reactions.[6,7] Such approaches, coupled with improved techniques of localizing and studying cellular damage,[8,9] should eventually make it possible to predict the sites of alkylation of an agent and to understand and modify the biologic consequences of such alkylations.

Types of Alkylating Agents Used Clinically

Nitrogen Mustards. The most clinically useful alkylating agents have been the bischloroethylamines or nitrogen mustards. The general structure of these compounds is shown in Figure 13–2. The first nitrogen mustard to be used extensively in the clinic was mechlorethamine (Fig. 13–5), sometimes referred to by its original code name HN2, or by the term "nitrogen mustard." The mechanism of alkylation by the nitrogen mustards is shown in Figure 13–6. In the initial step, chlorine is lost and the β-carbon reacts with the nucleophilic nitrogen atom to form the cyclic, positively charged, and very reactive aziridinium moiety. Reaction of the aziridinium ring with a nucleophile (electron-rich atom) yields the initial alkylated product. Formation of a second aziridinium by the remaining chloroethyl group allows for a second alkylation, which produces a crosslink between the two alkylated nucleophiles.

After the introduction of mechlorethamine a great many analogues were synthesized in which the methyl group was replaced by a variety of chemical groups. Most of these compounds proved to have less antitumor activity than mechlorethamine, but three derivatives appear to have a higher therapeutic index, have a broader range of clinical activity, and can be administered both orally and intravenously. These drugs, which for the most part have replaced mechlorethamine in clinical use, are melphalan (L-phenylalanine mustard), chlorambucil, and cyclophosphamide (Fig. 13–7).

As can be seen from the structures, these derivatives have electron withdrawing groups substituted on the nitrogen atom. This alteration reduces the nucleophilicity of the nitrogen and renders the molecules less reactive. Melphalan and chlorambucil retain alkylating activity and appear to be more selective than nitrogen mustard. Cyclophosphamide, on the other hand, possesses no alkylating activity and must be metabolized to produce alkylating compounds. Cyclophosphamide has been the most widely used alkylating agent and has activity against a wide variety of tumors.[10] In 1972 an isomeric analogue of cyclophosphamide, ifosfamide,[11] was introduced into clinical use and may have more activity against non-small cell lung cancer than cyclophosphamide.[12] Melphalan has been widely used in the treatment of ovarian cancer,[13] multiple myeloma,[14] and carcinoma of the breast.[15] Chlorambucil has been most widely used in the treatment of chronic lymphocytic leukemia,[16,17] lymphomas,[16,18] and ovarian carcinoma.[19]

Figure 13–4. S_N2 reaction. $RX + Y^- \longrightarrow [X \cdots R \cdots Y] \longrightarrow X^- + RY$

Aziridines. Compounds bearing two or more aziridine groups, such as those shown in Figure 13–8 (thio-TEPA,[20,21] triethylenemelamine,[22,23] and Trenimon[24]) have shown clinical activity against a variety of human tumors. The antitumor activity of these compounds appears to be comparable to that of the nitrogen mustards, and thio-TEPA in particular has been used in the therapy of carcinoma of the breast[25] and the ovary.[26] Thio-TEPA has also been used for the intrathecal therapy of meningeal carcinomatosis.[27] Trenimon has been widely employed in Europe. However, the aziridines do not appear to have a therapeutic advantage over the more commonly used nitrogen mustards, and thus have not been used and studied as extensively.

These compounds were originally tested for antitumor activity because the nitrogen mustards alkylate through an aziridine intermediate. Although the mechanism of action of these compounds has not been explored thoroughly, they presumably alkylate through opening of the aziridine rings as shown for the nitrogen mustards. The reactivity of the aziridine groups is increased by protonation, and thus is enhanced at low pH.

Epoxides. Epoxides, such as dianhydrogalactitol (Fig. 13–9), have antitumor activity against a variety of animal tumors. Dianhydrogalactitol has undergone Phase I trials,[28,29] and in Phase II trials has shown activity in patients with brain tumors.[30,31] The compound has demonstrated little antitumor effect in patients with sarcomas,[32] melanoma,[33] head and neck carcinomas,[34] or breast cancer.[35]

The epoxides are chemically similar to the aziridines, and presumably alkylate in a similar fashion. Like the aziridines and busulfan, the epoxides exhibit S_N2 alkylation kinetics. In the physiologic pH range the reactivity of the epoxides will be less pH-dependent than the aziridines, since the epoxides protonate less readily.

Halogenated polyhydroxyl compounds such as dibromodulcitol (Fig. 13–9) spontaneously produce the corresponding diepoxides in aqueous solution, and diepoxides are probably responsible for the antitumor activity that has been reported for these halogenated polyhydroxyl compounds.[36-38]

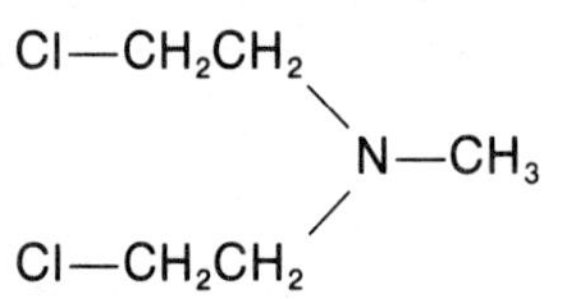

$$\begin{array}{l} Cl-CH_2CH_2 \\ \qquad\qquad\qquad \searrow \\ \qquad\qquad\qquad\quad N-CH_3 \\ \qquad\qquad\qquad \nearrow \\ Cl-CH_2CH_2 \end{array}$$

Figure 13–5. Mechlorethamine.

Alkyl Alkane Sulfonates. The major clinical representative of this class of alkylating agents is busulfan (Fig. 13–10), which is widely used for the treatment of chronic myelogenous leukemia.[39] Timmis and co-workers[40,41] have shown that compounds with one to eight methylene units between the sulfonate groups have antitumor activity, but that maximal activity is shown by the compound with four methylene units.

Busulfan alkylates as shown in Figure 13–11, and exhibits S_N2 alkylation kinetics. The compound reacts more extensively with thiol groups of amino acids and proteins[42] than do the nitrogen mustards, and these findings have prompted the suggestion that the alkyl alkane sulfonates may exert their cytotoxic activities through such thiol reactions rather than through interactions with DNA.[42,43] Brookes and Lawley were able to demonstrate the reaction of busulfan with the N-7 position of guanosine,[44] but Mitchell and Walker[45] were unable to show crosslinking of DNA in cells treated with busulfan.

In contrast to the nitrogen mustards and nitrosoureas, busulfan displays a more marked effect on myeloid cells than on lymphoid cells.[46] This specificity is manifest clinically in that busulfan is active against chronic myelogenous leukemia. Busulfan also is markedly cytotoxic to hematopoietic stem cells. This effect is seen clinically in the prolonged aplasia that may be seen after busulfan administration, and can be shown experimentally in stem cell cloning systems.[47] The pharmacologic bases for these properties of busulfan are not understood.

Nitrosoureas. The nitrosourea antitumor agents in current use were developed on the basis of the observations that methylnitrosoguanidine and methylnitrosourea exhibited modest antitumor activity in experimental animal tumor models.[48] Careful structure-function studies were carried out initially by Baker at the Stanford Research Institute[48,49] and subsequently under the direction of Montgomery at the Southern Research Institute.[50] These studies demonstrated that chloroethyl derivatives such as chloroethylnitrosourea (CNU) and bischloroethylnitrosourea (BCNU) (Fig. 13–12) possessed greater antitumor activity than methylnitrosourea and other alkyl deriva-

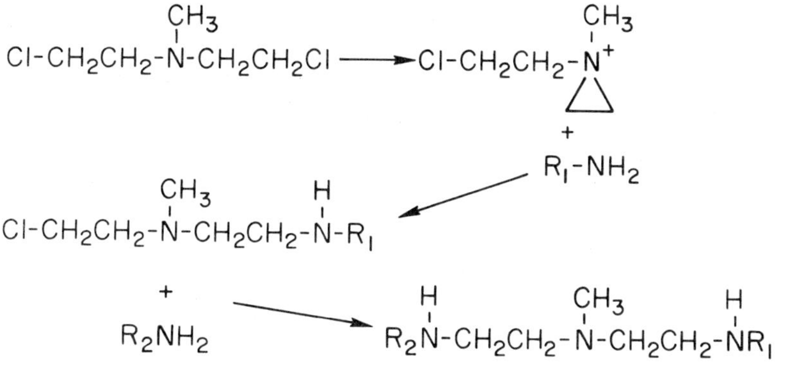

$$Cl\text{-}CH_2CH_2\text{-}\underset{}{\overset{CH_3}{N}}\text{-}CH_2CH_2Cl \longrightarrow Cl\text{-}CH_2CH_2\text{-}\overset{CH_3}{N^+}(\text{aziridine})$$

$$+ \; R_1\text{-}NH_2 \longrightarrow Cl\text{-}CH_2CH_2\text{-}\overset{CH_3}{N}\text{-}CH_2CH_2\text{-}\overset{H}{N}\text{-}R_1$$

$$+ \; R_2NH_2 \longrightarrow R_2\overset{H}{N}\text{-}CH_2CH_2\text{-}\overset{CH_3}{N}\text{-}CH_2CH_2\text{-}\overset{H}{N}R_1$$

Alkylation Mechanism via Aziridine Intermediate

Figure 13–6. (Reproduced with permission from Colvin M: *In* Cancer Chemotherapy, Vol. 3. Academic Press, New York, 1981, p. 291.)

tives, and the nitrosourea derivatives were found to be more active than the nitrosoguanidines.

Further study showed that these chloroethylnitrosoureas exhibited activity against intracranially inoculated tumors,[50] owing to their lipophilic character and ability to cross the blood-brain barrier. BCNU was the first of the chloroethylnitrosoureas to undergo clinical trial and has shown significant activity against a variety of human tumors.[51] Subsequently cyclohexylchloroethylnitrosourea (CCNU) and methylcyclohexylchloroethylnitrosourea (methyl-CCNU) (Fig. 13–12) have shown greater activity against solid tumors in experimental animals[52] and have been introduced into clinical use.

The nitrosoureas show some degree of cross-resistance with other alkylating agents.[50] Because of this fact and the structure of the compounds, the nitrosoureas were thought to be acting as alkylating agents. In the past few years a number of studies have confirmed that these drugs are indeed alkylating agents and the mechanism of the alkylation reaction has been established (Fig. 13–13).

At physiologic pH, proton abstraction by a hydroxyl ion initiates spontaneous decomposition of the molecule to yield an isocyanate compound[53] and diazonium hydroxide molecule.[54] The chloroethyl diazonium ion or the chloroethyl carbonium ion generated may then alkylate biologic molecules. Data from Ludlum et al.[55] and Kohn[56] indicate that the alkylation of nitrogens in cytidylate and guanylate units in DNA yields chloroethylamino groups on the nucleotide capable of a second alkylation to produce DNA-DNA and DNA-protein crosslinks.

The isocyanate produced from nitrosoureas has been shown to inhibit DNA polymerase,[57] the repair of DNA strand breaks,[58]and RNA synthesis and process-

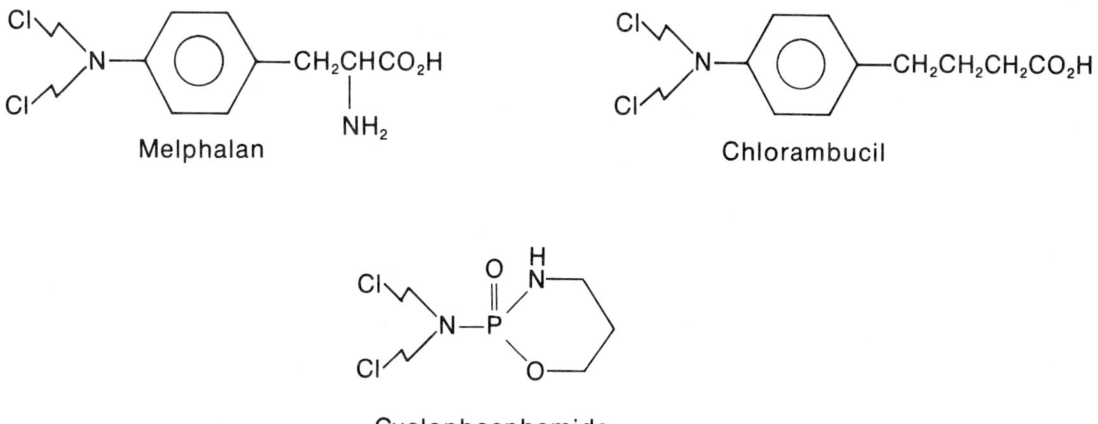

$$(ClCH_2CH_2)_2N\text{-}C_6H_4\text{-}CH_2CH(NH_2)CO_2H$$

Melphalan

$$(ClCH_2CH_2)_2N\text{-}C_6H_4\text{-}CH_2CH_2CH_2CO_2H$$

Chlorambucil

$$(ClCH_2CH_2)_2N\text{-}P(=O)(\text{-NH-CH}_2CH_2CH_2\text{-O-})$$

Cyclophosphamide

Figure 13–7. Nitrogen mustard derivatives in clinical use.

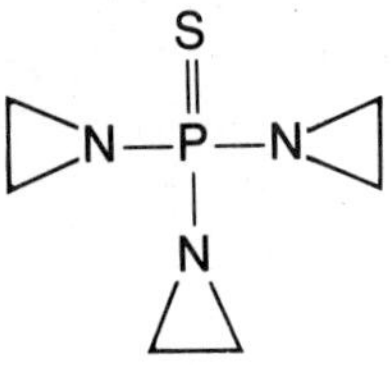

Thio-TEPA

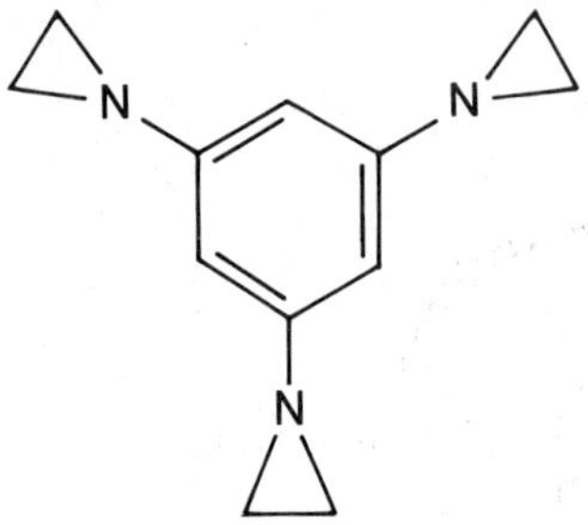

Triethylenemelamine

Trenimon

Figure 13–8. Aziridine antitumor agents.

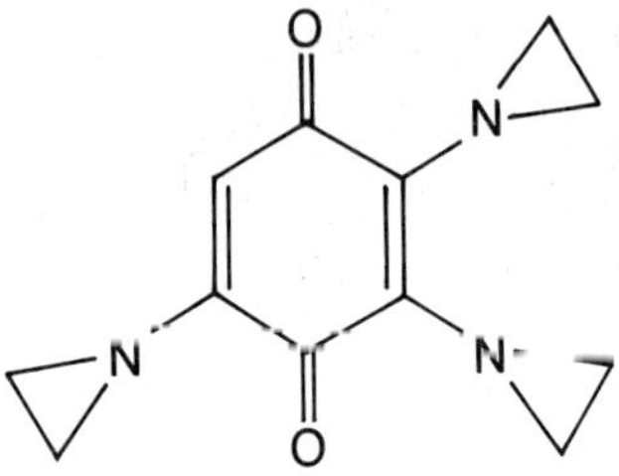

ing.[57] The alkylating activity, and not the isocyanate effects, appears to be responsible for the antitumor effects of the nitrosoureas. Nitrosoureas that lack carbamoylating activity, such as chlorozotocin, still retain potent cytotoxicity. However, the isocyanates may play a role in the toxic effects of these drugs.[54, 60, 61]

Streptozotocin (Fig. 13–14) is a methylnitrosourea derivative that was isolated from *Streptomyces* broth. This compound displays significant activity against the murine L1210 leukemia,[62] and is remarkable for its lack of bone marrow toxicity[63] and its strong diabetogenic effect in animals.[64] Because of this specific toxicity to pancreatic β cells, streptozotocin was tested against islet cell carcinoma of the pancreas in man and showed clinically significant activity.[65, 66] The dose-limiting toxicities in man have been gastrointestinal toxicity and nephrotoxicity, with considerably less hematopoietic toxicity than the other nitrosoureas.

In an effort to increase the antitumor effects of streptozotocin while preserving the bone marrow-sparing effect, chlorozotocin (in which the l-methyl group has been replaced by a chloroethyl group, Fig. 13–14) was synthesized and tested.[67, 68] This compound, and similar nitrosoureas bearing a glucose moiety, were shown to have reduced bone marrow toxicity in mice.[69] However,

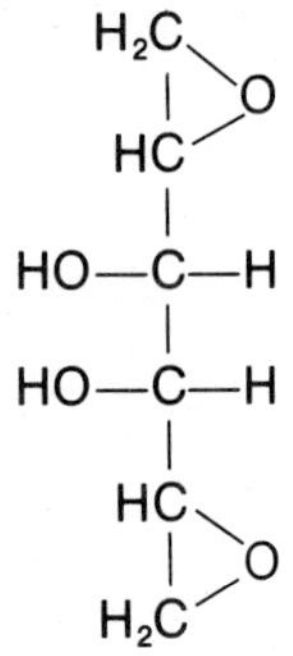

Dianhydrogalactitol

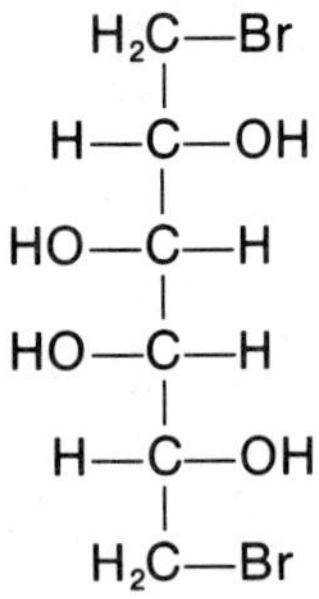

Dibromodulcitol

Figure 13–9.

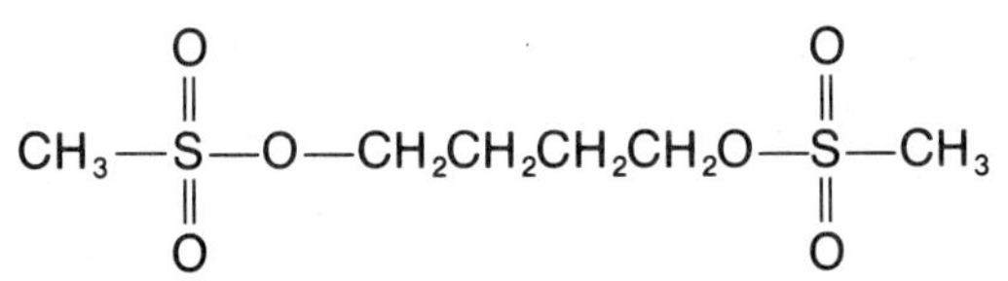

$$CH_3{-}\overset{\overset{O}{\|}}{\underset{\underset{O}{\|}}{S}}{-}O{-}CH_2CH_2CH_2CH_2O{-}\overset{\overset{O}{\|}}{\underset{\underset{O}{\|}}{S}}{-}CH_3$$

Figure 13–10. Busulfan.

the dose-limiting toxicity of chlorozotocin in man appears to be hematopoietic suppression.[70]

Currently, the nitrosoureas are used singly and in combination in the therapy of lymphomas,[71] lung cancer[72], colon cancer,[73] and drug-resistant multiple myeloma.[74] As predicted from the animal studies, the nitrosoureas have shown significant activity against brain tumors.[75] The severe hematopoietic depression (especially thrombocytopenia) produced by these agents is a significant limiting factor in their use.

CELLULAR PHARMACOLOGY

Sites of Alkylation

If a radioactive alkylating agent such as mechlorethamine is administered to an animal, the agent is found to be covalently bound to a wide variety of biologic molecules,[76] including nucleic acids, proteins, amino acids, and nucleotides. It is difficult to ascertain which of these alkylated sites represent the critical targets that are responsible for the cytotoxic actions of the alkylating agents. The action of these compounds could be due to inactivation of enzymes, depletion of critical amino acids or nucleic acid precursors, damage to nucleic acids, alteration of cell membranes, or a combination of these actions. Because the alkylating agents generally are active at very low doses, it seems unlikely that the antitumor effect is due to depletion of low-molecular-weight compounds such as amino acids, unless a particular target was present in very small quantities or specifically localized in tumors. Although these possibilities cannot be definitely eliminated, it seems more likely that the cytotoxicity is due to the inactivation of critical macromolecules such as enzymes or nucleic acids. Since one of the consistently observed biochemical effects of alkylating agents at cytotoxic levels is the inhibition of DNA synthesis,[77, 78] a number of studies have focused on the mechanism of this inhibition. Conflicting reports have appeared, but the evidence favors the hypothesis that the inhibition is due to damage to the nucleic acid template rather than to inactivation of DNA polymerase or other enzymes responsible for DNA synthesis.[79-83]

The DNA molecule presents a variety of potential sites for alkylation. The phos-

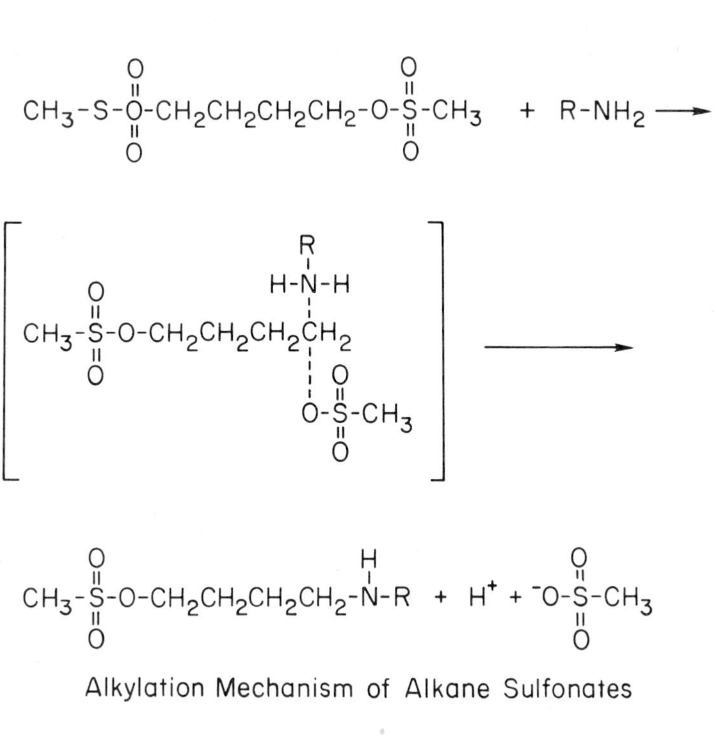

$$CH_3{-}\overset{\overset{O}{\|}}{\underset{\underset{O}{\|}}{S}}{-}O{-}CH_2CH_2CH_2CH_2{-}O{-}\overset{\overset{O}{\|}}{\underset{\underset{O}{\|}}{S}}{-}CH_3 + R{-}NH_2 \longrightarrow$$

$$\left[CH_3{-}\overset{\overset{O}{\|}}{\underset{\underset{O}{\|}}{S}}{-}O{-}CH_2CH_2CH_2\overset{\overset{\overset{R}{|}}{H-N-H}}{\underset{\underset{O-\overset{\overset{O}{\|}}{\underset{\underset{O}{\|}}{S}}-CH_3}{|}}{CH_2}} \right] \longrightarrow$$

$$CH_3{-}\overset{\overset{O}{\|}}{\underset{\underset{O}{\|}}{S}}{-}O{-}CH_2CH_2CH_2CH_2{-}\overset{\overset{H}{|}}{N}{-}R + H^+ + {}^-O{-}\overset{\overset{O}{\|}}{\underset{\underset{O}{\|}}{S}}{-}CH_3$$

Alkylation Mechanism of Alkane Sulfonates

Figure 13–11. (Reproduced with permission from Colvin M: *In* Cancer Chemotherapy, Vol. 3. Academic Press, New York, 1981, p. 292.)

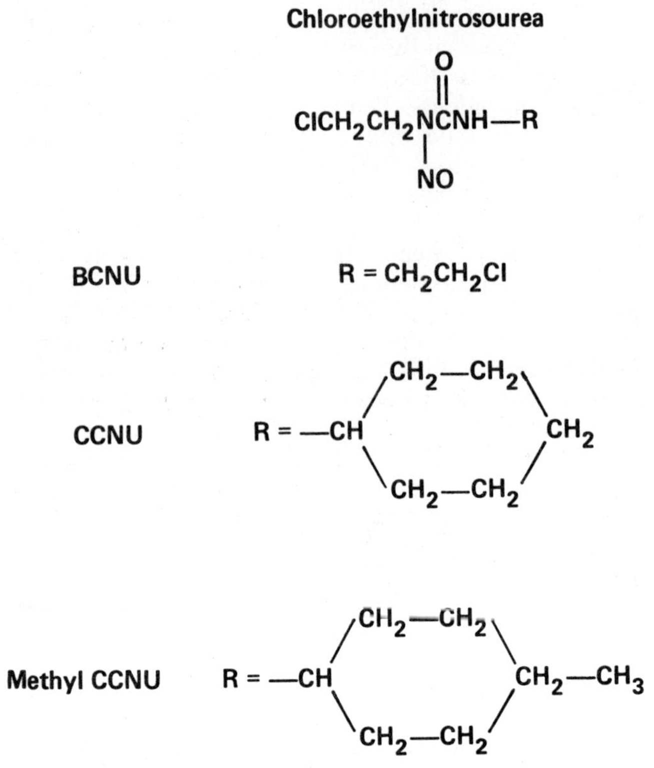

Chloroethylnitrosourea

$$\mathrm{ClCH_2CH_2N(NO)C(=O)NH{-}R}$$

BCNU $\quad R = CH_2CH_2Cl$

CCNU $\quad R = -CH$ (cyclohexyl: CH_2-CH_2, CH_2, CH_2-CH_2 ring)

Methyl CCNU $\quad R = -CH$ (cyclohexyl ring bearing CH_2-CH_3)

Figure 13–12. Structures of nitrosoureas.

phoryl oxygens of the sugar phosphate backbone are obvious electron-rich targets for alkylation. A number of studies have shown that alkylation of the phosphate groups does occur[84-86] and can result in strand breakages from hydrolysis of the resultant phosphotriesters. Although the biologic significance of the strand breakage due to phosphate alkylation remains uncertain, the process is so slow that it seems unlikely that it is a major determinant of cytotoxicity, even for monofunctional agents.[87]

Extensive studies with carcinogenic alkylating agents such as methyl methane sulfonate have shown that virtually all the oxygen and nitrogen atoms of the purine and pyrimidine bases of DNA can be alkylated, to varying degrees. The relative significance to carcinogenesis or cytotoxicity of alkylation of each of these sites remains uncertain.

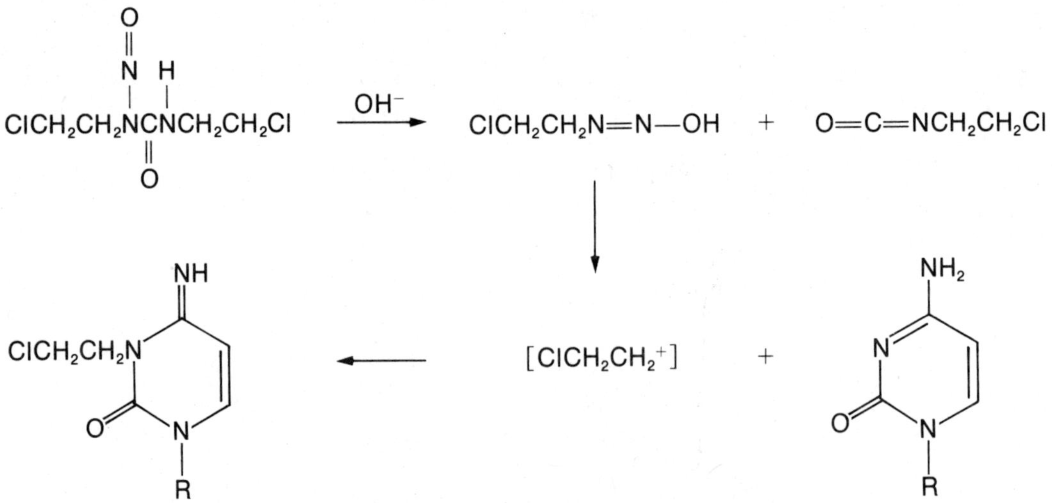

$$\mathrm{ClCH_2CH_2N(NO)C(=O)N(H)CH_2CH_2Cl \xrightarrow{OH^-} ClCH_2CH_2N{=}N{-}OH + O{=}C{=}NCH_2CH_2Cl}$$

$$\mathrm{ClCH_2CH_2N{=}N{-}OH \longrightarrow [ClCH_2CH_2^+] + \text{cytosine nucleoside (NH}_2\text{, N, O, N–R)} \longrightarrow \text{N-(ClCH}_2\text{CH}_2\text{)-alkylated nucleoside (=NH, O, N–R)}}$$

Figure 13–13. Alkylation of nucleoside by BCNU.

Figure 13–14.

Streptozotocin

Chlorozotocin

Various reports[88-90] have indicated that alkylation of the 0–6 atom and of the extracyclic nitrogen of guanosine may be of particular importance for carcinogenesis.

Studies of the base specificity of alkylation by the chemotherapeutic alkylating agents have been much less extensive. Brookes and Lawley[44] established that busulfan and mechlorethamine alkylate the N-7 position of guanosine and guanylic acid and that di(guanin-7-yl) derivatives (two guanine molecules bridged at the N-7 position by the alkylating agents) could be isolated from acid hydrolysates of the reaction mixtures. Ludlum and colleagues have recently confirmed this finding for busulfan.[91]

Price et al.[92] found that N,N-diethyl-2-chloroethylamine hydrochloride, a monofunctional nitrogen mustard, reacted with (in decreasing order of reactivity) the N-7 of guanosine, the N-1 of adenosine, the N-3 of deoxycytidine, and the N-3 of thymidine. Reaction of the nitrogen mustard with native DNA, however, produced initially only N-7 alkylated guanine, to an extent greater than would have been predicted from the guanosine studies. After there had been extensive alkylation and denaturation of the DNA considerable alkylation of N-1 of adenosine occurred. The reason for the enhanced alkylation of the N-7 position of deoxyguanosine when present in DNA is uncertain, but it has been suggested that base stacking and charge transfer may enhance the nucleophilic character of the N-7 position of the deoxyguanylic acid residue.[93]

DNA Crosslinking

On the basis of the finding of predominant alkylation of the N-7 position of guanosine and the isolation of the di(guanin-7-yl) products, Brookes and Lawley postulated that the bifunctional alkylating agents such as nitrogen mustards produced interstrand and intrastrand DNA-DNA crosslinks, and that these crosslinks were responsible for the inactivation of the DNA and for the cytotoxicity of the bifunctional alkylating agents.[93, 94] On the basis of the Watson-Crick DNA model, these authors suggested that the appropriate spatial relationship for crosslinking by nitrogen mustards or sulfur mustard between the N-7 positions of deoxyguanylic acid residues in complementary DNA strands occurred in the complementary base sequences shown in Figure 13–15.

This suggestion of the importance of crosslinking is supported by the fact that the bifunctional alkylating agents, with few exceptions, are much more effective antitumor agents than the analogous monofunctional agents, as originally described by Loveless and Ross.[95] Furthermore, increasing the number of alkylating units on the molecule beyond two does not usually increase the antitumor activity of the compound.

Direct evidence that DNA crosslinking occurs as the result of treatment of DNA and cells with bifunctional alkylating agents has been provided by a number of physical tech-

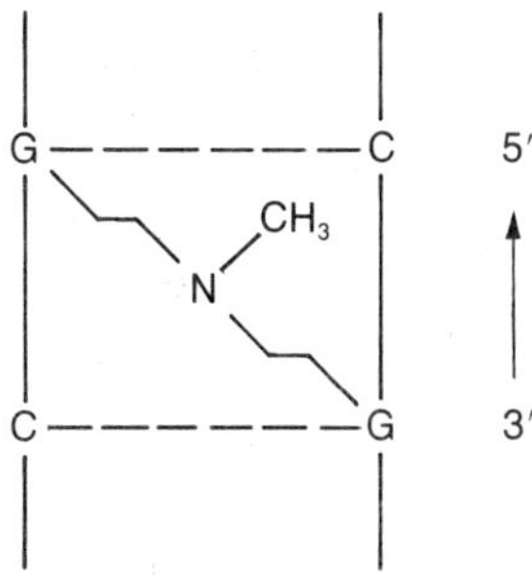

Figure 13–15. Crosslinking of DNA by nitrogen mustard. (Modified and reproduced with permission from Brookes P, and Lawley PD: The reaction of mono- and di-functional alkylating agents with nucleic acids. Biochem. J. 80:486, 1961.)

niques, including sedimentation velocity studies and denaturation-renaturation studies.[96-101] However, these techniques have not been sensitive enough to convincingly demonstrate DNA interstrand crosslinking in mammalian cells exposed to *therapeutic levels* of alkylating agents *in vitro*, or in tissues after *in vivo* drug administration. In 1976, a very sensitive assay for DNA interstrand crosslinking in cells was reported by Kohn et al.[102] This technique, the alkaline elution method, has the necessary sensitivity to detect DNA crosslinking in cells exposed to minimal cytotoxic levels of a variety of bifunctional alkylating agents.[8, 103] These studies have been extended to document DNA interstrand crosslinking in tumor cells and normal tissues of animals given therapeutic doses of alkylating agents.[104] Such studies have shown that DNA crosslinking by bifunctional alkylating agents correlates with cytotoxicity and that drug-resistant cells are not crosslinked.[105] Thus, a number of lines of evidence increasingly support the hypothesis that DNA interstrand crosslinking is the major mechanism of alkylating agent cytotoxicity.

Work by Ludlum et al.[55] and Kohn[56] suggests that the chloroethylnitrosoureas crosslink via a unique mechanism. The spontaneous decomposition of the chloroethylnitrosoureas generates a chloroethyldiazonium hydroxide entity,[54] which can alkylate either the N-3 position of deoxycytidylic acid residue or the N-7 position of a deoxyguanylic acid residue to produce an alkylating chloroethylamine group on the nucleotide in the DNA strand. This group could then alkylate an adjaceant nucleotide (presumably deoxycytidylate or deoxyguanylate) on the complementary DNA strand, producing an interstrand crosslink.

Studies using the alkaline elution technique have also established that DNA-protein as well as DNA-DNA crosslinks are formed by bifunctional alkylating agents.[106] This information supports data from previous investigators,[107-109] indicating that DNA-protein crosslinks were formed. The relative contribution of the two types of DNA crosslinks to cytotoxicity is not certain, but the studies of Kohn would indicate that DNA-protein crosslinks do not play a major role in cytotoxicity.

Although DNA-DNA crosslinks do appear to play a major role in the cytotoxic effects of alkylating agents, the monofunctional DNA alkylations produced greatly exceed crosslinks in number and must be considered to be cytotoxic. This hypothesis is supported by the fact that certain of the clinically effective agents, such as procarbazine and DTIC (see Chap. 15), chemically appear to be monofunctional alkylating compounds and do not produce crosslinks in experimental systems. The basis of the cytotoxic effects of monofunctional alkylation is probably single-strand DNA breaks. Although apurinic sites in the DNA will lead to spontaneous hydrolysis of an adjacent phosphodiester bond, this process is probably too slow to be of biologic significance.[87] However, endonucleases that will produce single-strand breaks at apurinic sites have been described,[110, 111] and may be responsible for the single-strand breaks that are produced by monofunctional agents and which probably produce the toxic and therapeutic effects of the monofunctional agents. It has been demonstrated that the presence of apurinic sites may produce crosslinks, but the low frequency of these crosslinks makes it unlikely that they are responsible for the antitumor activity of the monofunctional agents.[112]

It has usually been assumed that the alkylation of nucleic acids by alkylating agents is randomly distributed along the DNA molecule. However, specific regions of the DNA may be selectively susceptible to alkylation. Recent data from Tew and Schein have suggested that one determinant of regional specificity of DNA alkylations may be chromatin structure.[9, 113]

Intranuclear DNA exists in a tight complex with highly basic proteins (histones), other non-histone proteins, and RNA. This complex, called chromatin, has a beaded appearance in electron micrographs and is composed of tightly packed spheres of nucleic acid and protein, called nucleosomes, which contain highly active regions for transcription of RNA, and more linear intervening regions, called linker segments. Characteristic histones and non-histone proteins are associated with the nucleosome and linker regions, and are believed to modify the accessibility of DNA to alkylation and to enzymatic repair of alkylation. The nucleosome, containing the more "active region" of DNA, is more highly susceptible to alkylation by nitrosoureas and other alkylating agents, and less easily repaired than the linker region. Agents that preferentially alkylate transcriptionally active regions of nucleosomal DNA are thus believed to have greater toxicity for cells.

The glycosylated nitrosourea chlorozotocin, which has somewhat reduced myelotoxicity, has the interesting property of producing greater alkylation of nucleosomal DNA as compared with linker regions in tumor cells, and the opposite pattern in bone marrow cells.[114] This differential effect on tumor versus normal tissue may account for the improved therapeutic ratio of this new agent in preclinical studies. Lesser myelosuppression has also been observed in Phase I and II trials in man.[115] Although the significance of this regional specificity is not known, such localization of alkylation might play an important role in the cellular effect of the alkylating agents.

In summary, a substantial amount of evidence now supports the hypothesis that the major factor in the cytotoxicity of most of the clinically effective alkylating agents is interstrand DNA crosslinking, which results in inactivation of the DNA template, cessation of DNA synthesis, and ultimate cell death. The details of this interaction with DNA are still in the process of being elucidated, and may depend on the specific alkylating agent and on the target cell under consideration. As discussed above, monofunctional alkylations undoubtedly play a role in cytotoxicity, and the relative roles of crosslinks and monofunctional alkylations in the antitumor and toxic effects of the alkylating agents remain to be elucidated. An increased knowledge of alkylation mechanisms and targets may make it possible to improve the therapeutic index of these agents. For example, crosslinking activity appears in many instances to be associated with antitumor effect, whereas monofunctional alkylations are usually associated with general cytotoxicity and carcinogenicity. Thus, it seems likely that if the ratio of crosslinks to monofunctional alkylations produced by a drug can be increased, the carcinogenicity of the agent will be reduced, relative to the antitumor activity.

Cellular Uptake

The uptake of alkylating agents into cells is a critical step that is a potential determinant of cellular specificity. Despite the importance of such studies, the cellular uptake of only a few alkylating agents has been examined. Wolpert and Ruddon[116] and Goldenberg et al.[117] demonstrated that the uptake of mechlorethamine by Ehrlich ascites tumor cells and by L5178Y lymphoblasts is by active transport systems. These systems were found to be temperature-dependent, to accumulate drug against a concentration gradient, and to be sensitive to metabolic inhibitors. The natural substrate for the lymphoblast transport system appears to be choline.[118] whose structural resemblance to protonated mechlorethamine (the drug would be protonated at physiologic pH) is shown in Figure 13–16.

In 1977 Goldenberg and colleagues reported that melphalan is also actively transported into L5178Y lymphoblasts.[119] Subsequent studies by Vistica et al.[120] and further investigation by Goldenberg and colleagues[121] have shown that melphalan is transported into several cell types by at least two active transport systems, which also carry leucine and other neutral amino acids across the cell membrane. Vistica et al. showed that high levels of leucine in the medium will protect cells from the cytotoxic effects of melphalan by competing with melphalan for transport into the target cells.[122] Since appreciable levels of leucine are present in plasma and extracellular fluid, this competition may have pharmacologic significance. Although murine leukemia cells contain at least two transport systems for melphalan and L-leucine, one of these systems is lacking in murine granulocyte precursors (CFU-C's).[123] This system, missing in CFU-C's but present in leukemia cells, is identified by its capacity to transport the amino acid analogue 2-amino-bicyclo[2,2,]heptane-2-carboxylic acid (BCH). These unexpected findings have prompted a search for cytotoxic analogues of BCH that might be taken up by tumor cells, but not by normal granuloctye precursors.

In contrast to the active transport systems for mechlorethamine and melphalan, studies by Begleiter et al. demonstrated that the highly lipid-soluble nitrosoureas BCNU and CCNU enter cells by passive diffusion and

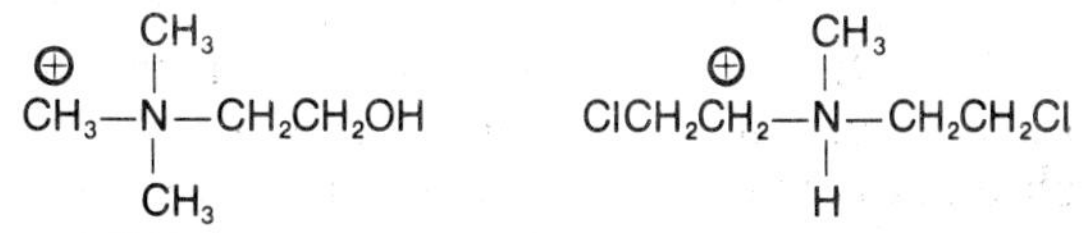

$$\overset{\oplus}{}CH_3-\underset{CH_3}{\overset{CH_3}{N}}-CH_2CH_2OH \qquad \overset{\oplus}{}ClCH_2CH_2-\underset{H}{\overset{CH_3}{N}}-CH_2CH_2Cl$$

Choline — Mechlorethamine

Figure 13–16.

not by active transport.[124] No accumulation of these drugs in excess of extracellular concentrations was seen. The unique cytotoxic properties and the delayed hematopoietic toxicity may be related to this mechanism of cell entry.

One potential mechanism by which selectivity for tumor cells over normal cells might be achieved is by the selective uptake of drugs into malignant cells. To the knowledge of this author, such a selective uptake by human tumor cells has not been demonstrated for any alkylating agent. However, the increased knowledge of the cell membranes and transport pathways of normal and malignant cells may make it possible to identify pathways through which such selectivity could be achieved. Correspondingly, the increased knowledge of the chemistry and structure-function relationships of the alkylating agents should allow the design of agents to capitalize on these leads.

Tumor Resistance

The emergence of alkylating agent-resistant tumor cells is a major problem that limits the clinical effectiveness of these drugs. One mechanism for drug resistance is that of decreased drug entry into the cell. Goldenberg et al. demonstrated that L5178Y lymphoblast cells resistant to mechlorethamine had decreased uptake of the drug.[125] A decreased uptake of drug by mechlorethamine-resistant cells was also reported by Klatt et al.,[109] Wolpert and Ruddon,[116] and Rutman et al.[126] Redwood and Colvin have recently reported that murine L1210 leukemia cells that are resistant to melphalan have a decreased transport of the drug.[127] These authors suggested that the resistant L1210 cells have specific mutation in the lower-affinity, higher-velocity L-transport system, which results in a decreased affinity of the carrier protein for leucine and melphalan.

Although decreased drug uptake is an obvious mechanism of cellular drug resistance, evidence for other mechanisms of resistance to alkylating agents has been presented. Hirono[128] demonstrated an increase in the nonprotein sulfhydryl content of Yoshida sarcoma cells resistant to mechlorethamine. Similarly, Calcutt and Connors[129] found that tumor cells resistant to alkylating agents possessed a higher ratio of protein-free to protein-bound thiol compounds, and suggested that the increased thiol content might function to react with and activate the alkylating agent intracellularly. The potential relationship of intracellular thiol content to alkylating agent resistance has not been further defined. Sladek[130] and Connors et al.[131] suggested that one mechanism of cellular resistance to cyclophosphamide might be enhanced metabolism of the primary metabolites to the inactive products 4-ketocyclophosphamide and carboxyphosphamide.

Another potential mechanism to explain resistance of cells to alkylating agents is that of enhanced repair of the lesions generated by alkylation. Since DNA appears to be the most critical target for the alkylating agents, the repair of DNA has been a major focus of study. Lawley and Brookes[100] and Kohn et al.[98] found that enhanced excision of alkylated nucleotides from DNA appeared to be responsible for the resistance of bacteria to alkylating agents. The fact that mammalian cells are capable of such excision repair of sulfur mustard alkylated nucleotides was demonstrated by Crathorne and Roberts.[132] More recently, Ewig and Kohn demonstrated that DNA interstrand crosslinks produced by alkylating agents could be repaired by mammalian cells.[8] Thus, although there has been no clear demonstration in mammalian cells of drug resistance due to enhanced excision repair of alkylated nucleotides, the existence of such a mechanism seems likely.

It is probable that multiple mechanisms of cellular resistance occur in a given tumor cell population and are responsible for the drug resistance seen clinically. Goldenberg[133] found that L5178Y lymphoma cells that are resistant to mechlorethamine are 18.5-fold more resistant to mechlorethamine than the wild-type sensitive cells, but are uniformly two- to threefold resistant to a variety of other alkylating agents. On this basis, Goldenberg suggested that resistance to specific alkylating agents occurred on the basis of decreased transport of these agents into the cell, whereas the general cross-resistance was due to nonspecific mechanisms, such as enhanced repair capacity. This hypothesis is consistent with the observation of Schabel et al.[134] in experimental animal tumors and with clinical experience. In both situations, varying degrees of cross-resistance between alkylating agents are seen, but a tumor that is resistant to one alkylating agent may remain significantly responsive to another.

DECOMPOSITION AND METABOLISM

Decomposition Versus Metabolism

A principal route of degradation of most of the reactive alkylating agents is spontaneous hydrolysis of the alkylating entity (i.e., alkylation by water). For example, mechlorethamine will rapidly undergo reaction to produce 2-hydroxyethyl-2-chloroethylmethylamine (Fig. 13–17*A*) and bis-2-hydroxyethylmethylamine (Fig. 13–17*B*).[135] Likewise, both melphalan[136] and chlorambucil[137] undergo similar hydrolysis to form the monohydroxyethyl and bishydroxyethyl products, although less rapidly than the aliphatic nitrogen mustards.

Most alkylating agents also undergo some degree of enzymatic metabolism. For example, if mechlorethamine radiolabeled in the methyl group is administered to mice, approximately 15 per cent of the radioactivity can be recovered as exhaled carbon dioxide, indicating that enzymatic demethylation is occurring.[76] A major route of metabolism of chlorambucil is oxidation of the butyric acid side chain to produce phenylacetic acid mustard (Fig. 13–18).[138, 139] Phenylacetic acid mustard undergoes hydrolysis to produce the mono- and bishydroxyethyl products[137] and is an active alkylating agent.[140] No enzymatic metabolic products of melphalan have yet been identified, and certainly most of the administered drug appears to degrade by hydrolysis of the mustard entity.

Cyclophosphamide

The alkylating agent whose metabolism has been most extensively studied is cyclophosphamide. This widely used drug is inactive *in vitro*, but is activated to alkylating and cytotoxic metabolites by the mixed function oxidases in hepatic microsomes.[141-144] The complex metabolic transformations that cyclophosphamide undergoes are illustrated in Figure 13–19 and have been reviewed by Friedman et al.[145] The initial metabolic step is the oxidation of the ring carbon adjacent to the ring nitrogen to produce 4-hydroxycyclophosphamide. The latter is a hemiaminal, which will spontaneously ring open and establish an equilibrium with the amino aldehyde, aldophosphamide.

4-Hydroxycyclophosphamide and aldophosphamide may be oxidized by soluble enzymes to produce 4-ketocyclophosphamide and carboxyphosphamide, respectively. These compounds have little cytotoxic activity and represent inactivated urinary excretion products, accounting between them for about 80 per cent of a dose of administered cyclophosphamide.[146, 147]

The aldophosphamide that has escaped enzymatic oxidation can spontaneously eliminate acrolein to produce phosphoramide mustard,[148] an active alkylating agent that appears to be responsible for the biologic effects of cyclophosphamide.[149, 150] 4-Hydroxycyclophosphamide/aldophosphamide is cytotoxic both *in vitro* and *in vivo*, but is not an alkylating agent. This compound appears to serve as a transport form to efficiently deliver the high polar phosphoramide mustard into cells, since 4-hydroxycyclophosphamide is cytotoxic at one fourth to one tenth the levels of phosphoramide mustard required for activity.[151] Furthermore, the amount of DNA crosslinking produced by the two compounds corresponds to their relative cytotoxic effects, and cytotoxicity from the two compounds occurs at similar degrees and types of DNA crosslinking.[152] The high therapeutic index and other unique properties of cyclophosphamide are most likely attributable to the properties of 4-hydroxycyclophosphamide, but circulating phosphoramide mustard may play a significant role in the effects of the drug.[145]

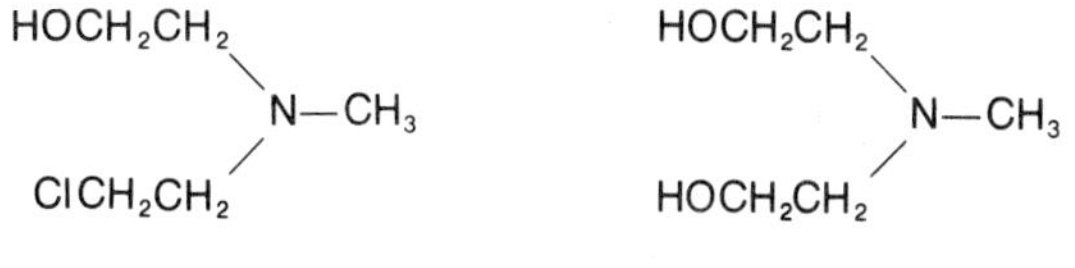

$HOCH_2CH_2(ClCH_2CH_2)N{-}CH_3$

A

$(HOCH_2CH_2)_2N{-}CH_3$

B

Figure 13–17. Hydrolysis products of mechlorethamine.

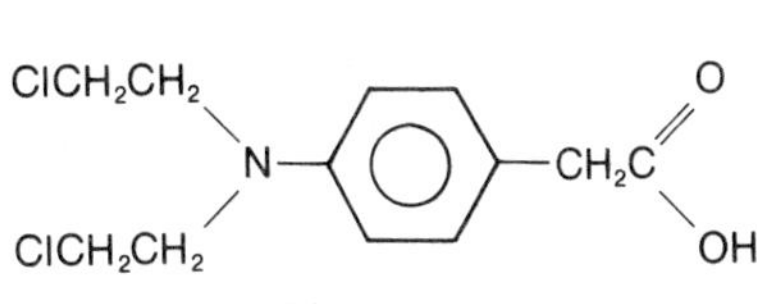

$(ClCH_2CH_2)_2N{-}C_6H_4{-}CH_2C(=O)OH$

Figure 13–18. Phenylacetic acid mustard.

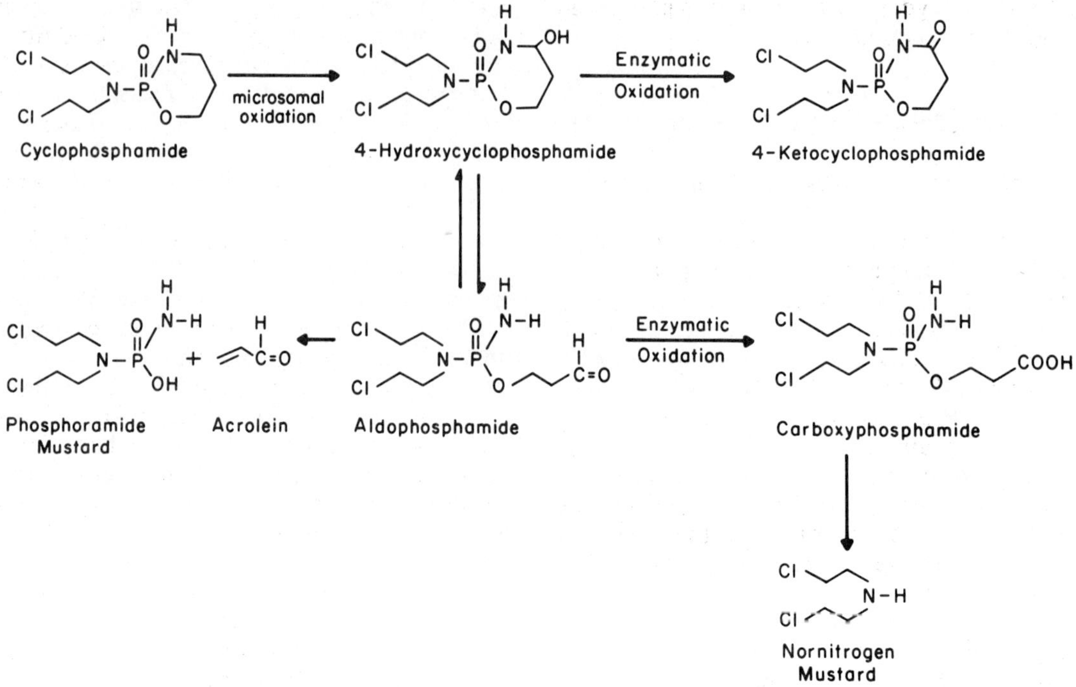

Figure 13–19. Metabolism of cyclophosphamide.

Nitrosoureas

The base catalyzed decomposition of nitrosoureas to generate the alkylating chloroethyldiazonium hydroxide entity[54] has been mentioned above, and the products generated by this decomposition in aqueous solution are illustrated in Figure 13–20. The nitrosoureas also undergo metabolic transformation. Hill et al.[153] demonstrated that BCNU is enzymatically denitrosated by hepatic microsomes. Data from Levin and colleagues[154] indicate that this metabolism may have clinical significance. These investigators found that enhancement of microsomal activity *in vivo* by phenobarbital abolished the therapeutic effect of BCNU against the 9L intracerebral rat tumor and decreased the

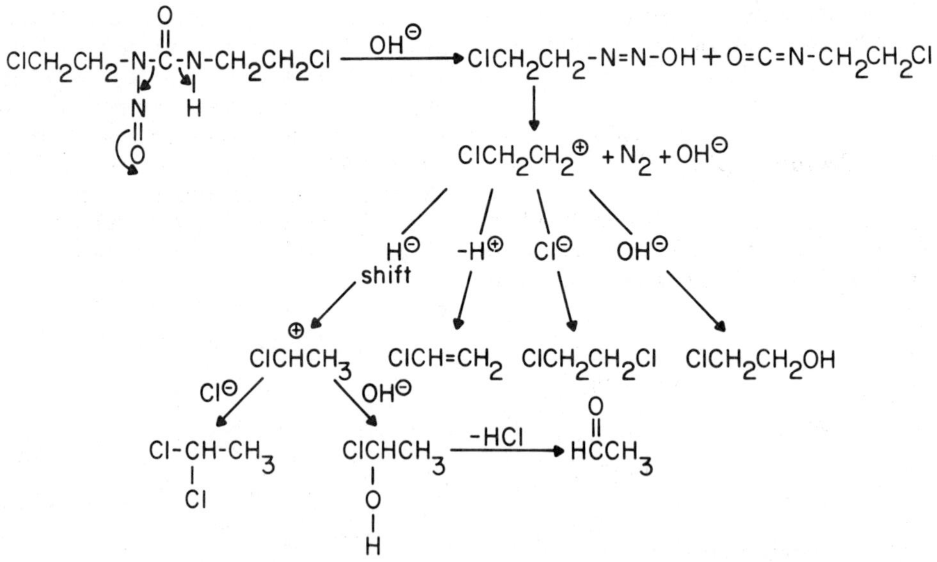

Figure 13–20. Decomposition of BCNU in buffered aqueous solution.

therapeutic activity of CCNU and BCNU against this tumor. The phenobarbital-treated rats were shown to have increased plasma clearance of BCNU, with lower plasma levels and lower area under the plasma curve values of BCNU. May et al.[155] and Hilton and Walker[156] showed that CCNU and methyl CCNU undergo hydroxylation of the cyclohexyl ring of the molecules to produce a series of hydroxylated metabolites that represent the major circulating species after treatment with these drugs. The antitumor properties of these metabolites are similar to those of the parent compounds.[157]

CLINICAL PHARMACOLOGY

Because of the lack of definitive techniques for measuring specific drug and metabolite molecules, the data on the clinical pharmacology of the alkylating agents have been relatively limited. Recently, however, techniques such as gas chromatography–mass spectrometry and high-pressure liquid chromatography (HPLC) have been applied to the study of several of the alkylating agents, and more definitive clinical pharmacologic data have been generated (Table 13–1).

Melphalan

The clinical pharmacology of melphalan has been examined by several groups. Alberts and colleagues studied the pharmacokinetics of melphalan in patients who received 0.6 mg/kg of the drug intravenously.[158] The peak levels of melphalan, as measured by HPLC, were found to be 4.5 to 13 nanomoles/ml (1.4 to 4.1 μg/ml) and the mean half-life ($t\frac{1}{2}\beta$) of the drug in the plasma was 1.8 hours. The 24-hour urinary excretion of the parent drug averaged 13 per cent of the administered dose.

Studies by Tattersall and Weinberg[159] and Alberts et al.[137] have shown that there is low and variable systemic availability of the drug after oral dosing. After oral administration of 0.6 mg/kg of melphalan, much lower peak levels of drug of about 1 nanomole/ml (0.3 μg/ml) were seen. The time to achieve peak plasma levels varied considerably in these patients and occurred as late as six hours after dosing.

In the report of Tattersall and Weinberg,[159] measurement of fecal excretion indicated that the low availability was due to incomplete absorption of the drug from the gastrointestinal tract, since 20 to 50 per cent of an oral dose could be recovered in the feces. No drug or drug products were found in the feces after intravenous administration.

Pallante and colleagues studied the plasma concentration of melphalan after the administration of more conventional oral doses of 0.15 to 0.25 mg/kg.[160] Peak plasma levels of 0.16 to 0.625 nanomole/ml (50 to 190 ng/ml) were found and occurred 0.7 to 2.3 hours after drug administration (Fig. 13–21). The same plasma levels were found after the initial dose of drug or after the second dose in a five-day schedule, indicating that no accumulation of plasma levels of the drug occurs with daily administration. In this

TABLE 13–1. Pharmacokinetics of Selected Alkylating Agents and Their Metabolites

Classical Alkylating Agents	*Dose (mg/kg)*	*Route*	*Peak Plasma Concentration (μM)*	*Plasma t½ (hrs)*	*Ref.*
Cyclophosphamide	60	IV	500	3–10	181
Aldophosphamide	10–20	IV	1.4–2.6	—	186, 187
Phosphoramide mustard	4–12	IV	3–18	8.68	184
	60–75	IV	50–100		
Nornitrogen mustard	4–9	IV	4–15	3.3	181
	60–75	IV	200–500		
Chlorambucil	0.6	PO	2.63	1.5	152
Phenylacetic acid mustard	0.6	PO	1.8–4.3	2.4	153
Melphalan	0.15–0.25	PO	0.16–0.63	—	178
	0.6	IV	4.5–13	1.8	176
Nitrosoureas					
BCNU	1.5–4.25	IV	5	1.13	201

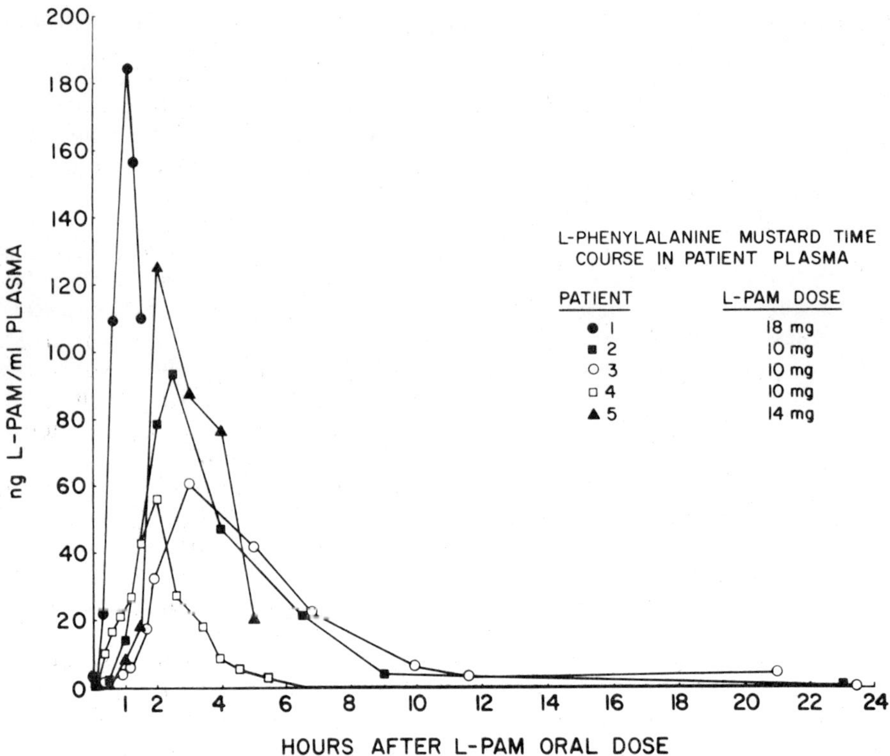

Figure 13–21. Plasma levels of melphalan after oral administration of 0.15 to 0.25 mg/kg.

study the magnitude and time of peak plasma levels appear to be more consistent than was seen with the higher doses reported by Alberts and co-workers.

Chlorambucil

Alberts et al. have also examined the pharmacokinetics of chlorambucil after the oral administration of 0.6 mg/kg.[137, 138] Peak levels of 2.0 to 6.3 nanomoles/ml (0.6 to 1.9 μg/ml) were found and occurred within one hour of administration of the drug. Peak plasma levels of phenylacetic acid mustard ranged from 1.8 to 4.3 nanomoles/ml (0.5 to 1.18 μg/ml), and the peak levels of this metabolite were achieved two to four hours after dosing. The terminal phase half-lives ($t\frac{1}{2}\beta$) of chlorambucil and phenylacetic acid mustard were 92 and 145 minutes, respectively. Less than 1 per cent of the administered dose of chlorambucil was excreted in the urine as either chlorambucil (0.54 per cent) or as phenylacetic acid mustard (0.25 per cent). Approximately 50 per cent of the radioactivity from ^{14}C-labeled chlorambucil administered orally was excreted in the urine in 24 hours. Of this material, over 90 per cent appeared to be the monohydroxy and dihydroxy hydrolysis products of chlorambucil and phenylacetic acid mustard. Thus, orally administered chlorambucil is absorbed more completely and more rapidly than melphalan and has a similar terminal phase half-life. Chlorambucil has an alkylating metabolite, phenylacetic acid mustard, whose peak levels approach those of the parent compound. Because of the longer half-life of the metabolite, the area under the curve or total exposure of tissue to the metabolite may be greater than that of chlorambucil. The potential role of phenylacetic acid mustard in the activities of chlorambucil is uncertain.

Cyclophosphamide

The study of the clinical pharmacology of cyclophosphamide has been complicated by the inactivity of the parent compound and by the complex array of metabolites. These metabolites have proved difficult to isolate and measure, and their properties are not yet completely established. The pharmacokinetics of the parent compound have been well established by a number of studies. After intravenous administration the peak plasma levels of the parent compound are dose-dependent, with peak levels of 4, 50, and 500 nanomoles/ml reported after the administration of 1 to 2,[161] 6 to 15,[162] and 60 mg/kg,[163] respectively. The terminal phase half-life of cyclophosphamide varies considerably between patients, with a range from three to ten hours reported by a number of authors.

Cyclophosphamide appears to be reasonably well absorbed after oral administration to man. D'Incalci et al.[161] found the systemic availability of the unchanged drug after oral administration of 100-mg doses (1 to 2 mg/kg) to be 97 per cent of that after intravenous injection of the same dose. Juma and colleagues[162] found the systemic availability of the drug to be somewhat less and more variable (mean = 74 per cent, range = 34 to 90 per cent) after oral administration of larger doses of 300 mg (3 to 6 mg/kg). A careful comparison of oral versus intravenous cyclophosphamide has not been carried out, but a great deal of clinical experience has indicated that doses of oral cyclophosphamide as high as 40 mg/kg produce the therapeutic effect and toxicities that would be expected from the same intravenous dose.

The pharmacokinetics of the metabolites are less well established. Until recently, methods for the quantitation of specific metabolites were not available, and the metabolites were quantitated as noncyclophosphamide radioactivity or as alkylating activity as measured by the nitrobenzyl pyridine technique. Measurements of plasma alkylating activity show considerable variation between patients, but similar ranges of alkylating activity of the equivalent of 10 to 80 nanomoles/ml of nitrogen mustard after doses of 40 to 60 mg/kg of cyclophosphamide have been found by several investigators.[162, 164, 165] Peak alkylating levels are achieved two to three hours after drug administration, and Juma found the t½ β of plasma alkylating activity to be 7.7 hours. All investigators have noted a plateau-like level of plasma alkylating activity maintained for at least six hours.

In 1978 Jardine et al.,[163] using gas chromatography–mass spectrometry, and Juma et al.,[166] using gas chromatography, measured the plasma concentrations of the metabolites phosphoramide mustard and nornitrogen mustard in patients who had received cyclophosphamide (Fig. 13–22). After doses of cyclophosphamide of 60 and 75 mg/kg, peak plasma levels of phosphoramide mustard of 50 to 100 nanomoles/ml occurred two to

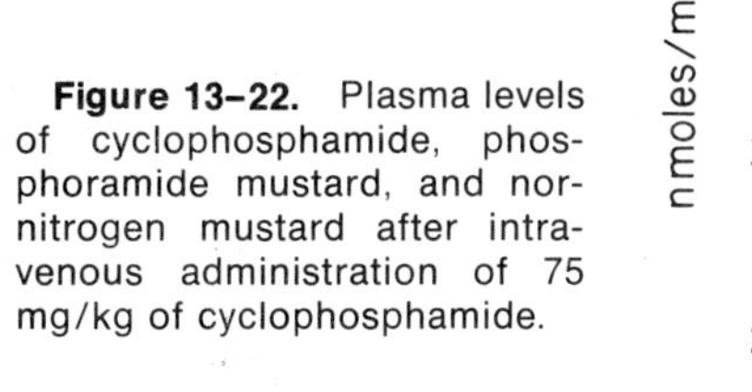

Figure 13–22. Plasma levels of cyclophosphamide, phosphoramide mustard, and nornitrogen mustard after intravenous administration of 75 mg/kg of cyclophosphamide.

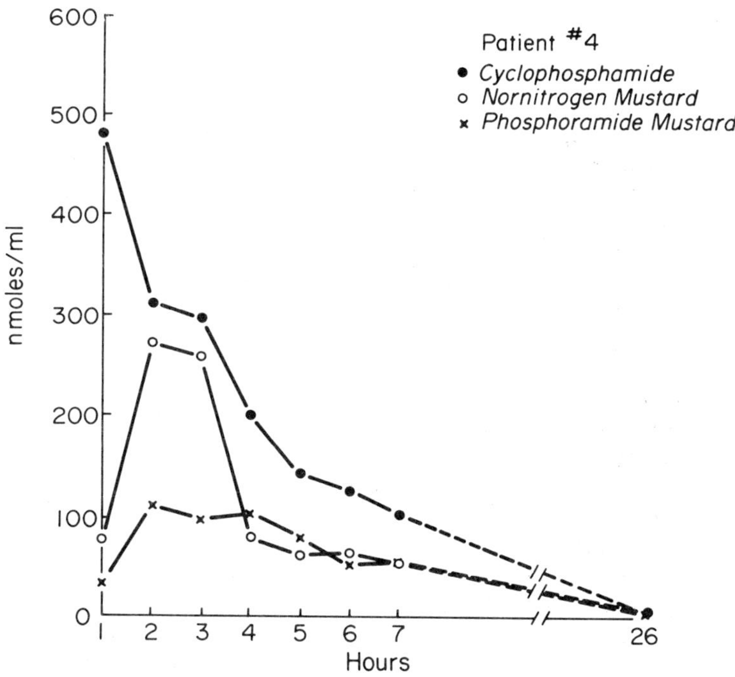

three hours after the beginning of a one-hour infusion. Sustained levels of phosphoramide mustard were seen for six to seven hours from the beginning of the infusion. Approximately 2 per cent of the administered dose of cyclophosphamide was excreted in the urine as phosphoramide mustard within 24 hours. After rapid injection of doses of cyclophosphamide of 4 to 12 mg/kg, peak levels of phosphoramide mustard of 3 to 18 nanomoles/ml were seen 0.25 to two hours (mean 0.9 hours) after injection.[166] In these patients the mean $t\frac{1}{2}\ \beta$ for phosphoramide mustard was 8.68 hours, and the area under the plasma concentration versus the time curve (AUC) for phosphoramide mustard was 40 to 100 nanomoles/ml × hours.

Both of these studies also measured nornitrogen mustard levels in the patients described. In patients receiving the infusions of 60 and 75 mg/kg of cyclophosphamide, peak plasma levels of nornitrogen mustard of 200 to 500 nanomoles/ml occurred two to three hours after the start of the infusion, but fell rapidly over the next three hours.[163] Between 10 and 15 per cent of the administered dose of cyclophosphamide was excreted in the urine within 24 hours as nornitrogen mustard. In patients who received the injections of 4 to 9 mg/kg of cyclophosphamide, Juma et al.[166] found peak levels of 4 to 15 nanomoles/ml of nornitrogen mustard 0.25 to two hours (mean 0.7 hours) after the drug injection. The mean $t\frac{1}{2}\ \beta$ for nornitrogen mustard was 3.31 hours, and the AUC varied from 11 to 28 nanomoles/ml × hours. Jardine et al.[163] found that carboxyphosphamide degraded to nornitrogen mustard in plasma, and suggested that the high levels of nornitrogen mustard found might be due at least in part to decomposition of carboxyphosphamide during storage and work-up of the sample.

Fenselau et al. identified aldophosphamide as the cyanohydrin derivative in the plasma of patients receiving cyclophosphamide,[167] and Wagner et al. identified a mercaptan derivative of 4-hydroxycyclophosphamide in the plasma of cyclophosphamide-treated patients.[168] Since the two primary metabolites are in equilibrium, the formation of either derivative should allow the measurement of the total of the two metabolites. Wagner et al. have recently used the mercaptan derivatization technique to estimate that peak plasma levels of 1.4 and 2.6 nanomoles/ml of 4-hydroxycyclophosphamide and aldophosphamide are achieved in man after injection of doses of 10 and 20 mg/kg of radiolabeled cyclophosphamide, respectively.[169] The AUC for 4-hydroxycyclophosphamide and aldophosphamide at these doses of drug ranged from 3 to 19 nanomoles/ml × hours.

The relative role of each of the known active metabolites, 4-hydroxycyclophosphamide/aldophosphamide, phosphoramide mustard, and nornitrogen mustard, in the therapeutic and toxic effects of the parent compound remains unclear. In our experience, greater than 100 nanomoles/ml concentrations (for 30 minutes, or greater than 50 nanomoles/ml × hours' exposure) of phosphoramide mustard and nornitrogen mustard are required *in vitro* to achieve a significant cytotoxic effect on murine L1210 leukemia cells. 4-Hydroxycyclophosphamide demonstrates significant cytotoxicity at levels of 10 to 30 nanomoles/ml (5 to 15 nanomoles/ml × hours' exposure). Also, the work of Sensenbrenner and colleagues indicates that phosphoramide mustard is considerably less immunosuppressive than cyclophosphamide, both on a molar basis and relative to the degree of hematopoietic suppression produced.[170] Furthermore, *in vivo,* phosphoramide mustard and nornitrogen mustard do not exhibit the characteristically high therapeutic index of cyclophosphamide, whereas 4-hydroxycyclophosphamide does.[171] Thus, the clinical pharmacologic data so far available suggest that the major antitumor and immunosuppressive effects of cyclophosphamide are mediated by 4-hydroxycyclophosphamide. However, even at the relatively low doses of cyclophosphamide studied by Juma et al.,[166] the total exposure of cells to phosphoramide mustard and to nornitrogen mustard should be sufficient to produce cytotoxicity. Thus, these compounds may well contribute to the antitumor effect of cyclophosphamide, and almost certainly play a role in the toxic effects of the drug.

Since the initial metabolism of cyclophosphamide is by the hepatic microsomal enzymes, it might be expected that modulation of the activity of these enzymes *in vivo* should alter the pharmacokinetics of the drug. Pretreatment with phenobarbital reduces the plasma half-life of the parent compound in both man and experimental animals.[172, 173] Also, with repeated doses of cyclophosphamide, the plasma half-life can be shown to become progressively shorter,[161] indicating that cyclophosphamide can induce the microsomal enzymes responsible for its metabolism. It is likely that the wide variation in the plasma half-life of cyclophosphamide seen in patients is due to differing previous drug exposure and the consequent differences in the hepatic microsomal activity. For example, Egorin et al.[174] found consistently short plasma half-lives of cyclophosphamide (less than two hours) in a group of brain tumor patients with chronic phenobarbital exposure.

In the mouse, phenobarbital pretreatment has been shown by Alberts and van Daalen Wetters to decrease the area under the plasma concentration curve for alkylating metabolites.[175] This alteration was associated with a decrease in toxicity of the cyclophosphamide dose. Sladek, however, was unable to find any effect of phenobarbital on the toxicity or therapeutic effect of cyclophosphamide in tumor-bearing rats.[176] Since the rate of cyclophosphamide metabolism in man is closer to the rate in the rat than to that in the mouse, the toxicity and therapeutic index of cyclophosphamide in man probably are not significantly altered by modulations of the rate of metabolism.

Two authors have reported increased and prolonged plasma levels of cyclophosphamide metabolites in patients with renal failure,[165, 177] and on this basis a reduction in dose has been recommended for such patients. However, it has not been established that these elevated metabolite levels are associated with increased toxicity; full doses of cyclophosphamide given to patients with severe renal impairment do not result in an increase in the hematologic or other toxicities.[178]

Isophosphamide

The clinical pharmacology of isophosphamide has been studied by Creaven and Allen.[179-181] After single doses of 3.8 to 5.0 gm/m^2, the t½ β of isophosphamide was found to be 15 hours, considerably longer than the previously cited values of three to ten hours of cyclophosphamide. However, at isophosphamide doses of 1.6 to 2.4 gm/m^2, the half-life of the drug was found to be similar to that of cyclophosphamide. Creaven et al.[179] found similar values for alkylating activity in plasma after administration of 3.8 gm/m^2 of isophosphamide or 1.1 gm/m^2 of cyclophosphamide. Also, the alkylating activity excreted in the urine was similar for these doses of the two analogues. These findings are consistent with the previous results of Allen and Creaven,[182] which indicate that microsomal activation of isophosphamide to alkylating metabolites proceeds more slowly than the activation of cyclophosphamide, in that the higher doses of isophosphamide appear to saturate the activation mechanism.

Norpoth[183] has reported that cleavage of the chloroethyl group from the side chain and ring nitrogens is a quantitatively more significant pathway for isophosphamide metabolism than for cyclophosphamide metabolism in man. Whereas less than 10 per cent of an administered dose of cyclophosphamide is dechlorethylated,[147] as much as 50 per cent of a dose of isophosphamide may be excreted in the urine as dechlorethylated products. These findings suggest that the less rapid oxidative activation at C-4 of isophosphamide allows the chloroethyl group cleavage to become a significantly competing pathway in the *in vivo* metabolism of the drug. While oxidation at C-4 of both cyclophosphamide and isophosphamide leads to ring opening and to compounds with alkylating activity, the products of side-chain cleavage have little alkylating activity. Thus, it appears that, at doses below 3.8 gm/m^2, the rates of metabolism and cyclophosphamide and isophosphamide are similar, but a lower proportion of the isophosphamide is converted into alkylating and biologically active metabolites.

Nitrosoureas

In the initial studies of the clinical pharmacology of BCNU, the unchanged compound could not be detected in plasma, even as early as five minutes after drug administration.[184] However, Levin et al. studied the pharmacokinetics of BCNU in man, using a sensitive and specific mass spectrometric assay.[185] After short-term infusion (15 to 75 minutes) of 60 to 170 mg/m^2, initial peak levels of up to 5 nanomoles/ml of BCNU were achieved. As shown in Figure 13–23, the plasma concentration curves were biexponential, with a distribution phase half-life of six minutes and second phase half-life of 68 minutes. Since the half-life for degrada-

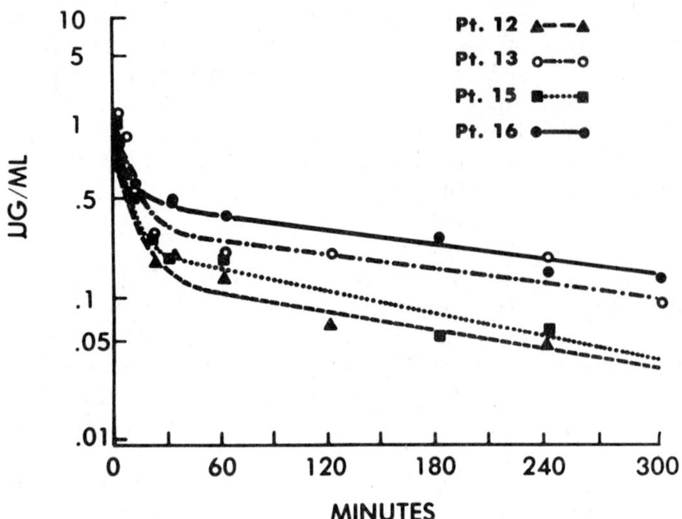

Figure 13-23. Plasma disappearance curves for BCNU in patients receiving 60 mg/m² (patient 16), 70 mg/m² (patients 12, 15), and 80 mg/m² (patient 13). BCNU administered over 30 to 45 minutes. (Reproduced with permission from Levin VA, Hoffman W, and Weinkam RJ: Pharmacokinetics of BCNU in man: a preliminary study of 20 patients. Cancer Treat. Rep. 62: 1305, 1978.)

tion of BCNU in plasma *in vitro* is approximately 15 minutes, the relatively long plasma half-life *in vivo* probably reflects return of BCNU to the plasma from a peripheral compartment.

TOXICITIES

Hematopoietic Suppression

The usual dose-limiting toxicity of the alkylating agents is suppression of hematopoiesis. Characteristically, this suppression includes all the formed elements of the blood — leukocytes, platelets, and red cells. However, the degree, time course, and cellular pattern of the hematopoietic suppression produced by the various alkylating agents differ. Figure 13–24*A* shows the pattern and time course of the decrease in circulating leukocytes and platelets after the administration of 0.4 mg/kg of mechlorethamine over four days.[186] In contrast to this pattern is that which occurs after 60 mg/kg of cyclophosphamide, also given over four days (Fig. 13–24*B*).[187] Although the depth of the leukocyte nadir is similar to that produced by nitrogen mustard, the return of the leukocyte count to normal is more rapid and the platelet count is not depressed to clinically hazardous levels. Clinically significant depression of the platelets may be seen when the dose of the drug exceeds 30 mg/kg, but a relative platelet sparing is very characteristic of cyclophosphamide. If platelet depression in the absence of significant leukocyte depression is seen in a patient treated with cyclophosphamide, another cause of the thrombocytopenia should be sought.

Even at the very high (200 mg/kg or greater) doses of cyclophosphamide used in preparation for bone marrow transplantation, some recovery of endogenous hematopoietic elements occurs within 21 to 28 days. This "stem cell–sparing" property of cyclophosphamide is further reflected in that cumulative damage to the bone marrow is rarely (if ever) seen with cyclophosphamide as a single agent, and repeated high doses of the drug can be given without progressive lowering of leukocyte and platelet counts. In contrast to cyclophosphamide, busulfan (Myleran) appears to be especially damaging to bone marrow stem cells,[47, 188] and prolonged hypoplasia of the bone marrow may be seen after busulfan administration. Phenylalanine mustard appears to be more damaging to hematopoietic stem cells than cyclophosphamide, in that a longer recovery period of hematopoietic cells is seen both in animals[189] and in man, and a cumulative bone marrow depression may be seen with repeated doses of melphalan.

The hematopoietic depression produced by the nitrosoureas is characteristically delayed. The onset of leukocyte and platelet depression occurs three to four weeks after drug administration and may last an additional two to three weeks.[190] Thrombocytopenia appears earlier and usually is more severe than leukopenia. Even if the nitrosourea is given at six-week intervals, hematopoietic recovery may not occur between courses and the drug dose often must be decreased when repeated courses are used.

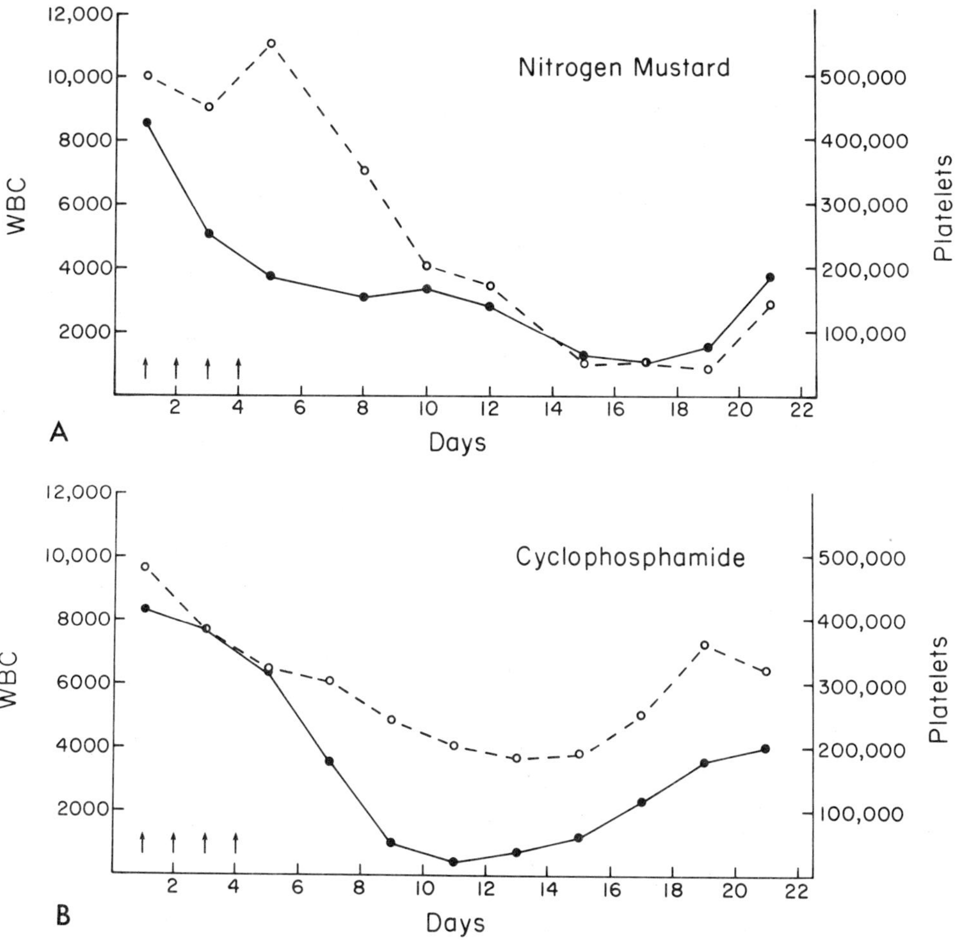

Figure 13–24. Leukopenia and thrombocytopenia after 0.1 mg/kg/day of mechlorethamine for four days (*A*) or 60 mg/kg/day of cyclophosphamide for four days (*B*). (•—• WBC; ∘ - - - ∘ platelets). (Modified and reproduced with permission from Nissen-Meyer R, and Host H: A comparison between the hematologic side effects of cyclophosphamide and nitrogen mustard. Cancer Chemother. Rep. 9:51, 1960.)

The differences in the time course and patterns of hematopoietic depression produced by the various alkylating agents are remarkable and indicate that these agents have selectivities for different hematopoietic precursors. Thus, cyclophosphamide appears to spare hematopoietic stem cells, busulfan is especially damaging to these stem cells, and the nitrosoureas appear to damage a hematopoietic precursor whose differentiation or maturation period is three to four weeks. The mechanistic and biochemical bases for these differences are not known.

Nausea and Vomiting

Although nausea and vomiting are not usually life-threatening toxicities, they are a frequent side effect of alkylating agent therapy and are poorly controlled by conventional antiemetics. These toxicities are a major source of patient discomfort, and a significant cause of lack of drug compliance and even discontinuation of therapy.[191] Some evidence has been presented that the nausea and vomiting produced by alkylating agents are centrally mediated and are not due to direct gastrointestinal toxicity.[192] The frequency and degree of this toxicity are highly variable among patients: some tolerate high doses of alkylating agents without nausea and vomiting, whereas others are severely incapacitated by low doses of these drugs. However, the overall frequency of nausea and vomiting increases as the dose of alkylating agent is increased. The time of onset of these side effects is also variable.

Some patients may experience nausea within a few minutes of administration of the drug, but in others the onset of this symptom is often delayed for several hours. In particular, the nausea and vomiting seen after cyclophosphamide is usually delayed and may occur as late as eight hours after drug administration. For this reason, it is important to see that the patient receives sustained antiemetic coverage.

Gonadal Atrophy

Alkylating agents have profound toxic effects on reproductive tissue, which are considered in greater detail in Chapter 6 and are briefly summarized in this chapter.

A depletion of testicular germ cells, but preservation of Sertoli cells, was described by Spitz[193] in the first extensive review of the histologic effects of mechlorethamine in patients. This toxic effect and its functional counterpart of aspermia have subsequently been well documented, both in animals[194] and man.[195, 196] Miller[196] found aspermia in nine of nine men under treatment for lymphoma with chlorambucil and two of two patients being treated with cyclophosphamide. Testicular biopsies in these patients demonstrated the germinal aplasia with preservation of Sertoli cells described by Spitz.[193] Fairley et al.[197] and Kumar et al.[198] made similar observations in men treated with cyclophosphamide. Sherins and DeVita studied reproductive capacity in men following treatment for lymphoma with drug combinations including either mechlorethamine or cyclophosphamide.[199] A very high incidence of aspermia (10/16) or oligospermia (2/16) was found in these patients, up to three years after cessation of therapy. In the patients with total absence of germ cells, an increase in plasma levels of follicle-stimulating hormone was found. However, four men, in remission and off therapy for from two to seven years, showed complete spermatogenesis, indicating that the testicular damage by alkylating agents is reversible. One of Sherins and DeVita's patients and at least two other men[200, 201] have fathered children after cyclophosphamide therapy.

Amenorrhea as a complication of busulfan therapy was reported by Galton et al.[202] Several reports subsequently documented the high incidence of amenorrhea and ovarian atrophy associated with cyclophosphamide therapy.[198, 199, 203, 204] The most extensive study, reported by Kyoma et al.,[205] was of 18 premenopausal women treated with prolonged daily cyclophosphamide after radical breast surgery. Seventeen of the patients (94 per cent) developed amenorrhea, and menstruation returned in only two of these. In this study and others,[199] amenorrhea developed after lower doses in older patients than in younger patients, and was less likely to be reversible in the older patients. A high incidence of amenorrhea after melphalan therapy has been established by Rose and Davis[206] and Fisher et al.[207] Pathologic examination of the ovaries after alkylating agent–induced amenorrhea reveals the absence of mature or primordial follicles. Endocrinologic studies demonstrate the decreased estrogen and progesterone levels and elevated serum FSH and LH typical of menopause.

Interstitial Pneumonitis and Pulmonary Fibrosis

Pulmonary fibrosis as a complication of long-term busulfan therapy was described initially by Ohner et al.[208] The characteristic clinical presentation of this syndrome is the gradual onset of a nonproductive cough and dyspnea, followed by tachypnea and cyanosis, progressing to severe pulmonary insufficiency and death.[209, 210] The chest roentgenogram shows a diffuse intra-alveolar or interstitial process, or a combination of these changes. The histologic changes include atypia of the alveolar and bronchiolar epithelia, hyperplasia of Type II pneumocytes, and interstitial and intra-alveolar edema and fibrosis.[211] The pulmonary diffusion capacity may be depressed before the onset of clinical symptoms.[212] If busulfan is stopped before the onset of clinical symptoms, the pulmonary function may stabilize, but if clinical symptoms are manifest the condition usually is rapidly fatal.[210]

A similar type of pulmonary damage has been described in occasional patients after treatment with cyclophosphamide[213-215] and after BCNU and methyl-CCNU in cumulative doses exceeding 1000 mg/m^2.[216-220] In addition, BCNU given in high single doses of 900 to 1500 mg/m^2, in association with autologous bone marrow transplantation, has been reported to cause the onset of pulmonary infiltrates, hyaline membrane formation, and fibrosis within three weeks of treatment in three of 14 patients.[220A] Respiratory failure supervened in two of these three patients, both of whom had received previous chest irradiation. Reports have also appeared of pulmonary fibrosis after melphalan,[221] chlorambucil,[222, 223] and mitomycin C.[224] Although the precise mechanism of the pulmonary toxicity is not known, this effect presumably is due to direct cytotoxicity of the alkylating agents to pulmonary epithelium, resulting in alveolitis and fibrosis.[210] The finding of a similar pulmonary toxicity as a major limitation of bleomycin therapy,[210] and reports of interstitial pulmonary damage after 6-mercaptopurine[225, 226] and azathioprine,[227] have demonstrated that such effects are not limited to the alkylating agents.

Renal and Bladder Toxicity

A toxicity that appears to be unique to cyclophosphamide and its analogues is that of hemorrhagic cystitis, which may range from a mild cystitis to severe bladder damage with massive hemorrhage.[228, 230] This toxicity is due to the excretion of toxic metabolites in the urine, with subsequent direct irritation of the bladder mucosa.[228, 231] Acrolein may be responsible for cyclophosphamide-induced cystitis, since in rats this complication is also produced by the cyclophosphamide analogue diethyl cyclophosphamide, which yields acrolein as its only alkylating metabolite.[232] The incidence and severity of the complication can be lessened by adequate hydration and frequent bladder emptying. In dogs the bladder damage from high doses of cyclophosphamide can be prevented by continuous irrigation of the bladder with a solution containing N-acetylcysteine,[233] and this technique has been used successfully in patients receiving high doses of cyclophosphamide and isophosphamide.[234] Parenteral administration of N-acetylcysteine and other sulfhydryl-containing compounds can be shown to prevent or diminish bladder damage in rodents,[235, 236] and this approach is now being used in man.[237] Experiments in animals indicate that the systemic administration of sulfhydryl compounds does not impair the antitumor or immunosuppressive effect of cyclophosphamide.[235, 236]

The danger of hemorrhagic cystitis increases with the magnitude of an acute dose of cyclophosphamide, and may occur in some patients receiving greater than 50 mg/kg despite adequate hydration. However, in our experience, some of the most severe cases of hemorrhagic cystitis have occurred suddenly in patients receiving daily oral cyclophosphamide who fail to maintain adequate hydration. It is important, therefore, to monitor such patients carefully. We have also seen patients who did not show evidence of bladder damage at the time of cyclophosphamide administration, but who developed bladder hemorrhage several months later on receiving a subsequent course of therapy with other antitumor agents such as cytosine arabinoside or methotrexate. Such patients presumably sustain subclinical bladder damage at the time of cyclophosphamide administration and have persistent abnormalities of the bladder mucosa as described by Forni et al.,[229] the bladder hemorrhage being precipitated by the mucosal irritation of the second drug. Various techniques of cauterization of the bladder have been used for severe hemorrhagic cystitis produced by cyclophosphamide, but we have found that continuous irrigation of the bladder to prevent intravesicular clots and transfusion to replace blood loss have usually been effective. In a few severe cases, vasopressin (Pitressin) administration has appeared to be useful in reducing the hemorrhage. Although the major urologic damage produced by cyclophosphamide is in the bladder, the damage in severe cases may extend up the ureters to the renal pelvices, and urinary epithelial casts may be seen after cyclophosphamide therapy.[238] The analogue isophosphamide produces a similar type of bladder damage, but is more likely than cyclophosphamide to produce renal damage. At high doses of isophosphamide, severe renal tubular damage with elevation of serum urea and creatinine has been seen,[234] and a Fanconi-like syndrome has been described after isophosphamide therapy.[239]

A toxicity of cyclophosphamide that is probably related to a renal tubular effect is that of water retention.[240] This syndrome is usually seen in patients receiving cyclophosphamide doses of 50 mg/kg or greater and is characterized by a marked fall in urinary output six to eight hours after drug administration, significant weight gain, a marked increase in urine osmolality, and a decrease in serum osmolality. In extreme cases, the patients may develop pleural and pericardial effusions. The onset of water retention coincides with the peak excretion of alkylating metabolites in the urine, an observation consistent with the hypothesis that the effect is due to a direct action of the metabolites on the renal tubules. The syndrome is self-limited, and by 12 to 16 hours fluid retention is reversed and excess fluid is excreted. In order to preserve high urinary output and at the same time avoid the possibility of inducing symptomatic hyponatremia, continuous infusion of furosemide is effective in maintaining a diuresis and promoting free water clearance, although K^+ supplementation is required to prevent hypokalemia.[240A] The complication of water retention has been seen most frequently in young children treated with high doses of cyclophosphamide,[241] especially those who have been hydrated with salt-free glucose solutions prior to treatment.

Preclinical toxicologic testing of the nitrosoureas disclosed nephrotoxicity in mice, dogs, and monkeys,[242] but initial clinical trials failed to confirm this complication in man. However, with more prolonged courses of treatment, it is now clear that all three commonly used nitrosoureas can produce a dose-related renal toxicity that can result in renal failure and death.[243-245] Total doses of greater than 1200 mg/m² of BCNU or methyl-CCNU caused renal toxicity in 14 of 17 patients reported by Schacht and Baldwin,[244] and Harmon et al.[245] found that all six children who received greater than 1500 mg/m² of methyl-CCNU either developed overt renal failure or had macroscopic evidence of renal damage (shrunken kidneys) at death. In patients developing clinical evidence of toxicity, increases in serum creatinine usually appear after the completion of therapy and may be first detected up to two years after treatment.

Renal biopsy findings in affected patients resemble those of radiation nephritis[245] and include prominent glomerulosclerosis, basement membrane thickening, and severe tubular loss, with varying amounts of interstitial fibrosis. Proteinurea and urinary sediment abnormalities are not consistently associated with nitrosourea-induced renal damage.

Alopecia

Alopecia was described by Bierman and colleagues in 1958[246] as a frequent complication of dimethyl busulfan therapy. This toxicity has not usually been seen with busulfan, and, of the alkylating agents, has been associated predominantly with cyclophosphamide. Marked alopecia is seen also with vincristine and with doxorubicin (Adriamycin), suggesting that this side effect is related to a penetrability property of a drug, rather than its mechanism of cytotoxicity.

Feil and Lamoureux[247] explored the structure-function requirements for depilation by cyclophosphamide, and found that at least two chloroethyl groups and the intact ring structure are required. Phosphoramide mustard has shown no depilatory effect, either in this study or in clinical trials.[248,249] This finding suggests that entry of the more lipophilic metabolites, 4-hydroxycyclophosphamide or aldophosphamide, into hair follicles is responsible for the depilatory action of cyclophosphamide.

The degree of alopecia following cyclophosphamide administration may be quite severe, especially when this drug is used in combination with vincristine or doxorubicin. Regrowth of the hair inevitably occurs after cessation of therapy, but may be associated with a change in the color and texture of the hair.[250] It has been reported that the use of a tourniquet[251] or ice pack applied to the scalp[252] during, and for a short period following, cyclophosphamide administration can prevent or significantly reduce the subsequent alopecia.

Allergic Reactions

Because of the ability of the alkylating agents to bind readily to biologic molecules, these compounds would be expected to act as haptenes and produce allergic reactions. An increasing number of reports have now appeared[253-257] of skin eruption, angioneurotic edema, urticaria, and anaphylactic reactions after systemic alkylating agent administration. Nitrogen mustard applied topically, as for treatment of mycosis fungoides, causes sensitization to subsequent applications of the same drug in many patients, and can also sensitize patients to other chloroethyl-containing agents administered systemically.[258] Although these complications occur infrequently, the clinician must observe patients carefully for evidence of sensitization and be aware of the possibility of an anaphylactic reaction when administering these drugs. There are as yet insufficient data to determine patterns of cross-reactivity between alkylating agents or to enable the possibility of desensitization to the alkylating agents to be predicted.

Teratogenesis

Nitrogen mustard was found to be teratogenic in the rat by Haskin[259] and Bodenstein and Goldin[260, 261] in 1948. Subsequent reports have demonstrated that virtually all the alkylating agents are teratogenic. These studies have been carried out in a number of systems, both *in vivo* and in embryo culture *in vitro.*[262-265] The teratogenic action appears to be due to direct cytotoxicity to the developing embryo by the same mechanisms operative in tumor cells,[266, 267] and the antimetabolites exhibit similar teratogenic effects.

Because of the demonstrated teratogenicity of the alkylating agents in animals, there has been appropriate concern about the potential effects of their administration to patients during pregnancy. In 1968 Nicholson reviewed the reports in the literature of women treated with cytotoxic agents during pregnancy.[268] In the 25 instances in which the alkylating agents were given during the first trimester of pregnancy and the status of the fetus recorded, there were four fetal malformations. The risk of fetal malformation after aminopterin administration during the first trimester was much higher. There were no reported instances of malformed fetuses when alkylating agents or other cytotoxic drugs were administered during the second or third trimester. This information would indicate that there is a definite risk of a malformed viable infant if alkylating agents are given during the first trimester, but the administration of such drugs during the second and third trimester does not increase the normal risk of fetal malformation. Information published since Nicholson's review is consistent with this conclusion, with reports of malformed children born to mothers who had received chlorambucil,[269] cyclophosphamide,[270] or nitrogen mustard and procarbazine[271] during the first trimester. Reports have continued to appear[272, 273] of normal infants born to mothers receiving alkylating agents during the second or third trimester, and there has been no report of a malformed infant born following such exposure.

Carcinogenesis

Case reports began appearing in the early 1970s of a fulminant acute leukemia developing in patients treated with alkylating agents. The initial reports described this association in patients with multiple myeloma[274, 275] and lymphomas,[276] and the possibility that the development of acute leukemia might be part of the natural history of these diseases had to be considered. However, a number of cases of acute leukemia following alkylating agent therapy have now been reported in patients with other malignancies and in patients treated for nonmalignant diseases. Most of the cases described have been in patients treated with melphalan,[275, 277] cyclophosphamide,[276, 278, 279] chlorambucil,[280, 281] and nitrosoureas.[282] This circumstance probably reflects the fact that these have been the most widely used of the alkylating agents, since the occurrence of acute leukemia has been reported after treatment with most of the known alkylating agents. Also, the preponderance of patients with multiple myeloma, Hodgkin's disease, and carcinoma of the ovary in the reports of leukemogenesis is probably due to the fact that patients with these diseases may have good responses and are often treated with alkylating agents for a number of years. Reimer et al.[283] have predicted that the rate of acute leukemia occurrence in patients with ovarian cancer who survive for ten years after treatment with alkylating agents might be as high as 5 to 10 per cent. Acute leukemia has been the most frequently described second malignancy, but other malignancies have also been reported to develop in patients treated with alkylating agents.[284] A more complete discussion of the carcinogenic effects of the alkylating agents and other types of antitumor drugs is contained in Chapter 6.

Gastrointestinal and Other Organ Toxicity

Bone marrow depression is the usual dose-limiting toxicity of the alkylating agents, and the gastrointestinal epithelial damage and other organ toxicities produced by many of the antimetabolites are not commonly seen. For this reason the alkylating agents have been used in high doses in conjunction with methods to protect or restore bone marrow function.[285, 286] At these high doses, toxicities that are not seen at lower doses become dose-limiting. Melphalan produces severe gut toxicity at high doses,[287] and at BCNU doses of 1200 mg/m^2 severe hepatic and central nervous system damage has been seen.[288, 289] In animals many of the alkylating agents produce convulsions.[290] At the usual clinical doses, convulsions have not been produced, but drowsiness and alterations of consciousness can occasionally be seen[291] and presumably are related to neurotoxicity. Severe eye pain and even blindness have been observed after the intracarotid infusion of BCNU.[292] Thus, with increased doses and direct CNS application of alkylating agents, more clinical evidence of neurotoxicity is likely to be seen.

The dose-limiting toxicity of cyclophosphamide appears to be cardiac toxicity.[293, 294] This toxicity has been reported at doses of over 100 mg/kg during a 48-hour period, and has been noted most often in patients receiving greater than 200 mg/kg preparatory to bone marrow transplantation. There is no evidence for cumulative damage to the heart following repeated moderate or low doses of cyclophosphamide.

Clinically, this toxicity may be characterized by the rapid onset of severe heart failure, which is intractable and fatal within 10 to 14 days. Although the fulminant syndrome is rare, decreased electrocardiographic voltage and a transient increase in heart size is seen in a significant number of high-dose patients. The hearts of patients who die with this toxicity are dilated and show patchy transmural hemorrhage and pericardial effusion. Histopathologic changes include interstitial hemorrhage and edema, myocardial necrosis and vacuolar changes, and characteristic changes in the intramural small coronary vessels.[295]

Immunosuppression

The immunosuppressive activity of alkylating agents was first described by Hektoen and Corper,[296] who reported that sulfur mustard would depress the serum antibody response of rabbits and dogs to heterologous red blood cells. In 1947, Philips et al.[297] reported that tris(β-chloroethyl)amine would delay and suppress the anamnestic antibody response of goats when given between the initial immunization and the antigenic challenge. The same year, Spurr described the immunosuppressive effect of mechlorethamine on rabbits immunized with typhoid vaccine.[298] Following these initial reports, numerous studies have shown the alkylating agents to suppress both humoral and cellular immunity in a variety of experimental systems.

The most immunosuppressive drug of any type, both on a molar basis and relative to other toxicities, is cyclophosphamide.[299, 300] Because of this property, the immunosuppressive effects of this agent have been extensively studied.[299, 301-304] Recently, selective effects of cyclophosphamide on different components of the lymphoid system have been described. *In vivo,* it has been reported to selectively suppress B-lymphocyte function and to deplete B lymphocytes morphologically.[305, 306] However, cyclophosphamide can suppress lymphocyte functions that are mediated by T cells, such as the graft-versus-host response and delayed hypersensitivity.[303, 307] It has also been established that appropriate doses of cyclophosphamide *in vivo,*[308] or of activated cyclophosphamide *in vitro,*[309] can enhance immunologic responses by selective inhibition of the function of suppressor T cells. Several lines of evidence suggest that at least some of the immunosuppressive effects of cyclophosphamide may involve mechanisms other than lethal damage to lymphocytes. Shand[310] has reported that induction of tolerance in B cells by cyclophosphamide *in vivo* or by activated cyclophosphamide *in vitro* occurs at noncytocidal drug concentrations, is reversible, and is associated with the failure of the cyclophosphamide-treated B cell to regenerate a surface immunoglobulin receptor after capping with anti-immunoglobulin serum. Also, Ozer et al.[311] have recently demonstrated that 4-hydroperoxycyclophosphamide, an "activated" analogue of cyclophosphamide, will block the differentiation of suppressor T cell precursors at drug levels that are not cytotoxic and do not produce demonstrable DNA cross-linking in drug-sensitive cell lines.

The clinical significance of the immunosuppression produced by alkylating agents (and other drugs) in the setting of cancer therapy is uncertain. The major concerns are the danger of increased susceptibility to infection in the immunosuppressed host and the potential interference with a host immune response to the tumor. Since it is not certain which immunologic measurements are most appropriate to estimate the risks, the degree and clinical importance of the immunosuppression resulting from antitumor therapy have not been well established. Mullins et al.[312] studied the immune responses of solid tumor patients treated with high-dose cyclophosphamide, 120 mg/kg over a two-day period. Six of the 12 patients studied became transiently anergic (for one to two weeks) to skin test antigens to which they had previously been responsive, but the response to these antigens recovered in all patients by four weeks after the cyclophosphamide therapy. Nine of the 12 showed an adequate antibody response to an antigenic challenge given 24 hours after the cyclophosphamide therapy, despite severe hematopoietic depression. Since most antitumor regimens would not be expected to be as immunosuppressive as the dose of cyclophosphamide used in this study, the results suggest that most intermittent antitumor regimens do not uniformly produce profound immunosuppression, and that recovery of the immune response is usually prompt. However, continuous drug therapy with cytotoxic agents is more likely to lead to severe lymphocyte depletion and profound immunosuppression, and to be associated with an increased frequency of viral, fungal, and protozoal infections.[313]

The immunosuppressive activity of alkylating agents, and of cyclophosphamide in particular, has been used for two types of clinical application. The first use has been for the suppression of the recipient immune response prior to organ transplantation. Since the demonstration by Santos and colleagues[314] that matched sibling bone marrow can be successfully transplanted into recipients who have been pretreated with large doses of cyclophosphamide, this drug has become the major immunosuppressive drug used for bone marrow transplantation. Cyclophosphamide has also been shown to be effective in controlling kidney graft rejection,[315] but has been less widely used for this application than the antimetabolite immunosuppressive agents.

The other use of alkylating agents in patients with nonmalignant disease has been in the therapy of immunologic disorders. Osborne et al., in 1947, reported the successful treatment of a systemic lupus erythematosus patient with nitrogen mustard.[316] Subsequently, the alkylating agents have been tried in a wide variety of diseases thought to be autoimmune in nature, with variable results. Cyclophosphamide has been shown to be an effective agent in the treatment of Wegener's granulomatosis,[317] rheumatoid arthritis,[318, 319] idiopathic thrombocytopenic purpura,[320] and membranous glomerulonephritis.[321, 322] However, because of the severe side effects, including carcinogenesis, the role of alkylating agents in the treatment of nonmalignant disease must be considered carefully.

References

1. Rhoads CP: Nitrogen mustards in treatment of neoplastic disease. J.A.M.A. 131:656, 1946.
2. Jacobson LP, Spurr CL, Barron ESQ, et al.: Studies on the effect of methyl-bis(beta-chloroethyl)amine hydrochloride on neoplastic diseases and allied disorders of the hemapoietic system. J.A.M.A. 132:263, 1946.
3. Goodman LS, Wintrobe MM, Dameshek W, et al: Use of methyl-bis(beta-chloroethyl)amine hydrochloride for Hodgkin's disease, lymphosarcoma, leukemia. J.A.M.A. 132:126, 1946.
4. Adair CPJ, and Bagg, HJ: Experimental and clinical studies on the treatment of cancer by dichloroethylsulphide (mustard gas). Ann. Surg. 93:190, 1931.
5. Ross WLJ: Alkylating agents. *In* Biological Alkylating Agents. Butterworths, London, 1962, pp. 3–18.
6. Colvin M, Brundrett RB, Kan MN, et al.: Alkylating properties of phosphoramide mustard. Cancer Res. 36:1121, 1976.
7. Brundrett RB, Cowens JW, and Colvin M: Chemistry of nitrosoureas. Decomposition of deuterated 1,3-bis(2-chloroethyl)-1-nitrosoureas. J. Med. Chem. 19:958, 1976.
8. Ewig RAG, and Kohn KW: DNA damage and repair in mouse leukemia L1210 cells treated with nitrogen mustard, 1,3-bis(2-chloroethyl)-1-nitrosourea, and other nitrosoureas. Cancer Res. 37:2114, 1977.
9. Sudhaker S, Tew KD, Schein PS, et al.: Nitrosourea interaction with chromatin and effect on poly (adenosine diphosphate ribose) polymerase activity. Cancer Res. 39:1411, 1979.
10. Friedman OM, Myles A, and Colvin M: Cyclophosphamide and certain structurally related phosphoramide mustards. *In* Rosowsky A (ed.): Advances In Cancer Chemotherapy, Vol. 1. Marcel Dekker, New York, 1979, p. 179.
11. Drings P, and Fritsch H: Erfahrungen mit Iphosphamide in hoher Einzeldosis bei metastasierten soliden Tumoren. Verh. Dtsch. Ges. Inn. Med. 78:166, 1972.
12. Costanzi JJ, Gagliano R, Loukas D, et al.: Ifosfamide in the treatment of recurrent or disseminated lung cancer. Cancer 41:1715, 1978.
13. Frick JC, Tretter P, Tretter W, et al.: Disseminated carcinoma of the ovary treated by L-phenylalanine mustard. Cancer 21:508, 1968.
14. Costa G, Engle RL Jr, Schilling A, et al.: Melphalan and prednisone: an effective combination for the treatment of multiple myeloma. Am. J. Med. 54:589, 1973.
15. Fisher B, Sherman B, Rockette H, et al.: L-Phenylalanine mustard (L-PAM) in the management of premenopausal patients with primary breast cancer. Cancer 44:847, 1979.
16. Goldin D, Israels L, Nabarro J, et al.: Clinical trials of p-(di-2-chloroethylamino)-phenylbutyric acid (CB 1348) in malignant lymphoma. Br. J. Med. 2:1172, 1955.
17. Rundles RW, Striggle J, Bell W, et al.: Comparison of

chlorambucil and Myleran in chronic lymphocytic and granulocytic leukemia. Am. J. Med. 27:424, 1959.
18. Zdink E, and Stutzman L: Chlorambucil therapy for lymphomas and chronic lymphocytic leukemia. J.A.M.A. 191:444, 1965.
19. Wiltshaw E: Chlorambucil in the treatment of primary adenocarcinoma of the ovary. J. Obstet. Gynaecol. Br. Commonw. 72:586, 1964.
20. Baterman JC: Chemotherapy of solid tumors with triethylene thiophosphoramide. N. Engl. J. Med. 252:879, 1955.
21. Ultmann JE, Hyman GA, Crandall C, et al.: Methylene thiophosphoramide thio-TEPA in the treatment of neoplastic disease. Cancer 10:902, 1957.
22. Rundles RW, and Barton WB: Triethylene melamine in the treatment of neoplastic disease. Blood 7:483, 1952.
23. Sykes MP, Rundles RW, Pierce VK, et al: Triethylene melamine in the management of far advanced ovarian cancer. Surg. Gynecol. Obstet. 101:133, 1955.
24. Morack G, Nissen E, Pockrandt H, et al.: Ergebnisse einer gezielten zytostatischen Behandlung des Ovarialkarzinoms. Zentralbl. Gynaekol. 100:367, 1978.
25. Perloff M, Hart RD, and Holland JF: Vinblastine, Adriamycin, thio-TEPA, and Halotestin (VATH). Cancer 42:2534, 1978.
26. Greenspan EM: Thio-TEPA and methotrexate chemotherapy of advanced ovarian carcinoma. J. Mount Sinai Hosp. N.Y. 35:52, 1968.
27. Gutin PH, Levi JA, Wiernik PH, et al.: Treatment of malignant meningeal disease with intrathecal thio-TEPA: a Phase II study. Cancer Treat. Rep. 61:885, 1977.
28. Haas CD, Stephens RC, Hollister M, et al: Phase I evaluation of dianhydrogalactitol (NSC-132313). Cancer Treat. Rep. 60:611, 1976.
29. Vogel CL, Winton EF, Moore MR, et al.: Phase I trial of dianhydrogalactitol administered IV in a weekly schedule. Cancer Treat. Rep. 60:895, 1976.
30. Espana P, Wiernik PH, and Walker M: Phase II study of dianhydrogalactitol in malignant glioma. Cancer Treat. Rep. 62:1199, 1978.
31. Chiuten DF, Rosencweig M, Von Hoff DD, et al.: Clinical trials with hexitol derivatives in the U.S. Cancer 47:442, 1981.
32. Thigpen JT, and Lamson MK: Phase II trial of dianhydrogalactitol in advanced soft tissue and bony sarcomas: a Southwest Oncology Group Study. Cancer Treat. Rep. 63:553, 1979.
33. Thigpen JT, Al-Serraf M, and Hewlett JS: Phase II trial of dianhydrogalactitol in metastatic malignant melanoma: a Southwest Oncology Group Study. Cancer Treat. Rep. 63:525, 1979.
34. Edmonson JH, Frytak S, Letendre L, et al.: Phase II evaluation of dianhydrogalactitol in advanced head and neck carcinomas. Cancer Treat. Rep. 63:2081, 1979.
35. Hoogstraten R, O'Bryan R, and Jones S: 1,2:5,6-Dianhydrogalactitol in advanced breast cancer. Cancer Treat. Rep. 62:841, 1978.
36. Elson LA, Jarman M, and Ross WCJ: Toxicity, haematological effects and antitumor activity of epoxides derived from disubstituted hexitols. Mode of action of mannitol, Myleran and dibromomannitol. Eur. J. Cancer 4:617, 1968.
37. Seller C, Ecklardt IP, Kralovanszky J, et al.: Clinical and pharmacologic experience with dibromodulcitol (NSC-104800), a new antitumor agent. Cancer Chemother. Rep. 53:377, 1969.
38. Andrews NL, Weiss AJ, Wilson W, et al.: Phase II study of dibromodulcitol (NSC-104800). Cancer Chemother. Rep. 58:653, 1974.
39. Galton D: Myleran in chronic myeloid Leukaemia. Lancet 264:208, 1953.
40. Haddow A, and Timmis GM: Myleran in chronic myeloid leukaemia — chemical constitution and biological action. Lancet 1:207, 1953.
41. Timmis GM, and Hudson RF: Part I. Chemistry of alkylating agents: discussion. Ann. N.Y. Acad. Sci. 68(3):727, 1958.
42. Roberts JJ, and Warwick GP: Mode of action of alkylating agents: formation of S-ethylcysteine from ethyl methanesulphonate *in vivo*. Nature 179:1181, 1957.
43. Roberts JJ, and Warwick GP: Metabolic and chemical studies of "Myleran": formation of 3-hydroxytetrahydrothiophene-1,1-dioxide *in vivo*, and reactions with thiols *in vitro*. Nature 184:1288, 1959.
44. Brookes P, and Lawley PD: The alkylation of guanosine and guanylic acid. J. Chem. Soc. 3923, 1961.
45. Mitchell MP, and Walker IG: Studies on the cytotoxicity of Myleran and dimethyl Myleran. Can. J. Biochem. 50:1074, 1972.
46. Elson LA: Hematological effects of the alkylating agents. Ann. N.Y. Acad. Sci. 68:826, 1958.
47. Fried W, Kede A, and Barone J: Effects of cyclophosphamide and of busulfan on spleen-colony–forming units and on hematopoietic stroma. Cancer Res. 37:1205, 1977.
48. Skinner WA, Gram HF, Greene MO, et al.: Potential anticancer agents — XXXI. The relationship of chemical structure to antileukemic activity with analogues. J. Med. Pharmaceut. Chem. 2:299, 1960.
49. Hyde KA, Acton E, Skinner WA, et al.: Potential anticancer agents — LXII. The relationship of chemical structure to antileukemia activity with analogues of 1-methyl-3-nitro-1-nitrosoguanidine (NSC-9369). II. J. Med. Pharmaceut. Chem. 5:1, 1962.
50. Schabel FM Jr, Johnston TP, McCaleb GS, et al.: Experimental evaluation of potential anticancer agents. VIII. Effects of certain nitrosoureas on intracerebral L1210 leukemia. Cancer Res. 23:226, 1963.
51. DeVita VT, Carbone PP, Owens AH Jr, et al.: Clinical trials with 1,3-bis(2-chloroethyl)-1-nitrosourea, NSC-409962. Cancer Res. 25:1876, 1965.
52. Schabel FM Jr: Nitrosoureas: A review of experimental antitumor activity. Cancer Treat. Rep. 60:665, 1976.
53. Montgomery J, Ruby J, McCaleb GS, et al.: The modes of decomposition of 1,3-bis(2-chloroethyl)-1-nitrosourea and related compounds. J. Med. Chem. 10:668, 1967.
54. Colvin M, Brundrett RB, Cowens JW, et al.: A chemical basis for the antitumor activity of chloroethylnitrosoureas. Biochem. Pharmacol. 25:695, 1976.
55. Ludlum DB, Kramer BS, Wang J, et al.: Reaction of 1,3-bis(2-chloroethyl)-1-nitrosourea with synthetic polynucleotides. Biochemistry 14:5480, 1975.
56. Kohn KW: Interstrand cross-linking of DNA by 1,3-bis(2-chloroethyl)-1-nitrosourea and other 1-(2-haloethyl)-1-nitrosoureas. Cancer Res. 37:1450, 1977.
57. Baril BB, Baril EF, Lazlo J, et al.: Inhibition of rat liver DNA polymerase by nitrosourea and isocyanates. Cancer Res. 35:1, 1975.
58. Kann HE Jr, Kohn KW, and Lyles JM: Inhibition of DNA repair by the 1,3-bis(2-chloroethyl)-1-nitrosoureas breakdown product, 2-chloroethyl isocyanate. Cancer Res. 34:398, 1974.
59. Kann HE Jr, Kohn KW, Widerlite L, et al.: Effects of 1,3-bis(2-chloroethyl)-1-nitrosourea and related compounds on nuclear RNA metabolism. Cancer Res. 34:1982, 1974.
60. Bowdon BJ, Grimsley J, and Lloyd HH: Interrelationships of some chemical, physicochemical, and biological activities of several 1-(2-haloethyl)-1-nitrosoureas. Cancer Res. 34:194, 1974.
61. Panasci LC, Green D, Nagourney R, et al.: A structure-activity analysis of chemical and biological parameters of chloroethylnitrosoureas in mice. Cancer Res. 37:2615, 1977.
62. Schein PS, Cooney DA, and Vernon ML: The use of nicotinamide to modify the toxicity of streptozotocin diabetes without loss of antitumor activity. Cancer Res. 27:2324, 1967.
63. Schein PS: 1-Methyl-1-nitrosourea and dialkylnitrosamine depression of nicotinamide adenine dinucleotide. Cancer Res. 29:1226, 1969.
64. Rakietan N, Rakietan M, and Nadkarni M: Studies on the diabetogenic action of streptozotocin (NSC-37917). Cancer Chemother. Rep. 29:91, 1963.
65. Broder LE, and Carter SK: Pancreatic islet cell carcinoma. Ann. Intern. Med. 79:108, 1973.
66. Moertel CG, Hanley JA, and Johnson LA: Streptozocin

alone compared with streptozocin plus fluorouracil in the treatment of advanced islet-cell carcinoma. N. Engl. J. Med. 303:1189, 1980.
67. Schein PA, O'Connell MJ, Blom J, et al.: Clinical antitumor activity and toxicity of streptozotocin (NSC-85998). Cancer 34:993, 1974.
68. Anderson T, McMenamim M, and Schein, P.: Chlorozotocin, 2-[3-(2-chloroethyl)-3-nitrosoureido]-D-glucopyranose, an antitumor agent with modified bone marrow toxicity. Cancer Res. 35:761, 1975.
69. Fox, PA, Panasci LC, and Schein PS: Biological and biochemical properties of 1-(2-chloroethyl)-3-(beta-D-glucopyranosyl)-1-nitrosourea (NSC-D-254157), a nitrosourea with reduced bone marrow toxicity. Cancer Res. 37:783, 1977.
70. Gralla RJ, Tan CTC, and Young CW: Phase I trial of chlorozotocin. Cancer Treat. Rep. 63:17, 1979.
71. Bennett JM, Bakemeier RF, Carbone PP, et al.: Clinical trials with BCNU (NSC-409962) in malignant lymphomas by the Eastern Cooperative Oncology Group. Cancer Treat. Rep. 60:739, 1976.
72. Wolt J: Nitrosoureas as single agents in the treatment of pulmonary cancer. Cancer Treat. Rep. 60:753, 1976.
73. Moertel CG, Schutt AJ, Reitemeier RJ, et al.: Therapy for gastrointestinal cancer with the nitrosoureas alone and in drug combination. Cancer Treat. Rep. 60:729, 1976.
74. Salmon SE: Nitrosoureas in multiple myeloma. Cancer Treat. Rep. 60:789, 1976.
75. Levin VA, and Wilson CB: Nitrosourea pharmacodynamics in relation to the central nervous system. Cancer Treat. Rep. 60:725, 1976.
76. Skipper HE, Bennett LL, and Langham WH: Overall tracer studies with C^{14}-labeled nitrogen mustard in normal and leukemic mice. Cancer 4:1025, 1951.
77. Drysdale RB, Hopkins A, Thompson RY, et al.: Some effects of nitrogen and sulphur mustards on the metabolism of nucleic acids in mammalian cells. Br. J. Cancer 12:137, 1958.
78. Wheeler GP: Studies related to the mechanism of action of cytotoxic alkylating agents: a review. Cancer Res. 22:651, 1962.
79. Goldstein NO, and Rutman RJ: The effect of alkylation on the *in vitro* thymidine-incorporating system of Lettré-Ehrlich cells. Cancer Res. 24:1363, 1964.
80. Tomisek AJ, and Simpson BT: Effect of *in vivo* cyclophosphamide treatment on the DNA-primary ability of DNA from Fortner plasmacytoma. Proc. Am. Assoc. Cancer Res. 7:71, 1966.
81. Ruddon RW, and Johnson JM: The effect of nitrogen mustard on DNA template activity in purified DNA and RNA polymerase systems. Mol. Pharmacol. 4:258, 1968.
82. Wheeler GP, and Alexander JA: Effects of nitrogen mustard and cyclophosphamide upon the synthesis of DNA *in vivo* and in cell-free preparation. Cancer Res. 29:98, 1969.
83. Roberts JJ, Brent TP, and Crathorn AR: Evidence for the inactivation and repair of the mammalian DNA template after alkylation by mustard gas and half mustard gas. Eur. J. Cancer 7:515, 1971.
84. Bannon P, and Verly W: Alkylation of phosphates and stability of phosphate triesters in DNA. Eur. J. Biochem. 31:103, 1972.
85. Lawley PD: Reaction of N-methyl-N-nitrosourea (MNUA) with P-labelled DNA: evidence for formation of phosphotriesters. Chem. Biol. Interact. 7:127, 1973.
86. Singer B, and Fraenkel-Courat H: Human pancreatic enzymes: purification and characterization of a nonelastolytic enzyme, protease E, resembling elastase. Biochemistry 14:722, 1975.
87. Verly WG: Monofunctional alkylating agents and apurinic sites in DNA. Biochem. Pharmacol. 23:3, 1974.
88. Loveless A: Possible relevance of O-6 alkylating of deoxyguanosine to the mutagenicity and carcinogenicity of nitrosamines and nitrosamides. Nature 233:206, 1969.
89. Gerchman LL, and Ludlum DB: The properties of O-6-methylguanine in templates for RNA polymerase. Biochim. Biophys. Acta 308:310, 1973.
90. Weinstein IB, Jeffrey AM, Jennette KW, et al.: Benzo[a]pyrene diol epoxides as intermediates in nucleic acid binding *in vitro* and *in vivo*. Science 195:592, 1976.
91. Tong WP, and Ludlum DB: Crosslinking of DNA by busulfan formation of diguanyl derivatives. Biochim. Biophys. Acta 608:174, 1980.
92. Price CC, Gaucher GM, Koneru P, et al.: Relative reactivities for monofunctional nitrogen mustard alkylation of nucleic acid components. Biochim. Biophys. Acta 166:327, 1968.
93. Brookes P, and Lawley PD: The reaction of mono- and di-functional alkylating agents with nucleic acids. Biochem. J. 80:486, 1961.
94. Brookes P, and Lawley PD: The action of alkylating agents on deoxyribonucleic acid in relation to biological effects of the alkylating agents. Exp. Cell. Res. 9(Suppl.):512, 1963.
95. Loveless A, and Ross WCJ: Chromosome alteration and tumour inhibition by nitrogen mustards: the hypothesis of cross-linking alkylation. Nature 166:1113, 1950.
96. Brookes P, and Lawley PD: Evidence for the action of alkylating agents on deoxyribonucleic acid. Exp. Cell. Res. 9(Suppl.):521, 1963.
97. Geiduschek EP: "Reversible" DNA. Proc. Natl. Acad. Sci. USA 47:950, 1961.
98. Kohn KW, Steigbigel NH, and Spears CL: Cross-linking and repair of DNA in sensitive and resistant strains of *E. coli* treated with nitrogen mustard. Proc. Natl. Acad. Sci. USA 53:1154, 1965.
99. Kohn KW, Spears CL, and Doty P: Intra-strand crosslinking of DNA by nitrogen mustard. J. Mol. Biol. 19:266, 1966.
100. Lawley PD, and Brookes P: Cytotoxicity of alkylating agents towards sensitive and resistant strains of *Escherichia coli* in relation to extent and mode of alkylation of cellular macromolecules and repair of alkylation lesions in deoxyribonucleic acid. Biochem. J. 109:433, 1968.
101. Venitt S: Interstrand cross-links in the DNA of *Escherichia coli* B/r and B_{S-1} and their removal by the resistant strain. Biochem. Biophys. Res. Commun. 31:355, 1968.
102. Kohn KW, Erickson LC, Ewig RAG, et al.: Fractionation of DNA from mammalian cells by alkaline elution. Biochemistry 15:4629, 1976.
103. Ross WE, Ewig RAG, and Kohn KW: Differences between melphalan and nitrogen mustard in the formation and removal of DNA cross-links. Cancer Res. 38:1502, 1978.
104. Thomas CB, Osieka R, and Kohn KW: DNA cross-linking by *in vivo* treatment with 1-(2-chloroethyl)-3-(4-methylcyclohexyl)-1-nitrosourea of sensitive and resistant human colon carcinoma xenografts in nude mice. Cancer Res. 38:2448, 1978.
105. Erickson CC, Bradley MO, Ducore JM, et al.: DNA cross-linking and cytotoxicity in normal and transformed human cells treated with antitumor nitrosourea. Proc. Natl. Acad. Sci. USA 77:467, 1980.
106. Ewig RAG, and Kohn KW: DNA-protein crosslinking and DNA interstrand crosslinking by haloethylnitrosourea in L1210 cells. Cancer Res. 38:3197, 1978.
107. Rutman RJ, Steele WJ, and Price CC: Experimental chemotherapy studies. I. Chemical and metabolic investigations of chloroquine mustard. Cancer Res. 21:1124, 1961.
108. Berenbaum MC: Histochemical evidence for crosslinking of DNA by alkylating agents *in vivo*. Biochem. Pharmacol. 11:1035, 1962.
109. Klatt P, Stehlin JS Jr, McBride C, et al.: The effect of nitrogen mustard treatment on the DNA of sensitive and resistant Ehrlich tumor cells. Cancer Res. 29:286, 1969.
110. Verly WG, and Paquette Y: An endonuclease for depurinated DNA in *Escherichia coli* B. Cancer J. Biochem. 50:217, 1972.
111. Hadi SM, and Goldthwait DA: Endonuclease II of *Escherichia coli*. Degradation of partially depurinated DNA. Biochemistry 10:4986, 1971.
112. Burnotte J, and Verly WG: Crosslinking of methylated

DNA by moderate heating at neutral pH. Biochim. Biophys. Acta 262:449, 1972.

113. Tew KD, Sudhakar S, Schein PS, et al.: Binding of chlorozotocin and 1-(2-chloroethyl)-3-cyclohexyl-1-nitrosourea to chromatin and nucleosomal fractions of HeLa cells. Cancer Res. 38:3371, 1978.

114. Tew KD, Smulson ME, and Schein PS: Molecular pharmacology of nitrosoureas. Recent Results Cancer Res. 76:130, 1981.

115. Gralla RJ, Tan CTC, and Young CW: Phase I trial of chlorozotocin. Cancer Treat. Rep. 63:17, 1979.

116. Wolpert MK, and Ruddon RW: A study on the mechanisms of resistance to nitrogen mustard (HN2) in Ehrlich ascites tumor cells: comparison of uptake of HN2-^{14}C into sensitive and resistant cells. Cancer Res. 29:873, 1969.

117. Goldenberg GJ, and Vanstone CL: Transport carrier for nitrogen mustard in HN2-sensitive and -resistant L5178Y lymphoblasts. Clin. Res. 17:665, 1969.

118. Goldenberg GJ, Vanstone CL, and Bihler I: Transport of nitrogen mustard on the transport-carrier for choline in L5178Y lymphoblasts. Science 172:1148, 1971.

119. Goldenberg GJ, Lee M, Lam H-YP, et al.: Evidence for carrier-mediated transport of melphalan by L5178Y lymphoblasts *in vitro*. Cancer Res. 37:755, 1977.

120. Vistica DT, Rabon A, and Rabinowitz M: Effect of L-alpha-amino-gamma-guanidinobutyric acid on melphalan therapy of the L1210 murine leukemia. Cancer Lett. 6(6):345, 1979.

121. Begleiter A, Lam, H-YP, Grover J, et al.: Evidence for active transport of melphalan by two amino acid carriers in L5178Y lymphoblasts *in vitro*. Cancer Res. 39:353, 1979.

122. Vistica DT, Toal JN, and Rabinowitz M: Amino acid conferred protection against melphalan. Characterization of melphalan transport and correlation of uptake with cytotoxicity in cultured L1210 murine leukemia cells. Biochem. Pharmacol. 27:2865, 1978.

123. Vistica DT: Cytotoxicity as an indicator for transport mechanism. Evidence that murine bone marrow progenitor cells lack a high affinity leucine carrier that transports melphalan in murine L1210 leukemia cells. Blood 56:427, 1980.

124. Begleiter A, Lam H-YP, and Goldenberg GJ: Mechanism of uptake of nitrosourea by L5178Y lymphoblasts *in vitro*. Cancer Res. 37:1022, 1977.

125. Goldenberg GJ, Vanstone CL, Israels LG, et al.: Evidence for a transport carrier of nitrogen mustard in nitrogen mustard-sensitive and -resistant L5178Y lymphoblasts. Cancer Res. 30:2285, 1970.

126. Rutman RJ, Chun EHL, and Lewis FA: Permeability differences as a source of resistance to alkylating agents in Ehrlich tumor cells. Biochem. Biophys. Res. Commun. 32:650, 1968.

127. Redwood WR, and Colvin M: Transport of melphalan by sensitive and resistant L1210 cells. Cancer Res. 40:1144, 1980.

128. Hirono I: Non-protein sulphydryl group in the original strain and subline of the ascites tumour resistant to alkylating reagents. Nature 186:1059, 1960.

129. Calcutt G, and Connors TA: Tumour sulphydryl levels and sensitivity to the nitrogen mustard Merophan. Biochem. Pharmacol. 12:839, 1963.

130. Sladek NE: Bioassay and relative cytotoxic potency of cyclophosphamide metabolites generated *in vitro* and *in vivo*. Cancer Res. 33:1150, 1973.

131. Connors TA, Cox PJ, Farmer PB, et al.: Some studies of the active intermediate formed in the microsomal metabolism of cyclophosphamide and isophosphamide. Biochem. Pharmacol. 23:115, 1974.

132. Crathorne AR, and Roberts JJ: Mechanism of the cytotoxic action of alkylating agents in mammalian cells and evidence for the removal of alkylated groups from deoxyribonucleic acid. Nature 211:150, 1966.

133. Goldenberg GJ: The role of drug transport in resistance to nitrogen mustard and other alkylating agents in L5178Y lymphoblasts. Cancer Res. 35:1687, 1975.

134. Schabel FM Jr, Trader MW, Laster WR Jr, et al.: Patterns of resistance and therapeutic synergism among alkylating agents. Antibiot. Chemother. 23:200, 1978.

135. Bartlett PD, Ross SD, and Swain CG: Kinetics and mechanisms of the reactions of tertiary β-chloroethylamines in solution. III. β-Chloroethyldiethylamine and tris-β-chloroethylamine. J. Am. Chem. Soc. 71:1415, 1949.

136. Chang SY, Alberts DS, Farquhar D, et al.: Hydrolysis and protein binding of melphalan. J. Pharm. Sci. 67:682, 1978.

137. Alberts DS, Chang SY, Chen H-SG, et al.: Comparative pharmacokinetics of chlorambucil and melphalan in man. Recent Results Cancer Res. 74:124, 1980.

138. Alberts DS, Chang SY, Chen H-SG, et al.: Pharmacokinetics and metabolism of chlorambucil in man: a preliminary report. Cancer Treat. Rev. 6(Suppl.): 9, 1979.

139. McLean A, Woods RC, Catovsky D, et al.: Pharmacokinetics and metabolism of chlorambucil in patients with malignant disease. Cancer Treat. Rev. 6(Suppl.):33, 1979.

140. Everett JC, Roberts, JJ, and Ross WCJ: Aryl-2-halogenoalkylamines. Part XII. Some carboxylic derivatives of N,N-di-2-chloroethylaniline. J. Chem. Soc. 2386, 1953.

141. Arnold H, Bourseaux F, and Brock N: Neuartige Krebs-Chemotherapeutika aus der Gruppe der zyklischen N-Lost-Phosphamidester. Naturwissenschaften 45:64, 1958.

142. Foley GE, Friedman OM, and Drolet BP: Studies on the mechanism of action of Cytoxan. I. Evidence of activation *in vivo*. Proc. Am. Assoc. Cancer Res. 3:111, 1960.

143. Brock N, and Hohorst H-J: Uber die Aktivierung von Cyclophosphamid *in vivo* und *in vitro*. Arzneim Forsch. 13:1021, 1963.

144. Cohen JL, and Jao JY: Enzymatic basis of cyclophosphamide activation by hepatic microsomes of the rat. J. Pharmacol. Exp. Ther. 174:206, 1970.

145. Friedman OM, Myles A, and Colvin M: Cyclophosphamide and related phosphoramide mustards: current status and future prospects. *In* Rosowsky A (ed.): Advances In Cancer Chemotherapy. Marcel Dekker, New York & Basel, 1979, pp. 159–164.

146. Struck RF, Kirk MC, Mellett LB, et al.: Urinary metabolites of the antitumor agent cyclophosphamide. Mol. Pharmacol. 7:519, 1971.

147. Bakke JE, Feil WJ, Fjelstul CE, et al.: Metabolism of cyclophosphamide by sheep. J. Agric. Food Chem. 20:384, 1972.

148. Colvin M, Padgett CA, and Fenselau C: A biologically active metabolite of cyclophosphamide. Cancer Res. 33:915, 1973.

149. Maddock CL, Handler AH, Friedman OM, et al.: Primary evaluation of alkylating agent cyclohexylamine salt of N,N-bis(2-chloroethyl)phosphorodiamidic acid (NSC-69945; OMF-59) in experimental antitumor assay systems. Cancer Chemother. Rep. 50:629, 1966.

150. Colvin M, Brundrett RB, Kan MN, et al.: Alkylating properties of phosphoramide mustard. Cancer Res. 36:1121, 1976.

151. Hohorst H-J, Draeger A, Peter G, et al.: The problem of oncostatic specificity of cyclophosphamide (NSC-27271): studies on reactions that control the alkylating and cytotoxic activity. Cancer Treat. Rep. 60:309, 1976.

152. Colvin M, and Hilton J: Pharmacology of cyclophosphamide and metabolites. Cancer Treat. Rep., 1981, in press.

153. Hill DL, Kirk, M. C., and Struck, R. F. Microsomal metabolism of nitrosoureas. Cancer Res. 35:296, 1975.

154. Levin VA, Stearns J, Byrd A, et al.: The effect of phenobarbital pretreatment on the antitumor activity of 1,3-bis(2-chloroethyl)-1-nitrosourea (BCNU), 1-(2-chloroethyl)-3-cyclohexyl-1-nitrosourea (CCNU) and 1-(2-chloroethyl)-3-(2,6-dioxo)-3-piperidy-1-nitrosourea (PCNU), and on the plasma pharmacokinetics and biotransformation of BCNU. J. Pharmacol. Exp. Ther. 208:1, 1979.

155. May HE, Boose R,. and Reed DJ: Hydroxylation of the

carcinostatic 1-(2-chloroethyl)-3-cyclohexyl-1-nitrosourea (CCNU) by rat liver microsomes. Biochem. Biophys. Res. Commun. 57:426, 1974.
156. Hilton J, and Walker MD: Hydroxylation of 1-(2-chloroethyl)-3-cyclohexyl-1-nitrosourea. Biochem. Pharmacol. 24:2153, 1975.
157. Wheeler GP, Johnston TP, Bowdon BJ, et al.: Comparison of the properties of metabolites of CCNU. Biochem. Pharmacol. 26:2331, 1977.
158. Alberts DS, Chang SY, Chen H-SG, et al.: Kinetics of intravenous melphalan. Clin. Pharmacol. Ther. 26:73, 1979.
159. Tattersall MHN, and Weinberg A: Pharmacokinetics of melphalan following oral or intravenous administration in patients with malignant disease. Eur. J. Cancer 14:507, 1978.
160. Pallante SL, Fenselau C, Mennel RG, et al.: Quantitation by gas chromatography–chemical ionization–mass spectrometry of phenylalanine mustard in plasma of patients. Cancer Res. 40:2268, 1980.
161. D'Incalci M, Bolis G, Facchinetti T, et al.: Decreased half-life of cyclophosphamide in patients under continual treatment. Eur. J. Cancer 19:7, 1979.
162. Juma FD, Rogers HJ, and Trounce JR: Pharmacokinetics of cyclophosphamide and alkylating activity in man after intravenous and oral administration. Br. J. Clin. Pharmacol. 8:209, 1979.
163. Jardine I, Fenselau C, Appler M, et al.: Quantitation by gas chromatography–chemical ionization mass spectrometry of cyclophosphamide, phosphoramide mustard, and nornitrogen mustard in the plasma and urine of patients receiving cyclophosphamide therapy. Cancer Res. 38:408, 1978.
164. Brock N, Gross R, Hohorst H-J, et al.: Activation of cyclophosphamide in man and animals. Cancer 27:1512, 1971.
165. Bagley CM Jr, Bostick FW, and DeVita VT Jr: Clinical pharmacology of cyclophosphamide. Cancer Res. 33: 226, 1973.
166. Juma FD, Rogers HJ, and Trounce JR: The pharmacokinetics of cyclophosphamide, phosphoramide mustard and nor-nitrogen mustard studied by gas chromatography in patients receiving cyclophosphamide therapy. Br. J. Clin. Pharmacol. 10:327, 1980.
167. Fenselau C, Kan M-NN, Subba Rao S, et al.: Identification of aldophosphamide as a metabolite of cyclophosphamide *in vitro* and *in vivo* in humans. Cancer Res. 37:2538, 1977.
168. Wagner T, Peter G, Voelcker G, et al.: Characterization and quantitative estimation of activated cyclophosphamide in blood and urine. Cancer Res. 37:2592, 1977.
169. Wagner T, Heydrich D, Voelcker G, et al.: Characterization and quantitative estimation of activated cyclophosphamide in blood and urine. Cancer Res. Clin. Oncol. 96:79, 1980.
170. Sensenbrenner LL, Marini JJ, and Colvin M: Comparative effects of cyclophosphamide, isophosphamide, 4-methylcyclophosphamide and phosphoramide mustard on murine hematopoietic and immunocompetent cells. J. Natl. Cancer Inst. 62:975, 1979.
171. Brock N: Comparative pharmacologic study *in vitro* and *in vivo* with cyclophosphamide (NSC-26271), cyclophosphamide metabolites, and plain nitrogen mustard compounds. Cancer Treat. Rep. 60:301, 1976.
172. Field RB, Gang M, Kline I, et al.: The effect of phenobarbital or 2-diethylaminoethyl-2,2-diphenylvalerate on the activation of cyclophosphamide *in vivo*. J. Pharmacol. Exp. Ther. 180:475, 1972.
173. Jao JY, Jusko WJ, and Cohen JL: Phenobarbital effects on cyclophosphamide pharmacokinetics in man. Cancer Res. 32:2761, 1972.
174. Egorin M, Kaplan R, Salcman M, et al.: Plasma and cerebrospinal fluid (CSF) pharmacokinetics of cyclophosphamide (CYC) in patients treated with and without dimethyl sulfoxide (DMSO). Proc. Am. Assoc. Cancer Res. 22:210, 1981.
175. Alberts DS, and van Daalen Wetters T: The effects of phenobarbital on cyclophosphamide antitumor activity. Cancer Res. 36:2785, 1976.
176. Sladek N: Therapeutic efficacy of cyclophosphamide as a function of its metabolism. Cancer Res. 32:535, 1972.
177. Mouridsen HT, and Jacobson E: Pharmacokinetics of cyclophosphamide in renal failure. Acta Pharmacol. Toxicol. 36:409, 1975.
178. Humphrey RL, and Kvols LK: The influence of renal insufficiency on cyclophosphamide-induced hematopoietic depression and recovery. Proc. Am. Assoc. Cancer Res. 15:84, 1974.
179. Creaven PJ, Allen LM, Alford DA, et al.: Clinical pharmacology of isophosphamide. Clin. Pharmacol. Ther. 16:77, 1974.
180. Allen LM, and Creaven PJ: Pharmacokinetics of ifosfamide. Clin. Pharmacol. Ther. 17:492, 1975.
181. Nelson RL, Allen LM, and Creaven PJ: Pharmacokinetics of divided-dose ifosfamide. Clin. Pharmacol. Ther. 19:365, 1976.
182. Allen LM, and Creaven PJ: *In vitro* activation of isophosphamide (NSC-109724), a new oxazaphosphorine, by rat liver microsomes. Cancer Chemother. Rep. 56:603, 1972.
183. Norpoth K: Studies on the metabolism of isophosphamide (NSC-109724) in man. Cancer Treat. Rep. 60:437, 1976.
184. DeVita VT, Denham C, Davidson JD, et al.: The physiological disposition of the carcinostatic 1,3-bis(2-chloroethyl)-1-nitrosourea (BCNU) in man and animals. Clin. Pharmacol. Ther. 8:566, 1965.
185. Levin VA, Hoffman W, and Weinkam RJ: Pharmacokinetics of BCNU in man: a preliminary study of 20 patients. Cancer Treat. Rep. 62:1305, 1978.
186. Nissen-Meyer R, and Host H: A comparison between the hematological side effects of cyclophosphamide and nitrogen mustard. Cancer Chemother. Rep. 9:51, 1960.
187. Mullins GM, and Colvin M: Intensive cyclophosphamide therapy in solid tumors. Cancer Chemother. Rep. 59:411, 1975.
188. Elson LA: Hematological effects of the alkylating agents. Ann. N.Y. Acad. Sci. 68:826, 1958.
189. Botnick LE, Hannon EC, and Hellman S: Multisystem stem cell failure after apparent recovery from alkylating agents. Cancer Res. 38:1942, 1978.
190. DeVita VT, Carbone PP, Owens AH Jr, et al.: Clinical trials with 1,3-bis(2-chloroethyl)-1-nitrosourea, NSC-409962. Cancer Res. 25:1876, 1965.
191. Penta JS, Poster DS, Bruno S, et al.: Clinical trials with antiemetic agents in cancer patients receiving chemotherapy. Cancer Clin. Pharmacol. 21:1981.
192. Borison HL, Brand ED, and Orkand RK: Emetic action of nitrogen mustard (mechlorethamine hydrochloride) in dogs and cats. Am. J. Physiol. 192:410, 1968.
193. Spitz S: The histological effects of nitrogen mustards on human tumors and tissues. Cancer 1:383, 1948.
194. DeRooij DG, and Kramer MR: The effects of three alkylating agents on the seminiferous epithelium of rodents. Virchows Arch. (Zellpathol.) 4:267, 1969.
195. Richter P, Calamera JC, Morgenfeld MC, et al.: Effect of chlorambucil on spermatogenesis in the human with malignant lymphoma. Cancer 25:1026, 1970.
196. Miller DG: Alkylating agents and human spermatogenesis. J.A.M.A. 217:1662, 1971.
197. Fairley KF, Barrie JU, and Johnson W: Sterility and testicular atrophy related to cyclophosphamide therapy. Lancet 1:568, 1972.
198. Kumar R, Biggart JD, McEvoy J, et al.: Cyclophosphamide and reproductive function. Lancet 1:1212, 1972.
199. Sherins RJ, and DeVita VT: Effect of drug treatment for lymphoma on male reproductive capacity. Ann. Intern. Med. 79:216, 1973.
200. Hinkes E, and Plotkin D: Reversible drug-induced sterility in a patient with acute leukemia. J.A.M.A. 223:1490, 1973.
201. Blake DA, Heller RH, Hsu SH, et al.: Return of fertility in a patient with cyclophosphamide-induced azoospermia. Johns Hopkins Med. J. 139:20, 1976.
202. Galton DAG, Till M, and Wiltshaw E: Busulfan (1,4-dimethyl-sulfonoxy-butane, Myleran): summary of clinical results. Ann. N.Y. Acad. Sci. 68:967, 1958.
203. Miller JJ, Williams GF, and Leissring JC: Multiple late

complications of therapy with cyclophosphamide, including ovarian destruction. Am. J. Med. 50:530, 1971.
204. Fosdick WM, Parson JL, and Hill DF: Long-term cyclophosphamide therapy in rheumatoid arthritis. Arthritis Rheum. 11:151, 1968.
205. Kyoma H, Wada T, Nishizawa T, et al.: Cyclophosphamide-induced ovarian failure and its therapeutic significance in patients with breast cancer. Cancer 39:1403, 1977.
206. Rose DP, and Davis TE: Ovarian function in patients receiving adjuvant chemotherapy for breast cancer. Lancet 1:1174, 1977.
207. Fisher B, Sherman B, Rockette H, et al.: L-Phenylalanine mustard (L-PAM) in the management of premenopausal patients with primary breast cancer. Cancer 44:847, 1979.
208. Ohner H, Schwartz R, Rubio F, et al.: Interstitial pulmonary fibrosis following busulfan therapy. Am. J. Med. 31:134, 1961.
209. Burn WA, McFarland W, and Matthews MJ: Busulfan-induced pulmonary disease. Am. Rev. Respir. Dis. 101:408, 1970.
210. Willson JKV: Pulmonary toxicity of antineoplastic drugs. Cancer Treat. Rep. 62:2003, 1978.
211. Koss, LG, Melamed MR, and Mayer K: The effect of busulfan on human epithelia. Am. J. Clin. Pathol. 44:385, 1965.
212. Littler WA, and Ogilvie C: Lung function in patients receiving busulphan. Br. Med. J. 4:530, 1970.
213. Mark GJ, Lehimgar-Zadeh A, and Ragsdale BD: Cyclophosphamide pneumonitis. Thorax 33:89, 1978.
214. Patel AR, Shah PC, Rhee HC, et al.: Cyclophosphamide therapy and interstitial pulmonary fibrosis. Cancer 38:1542, 1976.
215. Radin AE, Haggard ME, and Travis LB: Lung changes and chemotherapeutic agents in childhood. Am. J. Dis. Child. 120:337, 1970.
216. Bailey CC, Marsden HB, and Jones PH: Fatal pulmonary fibrosis following 1,3-bis(2-chloroethyl)-1-nitrosourea (BCNU) therapy. Cancer 42:74, 1978.
217. Crittenden D, Tranum BL, and Hunt A: Pulmonary fibrosis after prolonged therapy with 1,3-bis(2-chloroethyl)-1-nitrosourea. Chest 72:372, 1977.
218. Holoye PY, Jenkins DE, and Greenberg SD: Pulmonary toxicity in long-term administration of BCNU. Cancer Treat. Rep. 60:1691, 1976.
219. Lee W, Moore RP, and Wampler GL: Interstitial pulmonary fibrosis as a complication of prolonged methyl-CCNU therapy. Cancer Treat. Rep. 62:1355, 1978.
220. Hundley RF, and Lukens JN: Nitrosourea-associated pulmonary fibrosis. Cancer Treat. Rep. 63:2128, 1979.
220A. Litam JP, Dail DH, Spitzer G, et al.: Early pulmonary toxicity after administration of high-dose BCNU. Cancer Treat. Rep. 65:39, 1981.
221. Codling BW, and Chakera TM: Pulmonary fibrosis following therapy with melphalan for multiple myeloma. J. Clin. Pathol. 25:668, 1972.
222. Jacobs S: The Hamman-Rich syndrome following treatment of lymphoma with chlorambucil. J. La. State Med. Soc. 127:311, 1975.
223. Cole RC, Myers TJ, and Klatsky AU: Pulmonary disease with chlorambucil therapy. Cancer 41:455, 1978.
224. Orwoll ES, Kiessling PJ, and Patterson JR: Interstitial pneumonia from mitomycin. Ann. Intern. Med. 89:352, 1978.
225. Lampert F: Lungenveranderungen bei der akuten lymphoblastischen Leukamie. Radiologe 8:308, 1968.
226. Okita H, Ito L, Taketomi T, et al.: Four patients with leukemia who showed especially a typical type of interstitial pneumonia, probably caused following the administration of antileukemic drugs (author's translation). Jpn. J. Clin. Hematol. 15:764, 1974.
227. Rubin G, Baume P, and Vandenberg R: Azathioprine and acute restrictive lung disease. Aust. N.Z. J. Med. 2:272, 1972.
228. Philips FS, Sternberg SS, Cronin AP, et al.: Cyclophosphamide and urinary bladder toxicity. Cancer Res. 21:1577, 1961.
229. Forni AM, Koss LG, and Geller W: Cytological study of the effect of cyclophosphamide on the epithelium of the urinary bladder in man. Cancer 17:1348, 1964.
230. Rubin JS, and Rubin RT: Cyclophosphamide hemorrhagic cystitis. J. Urol. 96:313, 1966.
231. Bellin HJ, Cherry JM, and Koss LG: Effects of a single dose of cyclophosphamide. V. Protection effect of diversion of the urinary stream on dog bladder. Lab. Invest. 30:43, 1974.
232. Cox PJ: Cyclophosphamide cystitis — identification of acrolein as the causative agent. Biochem. Pharmacol. 28:2045, 1979.
233. Primack A: Amelioration of cyclophosphamide-induced cystitis. J. Natl. Cancer Inst. 47:223, 1971.
234. van Dyk JJ, Falkson HC, van Der Merwe AM, et al.: Unexpected toxicity in patients treated with iphosphamide. Cancer Res. 32:921, 1972.
235. Botta JA Jr, Nelson LW, and Weikel JN Jr: Acetylcysteine in the prevention of cyclophosphamide-induced cystitis in rats. J. Natl. Cancer Inst. 51:1051, 1973.
236. Kline I, Gang M, and Venditti JM: Protection with N-acetylcysteine (NAC) against isophosphamide (ISOPH, NSC-10924) host toxicity and enhancement of therapy in early murine leukemia L1210. Proc. Am. Assoc. Cancer Res. 13:29, 1972.
237. Scheef W, Klein HO, Brock N, et al.: Controlled clinical studies with an antidote against the urotoxicity of oxazaphosphorines: preliminary results. Cancer Treat. Rep. 63:501, 1979.
238. Fernbach DJ: Chemotherapy for acute leukemia in childron: comparison of cyclophosphamide (NSC 26271) and 6-mercaptopurine (NSC-755). Cancer Chemother. Rep. 51:381, 1967.
239. DeFronzo RA, Abeloff M, Braine H, et al.: Renal dysfunction after treatment with isophosphamide (NSC-109724). Cancer Chemother. Rep. (Pt. 1) 58:375, 1974.
240. DeFronzo RA, Braine HG, Colvin M, et al.: Water intoxication in man after cyclophosphamide therapy. Ann. Intern. Med. 78:861, 1973.
240A. Green TP, and Mirkin BL: Prevention of cyclophosphamide-induced antidiuresis by furosemide infusion. Clin. Pharmacol. Ther. 29:634, 1981.
241. Harlow PJ, DeClerck YA, Shore NA, et al.: A fatal case of inappropriate ADH secretion induced by cyclophosphamide therapy. Cancer 44:896, 1979.
242. Carter SK, and Newman JW: Nitrosoureas: 1,3-bis(2-chloroethyl)-1-nitrosourea (NSC-409962; BCNU) and 1-(2-chloroethyl)-3-cyclohexyl-1-nitrosourea (NSC-70937; CCNU) — clinical brochure. Cancer Chemother. Rep. (Pt. 3) 1:115, 1968.
243. Silver HKB, and Morton DL: CCNU nephrotoxicity following sustained remission in oat cell carcinoma. Cancer Treat. Rep. 63:226, 1979.
244. Schacht RG, and Baldwin DS: Chronic interstitial nephritis and renal failure due to nitrosourea (NU) therapy. Kidney Int. 14:661, 1978.
245. Harmon WE, Cohen HJ, Schneeberger EE, et al.: Chronic renal failure in children treated with methyl CCNU. N. Engl. J. Med. 300:1200, 1979.
246. Bierman HR, Kelly KH, Knudson AG Jr, et al.: The influence of 1,4-dimethylsulfonoxy-1,4-dimethylbutane (CB 2348, dimethyl Myleran) in neoplastic disease. Ann. N.Y. Acad. Sci. 68:1211, 1958.
247. Feil VS, and Lamoureux CJH: Alopecia activity of cyclophosphamide metabolites and related compounds in sheep. Cancer Res. 34:2596, 1974.
248. Nathanson L, Hall TC, Rutenberg A, et al.: Clinical toxicologic study of cyclohexylamine salt of N,N-bis(2-chloroethyl)-phosphorodiamidic acid (NSC-69945; OMF-59). Cancer Chemother. Rep. 51:35, 1967.
249. Frei E III: Personal communication, 1975.
250. Ganci L, and Serrou B: Changes in hair pigmentation associated with cancer chemotherapy. Cancer Treat. Rep. 64:193, 1980.
251. Hennessy JD: Alopecia and cytotoxic drugs. Br. Med. J. 2:1138, 1966.
252. Dean JC, Salmon SE, and Griffith KS: Prevention of doxorubicin-induced hair loss with scalp hypothermia. N. Engl. J. Med. 301:1427, 1980.

253. Lakin JD, and Cahill RA: Generalized urticaria to cyclophosphamide: type I hypersensitivity to an immunosuppressive agent. J. Allergy Clin. Immunol. 58:160, 1976.
254. Ross, WE, and Chabner BA: Allergic reaction to cyclophosphamide in a mechlorethamine-sensitive patient. Cancer Treat. Rep. 61:495, 1977.
255. Karchmer RK, and Hansen BL: Possible anaphylactic reaction to intravenous cyclophosphamide. J.A.M.A. 237: 475, 1977.
256. Legha SS, and Hall S: Acute cyclophosphamide hypersensitivity reaction: possible lack of cross-sensitivity to mechlorethamine and isophosphamide. Cancer Treat. Rep. 62:180, 1978.
257. Cornwell GG III, Pajak TF, and McIntyre OR: Hypersensitivity reactions to i.v. melphalan during treatment of multiple myeloma: cancer and leukemia group B experience. Cancer Treat. Rep. 63:399, 1979.
258. Weiss RB, and Bruno S: Hypersensitivity reactions to cancer chemotherapeutic agents. Ann. Intern. Med. 94:66, 1981.
259. Haskin D: Some effects of nitrogen mustard on the development of external body form in the fetal rat. Anat. Record 102:493, 1948.
260. Bodenstein D: The effects of nitrogen mustard on embryonic amphibian development. J. Exp. Zool. 108:93, 1948.
261. Bodenstein D, and Goldin A: A comparison of the effects of various nitrogen mustard compounds on embryonic cells. J. Exp. Zool. 108:75, 1948.
262. Murphy ML, and Karnofsky DA: Effect of azaserine and other growth-inhibiting agents on fetal development of the rat. Cancer 9:955, 1956.
263. Murphy ML, Del Moro A, and Lacon C: The comparative effects of five poly-functional alkylating agents on the rat fetus, with additional notes. Ann. N.Y. Acad. Sci. 68:762, 1958.
264. Klein NW, Vogler MA, Chatot CL, et al.: The use of cultured rat embryos to evaluate the teratogenic activity of serum: cadmium and cyclophosphamide. Teratology 21:199, 1958.
265. Gibson JE, and Becker BA: Teratogenicity of structural truncates of cyclophosphamide in mice. Teratology 4:141, 1971.
266. Sadler TW, and Kochhar DM: Chlorambucil-induced cell death in embryonic mouse limb buds. Toxicol. Appl. Pharmacol 37:237, 1976.
267. Brummett ES, and Johnson EM: Morphological alterations in the developing fetal rat limb due to maternal injection of chlorambucil. Teratology 20:279, 1979.
268. Nicholson HO: Cytotoxic drugs in pregnancy. J. Obstet. Gynaecol. Br. Commonw. 75:307, 1968.
269. Steege JF, and Caldwell DS: Renal agenesis after first trimester exposure to chlorambucil. South. Med. J. 73:1414, 1980.
270. Toledo TM, Harper RC, and Moser RH: Fetal effects during cyclophosphamide and irradiation therapy. Ann. Intern. Med. 74:87, 1971.
271. Garrett MJ: Teratogenic effects of combination chemotherapy. Ann. Intern. Med. 80:667, 1974.
272. Ortega J: Multiple agent chemotherapy including bleomycin of non-Hodgkin's lymphoma during pregnancy. Cancer 40:2829, 1977.
273. Lergier JE, Jiminez E, Maldonado N, et al.: Normal pregnancy in multiple myeloma treated with cyclophosphamide. Cancer 34:1018, 1974.
274. Kyle RA, Pierce RV, and Bayrd ED: Multiple myeloma and acute myelomonocytic leukemia. N. Engl. J. Med. 283:1121, 1970.
275. Rosner F, and Grunwald H: Multple myeloma terminating in acute leukemia. Am. J. Med. 57:927, 1974.
276. Rosner F, and Grunwald H: Hodgkin's disease and acute leukemia. Am. J. Med. 58:339, 1975.
277. Einhorn N: Acute leukemia after chemotherapy (melphalan). Cancer 41:444, 1978.
278. Seiidenfeld AM, Smythe HA, Ogryzlo MA, et al.: Acute leukemia in rheumatoid arthritis treated with cytotoxic agents. J. Rheumatol. 3:295, 1976.
279. Hochberg MC, and Shulman LE: Acute leukemia following cyclophosphamide therapy for Sjögren's syndrome. Johns Hopkins Med. J. 142:211, 1978.
280. Steigbigel RT, Kim H, Potolsky A, et al.: Acute myeloproliferative disorder following long-term chlorambucil therapy. Arch. Intern. Med. 134:728, 1974.
281. Cardamone JM, Kimmerle RI, and Marshall EY: Development of acute erythroleukemia in B-cell immunoproliferative disorders after prolonged therapy with alkylating drugs. Am. J. Med. 57:837, 1974.
282. Cohen RJ, Wiernik PH, and Walker MD: Acute nonlymphocytic leukemia associated with nitrosourea chemotherapy: report of two cases. Cancer Treat. Rep. 60:1257, 1976.
283. Reimer RR, Hoover R, Fraumeni JF Jr, et al.: Acute leukemia after alkylating-agent therapy of ovarian cancer. N. Engl. J. Med. 297:177, 1977.
284. Penn I: Second malignant neoplasms associated with immunosuppressive medications. Cancer 37:1024, 1976.
285. Tobias JS, Weiner RS, Griffiths CT, et al.: Cryopreserved autologous marrow infusion following high dose cancer chemotherapy. Eur. J. Cancer 13:269, 1977.
286. McElwain TJ, Hedley DW, Burton G, et al.: Marrow autotransplantation accelerates haematological recovery in patients with malignant melanoma treated with high-dose melphalan. Br. J. Cancer 40:72, 1979.
287. McElwain TJ, Hedley DW, Gordon MY, et al.: High dose melphalan and non-cryopressed autologous bone marrow treatment of malignant melanoma and neuroblastoma. Exp. Hematol. 7(Suppl. 5):360, 1979.
288. Phillips GL, Fay JW, Wolff SN, et al.: 1,3-bis(2-chloroethyl)-1-nitrosourea (BCNU) and autologous bone marrow transplantation (BMTX) for refractory malignancy. Proc. Am. Assoc. Cancer Res. 21:180, 1980.
289. Takvorian T, Parker LM, Hochberg FH, et al.: Single high dose of BCNU with autologous bone marrow (ABM). Proc. Am. Soc. Clin. Oncol. 21:341, 1980.
290. Steinberg SS, Philips FS, and Scholler J: Pharmacological and pathological effects of alkylating agents. Ann. N.Y. Acad. Sci. 68:811, 1958.
291. Bethlenfalvay NC, and Bergin JJ: Severe cerebral toxicity after intravenous nitrogen mustard therapy. Cancer 29:366, 1972.
292. Yamada K, Bremer AM, West CR, et al.: Intra-arterial BCNU therapy in the treatment of metastatic brain tumor from lung carcinoma. Cancer 44:2000, 1979.
293. Colvin M, and Santos GW: High dose cyclophosphamide administration in man. Proc. Am. Assoc. Cancer Res. 11:17, 1970.
294. Buckner CD, Rudolph RJ, Fefer A, et al.: High dose cyclophosphamide therapy for malignant disease. Cancer 29:357, 1972.
295. Slavin RE, Millan JC, and Mullins GM: Pathology of high dose intermittent cyclophosphamide therapy. Hum. Pathol. 6:693, 1975.
296. Hektoen L, and Corper HJ: The effect of mustard gas (dichloroethyl-sulphid) on antibody formation. J. Infect. Dis. 28:279, 1921.
297. Philips FS, Hopkins FH, and Freeman MLH: Effects On tris(beta-chloroethyl)amine on antibody-production in goats. J. Immunol. 55:289, 1947.
298. Spurr CL: Influence of nitrogen mustards on the antibody response. Proc. Soc. Exp. Biol. Med. 64:259, 1947.
299. Makinodan T, Santos GW, and Quinn RP: Immunosuppressive drugs. Pharmacol. Rev. 22:189, 1970.
300. Sensenbrenner LL, Owens AH Jr, Heiby JR, et al.: Comparative effects of cytotoxic agents on transplanted hematopoietic and antibody-producing cells. J. Natl. Cancer Inst. 50:1027, 1973.
301. Berenbaum CC, and Brown IN: Dose-response relationships for agents inhibiting the immune response. Immunology 7:65, 1964.
302. Santos GW, and Owens AH Jr: 19S and 7S antibody production in the cyclophosphamide- or methotrexate-treated rat. Nature 209:622, 1966.
303. Owens AH Jr, and Santos GW: The effect of cytotoxic drugs on graft-versus-host disease in mice. Transplantation 11:378, 1971.
304. Many A, and Schwartz RS: On the mechanisms of immu-

nological tolerance in cyclophosphamide-treated mice. Clin. Exp. Immunol. 6:87, 1970.
305. Lerman SP, and Weidanz WO: The effect of cyclophosphamide on the ontogeny of the humoral immune response in chickens. J. Immunol. 105:614, 1970.
306. Turk JL, and Paulter LW: Selective depletion of lymphoid tissue by cyclophosphamide. Clin. Exp. Immunol. 10:285, 1972.
307. Turk JL: Studies on the mechanism of action of methotrexate and cyclophosphamide on contact sensitivity in the guinea pig. Int. Arch. Allergy 24:191, 1964.
308. Maguire HC, and Ettore VL: Enhancement of dinitrochlorobenzene (DNCB) contact sensitization by cyclophosphamide in the guinea pig. J. Invest. Dermatol. 48:39, 1967.
309. Stevenson HC, and Fauci AS: XII. Differential effects of *in vitro* cyclophosphamide on human lymphocyte subpopulations involved in B-cell activation. Immunology 39:391, 1980.
310. Shand FL, and Howard JG: Cyclophosphamide inhibited B-cell receptor regeneration as a basis for drug-induced tolerance. Nature 271:255, 1978.
311. Ozer H, Cowens JW, Nussbaum A, et al.: Human immunoregulatory T subset function defined *in vitro* by cyclophosphamide metabolites. Fed. Proc. 40:1075, 1981.
312. Mullins GM, Anderson PN, and Santos GW: High dose cyclophosphamide therapy in solid tumors. Cancer 36:1950, 1975.
313. Santos GW: Immunological toxicity of cancer chemotherapy. Recent Results Cancer Res. 10:20, 1974.
314. Santos GW, Sensenbrenner LL, Anderson PN, et al.: HL-A-identical marrow transplants in aplastic anemia, acute leukemia, and lymphosarcoma employing cyclophosphamide. Transplant. Proc. 8:607, 1976.
315. Starzl TE, Groth CG, Putman CW, et al.: Cyclophosphamide for clinical renal and hepatic transplantation. Transplant. Proc. 5:511, 1973.
316. Osborne EO, Jordon JW, Hoak FC, et al.: Nitrogen mustard therapy in cutaneous blastomatous disease. J.A.M.A. 135:1123, 1947.
317. Reza MJ, Dornfield L, Goldberg LS, et al.: Long-term follow-up of patients treated with cyclophosphamide. Arthritis Rheum. 18:501, 1975.
318. Cooperating Clinics Committee of The American Rheumatism Association: A controlled trial of cyclophosphamide in rheumatoid arthritis. N. Engl. J. Med. 283:883, 1970.
319. Townes AS, Sowa JM, and Schulman LE: Controlled trial of cyclophosphamide in rheumatoid arthritis (RA): an 11-month double-blind crossover study. Arthritis Rheum. 15:129, 1972.
320. Laros RK Jr, and Penner JA: "Refractory" thrombocytopenic purpura treated successfully with cyclophosphamide. J.A.M.A. 215:445, 1971.
321. Weinerman B, Maxwell I, and Hryniuk W: Intermittent cyclophosphamide treatment of autoimmune thrombocytopenia. Can. Med. Assoc. J. 111:1100, 1974.
322. Barratt TM, and Soothill JF: Controlled trial of cyclophosphamide in steroid-sensitive relapsing nephrotic syndrome of childhood. Lancet 2:479, 1970.

PLATINUM COMPLEXES

Leonard A. Zwelling

Kurt W. Kohn

14

HISTORY

The development of *cis*-diamminedichloroplatinum (II) (*cis*-DDP, Platinol) for the first time brought inorganic chemistry in a major way into the field of cancer chemotherapy. A compound with the formula $Pt(NH_3)_2Cl_2$ was first described by Reiset in 1844, and another compound with the same formula was reported by Peyrone one year later. In 1893 Werner suggested that the compounds were geometric isomers; it is now known that Reiset's chloride was the *trans* isomer and Peyrone's the *cis* isomer of a planar complex (Fig. 14–1).[1]

The discovery of the biologic actions of the platinum complexes developed from a fortuitous observation by Rosenberg et al.[2] during a study of the effect of electric current on growing bacteria. It was noted that alternating current delivered through platinum electrodes into a bacterial culture inhibited cell division and caused the bacteria to grow into long filaments. The same result was seen when an attempt was made to grow the bacteria in medium that had previously been subjected to the electric current. The result was notable because similar effects on bacteria were known to be produced by a variety of DNA damaging agents, including radiation and alkylating agents. Subsequent study showed that platinum atoms from the electrodes entered the medium in the form of hexachloroplatinate anions that, in the presence of light, reacted with ammonia ions in the medium to form complexes containing both chloride and ammonia. Examination of several complexes of this type showed that bacterial growth into filaments was effectively produced by the *cis* isomer of $Pt(NH_3)_2Cl_2$.

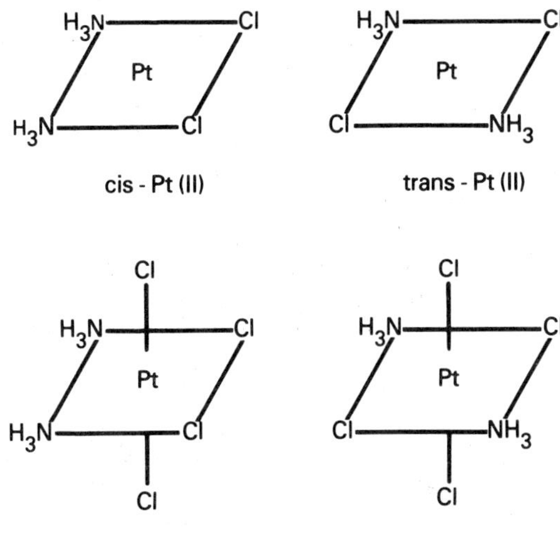

Figure 14–1. Steric configuration of Pt complexes.

In 1969 Rosenberg et al.[3] reported that the *cis* isomer had potent antitumor activity against sarcoma 180 and leukemia L1210 in mice. In addition to the planar complex, in which the platinum has the oxidation state Pt(II), the *cis* form of the octahedral $Pt(IV)(NH_3)_2Cl_4$ complex was also active. The *trans* isomers, however, were inactive.

Phase I clinical studies of *cis*-DDP were begun in 1971.[4-7] The toxicities and antineoplastic effects[8] predicted in animal models were also evident in man. The successful incorporation of *cis*-DDP into several combination chemotherapy regimens soon followed, the most notable achievement being in the treatment of advanced testicular cancer.[9] In late 1978 the Food and Drug Administration approved the use of *cis*-DDP for the treatment of malignant disease in the United States.

CHEMISTRY

Covalent Bond Character

Platinum is in the third row of transition metals in the Periodic Table and has eight electrons in the outer *d* shell. Palladium and nickel, which occupy analogous positions in the second and first transition series, have similar configurations of outer electrons, but little or no antitumor activity. However, since the platinum atom has a much larger total number of electrons, the orbitals of its outer electrons are more polarizable, and bonds involving these orbitals have a highly covalent character.

Covalent bond character provides two essential properties: stereospecificity of the bonds and energy barriers to exchange reactions. The steric arrangement of the bonds depends on the oxidation state, which in the case of the compounds of these metals can be +2 or +4. In the +2 oxidation state the metal has four bonds that point to the corners of a square with a metal atom at the center, thus producing a planar complex. In the +4 state there are an additional two bonds directed 90° above and below the plane, producing an octahedral configuration. The complexes of Pt are stereospecific in that bound ligands remain fixed in position, thereby producing distinct isomers such as *cis*- and *trans*$Pt(II)(NH_3)_2Cl_2$ (Fig. 14–1).

The high stability of these distinct isomers implies an energy barrier to exchange between ligands. The energy barrier limits the rate of replacement of one ligand by another, even when this displacement would lead to a product having higher stability. The covalent character of the bonding makes reactions of Pt complexes similar in some respects to substitution reactions at carbon, in particular to alkylation reactions. As in the case of bimolecular nucleophilic (SN2) alkylation reactions, the rate of substitution at Pt (II) is sensitive to the concentration and character of the entering group. However, unlike SN2 alkylations, which occur with inversion of steric configuration, displacement at Pt (II) occurs with retention of configuration.

Oxidation States

Although complexes of Pt(II) and Pt(IV) (i.e., platinum in oxidation states +2 and +4) both can have antitumor activity, the activity of Pt (IV) complexes may be due to conversion of the +2 state in the cell. The oxidation reduction potential, approximately −0.7 volt, is not far from the oxidation reduction potential supposed to exist in cells[10]; hence, reduction to Pt(II) is possible. Pt(IV) *per se* in fact may be generally unreactive because access to the Pt atom is blocked by ligands from all directions. Pt(II) complexes, on the other hand, are accessible to attack from above and below the plane where the additional two Pt orbitals can be directed for bond formation. Combined or intermediate states of oxidation occur in the Pt pyrimidine blue complexes,[11, 12] which are potentially interesting new antitumor agents.

Displacement Reactions

The Pt(II) reactions of greatest interest from a biologic viewpoint involve the replacement of one ligand by another. The important considerations are the stability (equilibrium constant for binding) of a given ligand and the rate at which it can enter or be displaced from a complex. Table 14–1 shows the relative order of stability and the rate effects for several types of ligands.[13] The stability and the relative leaving rates are seen to be inversely related, the most stable ligands being displaced most slowly. In general, the stability increases with the polarizability of the ligand (thus $I^- > Br^- > Cl^-$). However, NH_3 and OH^- form strong bonds despite having low polarizabilities. The entry rates, on the other hand, are more completely dominated by polarizability, so that NH_3 is low on this list.

The leaving rates also depend on the identity of the other ligands in the complex, especially the ligand located *trans* to the leaving ligand. The *trans* effect, like the entry rate, is dominated by polarizability. Thus, amines are strongly bound, but the rate of ligand entry is relatively slow, and amines do not enhance the ability of a *trans* ligand to be displaced. Sulfur ligands, on the other hand, not only are strongly bound but also form rapidly and have a strong tendency

TABLE 14–1. Relative Stability and Kinetic Effects of Various Ligands in Pt(II) Complexes

Stability	Kinetics: LEAVING RATE	Kinetics: *Trans* EFFECT	Kinetics: ENTRY RATE
high ↑	low ↓	high ↑	high ↑
CN^-	CN^-	CN^-	$S_2O_3^=$
RS^-, R_2S		R_2S, thiourea	thiourea
OH^-	NO_2^-	NO_2^-	RS^-
NH_3		SCN^-, I^-	I^-
SCN^-	SCN^-	Br^-	Br^-
I^-	I^-	Cl^-	NO_2^-
Br^-	Br^-	NH_3, RNH_2, pyridine	NH_3
Cl^-	Cl^-	OH^-	Cl^-
H_2O	H_2O	H_2O	RO^-
low	high	low	low

From data in Thomson AJ, Williams RJP, and Reslova S: Struct. Bond. 11:1, 1972.

to labilize the *trans* ligand. The kinetic *trans* effect could make some types of biologically significant Pt(II) binding reversible.

Reactions in Water and Biologic Fluids

The reactions of *cis*-DDP with water, summarized in Figure 14–2, must be taken into account in considerations of pharmacology and mechanism of action. Indeed, it is probably the aquated Pt species that reacts with the critical cellular targets. Although the Pt-water bond is weaker than the Pt-Cl bond, the overwhelming concentration of H_2O molecules can override the difference in bond stability. This can occur, however, only when the Cl^- concentration is very low, since Cl^- will shift the equilibrium away from the aquo forms. The chlorides of *cis*-DDP can be replaced by water molecules in a sequence of two steps: reactions 1 and 2 in Figure 14–2. Each of the bound water molecules can dissociate a proton, with acid dissociation constants (pKa values) as shown in Figure 14–2. In addition, two Pt complexes can combine to form dimers (reaction 7) and higher polymers. The Pt species connected by this network of reactions would be expected to differ in their pharmacokinetic behavior and in their reactivity with biomolecules. It is possible (al-

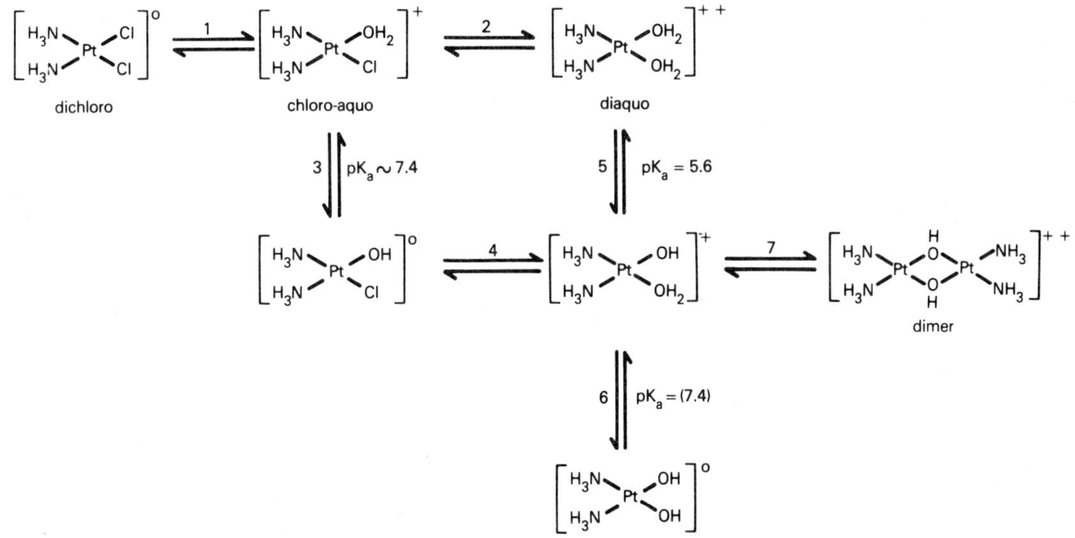

dichloro ⇌(1) chloro-aquo ⇌(2) diaquo

3: $pK_a \sim 7.4$ 5: $pK_a = 5.6$

4 ⇌ 7 ⇌ dimer

6: $pK_a = (7.4)$

Figure 14–2. Reactions of *cis*-DDP with water. (pKa values from Harrison and McAuliffe.[15])

though still unproved) that the neutral species can penetrate membrane barriers by passive diffusion and that the charged species are excluded from cells. For these reasons, it is important to know the relative concentrations of the different Pt species under various conditions.

A complicating feature is that the displacement reactions of Cl^- by H_2O are slow, so that one must consider the kinetics of these reactions, as well as the equilibrium constants. Some currently accepted values for the kinetic and equilibrium constants are summarized in Table 14–2.[14, 15, 17, 18]

The first point to be noted is the equilibrium constant of reaction 1 (4.4×10^{-3}M at 35°C). Thus, at $[Cl^-] = 4.4 \times 10^{-3}$M (which is close to the intracellular Cl^- concentration), the concentrations of the dichloro and chloro-aquo species are theoretically equal. However, this is true only at equilibrium, which is not likely to be achieved in practice, because the half-life for this reaction alone is 2.5 hours, which is considerable in relation to the excretion rate or the rate of binding to proteins.

The positively charged chloro-aquo form can undergo a rapid acid-base equilibrium (reaction 3) in which the deprotonated form is uncharged. At physiologic pH, both the protonated and unprotonated forms are probably present.

The second equation (reaction 2) is a slow reaction with equilibrium constant 1.9×10^{-4}M. At an intracellular Cl^- concentration of 4 mM, the equilibrium concentration of the diaquo form would be $1.9 \times 10^{-4}/4 \times 10^{-3} = 4.8$ per cent of the chloro-aquo concentration. The diaquo species, however, dissociates a proton at pKa = 5.6 and a second proton at pKa = 7.4. At physiologic pH, the concentration of the diaquo form would be exceeded about 25-fold by the combined concentration of its deprotonated forms. At the Cl^- concentration in the cell, the equilibrium distribution would consist of comparable concentrations of dichloro, chloro-aquo, and deprotonated diaquo species. This analysis, however, neglects other intracellular anions, such as carboxylate and phosphate, which could participate in the equilibrium.

The equilibrium concentration of dimer, formed by reaction 7, would increase with the square of the concentration of the aquo-hydroxo form; at an aquo-hydroxo concentration of 1 μM, the equilibrium concentration of dimer would be about 0.05 μM. However, at this low concentration of monomer, the rate of dimer formation would probably be too slow for any pharmacologically significant accumulation of dimer.

These equilibria are of major importance, because the chloride ligand is not displaced by nitrogen target sites in the cell, whereas the OH_2 ligand, which is less strongly bound, can be displaced by various types of amines and nitrogen-containing heterocyclic rings. *Cis*-DDP does not react with such targets until one or both chlorides have been replaced by water molecules. Since the aquation reactions require several hours to approach equilibrium, most of the drug would, at early times, remain in the relatively unreactive dichloro form. The dichloro form, however, could react directly with target sites that are more potent than nitrogen compounds as entering ligands. In particular, thio groups might directly displace chloride at significant rates.

Our considerations have so far centered on intracellular conditions. In plasma, the Cl^-

TABLE 14–2. Reactions of *cis*-DDP with Water

			Rate of Forward Reaction			
*Reaction**	*Equilibrium Constant*		*k (sec^{-1})*		*t½ (hrs)*	
	25°	*35°*	*25°*	*35°*	*25°*	*35°*
1	3.6×10^{-3}M§	4.4×10^{-3}M§	2.5×10^{-5}‖	7.6×10^{-5}‖	7.7	2.5
2	1.1×10^{-4}M§	1.9×10^{-4}M§	3.3×10^{-5}‖		5.8	
7	$4.8 \times 10^{-}M^{-1}$†		$6.1 \times 10^{-3}M^{-1}sec^{-1}$†			

*See Figure 14–2.
†Chikuma et al.[14]
§Lim and Martin[16]; LeRoy et al.[18]
‖Reishus and Martin.[17]

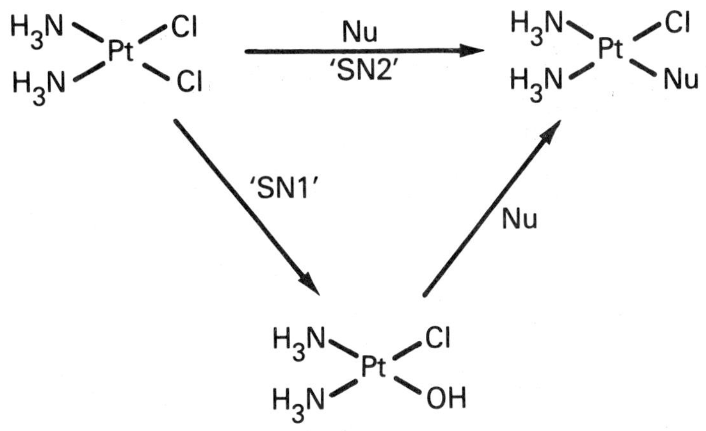

Figure 14–3. Direct and indirect reactions with nucleophile (Nu); analogy to SN2 and SN1 alkylation mechanisms.

concentration is high enough to prevent more than a low percentage replacement of chloride by water, even at equilibrium. *Cis*-DDP in plasma nevertheless binds to plasma proteins over a period of a few hours,[18] possibly by reacting directly with protein sulfyhydryl groups.

In general, *cis*-DDP may bind to a nucleophile either by direct chloride displacement or via an aquo-intermediate (Fig. 14–3). The direct reaction may be significant only for thio compounds, whereas amines may react exclusively through the aquo path. The direct chloride displacement is analogous to an SN2 alkylation mechanism, in that its rate is sensitively dependent on the concentration and reactivity of the nucleophile. The aquo path is analogous to an SN1 alkylation path, in that a slow first-order reaction is the rate-limiting step leading to an intermediate that reacts relatively rapidly and somewhat indiscriminately with nucleophiles.

EFFECTS ON MACROMOLECULES

DNA as Target

The role of DNA as target in the action of Pt complexes was already suggested by the initial observation of Rosenberg et al. that electrolytic products derived from platinum electrodes inhibited cell division in bacteria, causing the organisms to grow into long filaments.[19, 20] This type of effect is characteristic for some classes of DNA-damaging agents, particularly bifunctional alkylating agents. *Cis*-DDP selectively inhibits bacterial DNA synthesis, as is the case with alkylating agents.[21]

A clear indication of the biologic role of DNA damage in *cis*-DDP–treated bacteria was the finding that mutants defective in DNA excision or recombination repair have increased sensitivity to the drug.[22-24] Furthermore, *cis*-DDP is mutagenic, producing both base substitution[25-29] and frame-shift mutations.[30] *Cis*-DDP inactivates transforming DNA by inhibiting the integration of the treated DNA into the recipient bacterial genome.[31]

As is commonly the case with DNA-damaging agents, *cis*-DDP induces prophage in lysogenic bacteria.[32] In mammalian cells bearing Epstein-Barr virus, *cis*-DDP has been reported to increase the number of virus-positive cells as well as actual virus particles in the culture,[33, 34] suggesting that the drug can induce viruses in human cells. *Cis*-DDP treatment of DNA viruses causes their inactivation.[35-37] *Cis*-DDP is also mutagenic in mammalian cells,[38-41] carcinogenic in whole animals,[42] teratogenic,[43] and produces sister-chromatid exchanges in mammalian cells.[39, 44, 45]

Recent electron microscopic evidence has localized Pt to the nucleolus and inner nuclear membrane in *cis*-DDP–treated HeLa cells.[46]

Although reactions with other sites can be hypothesized to contribute to the cytotoxicity of cis-Pt(II) complexes, reactions with DNA are at present the most concrete and most plausible source of the major effects.

Sites of Reaction with Nucleic Acids

The nitrogen atoms of the DNA bases would be expected to be the major sites of Pt binding. Some of the nitrogens, however, are much more readily complexed than others, either because of the ease with which they can donate an electron pair or because of steric factors. The DNA site of greatest intrinsic reactivity with Pt is the guanine-N_7 position, because of the high nucleophilicity of the imidazole ring, which also makes this the most easily alkylated site.[47, 48]

The ability of nucleic acids to bind Pt increases with guanine content.[31, 49-51] Pt(II)enCl_2 (an active analogue of *cis*-DDP in which an ethylenediamine bridge replaces the two *cis*-NH_3 groups)[52] reacts an order of magnitude faster with guanosine than with adenosine or cytidine, and does not react at all with thymidine or uridine. The preferential reaction with guanosine, however, appears not to be due to any greater thermodynamic bond stability as compared to bonds with adenosine or cytidine.[53] Rather, the preference for guanine is a kinetic one: the reaction is faster, probably because the high polarizability at the N_7 position allows the electrons to move more easily into positions that favor bond formation.

The rate of binding, however, depends not only on the primary binding site at base nitrogens, but also on charge and hydrogen bonding effects. The reaction of Pt(II)enCl_2 (en = ethylenediamine) with the adenine ring, for example, is greatly enhanced by a phosphate moiety, as in AMP,[54] the order of reactivity being poly A > AMP > ApA > poly d(AT) > adenosine.

Clues to the nature of the secondary interactions that influence reaction rate and specificity are revealed by structure analysis. The structure of several Pt(II)-nucleoside or -nucleotide complexes has been determined by x-ray crystallography. The structure of the complex of Pt(II) en with two guanosine molecules is shown in Figure 14–4. *Cis*-Pt(II) $(NH_3)_2$ produces a similar structure with slightly different bond distances.[56] The first point of interest is the short distance between the two guanine N_7 atoms, about 2.7 Å, compared with the 3.4 Å separation between parallel base-pair layers in the DNA helix. The shortness of the distance, together with the fact that the angle between the two guanine rings in the complex is about 74°, means that the DNA helix must be greatly distorted if G-G binding is to take place. Another important observation is the H-bonding of the amine hydrogen to an O_6 atom of an adjacent molecule. H-bonding from the amine group is seen repeatedly in the x-ray structures that have been determined. It is interesting that *cis*-Pt(II) complexes in which the amine hydrogens have all been replaced by alkyl substituents, so that no H-bonding is possible, have no antitumor activity.[57]

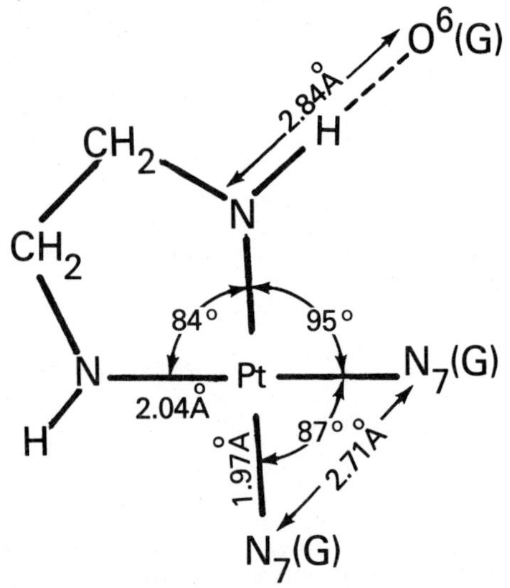

Figure 14–4. Structure, bond angles, and bond distances of Pt(II)en and 2 guanosine molecules. (Taken from data of Bau et al.: Crystallographic studies on platinum-nucleoside and platinum-nucleotide complexes. J. Clin. Hematol. Oncol. 7:51, 1977.)

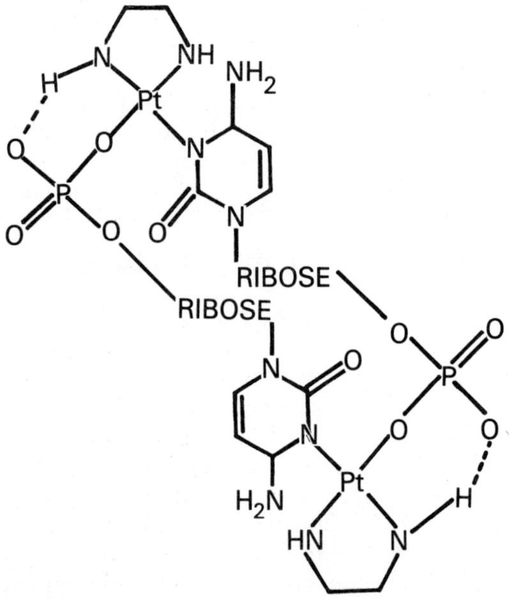

Figure 14–5. Structure of Pt(II)en and 5′-CMP. (Taken from data of Louie S, and Bau R: Structure of $[Pt(en)(5'-CMP)]_2 \cdot 2H_2O$. An example of direct platinum-phosphate bonding. J. Am. Chem. Soc. 99:3874, 1977.)

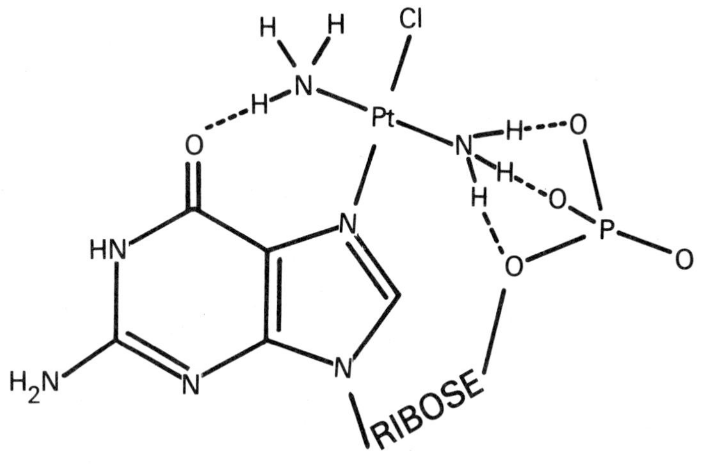

Figure 14–6. Reaction product of *trans*-DDP and guanine-N_7 in t-RNA. (Taken from data of Jack et al.: A crystallographic study of metal-binding to yeast phenylalanine transfer RNA. J. Mol. Biol. 111:315, 1977.)

Figure 14–5 shows the binding of Pt(II) en with 5′-CMP.[58] The Pt atom is bound to the cytosine-N_3 and to a phosphate oxygen. A second phosphate oxygen forms a strong H-bond (2.75 Å) to an amine of the Pt complex. A pair of Pt(II)en-5′-CMP molecules are linked together in head-to-tail fashion with the cytosine rings approximately parallel and 3.51 Å apart. The bonding to phosphate revealed by this structure could occur with a variety of molecules in the organism.

It has been proposed that *cis*-Pt(II) may bind to the N_7 and O_6 positions of the same guanine base, but confirmation of the existence of this type of binding is still lacking.[59]

Trans-Pt(II)$(NH_3)_2$ reacts with t-RNA at a specific guanine-N_7 (Fig. 14–6).[60] One of the amines of the complex is H-bonded to the O_6 of the same guanine; the other amine forms three H-bonds to the phosphate group. The *cis* complex does not react in a specific manner with t-RNA, suggesting that the H-bonding geometry may determine the ability of particular Pt complexes to react at specific sites.

Effect of Pt Binding on DNA Conformation

Both *cis*- and *trans*-Pt(II) complexes have marked effects on the conformation of purified DNA, characterized by unwinding of the helix and shortening of the molecules.[61] The detailed nature of the conformational change produced by these two isomeric complexes, however, is different (see below).

The DNA unwinding effect is similar to that produced by intercalation, and the extent of unwinding is similar for the *cis* and *trans* complexes.[61] Contrary to the effects of intercalation, however, there are reductions in intrinsic viscosity and electric birefringence,[62] and the net length of the DNA molecules, as seen by electron microscopy, is shortened.

The difference between the conformational effects of the different complexes has been best shown by circular dichroism spectra.[63, 64] Both the *cis* and *trans* complexes produce marked effects on circular dichroism. The *cis* complex increases ellipticity, which peaks at a binding ratio of 1 Pt per 10 nucleotides; the ellipticity then falls markedly as the extent of binding is further increased. The *trans* complex only causes a fall in ellipticity. The marked changes in ellipticity appear to require bifunctional binding, since Pt(II)dienCl, which can bind only monofunctionally, produces little effect on circular dichroism. The precise nature of the high-ellipticity conformation that is unique for the *cis* complex is not known, but it is possible that this type of DNA binding is responsible for the antitumor effect, since it is not produced by the inactive *trans* and monofunctional complexes. The change in circular dichroism reflects a change in conformation of the DNA helix, since this change is not produced in denatured DNA.

Interstrand and Intrastrand Crosslinking

Interstrand crosslinking of purified DNA has been demonstrated to be produced by both *cis* and *trans* complexes.[65-67] The crosslinking effect is inhibited by Cl^-, indicating that only the aquated complexes can react to produce this effect. There is, however, a difference between the isomeric complexes in that the aquated *cis* complex produces crosslinks much faster than does the aquated *trans* complex.[65] It may be that the DNA conformational distortion required to permit interstrand crosslinking by the *trans* complex is greater or of a less probable nature than the conformational change that permits interstrand crosslinking by the *cis* complex.

It is clear from the geometry of the Pt complexes that a large conformational distortion in the DNA is necessary for interstrand crosslinking. The distance between ligated bases, in the case of *cis*-Pt(II) binding to two guanine-N_7 positions, for example, is only 2.7 Å,[68] which is much shorter than the separation between these positions in the helix. To accomplish this binding, the guanines must be tilted far from parallel, producing a kink in the DNA helix. Such kinking may be the reason for the shortening of the net length of the DNA molecules.[61] Although DNA may well be able to undergo the distortion necessary to permit crosslinking between guanine-N_7 positions, an alternative possibility is that interstrand crosslinking occurs between adenine-N_6 positions that can be as close as 3.4 Å.[69-71]

The role of interstrand crosslinks in the inactivation of bacteriophage λ DNA was studied by Filipski et al.[72, 73] The inactivation by *trans*-DDP was fully accounted for on the basis of interstrand crosslinks: those λ DNA molecules that had one or more interstrand crosslinks were inactive, whereas those without interstrand crosslinks retained their transfection activity. In the case of *cis*-DDP, however, less than 25 per cent of inactivation could be attributed to interstrand crosslinks: most of the DNA molecules lacked interstrand crosslinks but yet were inactive, in accord with similar observations by Shooter et al.[37] The inactivity was due to the presence of Pt adducts, because the activity could be restored by removing the Pt adducts by means of thiourea.[72, 73] The inactivating Pt adducts were probably bifunctional, because delayed inactivation was demonstrated, consistent with a delayed conversion of Pt-DNA monoadducts to diadducts, i.e., crosslinks. It was therefore inferred that most of the inactivation produced by *cis*-DDP was due to *intrastrand* crosslinks.

This conjecture implies that *cis*-DDP should have a greater propensity for producing intrastrand crosslinks than does *trans*-DDP. Support for this presumption is given by the findings of Roos et al. that *cis*-DDP can link together the two bases of a dinucleotide, whereas *trans*-DDP cannot, probably because the geometry is unfavorably.[71] Newer support for *cis*-DDP intrastrand crosslinking has demonstrated that the production of such lesions could be more favored in left-handed DNA.[74]

Indirect evidence for the production of intrastrand crosslinks does exist. *Cis*-DDP greatly increased the buoyant density of the synthetic polynucleotide poly dG.poly dC although not poly dG.dC. The former has adjoining guanine bases that were hypothesized to be crosslinked by *cis*-DDP.[51] Kelman and Buchbinder have reported that the ability of a restriction endonuclease that cleaves DNA between adjoining guanine bases to generate DNA fragments was prevented by pretreating the DNA with *cis*-Pt(en)Cl_2. DNA fragments, however, could be generated by removing the Pt adducts with KCN. It was hypothesized that a Pt-bridge joining adjacent guanines within one DNA strand had prevented detection of the fragments. The fragment pattern then could be regenerated once the Pt-intrastrand bridges were removed.[75, 76] Recent work by Cohen et al. also indicated the possibility that the binding of *cis*-DDP to DNA may be sequence-specific.[77]

These observations indicate that intrastrand, as well as interstrand, crosslinks must be considered as likely inactivating lesions in cells treated with *cis*-DDP, although the presence of intrastrand crosslinks in cells still requires direct confirmation.

RNA and Protein

Both *cis*- and *trans*-DDP have been found to inactivate DNA as a template for RNA polymerase.[64] The enzyme itself was not inactivated. *Cis*-DDP was a more potent inhibitor than *trans*-DDP.

Both *cis*- and *trans*-DDP also have been demonstrated to inhibit the function of various enzymes. There is, however, no clear superiority of *cis*- over *trans*-DDP in enzyme inactivation, thus making this an unlikely explanation for the relative antineoplastic actions of these compounds.[78] The propensity of *trans*-DDP to bind to DNA-associated protein in cells[79, 80] and chromatin has generated interest in this compound as a probe for the study of chromosomal structure.[81] Additionally, *cis*-DDP altered the electron spin resonance of membrane ghosts in a manner that suggested an alteration in the configuration of membrane proteins.[82]

DNA CROSSLINKING AND CYTOTOXICITY

As in the case of alkylating agents, the major factor in the cytotoxicity of *cis*-DDP probably is the formation of DNA crosslinks of some kind. This is inferred from the long-known dependence of the high cytotoxic and antitumor potencies of these agents on the presence of two functional groups, each capable of forming covalent bonds. Three types of Pt diadducts (crosslinks) involving DNA have been identified: interstrand, intrastrand, and DNA-protein crosslinks.[83]

Although bifunctional reactions with macromolecules are probably the main source of cytotoxicity, the predominant form of *cis*-DDP binding to macromolecules is monofunctional. The second reactive site of the Pt complex may be ligated to low-molecular-weight nucleophiles, e.g., amines and thiols, in the cell. Pascoe and Roberts[84] noted intracellular binding of both *cis*- and *trans*-DDP to RNA>DNA> protein (based on moles of Pt bound per gm of macromolecule). The cytotoxicity produced at a given extent of DNA binding was much greater for *cis*-DDP than for the *trans* isomer. This can be explained on the basis of a much greater formation of interstrand crosslinks by *cis*- than by *trans*-DDP.[80, 84] DNA-protein crosslinks, on the other hand, were prominently produced by both isomers.[80] These findings point to interstrand crosslinks but not DNA-protein crosslinks as major cytotoxic lesions. (The possibly important role of intrastrand crosslinks was not excluded, since these lesions could not be measured by the methods used.)

Cis-DDP selectively inhibits DNA synthesis in mammalian cells, whereas RNA and protein syntheses are inhibited only at high drug concentrations.[85-88] The inhibition of DNA synthesis by *cis*-DDP was delayed for several hours, perhaps because of the time required for the formation of interstrand crosslinks.[80] Further evidence for a possible role for crosslinking in the cytotoxic action of *cis*-DDP comes from recent work that demonstrated a parallel enhancement of crosslink formation and cytotoxicity in cells treated with *cis*-DDP at elevated temperature (up to 43°C).[89, 90]

Crosslink Formation and Removal

Cis-DDP–induced interstrand crosslinking in mammalian cells was first demonstrated by Roberts and Pascoe.[91] The standard techniques for interstrand crosslink detection were relatively insensitive, however, so that drug dosage far in excess of pharmacologic levels had to be used.[84] The earlier work measured DNA crosslinking only at early times after drug treatment, and led to the conclusion that interstrand crosslinking is unlikely to be a major cytotoxic lesion.[88] This conclusion must now be reconsidered in the light of the finding that interstrand crosslinking increases markedly for several hours after treatment of cells with *cis*-DDP.[40, 80]

Crosslinking measurements in the pharmacologic range of dosage are now obtainable by means of the alkaline elution technique,[92, 93] which permits the sensitive measurement of both interstrand and DNA-protein crosslinking. Intrastrand crosslinking cannot be measured by this technique and as yet has not been studied directly in cells.

We have recently studied the kinetics of crosslink formation and removal in mouse leukemia cells, using the alkaline elution technique[80] (Fig. 14–7). Cells were exposed to drug for one hour and crosslinking was measured as a function of time following drug removal. Immediately following treatment with *cis*-DDP, some DNA-protein crosslinking was evident, but interstrand crosslinking was not detectable. Upon further incubation in the absence of drug, interstrand crosslinking rises to a peak after six to 12 hours. Both types of crosslinks are then eliminated, probably through the action of DNA repair mechanisms.

In the case of *trans*-DDP, DNA-protein crosslinking is the major effect, whereas interstrand crosslinks are barely detectable.[79] These DNA-protein crosslinks form relatively quickly and are gradually removed over a 24-hour period (Fig. 14–7). These lesions are not highly cytotoxic, because a concentra-

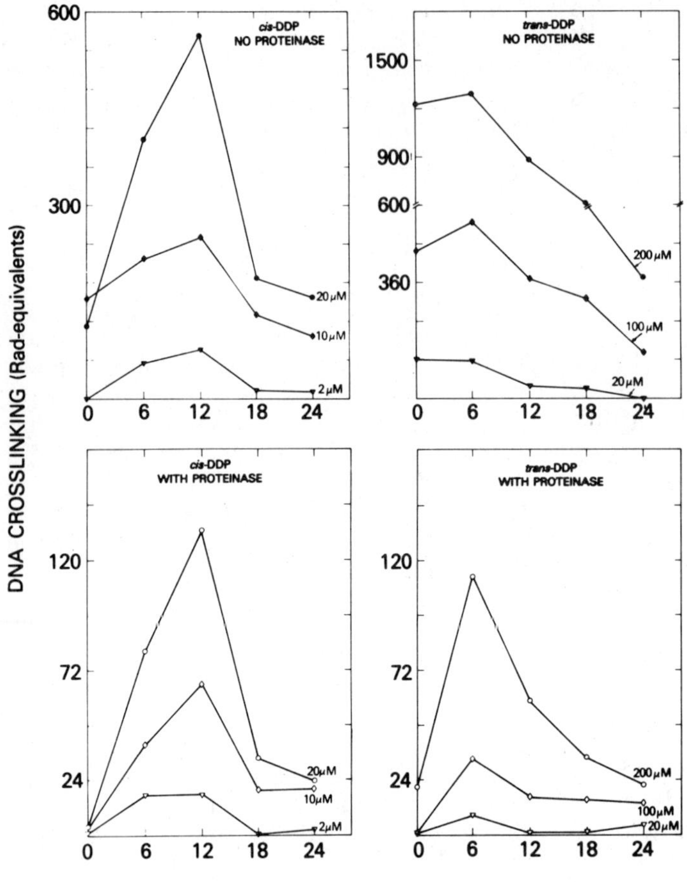

Figure 14–7. The kinetics of formation and removal of DNA-protein *(upper panels)* and DNA interstrand *(lower panels)* crosslinks in mouse leukemia cells treated with *cis-* or *trans*-DDP. (Reproduced with permission from Zwelling et al.: DNA-protein and DNA interstrand cross-linking by *cis-* and *trans*-platinum(II)diamminedichloride in L1210 mouse leukemia cells and relation to cytotoxicity. Cancer Res. 39:365, 1979.)

tion of 100 μM — which would produce about 1.4 DNA-protein crosslinks per 10^6 nucleotides[79] or about 2.8×10^4 per cell — still permitted 70 per cent of the cells to survive and form colonies.[93] Hence, cells are capable of successfully repairing DNA-protein crosslinks, at least of the type produced by *trans*-DDP.

Differences between the types of crosslinks produced by *cis-* or *trans*-DDP in mammalian cells have also been studied in isolated mammalian nucleosomal cores. *Cis*-DDP was found to bind preferentially to the DNA of nucleosomal cores with little interference from histones, whereas *trans*-DDP rapidly formed DNA-protein and protein-protein (histone-to-histone) crosslinks.[81]

Prevention of Interstrand Crosslink Formation by Thiourea

A potentially new approach in the pharmacologic application of Pt complexes is presented by the possibility of using avid Pt binders such as thiourea to prevent or possibly reverse some of the chemical actions of these drugs. The binding of thiourea to Pt is very stable and should irreversibly inactivate the bound Pt site.[72, 73, 94, 95] The possible ways in which thiourea may interfere with the crosslinking reactions of *cis*-Pt(II) complexes is schematized in Figure 14–8.[95] Three kinds of effects are possible.

1. Thiourea may react with free Pt(II) species — either in the chloride or aquo form — and thereby prevent any possibility of crosslink formation (Fig. 14–9, reactions 5 and 5′). Concentrations as low as 1 mM can prevent the cytotoxicity of *cis*-DDP when the thiourea is present at the time of *cis*-DDP addition.[94]

2. After one reactive Pt site has reacted with a macromolecular site (such as a DNA base) to form a monoadduct (Fig. 14–8, reaction 2), the second reactive Pt site may bind to thiourea (reactions 6 and 6′) before it reacts with another DNA base to form a

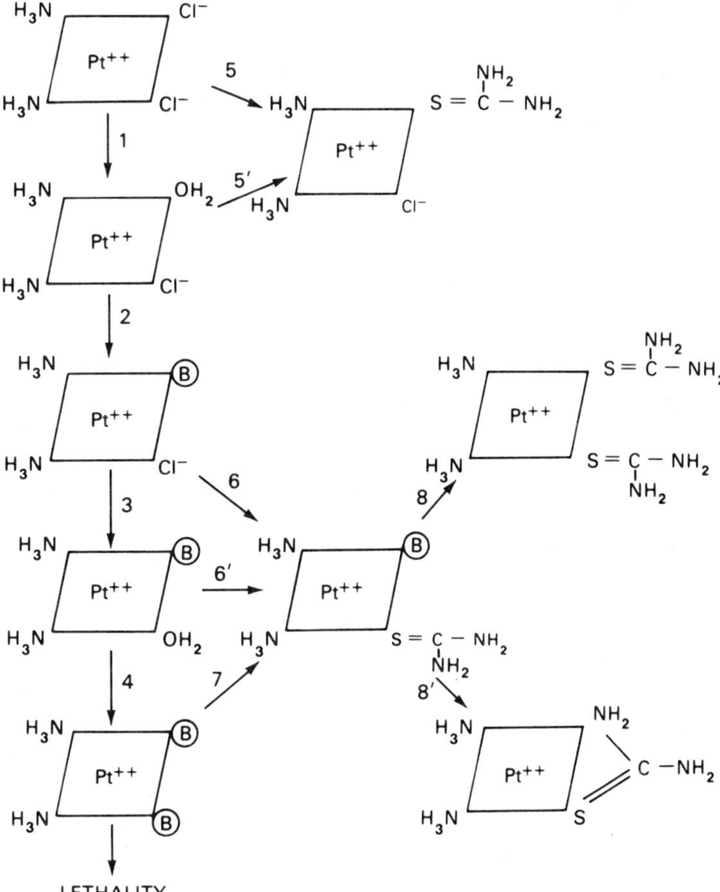

Figure 14–8. Possible ways in which thiourea may interfere with DNA crosslink formation by *cis*-DDP. (Reproduced with permission from Zwelling et al.: Effects of thiourea on survival and DNA cross-link formation in cells treated with platinum(II) complexes, L-phenylalanine mustard and bis(2-chloroethyl)methylamine. Cancer Res. 39:4989, 1979.)

crosslink (reaction 4). This monoadduct inactivation process is favored by the slowness of the crosslinking step (reaction 4), which is delayed about 6 hours. If thiourea is added during the latent period, interstrand crosslinking is prevented and considerable rescue of cells can be demonstrated (Fig. 14–9).[95] The crosslink prevention and survival enhancement occur in parallel fashion with respect to thiourea concentration or time of addition, as would be expected if crosslinking were causally related to cell killing.

3. Thiourea has been shown to reverse interstrand crosslinks and other lethal lesions in isolated DNA.[67, 72, 73] The thiourea concentrations required for this effect, however, were not attainable in viable cells.[95]

The point of pharmacologic interest is that the cytotoxicity of *cis*-Pt(II) complexes can be reduced by thio compounds, even if these are administered a short time after the Pt complex.

Role of DNA Repair Mechanisms

The various types of Pt adducts to DNA, including interstrand and DNA-protein crosslinks, are removed through the action of cellular DNA repair mechanisms.[83, 88]

Prokaryotes and eukaryotic cells have a multiplicity of DNA repair mechanisms to deal with various types of DNA damage. The repair mechanisms that obtain in enhancing survival differ, depending on the DNA-damaging agent. In *E. coli*, the ability to survive *cis*-Pt(II) treatment depends mainly on the excision repair function, *exr* (now called *lex*), and to a lesser degree on the host cell reactivation function, *hcr*. This dependence differs from those of other DNA-damaging agents, such as ultraviolet (UV) light, methylating agents, and x-ray[24] (Table 14–3).

The role of the various DNA repair mechanisms of mammalian cells in protecting

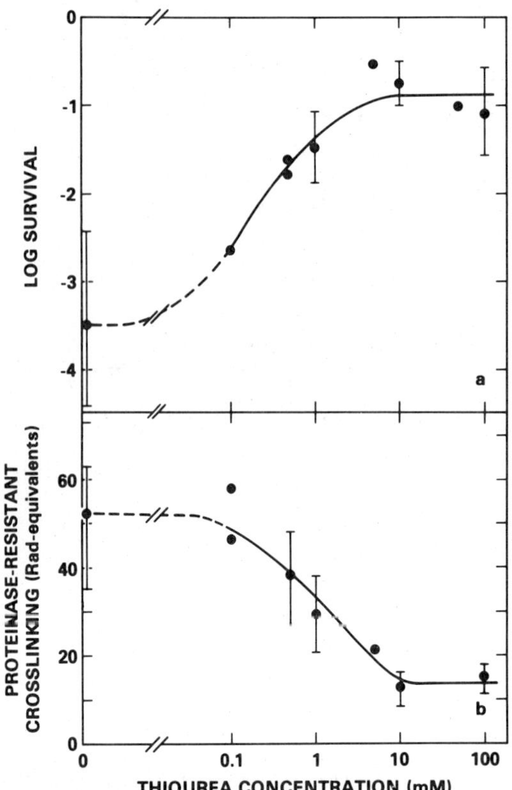

Figure 14–9. Thiourea prevention of crosslink formation *(b)* and enhancement of cell survival *(a)* in L1210 cells following *cis*-DDP treatment. (Reproduced with permission from Zwelling et al.: Effects of thiourea on survival and DNA cross-link formation in cells treated with platinum(II) complexes, L-phenylalanine mustard and bis(2-chloroethyl)methylamine. Cancer Res. 39:4989, 1979.)

TABLE 14–3. Effects of DNA Repair Defects on Sensitivity of *E. coli* to DNA Damaging Agents*

Agent†	*exr*	*hcr*	*fil*
UV	3–6	4–17	4–12
MNNG	3–3.6	1–1.2	3
X-ray	1.6–1.9	–	–
cis-DDP	13–23	1.8–5	1.0

*Given as sensitivity increase factor due to a defect in each phenotype.

†UV, ultraviolet light; MNNG, 1-methyl-nitroso-3-nitroguanidine.

Modified from data in Drobnik et al.[24]

cells against the lethal effects of Pt complexes is still not clear. Fraval et al.[96] found that a UV-repair defective strain of xeroderma pigmentosum cells was almost equally sensitive to *cis*-DDP, as compared with a strain of human fetal lung cells. However, when differences between Pt binding to DNA in these two cell strains were taken into account, the xeroderma cells appeared to be more sensitive than the fetal lung cells. These authors also reported a difference between the repair of UV and *cis*-DDP lesions in that a UV-specific endonuclease from *Micrococcus luteus,* which cleaved DNA strands extracted from UV-irradiated Chinese hamster cells, had no effect on DNA from cells treated with *cis*-DDP. Changes in the DNA sedimentation and DNA alkaline elution profiles from *cis*-DDP–treated cells with time following drug treatment have demonstrated crosslink formation and subsequent removal. The crosslink removal effect may be that of crosslink repair.[40, 80, 93, 95, 97] Additionally, a form of repair that may be unique to rodent cells, caffeine-sensitive postreplication repair, is induced by *cis*-DDP (see below).[88, 98, 99]

It would seem, then, that both the cell's ability to repair *cis*-DDP damage and the magnitude of this damage could determine the cell's ultimate survival. Recent work with mammalian cells resistant to *cis*-DDP supports this concept. Zwelling et al. have noted a relationship between *cis*-DDP DNA crosslinking and *in vitro* and *in vivo* cell survival. The survival of sensitive/resistant murine leukemia lines to *cis*-DDP treatment correlated with DNA interstrand crosslinking as measured by alkaline elution.[100] Similar findings in human Burkitt's lymphoma cells[101] and normal and SV-40-transformed human fibroblasts[102] have also been reported. However, several exceptions were found to a simple correlation between the absolute level of crosslinking produced by a given *cis*-DDP dose and the resultant cytotoxicity.[100, 101, 103] These deviations from the expected relationship between interstrand crosslinking and cytotoxicity could derive from lesions not measured by techniques that quantitate interstrand crosslinks (e.g., intrastrand crosslinks) or differences among cell lines in regard to their ability to tolerate interstrand crosslinks, including differences in repair capacity. As an example, Micetich et al. have characterized a *cis*-DDP–resistant cell line in which *cis*-DDP crosslinks form at a reduced rate, owing either to intracellular inactivation or to rapid repair of DNA-Pt monoadducts.[104]

Cell Cycle Relationships

The cell cycle phase-dependence of *cis*-DDP cytotoxicity is unusual in that some cell types are much more sensitive in G_1 phase than in S phase. This was demonstrated by Roberts and Fraval[105, 106] in both Chinese hamster cells and HeLa cells, and was verified by measurements of colony survival as a function of Pt binding to cell DNA. (In human lymphoma cells this phase-dependence was less dramatic.[107])

This phase-dependence may be influenced by the time delay inherent in DNA crosslink formation. Thus, treatment of cells in G_1 would lead to maximal crosslinking about six hours later, at which time the cells would be in S phase. Hence, although cells are most sensitive to drug exposure during G_1 phase, it would appear that they may be most sensitive to DNA crosslink formation during S phase.

When Chinese hamster cells are exposed to *cis*-DDP for one hour during G_1 phase, the subsequent S phase and cell division are delayed for several hours, the magnitude of the delay increasing with drug dose.[108] It appears that the Pt-induced DNA damage interferes with DNA synthesis, and that the block is overcome with time, possibly owing to some form of lesion repair or to some process that circumvents the DNA lesions. The recovery of DNA synthesis however, is not accounted for by overall removal of Pt adducts from the DNA, because this removal appears to be too slow,[105, 109] although recent work with human fibroblasts indicated that interstrand crosslink removal occurred more rapidly than the removal of Pt adducts.[110]

If the Pt dose is not too high, the second S phase and cell division following G_1 treatment occur after a normal cycle time, suggesting that the DNA block has by this time been overcome.[108] Despite the removal of the immediate DNA block, however, most of the cells fail to continue proliferation into colonies.

Caffeine, a known inhibitor of certain DNA repair processes in rodent cells, prevents the delay in DNA synthesis that occurs during the first S phase after treatment of Chinese hamster cells with *cis*-DDP. However, the DNA synthesized under these conditions is in the form of relatively short segments whose joining into long strands is delayed.[99] This can be interpreted in terms of the ability of caffeine to inhibit a repair process that permits replication past lesions existing on the DNA template strand.

In contrast to the case of Chinese hamster cells, the human HeLa cell line did not show a delay in the onset of S phase following *cis*-DDP treatment in G_1 phase.[111] Instead, the amount of ^{3}H-thymidine incorporation during S — or the fraction of cells going through S — was diminished: whereas the rodent cells exhibited a delayed S phase followed by a normal cell cycle duration, the human cells entered the first S phase at the normal time but were delayed in entering the second S phase. The human cells also differed in that they did not show the effects of caffeine seen in the rodent cells. This is not unexpected, since human cells generally do not exhibit the caffeine-sensitive post-replication repair that is usual for rodent cells.

In addition to phase-specificity differences in cell sensitivity to *cis*-DDP, cycle-specificity has been described in two studies in which exponentially growing cells were less sensitive than stationary cells to *cis*-DDP.[109, 112] In one of these studies, this difference was attributed to a greater ability of exponentially growing cells to excise Pt adducts from their DNA.[109]

These species differences in cell physiologic response to *cis*-DDP suggest that drug effects on tumor and normal cells in rodents do not necessarily predict the effects in humans.

EFFECTS ON THE IMMUNE SYSTEM

Most of the agents used to treat human malignancy are immunosuppressive, and several have been used in the therapy of nonmalignant disorders of immunologic origin.[113] Initial evidence appeared to classify *cis*-DDP among these agents as an immunosuppressive. Antibody-mediated spleen-plaque formation,[114, 115] skin graft rejection,[116, 117] adjuvant-induced arthritis,[118] and graft-versus-host responses[119] were all suppressed in animals treated with *cis*-DDP. DNA synthesis in phytohemagglutinin-stimulated lymphocytes was suppressed by *cis*-DDP, much as it had been in other cell types[87] (see above). The growth of B and T cells in culture was inhibited by *cis*-DDP.[120]

Mally et al. measured the effects of *cis*-DDP on several functions of human peripheral blood lymphocytes and malignant human lymphoblasts.[121] *Cis*-DDP also inhibited DNA and protein synthesis by the lymphoblast line. Most important, malignant lymphoblast target cells treated with *cis*-DDP displayed a decreased ability to stimulate ^{3}H-thymidine uptake by normal responder T lymphocytes as compared with *trans*-DDP–treated or untreated malignant targets. This immune recognition by T lymphocytes was not suppressed when mitogen-stimulated normal lymphoblast targets were substituted for the malignant lines. *Cis*-DDP was thought to lower tumor antigenicity.

In addition to immunosuppressive actions, recent work suggests that *cis*-DDP may also function to stimulate certain immune processes. Kleinerman et al. have shown that both *cis*-DDP[122] and x-rays[123] can stimulate spontaneous monocyte-mediated cytotoxicity (SMMC), an *in vitro* measure of the ability of human peripheral blood monocytes to lyse ^{51}Cr-labeled red cell targets. The ability of the monocyte effector cell to lyse the target is held in check by a lymphocyte suppressor cell that loses its suppressive effect over five to seven days in culture, then allowing the monocyte killer function to be expressed. X-irradiation enhanced this monocyte killer function by inhibiting the suppressor lymphocyte. By contrast, *cis*-DDP had no effect on the lymphocyte population, but instead directly stimulated the monocyte population, even at concentrations as low as 10^{-9}M. Mally et al., using a different measure of spontaneous cytotoxicity in which effector cells were lymphocytes, also noted an enhancement in immune function produced by *cis*-DDP. This appeared to be mediated through an effect on the target rather than the effector cell.[124]

In vitro tests like SMMC may correlate with *in vivo* immune function.[125] Patients with various neoplasms have been shown to have significantly depressed SMMC.[126] In a small group of eight patients with ovarian cancer, SMMC was followed during chemotherapy with a *cis*-DDP–containing regimen (cyclophosphamide, hexamethylmelamine, 5-fluourouracil) or with *cis*-DDP alone. All these patients had depressed SMMC when measured within two months of initiation of therapy. Only seven received six full months of therapy, but in those seven, all raised their SMMC at least threefold above initial values during therapy. Six of seven had objective tumor regression. Current investigations are aimed at discerning whether this preliminary clinical correlation is due to a direct effect of chemotherapy on immune function *in vivo* or a secondary phenomenon associated with improved disease status. *Cis*-DDP may not be unique in this regard, and future work will explore the effects of other antineoplastic compounds on immune functions like SMMC *in vitro* and *in vivo*. The enhancement of naturally occurring immune function is another possible mechanism by which *cis*-DDP, as well as other antineoplastic agents, produce tumor regression *in vivo*.

PHARMACOKINETICS

Introduction

Pharmacokinetics is the time-dependence of the concentrations of drug and its chemical and metabolic products in various body compartments following drug administration by a given route and schedule. Pharmacokinetic information is useful in so far as concentration *versus* time of relevant drug species at certain sites can be related to therapeutic activity or toxicity. The ideal of acquiring this information directly is rarely achieved, however, and judgments often must be based on incomplete information.

The chemical transformations of Pt(II) complexes in aqueous media are now fairly well known and the available information was summarized on p. 311 and Figure 14–2. The important question of the ability of the particular species to penetrate into cells is still mainly subject to conjecture. We can be reasonably confident that we know at least some of the active chemical species and the general types of reactions at target sites (see pp. 310–314). However, it has only recently been possible, in principle, to obtain pharmacokinetic information for the presumed active chemical species as distinguished from unreactive products.

Measurement of Pt Complexes in Biologic Samples

The inorganic nature of *cis*-DDP provides the clinical pharmacologist with a unique problem. The usual methods of radioactive drug labeling (^{14}C, ^{3}H, and so on) for distribution and pharmacokinetic studies are not applicable to *cis*-DDP *per se*, although these labels can be incorporated in *cis*-Pt(II) complexes having alkylamine ligands. Since the amine ligand remains firmly bound to the Pt atom under physiologic conditions, a labeled ethylenediamine moiety, for example, can be used as a tracer. Ethylenediamine Pt(II) dichloride is an active antitumor compound, and valuable pharmacologic data have been obtained using a ^{14}C-ethylenediamine label.[127]

Radioactive forms of Pt can be used in pharmacologic studies, but these γ-emitting Pt isotopes have half-lives of only about four days.[128-132]

A powerful, nonradioactive method for Pt analysis in biological samples is flameless atomic absorption spectroscopy (FAAS). Samples are atomized at 2700°C and absorbance is measured at 265.9 nm. Urine and blood samples can be measured directly and tissue samples can be measured after lyophilization.[133, 134] Typical Pt sensitivities were 0.35 μg per ml of plasma and 0.3 to 0.5 mg per kg of tissue. High-performance liquid chromatography (HPLC) has recently been used to detect Pt at 0.025 μg per ml in urine.[135] The major disadvantages of FAAS are the expense and complexity of the required apparatus and the long time required for sample preparation.

Another physical technique for Pt analysis is x-ray fluorescence spectroscopy, which is less time-consuming than FAAS, but has a substantially lower sensitivity.[136, 137]

Pt concentrations in plasma have also been measured colorimetrically after precipitation of plasma protein with sulfosalicylic acid.[138]

Free Pt can be separated from protein-bound Pt in plasma by centrifuge ultrafiltration. The ultrafiltrate can be converted to a cationic complex by reaction with ethylenediamine, collected on a paper disk impregnated with a cation-exchange resin, sonicated, dried, and prepared for atomic absorption assay by the addition of HCl.[139]

Recent applications of HPLC techniques have allowed analysis of the various *cis*-DDP aquation products. These techniques now permit studies of the distribution and pharmacokinetics of *cis*-DDP and its various derivatives.[135, 140-142]

Drug Administration

Cis-DDP is administered intravenously in an isotonic solution containing enough NaCl to avoid drug decomposition (see p. 000). Dilution in 5 per cent dextrose/water, however, has been reported to lead to the appearance of new products over several hours.[143] Repta et al.[144] report that, in the absence of Cl^-, 10 per cent of the *cis*-DDP (analyzed by HPLC) is lost in 40 to 60 minutes at 25° C, but that in the presence of as little as 0.1 per cent NaCl, 10 per cent loss occurs only after six hours. In 0.45 per cent NaCl (one half physiologic saline), less than 5 per cent of the *cis*-DDP was lost over a 48-hour period. The rates of loss were stated to be unaffected by the presence of 5 per cent dextrose or mannitol. LeRoy,[145] however, reports at least 15 per cent loss in four hours at 25° C in 0.45 per cent NaCl plus 5 per cent dextrose. In view of these uncertainties, *cis*-DDP should not be kept in solutions of low Cl^- concentration for prolonged periods before administration. If NaCl administration must be limited for clinical reasons, the time between dilution into low-chloride media and completion of the infusion should probably be kept to less than one hour. Alternatively, a slow infusion pump can be used to administer the saline drug solution over a prolonged period. Since a precipitate of Pt can be formed in intravenous solutions containing bicarbonate, such solutions should be avoided.[142]

The infusion equipment used for the administration of *cis*-DDP must not include aluminum needles, because the Pt(II) undergoes an oxidation displacement reaction with aluminum metal, yielding a brownish or black precipitate accompanied by a loss of *cis*-DDP from the solution.[146, 147] Stainless steel needles appear to be satisfactory.

Clinical Usage

The clinical spectrum in which *cis*-DDP has proven efficacy is narrower than some of the alkylating agents. However, it is clearly active in the treatment of germinal neoplasms of the testes, advanced ovarian carci-

TABLE 14–4. Some Typical Doses and Schedules of *cis*-DDP

2–3 mg/kg	every 3–4 wks
20 mg/m²/day × 5 days	every 3–4 wks
100–120 mg/m²	every 3–4 wks
80 mg/m² (24-hr infusion)	every 3–4 wks

noma, and head and neck cancer. Detailed reviews compiling the data from many clinical trials have recently been published.[148-150] Response rates of up to 100 per cent have been reported in patients with testicular cancer treated with a combination of *cis*-DDP, bleomycin, and vinblastine,[9] and some of the complete remissions have translated into increased survival time. *Cis*-DDP has also demonstrated single-agent activity in the treatment of bladder cancer, and variable degrees of success have been achieved with regimens containing *cis*-DDP in the treatment of patients with cervical cancer and possibly lung cancer and osteogenic sarcoma. *Cis*-DDP has no activity in the treatment of breast or colorectal malignancies.

Some of the *cis*-DDP doses commonly used are listed in Table 14–4. *Cis*-DDP should be given by oncologists or oncology nurses skilled in its use and in the use of techniques to counter its nephrotoxicity (see below). Some of the drugs frequently used in combination with *cis*-DDP are listed in Table 14–5.

Reactions in Plasma

The Cl^- concentration of plasma tends to prevent the aquation reaction and therefore maintains the drug in the relatively unreactive dichloro form. The conclusion that the drug is totally unreactive in plasma must be reconsidered, however, because of a progressive binding of Pt to plasma proteins,[130, 131] which could be the result of covalent reaction.

TABLE 14–5. Other Antineoplastic Agents Commonly Used with *cis*-DDP

Testicular Cancer
- Vinblastine
- Bleomycin
- Actinomycin D

Ovarian Cancer
- Cyclophosphamide
- Doxorubicin (Adriamycin)
- Hexamethylmelamine
- 5-Fluorouracil

Head and Neck Cancer
- Bleomycin
- Methotrexate

The first question is whether the aquation reaction in fact is completely prevented in plasma. From the equilibrium constants given in Table 14–2, it can be concluded that, at equilibrium in 0.15 M Cl^-, the concentration of the chloro-aquo form would be about 3 per cent that of the dichloro form. Assuming a half-life of two hours at 37° C for this aquation reaction, about 1 per cent of the drug would be in the reactive chloro-aquo form after one hour. Whether this small extent of conversion could have biologic significance is questionable.

As was explained on p. 323, the chloride ligand is firmly enough bound to the Pt atom so that it is unlikely to be displaced by amines, including the probable nucleic acid binding sites. Chloride ligands, however, could be directly displaced by sulfur-containing compounds, such as sulfhydryl groups of proteins or other molecules in plasma.

Protein binding of *cis*-DDP was first noted by DeConti et al.[128] in human serum. Since the binding was not inhibited by NaCl concentrations up to 2 M, these authors felt that covalent binding was unlikely. However, the possibility of direct displacement of chloride ligands by sulfhydryl groups also should be considered.

The findings of Litterst et al.[151] and LeRoy et al.[18] that the reaction has exponential kinetics suggest that the protein binding in fact may be covalent. After addition of *cis*-DDP to dog plasma, the concentration of nonprotein-bound Pt (measured by the ability of Pt to pass through a 50,000 MW cut-off ultrafilter) declined with a half-life of 2.7 hours. In the intact dog, Manaka and Wolf[131] found the rate of decline of unbound drug to be much faster: the protein binding of Pt was 22 per cent after two minutes, 49 per cent after 15 minutes, and 89 per cent after 60 minutes. This apparently more rapid rate can be explained on the basis of selective urinary excretion and tissue uptake of free drug. The bound Pt was precipitable with the plasma proteins by means of ammonium sulfate, and migrated with the plasma proteins, especially with serum albumin, in gel electrophoresis.

This is in accord with an irreversible covalent bond. After binding to plasma proteins, the drug is no longer cytotoxic to cells in culture.[152] The binding to plasma proteins thus may irreversibly remove the drug from any further possibility of pharmacologic action.[153]

LeRoy et al. believed that protein binding occurred only after aquation of the drug, and that it is the aquation rate that limits the rate of protein binding.[18] They did not consider the possibility of direct binding of unchanged drug to protein at reactive sulfhydryl sites.

Gullo et al.[154] observed *cis*-DDP binding to a variety of proteins in human plasma. High levels of Pt were noted in the γ-globulin and albumin-transferrin fractions (Sephadex G-200 chromatography). Incubation of *cis*-DDP with purified transferrin or serum albumin resulted in Pt binding to each of these proteins.

Serum albumin could well be a major Pt-binding site, since this protein molecule contains a reactive sulfhydryl group. The albumin concentration in plasma (about 0.8 mM) is well in excess of the maximal plasma levels of Pt expected in man (e.g., 0.03 mM after 70 mg/m^2).[152] The binding of Pt to albumin through a sulfhydryl group would be expected to be irreversible, and the Pt would remain in the plasma as long as the protein molecule to which it is bound.

In addition to binding to plasma proteins, *cis*-DDP may well react directly with small molecules containing sulfhydryl groups. Such products could be filterable and yet represent inactivated drug products. The chemical nature of Pt species in plasma and urine as a function of time still remains to be determined.

Transport into Cells

Little direct information is available on the transport of *cis*-DDP species into cells. It is generally supposed that the uncharged species — e.g., dichloro, chloro-hydroxy, dihydroxy (see Fig. 14–2) — can penetrate cell membranes by passive diffusion and that the charged species are excluded.[155, 156] The drug, however, penetrates only to a small extent into cerebrospinal fluid or brain,[157, 158] which argues against the free diffusion of any of the major drug species through membrane barriers.

Fate, Distribution, and Excretion

Most studies of distribution and excretion have measured only the total Pt concentrations or have distinguished only between free and protein-bound Pt. The *in vivo* drug transformations into various chemical species and reactions with various body constituents are key factors awaiting further study.

Plasma Disappearance

After intravenous administration of *cis*-DDP in various animal species, including man, the plasma concentration of Pt falls relatively quickly for one to four hours and then levels off as the drug becomes bound to plasma proteins.[159] Estimates of the initial plasma disappearance rate differ widely, probably because two or more rate processes are encompassed within the early events. There must be at least two early processes contributing to the fall in plasma Pt concentration: (1) entry into tissues, and (2) renal excretion. These two processes have not been experimentally distinguished and may contribute to the variability of the plasma half-life estimates, which range from less than 10 to more than 40 minutes. (It can be assumed that entry into tissues and renal excretion is possible only for nonprotein-bound forms of Pt.)

During the first few hours after drug administration, the proportion of Pt in the plasma that is bound to protein increases until very little unbound Pt remains. The plasma Pt level then falls extremely slowly, with half-lives usually estimated in the range of one to five days.

In man, the plasma clearance of total Pt was reported by DeConti et al.[128] to be 25 to 49 minutes for the fast phase, followed by 58 to 73 hours during the slow phase. At the time when the slow phase was reached (about four hours after injection), more than 90 per cent of the plasma Pt was protein-bound, as indicated by gel filtration studies. During the rapid phase of plasma clearance, urinary excretion of Pt was rapid, and then it decreased to a very slow rate.

Since the protein-bound Pt is not cytotoxic,[152, 160] the most pertinent pharmacologic parameter is the plasma concentration of unbound Pt as a function of time. The fall in the plasma concentration of nonprotein-bound Pt depends on (1) its rate of urinary excretion, (2) its rate of entry into and binding in tissue, (3) its rate of binding to blood cells, and (4) its rate of binding to plasma proteins. Although some of the Pt may become bound to small molecules in plasma, and thereby become inactivated, the nonprotein-bound Pt concentration *versus* time is at present the best measure of effective dosage. This means that plasma Pt determinations are likely to have therapeutic significance only during the first few hours after the drug enters the circulation, and the most significant values would be those obtained at the earliest times.

Patton et al.[160] determined plasma disappearance of filterable (nonbound) Pt in patients following intravenous *cis*-DDP administration. Following an initial rapid decline, free drug concentration fell with a half-life in the range of 23 to 54 minutes, depending on the mode of administration. When the dose (100 mg/m^2) was given quickly, the maximal plasma concentration of filterable Pt was 2.9 to 4.9 μg per ml (14.5 to 24.5 μM) (three patients) and the plasma half-life was 32 to 54 minutes. When the same dose was given in a 6-hour infusion, the maximal concentration achieved was 0.46 to 0.54 μg per ml (2.3 to 2.7 μM) (three patients) and the half-life was 17 to 37 minutes. The difference in half-lives was significant and resulted in a substantial difference in the fraction of the administered Pt recovered in the urine in 24 hours: following bolus injection 50 $\pm$ 5 per cent of the dose was recovered, whereas following infusion 75 $\pm$ 3 per cent of the dose was recovered. The origin of this difference is not clear, but one may suppose that the effective dose would generally be in proportion to the amount of Pt retained in the body.

When plasma protein binding is nearly complete, Pt elimination becomes very slow. The consequences of the slow fall in plasma Pt over a period of days or weeks is unknown, but the possibility of chronic toxicity due to prolonged retention of unreactive Pt is not eliminated. The rate of fall of total plasma Pt is probably governed by the rate of degradation of plasma proteins bearing bound Pt. The normal turnover rate of serum albumin, for example, is $t\frac{1}{2}$ = four days.[161] In addition, degradation products of Pt-containing tissue macromolecules would be expected to enter the circulation and be excreted in the urine or bile.[18, 162, 163]

Tissue Distribution

Cis-DDP rapidly enters a variety of tissues, and a fraction of the administered Pt is retained in tissues for long periods. The initial tissue distribution, occurring perhaps during the first 30 minutes following intravenous administration, gives an indication of the distribution of unchanged *cis*-DDP that can then react intracellularly. As time progresses, an increasing fraction of the drug becomes bound to plasma and tissue proteins, yielding inactive bound Pt species. As already suggested, the binding to certain reactive protein sites might not require aquation of the drug, whereas binding to nucleic acids does require such activation. Some of the administered Pt remains in tissues, presumably in a bound inactive form, for many days or weeks.

Litterst et al.[151] and LeRoy et al.[18] measured tissue Pt concentrations in the dog at various times following intravenous injection of 1 mg per kg *cis*-DDP. At early times (10 to 60 minutes), which may reflect the distribution of active drug species, the highest concentrations appeared in kidney > liver, ovary, uterus, and lung. Except for the higher kidney concentrations, the Pt concentrations in these tissues at these times were in the range of 0.7 to 1.8 μg per gm of wet tissue. Low initial concentrations (<0.4 μg/gm) were found in muscle, heart, intestine, pancreas, and spleen. Intermediate results were obtained for skin, adrenal gland, and colon. For essentially all tissues, 25 to 100 per cent of the Pt content noted at 60 minutes was still present after four days. LeRoy et al.[18] simulated the tissue distribution curves by means of a pharmacokinetic model based on several assumptions (LeRoy et al.,[18] Fig. 5).

The distribution of Pt in various tissue compartments in rats was studied by Wolf and Manaka.[164] The data were reported as the fraction of administered dose present in each organ. Thus, although Pt concentration in skin was relatively low, the large total quantity of this tissue made it the major site of Pt deposition (Fig. 14–10). It is remarkable that, in all the major sites of Pt deposition (skin > bone, muscle > liver > blood, kidney), there was relatively little loss of Pt between one hour and three days. At one hour about 40 per cent of the administered Pt was accounted for in these tissues; most of the rest had

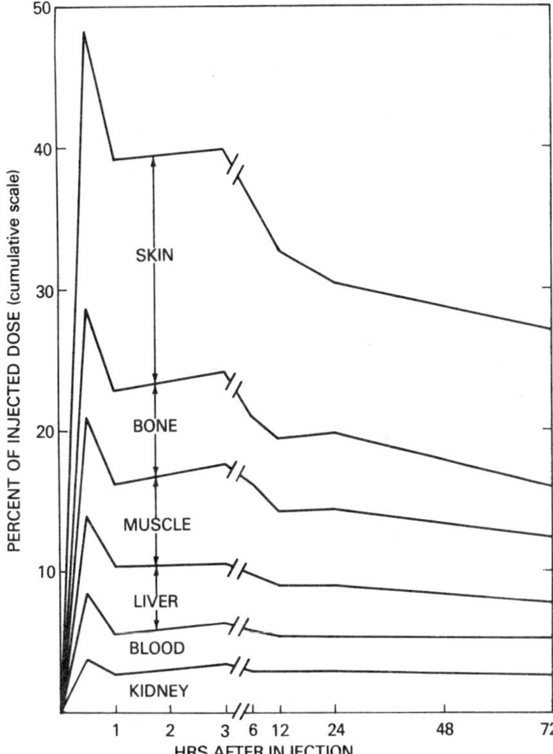

Figure 14–10. Tissue distribution of Pt in rats following intravenous injection of 1 mg/kg *cis*-DDP. (Plotted from data of Wolf W, and Manaka RC: Synthesis and distribution of ^{196m}Pt *cis*-dichlorodiammine platinum(II). J. Clin. Hematol. Oncol. 7:79, 1977.)

presumably been excreted in the urine. After three days 27 per cent of the administered Pt was still in these tissues. In bone the uptake apparently was mainly in the matrix, since the Pt concentration in bone marrow was stated to be low.

Wolf and Manaka[164] measured Pt content in skin biopsies obtained 18 days following therapy in patients receiving *cis*-DDP, and estimated that 13 per cent of the administered Pt was still present in the skin.

Cis-DDP does not readily penetrate into the cerebrospinal fluid or brain,[151, 152, 159, 160] even though the unchanged drug and some of its hydrolytic products are neutral molecules. Gormley et al.[157] observed cerebrospinal fluid Pt concentrations in monkeys to increase to a maximum 30 to 40 minutes after a rapid intravenous dose of *cis*-DDP, but the CSF/plasma concentration ratio never exceeded 0.04. Three other *cis*-Pt(II) complexes were tested, but showed no improvement in CSF/plasma ratios; the complexes tested were the malonato, sulfato, and 4-carboxyphthalato derivatives of 1,2-diaminocyclohexane-Pt(II). In one patient the CSF/plasma ratio was 0.025 to 0.05.[158]

Platinum has also been detected in pleural[165] and ascitic fluid.[166] This latter third space, common among patients with ovarian cancer, has been postulated to be a potential Pt reservoir.[166] The inference was based on measurements of filterable Pt concentrations in ascites and plasma. It is not known whether the Pt is in pharmacologically active species, however.

The retention of Pt in various tissues would be expected to depend on multiple factors, including (1) rates of Pt uptake into cells, (2) rates of Pt binding to small molecules that can be exported from cells, (3) rates of Pt binding to macromolecules (or to small molecules) that are retained in cells, and (4) rates of turnover of retained molecules bearing bound Pt. It is not surprising, therefore, that, with the exception of kidney, no correlation has been discerned between Pt concentrations in normal or tumor tissues and the observed biologic responses.[167]

The selective retention in kidney appears to be less in the case of certain *cis*-DDP analogues than for *cis*-DDP itself,[167] suggesting the possibility that this criterion may permit the identification of analogues having reduced renal toxicity.

Excretion

In various animal species, including man, the kidney is the major route of excretion of *cis*-DDP or its chemical products, accounting for the eventual excretion of perhaps 70 to 90 per cent of the administered Pt. Renal excretion of Pt is most rapid immediately after entry of the drug into the circulation. The renal excretion rate then falls markedly as the concentration in plasma declines and as the drug binds to plasma proteins. Only a fraction of the administered Pt (typically 15 to 60 per cent) is excreted during the first few hours, and the remainder may be excreted very slowly over a period of several weeks. The renal excretion is of low-molecular-weight Pt species, probably at first mainly unchanged drug, which are filtered freely through the glomerulus.

However, Jacobs et al.[168] have shown that free-Pt clearance can exceed glomerular filtration rate (GFR) (simultaneously measured creatinine clearance) by as much as 50 per cent, implying that *cis*-DDP or a metabolite may also be secreted by the renal tubule. In animals the major area of tubular secretion is the pars recta of the proximal tubule in the outer medulla. This area has been shown to be the site of greatest Pt accumulation and damage in Pt nephropathy in animals. It has recently been found that the nephrotoxicity of Pt can be decreased by probenecid.[169] This protection may be due to inhibition by probenecid of this proximal tubular secretion.

At later times the excreted Pt presumably is in chemically altered form, perhaps in the form of reaction products of *cis*-DDP with small molecules containing sulfhydryl or amino groups. The chemical nature of the Pt compounds excreted at various times remains to be investigated.

Aside from the renal route, a small percentage of Pt excretion occurs in bile[18, 162, 163] and perhaps also in saliva.[170] The excretion in bile is slight at early times after drug administration and then increases with time, indicating that only chemically or metabolically altered forms of the drug are excreted by this route.

LeRoy et al.[18] estimated the initial renal clearance of Pt in the dog to be of the same order as the GFR, which would suggest that Pt is excreted by glomerular filtration without tubular secretion in this case. Pt clearance fell rapidly for one to two hours after an intravenous dose and then continued at about 1 per cent of the initial clearance for many days. During the slow and prolonged phase of Pt excretion some Pt appeared in the bile, but the rate of biliary excretion was only about 6 per cent of the slow rate of renal excretion. The Pt concentration in the bile increased for 24 hours, perhaps reflecting the formation of chemical forms of Pt that can be expected by this route.

Urinary excretion in rats accounted for 30 to 40 per cent of the administered dose in four hours, following 5 mg per kg of *cis*-DDP IV.[159] Urinary excretion of Pt continued at a decreasing rate for at least 30 days, at which time about 75 per cent of the administered Pt had been eliminated in the urine (Litterst et al.,[159] Fig. 1).

DeConti et al.[128] found that urinary excretion in man following a rapid IV dose of *cis*-DDP occurred rapidly at first, 15 to 27 per cent of the administered Pt being eliminated in six hours, and then much more slowly, so that a total of only 27 to 45 per cent of the administered Pt was recovered in the urine by five days. Chromatographic analysis in three patients indicated that 33 to 72 per cent of the Pt excreted during the first six hours was not in the form of *cis*-DDP, but the nature of the alteration — whether aquation or reaction with other small molecules — was not determined.[128]

Gormley et al.[152] studied plasma disappearance and renal excretion of Pt in patients treated with *cis*-DDP together with diuretics and hydration to protect the kidney. *Cis*-DDP (70 mg/m^2) was given as an IV infusion over a period of one hour. Patients were hydrated intravenously, and given a six-hour infusion of 10 per cent mannitol beginning one hour before drug and an injection of 40 mg furosemide just before the start of the *cis*-DDP infusion. The peak plasma concentration of total Pt was 30 $\pm$ 6 μM at the end of the *cis*-DDP infusion, and then fell, stabilizing three hours later at about 14 μM. (Plasma Pt levels then fell slowly with a half-life of 2.8 days, but 21 days later the Pt levels were still 1.6 $\pm$ 0.5 μM.) Renal excretion was rapid for about three hours, during which time about 16 per cent of the administered Pt was excreted. Excretion then slowed markedly, and the total excretion at the end of 24 hours was only 23 $\pm$ 4 per cent. The fall in renal excretion rate during the first three hours was in proportion to the extent of protein binding that occurred during this time. This was as expected if only nonprotein-bound Pt was excreted in the urine. The renal clearance of Pt initially approximated the GFR (estimated on the basis of pretreatment creatinine clearance values), and then fell exponentially with a half-life of about 50 minutes. These results are in accord with the simple picture that excretion proceeds primarily by glomerular filtration of nonprotein-bound Pt and is curtailed by the binding of Pt to plasma proteins. The possibility of tubular secretion, however, is not excluded.[168, 169]

TOXICOLOGY

Until recently the major toxicity limiting the clinical use of *cis*-DDP was renal. It appears now that the kidney can be partially protected by the use of hydration and diuretics, and the emerging limiting toxicities now appear to be myelosuppression and nausea.

Although Pt is excreted to some extent in the bile, there appears to be no significant hepatic toxicity.[171] Litterst et al.[159] found no effect of *cis*-DDP on hepatic drug metabolism in the rat. The toxicities discussed below are listed in Table 14–6.

Renal Toxicity

The earlier experience with Pt nephrotoxicity in animals and man has been summarized by Madias and Harrington.[172] The evidence surveyed indicated that renal toxicity occurs in about 30 per cent of patients receiving a single dose of *cis*-DDP in the range of 2 mg per kg or 50 to 75 mg per m^2. A similar incidence was noted for a five-day course of 15 to 20 mg per m^2 per day. However, the toxicity produced by a single course of either of these two regimens was usually mild-to-moderate and reversible. Following higher doses or repeated courses, the nephrotoxicity increases in frequency and severity and may become irreversible.

More recent experience indicates that the nephrotoxicity can be reduced by physiologic and pharmacologic means that will be discussed.

Madias and Harrington note that the nephrotoxicity produced by *cis*-DDP is in some respects similar to the effects of heavy metal poisoning by mercury salts.[172]

TABLE 14–6. Toxicities of *cis*-DDP in Humans

Toxicity
Renal tubular damage
Nausea and vomiting
Myelosuppression, hemolytic anemia (2 cases)
Decreased hearing and deafness
Peripheral neuropathy
Hypomagnesemic tetany
Seizures
Allergic reactions, including anaphylaxis
Toxic liver damage (1 case)
Coronary artery disease (2 cases)
Platinum gum line (1 case)

Morphologic and Chemical Changes in the Kidney

The main sites of morphologic changes due to *cis*-DDP are in the renal tubules, while the glomeruli remain unaffected. Proximal tubular necrosis has been reported in rat, mouse, marmoset monkey,[173-175] and dog.[176] The proximal tubules in the rat showed an early loss of the brush border of the microvilli.[174] Necrotizing and degenerative lesions then developed in the pars recta of the proximal tubules located in the outer medullary stripe. These lesions reached a maximum at five days, and were accompanied by peaks in BUN and greatest weight loss.[174, 177, 178]

Some of the effects of *cis*-DDP resemble those of mercury salts.[172] Mercury and platinum are both heavy metals having a specific affinity for sulfhydryl groups. Levi et al.[179, 180] reported a decrease of protein-bound sulfhydryl groups in kidney of *cis*-DDP–treated rats. A simple reaction with a sulfhydryl group, however, may not fully explain the renal toxicity of *cis*-DDP, because no such toxicity is produced by the *trans*-Pt(II) isomer.[173]

Dentino et al.,[181] however, noted that, unlike victims of heavy metal poisoning, *cis*-DDP–treated patients did not exhibit renal tubular acidosis or prominent proteinuria. Urinary beta-glucuronidase, N-acetyl beta-glucosaminidase, and beta$_2$-microglobulin, however, may be elevated following *cis*-DDP therapy and may be useful monitors for Pt nephrotoxicity.[182, 183]

Pathologic examination of kidneys of patients dying at various times following administration of *cis*-DDP as the last single-agent therapy revealed focal coagulative necrosis of epithelium, which affected chiefly the *distal* convoluted tubules and collecting ducts.[184] These patients had normal BUN and creatinine levels prior to *cis*-DDP therapy, and these values became elevated after therapy. In support of the view that *cis*-DDP was the cause of the renal damage, it was noted that nuclear changes, affecting primarily the large renal collecting ducts, were a major feature. Similar alterations in nuclei have been observed following cyclophosphamide therapy in epithelium of bladder and esophagus, and are also produced by *cis*-DDP in intestinal epithelium.

Effects on Renal Blood Flow and Glomerular Filtration Rate

Animal studies of the acute nephrotoxicity produced by heavy metals, including mercuric chloride, suggested that the acute renal failure was due to marked reductions in GFR and renal blood flow.[172] The reduced renal blood flow, especially to the cortex and outer medulla, was thought to be mediated through activation of the renin-angiotensin system. In accord with this hypothesis, saline-loaded rats had less reductions in GFR and less azotemia despite similar degrees of tubular necrosis following the administration of mercuric chloride.[172]

Dentino et al.[181] reported that *cis*-DDP therapy in 15 patients with testicular carcinoma resulted in a regular and persistent decrease in GFR. Patients received three or more courses of 20 mg per m^2 per day for five days at three-week intervals without hydration or diuretics. Creatinine clearance fell from 112 ± 12 ml per min before therapy to 69 ± 12 ml per min six months later. At the same time there were only mild elevations in BUN. Renal biopsies in three of these patients revealed regions of cellular necrosis, hydropic degeneration, and nuclear atypia in *both proximal* and *distal* tubules three to six weeks following chemotherapy. At five months, focal interstitial fibrosis was evident, as well as tubular atrophy and dilatation.

Magnesium Loss

Recent clinical observations suggest that *cis*-DDP may interfere with the renal tubular reabsorption of magnesium.[185-187] Hypomagnesemia was observed in more than 50 per cent of evaluable patients following *cis*-DDP therapy. In some patients, inappropriate renal magnesium wasting was documented. *Cis*-DDP conceivably may inhibit a magnesium-transport system in the renal tubule.[188] In addition, potassium, phosphate, and calcium may be inappropriately excreted during or after *cis*-DDP treatment.[189]

Protection

Hydration and Diuretics. Attempts have been made during the last few years to protect the kidneys by increasing the urine flow during the period of rapid Pt excretion. This has been done by means of pretreatment hydration or the use of diuretics, particularly mannitol and furosemide. These procedures probably have little effect on the Pt concentration in the proximal tubules, since the fluid they contain is mainly an ultrafiltrate of plasma. The Pt concentrations in the more distal regions of the nephron, however, could be reduced by the maintenance of high fluid volumes.[190-193]

An additional protective mechanism that might be supposed to act in the distal nephron is the maintenance of high chloride concentrations that would retard Pt aquation. However, aquation could only be significant if the chloride concentration were sufficiently low and the transit time through the nephron sufficiently long.[194, 195]

The mechanism of renal protection is difficult to analyze at this time, because the mechanism of renal toxicity is not known. In particular, we do not know whether Pt must enter the renal tubule cells or whether toxicity may result from reactions at the cell surface. Pt damage may occur as a consequence of tubular secretion of *cis*-DDP or its metabolites.

Renal protection by diuresis may be particularly effective in man because, unlike its effect in several animal species, there may be relatively little effect on the proximal convoluted tubules: the major toxicity in man occurs in the distal parts of the nephron,[184] where the opportunity exists for protection by increased urine volume.

Reduction of *cis*-DDP–induced renal toxicity by means of diuresis was first reported by Cvitkovic et al.[191] Induction of diuresis by means of pretreatment hydration and mannitol administration to dogs prevented the increases in BUN and serum creatinine levels that were otherwise seen after *cis*-DDP treatment.

The induced diuresis, however, did not affect the plasma Pt concentration curve, and there was no significant protection against *cis*-DDP–induced leukopenia and thrombocytopenia.

Ward et al.[192, 193] found that rats could be partially protected against nephrotoxicity by administration of furosemide 30 minutes before *cis*-DDP. The pretreatment with furosemide diminished the renal tubular necrosis and the azotemia. However, furosemide did not reduce the gastrointestinal toxicity or the cellular depletion of the bone marrow, thymus, and spleen, and the survival of the rats was not significantly enhanced.

On the other hand, LeHane et al.,[196] using a different strain of rats, were unable to confirm the renal protective effect of diuresis, and in fact found that diuresis aggravated the nephrotoxicity of *cis*-DDP.

Pera et al.[197] studied the effects of furosemide and mannitol on *cis*-DDP–induced nephrotoxicity in rats. Either of the diuretics greatly reduced the impairments of renal function — as measured by increased BUN, decreased GFR, and decreased para-aminohippurate clearance — that followed *cis*-DDP administration. The diuretics, however, did not prevent the renal tubular necrosis (proximal convoluted tubules). Furosemide in fact seemed to increase and prolong the damage, perhaps owing to its own renal toxic effect. Mannitol appeared to reduce the duration of morphologic damage. Furosemide increased the amount of Pt deposited in the kidneys (at one or four days after *cis*-DDP), whereas mannitol tended to reduce this value. The diuretics, however, did not affect the plasma Pt level of disappearance rate or the urinary excretion of Pt.

In further studies, Pera and Harder[198] found that mannitol, but not furosemide, was able to protect rats against acute lethal toxicity. Mannitol, but not furosemide, also reduced the magnitude or duration of the *cis*-DDP–induced depression of proliferative cells in bone marrow, gastrointestinal mucosa, spleen, and thymus. Mannitol, however, did not impair the *cis*-DDP–induced enhancement of survival time in leukemic rats.

The possibility must be considered that the effects of mannitol may be partly due to a direct interaction with Pt(II) species, since complex formation between mannitol and Pt(II) has been demonstrated.[199] It is not clear, however, whether this interaction would occur to a significant extent under the conditions of mannitol diuresis.

The clinical use of hydration and diuretics can give at least partial protection of the kidneys, and permits the use of higher *cis*-DDP doses.[200-202] In the study by Chary et al.,[200] patients were hydrated with 1 liter of 5 per cent dextrose; *cis*-DDP was then infused over a six-hour period in 2 liters of 5 per cent dextrose, 0.33 per cent normal saline, and 40 mEq KCl, and 40 mg furosemide was injected at the beginning of the infusion. A transient fall in creatinine clearance was noted in some patients, but could have been related to the diuretic rather than the *cis*-DDP. Instead of renal toxicity, the limiting toxicities were myelosuppression, nausea, and emesis.

Stark and Howell[203] studied renal function following treatment of ten patients with 20 mg per m^2 per day for five days, with saline hydration as the only nephroprotective measure. They concluded that, with moderate saline hydration alone, patients can be treated with several courses of *cis*-DDP without significant nephrotoxicity but with retention of antitumor activity. Saline hydration was also the sole protection used in a recent trial of continuous 24-hour *cis*-DDP infusion. Antitumor activity was maintained without significant nephrotoxicity.[204]

Rescue by Thio Compounds. Borch and Pleasants[205] recently hypothesized that *cis*-DDP nephrotoxicity could be inhibited by means of a rescue stratagem using thio compounds. Their hypothesis was based on considerations of the probable action mechanisms of Hg(II). Hg(II) has a high binding affinity for sulfhydryl groups, which are abundant on the brush border of the proximal tubules. Hg(II) is postulated to induce diuresis by binding reversibly to the sulfhydryl group of a membrane-bound transport enzyme. Pt(II) may also bind to such sulfhydryl groups, but the binding would ordinarily be irreversible. The binding might, however, be reversed in the presence of thio compounds having a very high affinity for Pt.

The hypothesis was tested by the use of diethyldithiocarbamate ($Et_2NCS_2^-$), which has two sulfur atoms capable of chelating Pt. Since this is a charged molecule, it perhaps is excluded from cells, and hence would not interfere with the intracellular actions of *cis*-DDP. It would be filtered through the glomerulus, however, and could have access to Pt bound to the surface of the renal tubular cells.

When administered to rats one to four hours after *cis*-DDP, $Et_2NCS_2^-$ markedly reduced the azotemia, weight loss, and tubular necrosis seen five days later. In addition, the gastrointestinal toxicity, as indicated by the incidence of diarrhea, was ameliorated.

Since 95 per cent of Pt excretion by the kidney takes place within 1.5 hours, the effectiveness of $Et_2NCS_2^-$ administered at later times suggests that a rescue mechanism must be involved. $Et_2NCS_2^-$ is rapidly metabolized to the S-glucoimide, for example, and the compound also decomposes rapidly at pH < 7. Significant concentrations of the dithio compound in urine are likely to occur only if the urine is alkaline. The short lifetime of the dithio compound can explain the dependence of its effectiveness on the time of administraion. If the compound is administered too soon, it will have disappeared before Pt fixation in the kidney is complete. There appears to be a window of several hours during which fixed Pt might be removed, or a Pt lesion that is formed in a delayed fashion could be blocked by the dithio compound before the time that the injury to the renal tubule cells becomes irreversible. Of equal importance, this beneficial rescue could be effected while the antineoplastic potency of *cis*-DDP was maintained.[206, 207]

Other Toxicities

A major problem for patients receiving *cis*-DDP is intense nausea and vomiting, which tends to be refractory to conventional treatment. Some newer antiemetics, such as metoclopramide or Nabilone, may prove useful.[208-210] Administration of *cis*-DDP by slow infusion or by dose-splitting over several days[211, 212] has been reported to reduce nausea and vomiting by some studies,[213-215] but not by others.[216, 217]

Myelosuppression has become a more commonly encountered toxicity of *cis*-DDP. In the past, the renal damage was the major dose-limiting toxicity. With hydration and diuretics ameliorating most acute nephrotoxicity and with the inclusion of *cis*-DDP in regimens containing other myelotoxic drugs (see Table 14–5), this side effect assumes greater importance[218, 219] Granulocytopenia and, to a lesser extent, thrombocytopenia occur. Anemia is a common finding, but may have multiple origins: (1) direct bone marrow toxicity; (2) indirect marrow effects due to renal damage mediated through erythropoietin;[6, 199, 219] or (3) hemolysis with positive direct antiglobulin test, probably due to IgG antibody directed against membrane-bound *cis*-DDP.[220] Thrombocytopenia may also be immunologically mediated in patients receiving *cis*-DDP. The precise cell population depressed, the onset, and the duration of depression are variable; these therefore, as with renal function, warrant careful monitoring.

Neurologic dysfunction of several types has been seen in patients receiving *cis*-DDP. A peripheral neuropathy has been described, primarily distal and sensory, with paresthesias of hands and feet, abnormal vibration and position sense, and diminished light touch.[221, 222] Nerve conduction studies in affected patients are abnormal. Biopsies revealed destruction of the myelin sheath with segmental demyelination. The clinical resemblance to vitamin B_{12} deficiency has prompted the proposal that the Pt interferes with the bioavailability of cobalt, the metal in vitamin B_{12}. This is as yet unproved.[224]

Tetany has been described in several patients receiving *cis*-DDP and is thought to be secondary to hypomagnesemia and hypocalcemia resulting from renal loss of these cations, or renal loss of magnesium with secondary abnormal Ca^{++} metabolism.[185, 187] This may be particularly severe in children. Seizures have also been reported to occur in patients receiving *cis*-DDP.[148-150]

Cis-DDP can produce ototoxicity with high-frequency hearing loss, tinnitus, and even deafness.[225, 226] These changes tend to be bilateral and more detectable in patients over 46 years of age. Ototoxicity is unaffected by the hydration and diuretic maneuvers used to decrease nephrotoxicity. There appears to be no concomitant damage to vestibular function.[227] Studies in rhesus monkeys support the concept that *cis*-DDP produces its ototoxicity through hair cell loss in the organ of Corti within the cochlea.[225]

Allergic reactions to Pt compounds were first reported in 1911[228] in platinum workers. Allergic reactions to *cis*-DDP, including anaphylaxis,[229, 230] have also been noted. Allergic reactions to *cis*-DDP or other Pt salts may not be mediated through a single determinant, since platinum workers who react to hexachloroplatinate ($[PtCl_6]^{-2}$) do not cross-react to *cis*- or *trans*-DDP.[231] However, a single patient who had an anaphylactic reaction following his eighth dose of *cis*-DDP had a positive wheal and flare reaction not only to intracutaneous *cis*-DDP, but also to *cis*-diiododiammineplatinum(II), potassium chloroplatinate (K_2Cl_6Pt), potassium chloroplatinite (K_2Cl_4Pt), and $Pt(NH_3)_2(H_2O)_2^{2+}$. Potassium chloropalladite (K_2Cl_4Pd), Pt(II)ethylenediamine malonate, and Pt(II) 1,2-diaminocyclohexane malonate did not produce a wheal and flare. This patient's leukocytes also released histamine in response to *cis*-DDP. Treatment with Pt(II) 1,2-diaminocyclohexane malonate produced no anaphylaxis in this patient.[229] Patients who have reacted adversely to *cis*-DDP have been successfully retreated by the concurrent administration of diphenhydramine.[232] Pyrexia, distinguishable from anaphylaxis, has recently been reported to follow *cis*-DDP administration in three patients.[233]

In addition to these toxicities, a single instance of hepatotoxicity in the absence of nephropathy has been reported.[234] Two young males receiving *cis*-DDP with vinblastine and bleomycin were noted to have isolated coronary artery atherosclerosis at autopsy.[235] A gum line thought to be secondary to the reaction of salivary Pt with areas of poor dental hygiene in a patient receiving *cis*-DDP has been described.[170]

CONCLUSION

The biologically relevant reactions available to *cis*-DDP must derive from the unique chemistry and structure of this inorganic compound. Among these possible reactions, those with various intracellular macromolecules, particularly DNA, seem most likely to explain the ability of *cis*-DDP to kill neoplastic cells. In whole animals and man, these reactions may play a major role in the ability of this compound to cause malignant tumors to regress. Additionally, interactions with non-neoplastic cell and organ systems may be of great consequence to both the beneficial and the detrimental effects of *cis*-DDP. We have tried to explain the pharmacology of *cis*-DDP by building on a foundation of inorganic chemistry and reactions in aqueous solutions, by considering potential interactions with molecules known to be present within the biologic milieu, through studies in whole cells, and finally through pharmacologic and toxicologic data obtained in whole organisms, including man. The pharmacology and toxicology must follow from the chemistry. The framework in which lie the answers to the remaining questions of the molecular and clinical pharmacology of *cis*-DDP has been erected. Future efforts will be needed to complete the structure.

Acknowledgments

Thanks to our research assistants Stephen T. Michaels, Ronald Schwartz, and Howard Schwartz. Thanks to Madie Tyler and Kathy Moore for typing the manuscript. Special thanks to Dr. Eugenie S. Kleinerman for valuable contributions and criticisms.

References

1. Basolo F, and Pearson RG: The trans effect in metal complexes. Prog. Inorg. Chem. 4:381, 1962.
2. Rosenberg B, Van Camp L, and Krigas T: Inhibition of cell division in *Escherichia coli* by electrolysis products from a platinum electrode. Nature 205:698, 1965.
3. Rosenberg B, Van Camp L, Trosko JE, et al.: Platinum compounds: a new class of potent antitumour agents. Nature 222:385, 1969.
4. Higby DJ, Wallace HJ Jr, and Holland JF: *Cis*-diamminedichloroplatinum (NSC-119875): a phase I study. Cancer Chemother. Rep. 57:459, 1973.
5. Higby DJ, Wallace HJ Jr, Albert DJ, et al.: Diamminodichloroplatinum: a phase I study showing responses in testicular and other tumors. Cancer 33:1219, 1974.
6. Rossof AH, Slayton RE, and Perlia CP: Preliminary clinical experience with *cis*-diamminedichloroplatinum(II) (NSC-119875, CACP). Cancer 30:1451, 1972.
7. Talley RW, O'Bryan RM, Gutterman JU, et al.: Clinical evaluation of toxic effects of *cis*-diamminedichloroplatinum (NSC-119875) — a phase I clinical study. Cancer Chemother. Rep. 57:465, 1973.
8. Wolpert-DeFilippes MK: Antitumor activity of *cis*-dichlorodiammineplatinum(II). Cancer Treat. Rep. 63: 1453, 1979.
9. Einhorn LH, and Donohue J: *Cis*-diamminedichloroplatinum, vinblastine, and bleomycin combination chemotherapy in disseminated testicular cancer. Ann. Intern. Med. 87:293, 1977.
10. Cleare MJ: Some aspects of platinum complex chemistry and their relation to anti-tumor activity. J. Clin. Hematol. Oncol. 7:1, 1977.
11. Lippard SJ: Platinum complexes: probes of polynucleotide structure and antitumor drugs. Acc. Chem. Res. 11:211, 1978.
12. Barton JK, and Lippard SJ: A crystalline platinum blue: its molecular structure, chemical reactivity, and possible relevance to the mode of action of antitumor platinum drugs. Ann. N.Y. Acad. Sci. 313:686, 1978.
13. Thomson AJ, Williams RJP, and Reslova S: The chemistry of complexes related to *cis*-$Pt(NH_3)_2Cl_2$. An anti-tumor drug. Struct. Bond. 11:1, 1972.
14. Chikuma M, Pollock RJ, Ott KC, et al.: Hydroxo-bridged platinum(II) complexes. V. Kinetic studies on olation reaction of *cis*-diaquodiammineplatinum(II) by ^{195}Pt fourier transform nuclear magnetic resonance. J. Am. Chem. Soc., submitted.
15. Harrison RC, and McAuliffe CA: Platinum(II) complexes of DNA constituents. Inorg. Perspect. Biol. Med. 1:261, 1978.
16. Lim MC, and Martin RB: The nature of cis amine Pd(II) and antitumor cis amine Pt(II) complexes in aqueous solutions. Inorg. Nucl. Chem. 38:1911, 1976.
17. Reishus JW, and Martin DS Jr: *Cis*-dichlorodiammineplatinum(II) acid hydrolysis and isotopic exchange of the chloride ligands. J. Am. Chem. Soc. 83:2457, 1961.
18. LeRoy AF, Lutz RJ, Dedrick RL, et al.: Pharmacokinetic study of *cis*-dichlorodiammineplatinum in the beagle

dog: thermodynamic and kinetic behavior of DDP in a biological milieu. Cancer Treat. Rep. 63:59, 1979.
19. Rosenberg B, Van Camp L, Grimley EB, et al.: The inhibition of growth or cell division in *Escherichia coli* by different ionic species of platinum(II) complexes. J. Biol. Chem. 242:1347, 1967.
20. Rosenberg B, Renshaw E, Van Camp L, et al.: Platinum-induced filamentous growth in *Escherichia coli*. J. Bacteriol. 93:716, 1967.
21. Shimizu M, and Rosenberg B: A similar action to UV-irradiation and a preferential inhibition of DNA synthesis in *E. coli* by antitumor platinum compounds. J. Antibiot. 26:243, 1973.
22. Beck DJ, and Brubaker RR: Effect of *cis*-platinum(II) diamminodichloride on wild type and deoxyribonucleic acid repair-deficient mutants of *Escherichia coli*. J. Bacteriol. 116:1247, 1973.
23. Beck DJ, Vazquez D, and Cook R: Effect of *cis*-platinum(II) diamminedichloride on wild type and a recA mutant of *Escherichia coli*. J. Clin. Hematol. Oncol. 7:726, 1977.
24. Drobnik J, Urbankova M, and Krekulova A: The effect of *cis*-dichlorodiammineplatinum(II) on *Escherichia coli*. B. The role of fil, exr and hcr markers. Mutat. Res. 17:13, 1973.
25. Beck DJ, and Brubaker RR: Mutagenic properties of *cis*-platinum(II)diamminodichloride in *Escherichia coli*. Mutat. Res. 27:181, 1975.
26. Benedict WF, Baker MS, Haroun L, et al.: Mutagenicity of cancer chemotherapeutic agents in the *Salmonella*/microsome test. Cancer Res. 37:2209, 1977.
27. LeCointe P, Macquet FP, Butour J-L, et al.: Relative efficiencies of a series of square-planar platinum(II) compounds on *Salmonella* mutagenesis. Mutat. Res. 48:139, 1977.
28. LeCointe P, Macquet J-P, and Butour J-L: Correlation between the toxicity of platinum drugs to L1210 leukemia cells and their mutagenic properties. Biochem. Biophys. Res. Commun. 90:209, 1979.
29. Monti-Bragadin C, Tamaro M, and Banfi E: Mutagenic activity of platinum and ruthenium complexes. Chem. Biol. Interact. 11:469, 1975.
30. Anderson KS: Platinum(II) complexes generate frame-shift mutations in test strains of *Salmonella typhimurium*. Mutat. Res. 67:209. 1979.
31. Muchausen L: The chemical and biological effects of *cis*-dichlorodiammine platinum(II), an antitumor agent on DNA. Proc. Nat. Acad. Sci. USA 71:4519, 1974.
32. Reslova S: The induction of lysogenic strains of *Escherichia coli* by *cis*-dichlorodiammineplatinum (II). Chem. Biol. Interact. 4:66, 1971.
33. Anisimova E, Roubal J, Vlckova I, et al.: Electron-microscopic findings in EB-3 lymphoblastoid cell line exposed to *cis*-dichloro-diammine-platinum(II). Acta Virol. 18:203, 1974.
34. Vonka V, Kutinova L, Drobnik, J, et al.: Increase of Epstein-Barr–virus-positive cells in EB3 cultures after treatment with *cis*-dichlorodiammineplatinum(II). J. Nat. Cancer Inst. 48:1277, 1972.
35. Drobnik J, Blahuskova A, Vasilukova S, et al.: Inactivation of bacteriophages with *cis*-platinum(II)diamminedichloride. Chem. Biol. Interact. 11:365, 1975.
36. Kutinova L, Vonka V, and Drobnik T: Inactivation of papovavirus SV 40 by *cis*-dichlorodiammineplatinum(II). Neoplasma 19:453, 1973.
37. Shooter KV, Howse R, Merrifield RK, et al.: The interaction of platinum II compounds with bacteriophages T7 and R17. Chem. Biol. Interact. 5:289, 1972.
38. O'Neill JP, Couch DB, Machanoff R, et al.: A quantitative assay of mutation induction at the hypoxanthine-guanine phosphoribosyl transferase locus in Chinese hamster ovary cells (CHO/HGPRT system): utilization with a variety of mutagenic agents. Mutat. Res. 45:103, 1977.
39. Turnbull D, Popescu NC, DiPaolo JA, et al.: *Cis*-platinum(II) diamine dichloride causes mutation, transformation, and sister-chromatid exchanges in cultured mammalian cells. Mutat. Res. 66:267, 1979.
40. Zwelling LA, Bradley MO, Sharkey NA, et al.: Mutagenicity, cytotoxicity and DNA crosslinking in V79 Chinese hamster cells treated with *cis*- and *trans*-Pt(II)diamminedichloride. Mutat. Res. 67:271, 1979.
41. Johnson NP, Hoeschele JD, Rahn RO, et al.: Mutagenicity, cytotoxicity, and DNA binding of platinum(II)-chloroamines in Chinese hamster ovary cells. Cancer Res. 40:1463, 1980.
42. Leopold WR, Miller EC, and Miller JA: Carcinogenicity of antitumor *cis*-platinum(II) coordination complexes in the mouse and rat. Cancer Res. 39:913, 1979.
43. Lazar R, Conran PC, and Damjanov I: Embryotoxicity and teratogenicity of *cis*-diamminedichloroplatinum. Experientia 35:647, 1979.
44. Bradley MO, Hsu IC, and Harris CC: Relationships between sister chromatid exchange and mutagenicity, toxicity and DNA damage. Nature 282:318, 1979.
45. Wiencke JK, Cervenka J, and Paulus H: Mutagenic activity of anticancer agent *cis*-dichlorodiammine platinum(II). Mutat. Res. 68:69, 1979.
46. Khan MUA, and Sadler PJ: Distribution of platinum antitumor drug in HeLa cells by analytical electron microscopy. Chem. Biol. Interact. 21:227, 1978.
47. Johnson NP, Hoeschele JD, and Rahn RO: Kinetic analysis of the *in vitro* binding of radioactive *cis*- and *trans*-dichloroammineplatinum(II) to DNA. Chem. Biol. Interact. 30:151, 1980.
48. Macquet JP, Jankowski K, and Butour JL: Mass spectrometry study of DNA-cisplatin complexes: perturbation of guanine-cytosine base pairs. Biochem. Biophys. Res. Commun. 92:68, 1980.
49. Munchausen LL, and Rahn RO: Physical studies on the binding of *cis*-dichlorodiammineplatinum(II) to DNA and homopolynucleotides. Biochim. Biophys. Acta 414:242, 1979.
50. Stone PJ, Kelman AD, and Sinex FM: Specific binding of antitumour drug *cis*-$Pt(NH_3)_2Cl_2$ to DNA rich in guanine and cytosine. Nature 251:736, 1974.
51. Stone PJ, Kelman AD, Sine FM, et al.: Resolution of α, β and γ DNA of *Saccharomyces cerevisiae* with the antitumor drug *cis*-$Pt(NH_3)_2Cl_2$. Evidence for preferential drug binding by GpG sequences of DNA. J. Mol. Biol. 104:793, 1976.
52. Robins AB: The reaction of ^{14}C-labelled platinum ethylenediammine dichloride with nucleic acid constituents. Chem. Biol. Interact. 6:35, 1973.
53. Scovell WM, and O'Connor T: Interaction of aquated *cis*-$[(NH_3)_2PtII]$ with nucleic acid constituents. 1. ribonucleosides. J. Am. Chem. Soc. 99:120, 1977.
54. Robins AB: The reaction of ^{14}C-labelled platinum ethylenediamine dichloride with adenine compounds and DNA. Chem. Biol. Interact. 7:11, 1973.
55. Bau R, Gellert RW, Lehovec SM, et al.: Crystallographic studies on platinum-nucleoside and platinum nucleotide complexes. J. Clin. Hematol. Oncol. 7:51, 1977.
56. Cramer RE, and Dahlstrom PL: The crystal and molecular structure of *cis* $(pt(NH_3)_2(Guo)_2\ Cl_{3/2}(Cl0)_4)_{1/2} \cdot 7H_2O$. J. Clin. Hematol. Oncol. 7:330, 1977.
57. Cleare MJ, and Hoeschele JD: Studies on the antitumor activity of group VIII transition metal complexes. Part I. Platinum(II) complexes. Bioinorg. Chem. 2:187, 1973.
58. Louie S, and Bau R: Structure of $[Pt(en)(5'\text{-}CMP)]_2.2H_2O$. An example of direct platinum-phosphate bonding. J. Am. Chem. Soc. 99:3874, 1977.
59. Macquet J-P, and Butour J-L: Modifications of the DNA secondary structure upon platinum binding: a proposed model. Biochimie 60:901, 1978.
60. Jack A, Ladner JE, Rhoder D, et al.: A crystallographic study of metal-binding to yeast phenylalanine transfer RNA. J. Mol. Biol. 111:315, 1977.
61. Cohen GL, Bauer WR, Barton JK, et al.: Binding of *cis*- and *trans*-dichlorodiammineplatinum(II) to DNA: evidence for unwinding and shortening of the double helix. Science 203:1014, 1979.
62. DePauw-Gillet M-C, Houssier C, and Fredericq E: Interaction of DNA and purine nucleosides with *cis*-

dichlorodiammineplatinum(II) and antimitotic activity of the complexes on meristematic root cells. Chem. Biol. Interact. 25:87, 1979.

63. Macquet J-P, and Butour J-L: A circular dichroism study of DNA platinum complexes. Differentiation between monofunctional, *cis*-bidentate and *trans*-bidentate platinum fixation on a series of DNA's. Eur. J. Biochem. 83:375, 1978.

64. Srivastava RC, Froelich J, and Eichhorn GL: The effect of platinum binding on the structure of DNA and its function in RNA synthesis. Biochimie 60:879, 1979.

65. Drobnik J, and Horacek P: Specific biological activity of platinum complexes. Contribution to the theory of molecular mechanism. Chem. Biol. Interact. 7:223, 1973.

66. Harder HC: Renaturation effects of *cis*- and *trans*-platinum II and IV compounds on calf thymus deoxyribonucleic acid. Chem. Biol. Interact. 10:27, 1975.

67. Deutsch WA, Spiering AL, and Newkome GR: An *in vitro* characterization of interstrand cross-links in DNA exposed to the antitumor drug *cis*-dichlorodiammineplatinum(II). Biochem. Biophys. Res. Commun. 97:1220, 1980.

68. Gellert RW, and Bau R: The structure of the [platinum(ethylenediamine)(guanosine)$_2$]$^{2+}$ cation. J. Am. Chem. Soc. 97:7379, 1975.

69. Harder HC, Smith RG, and LeRoy AF: Template primer inactivation by *cis*- and *trans*-dichlorodiammine platinum, for human DNA polymerase α, β, and Rauscher murine leukemia virus reverse transcriptase, as a mechanism of cytotoxicity. Cancer Res. 36:3821, 1976.

70. Mansy S, Rosenberg B, and Thomson AJ: Binding of *cis*- and *trans*-dichlorodiammineplatinum(II) to nucleosides. I. Location of the binding site. J. Am. Chem. Soc. 95:1633, 1973.

71. Roos IAG, Thomson AJ, and Mansy S: Interaction of platinum compounds with dinucleotides. J. Am. Chem. Soc. 96:6484, 1974.

72. Filipski J, Kohn KW, and Bonner WM: The nature of inactivating lesions produced by platinum(II) complexes in phage λ DNA. Chem. Biol. Interact. 32:321, 1980.

73. Filipski J, Kohn, KW, Prather R, et al.: Thiourea reverses cross-links and restores biological activity in DNA treated with dichlorodiamminoplatinum(II). Science 204:181, 1979.

74. Chottard JC, Girault JP, Chottard G, et al.: Interaction of *cis*-$[Pt(NH_3)_2(H_2O)_2](NO_3)_2$ with ribose dinucleoside monophosphates. J. Am. Chem. Soc. 102:5565, 1980.

75. Kelman AD, and Buchbinder M: Platinum-DNA crosslinking: platinum antitumor drug interactions with native λ-bacteriophage DNA studied using a restriction endonuclease. Biochimie 60:893, 1978.

76. Kelman AD, and Peresie HJ: Mode of binding of *cis*-platinum antitumor drugs: a base sequence dependent mechanism is proposed. Cancer Treat. Rep. 63:1445, 1979.

77. Cohen GL, Ledner JA, Bauer WR, et al.: Sequence-dependent binding of *cis*-dichlorodiammineplatinum (II) to DNA. J. Am. Chem. Soc. 102:2487, 1980.

78. Melius P, and Friedman ME: Complexes of platinum with polypeptides and proteins. Inorg. Perspect. Biol. Med. 1:1, 1977.

79. Kohn KW, and Ewig RAG: DNA-protein crosslinking by *trans*-platinum(II) diamminedichloride in mammalian cells, a new method of analysis. Biochim. Biophys. Acta 562:32, 1979.

80. Zwelling LA, Anderson T, and Kohn KW: DNA-protein and DNA interstrand cross-linking by *cis*- and *trans*-platinum(II)diamminedichloride in L1210 mouse leukemia cells and relation to cytotoxicity. Cancer Res. 39:365, 1979.

81. Lippard SJ, and Hoeschele JD: Binding of *cis*- and *trans*-dichlorodiammineplatinum(II) to the nucleosome core. Proc. Natl. Acad. Sci. USA 76:6091, 1979.

82. Sinha BK, and Chianell CF: Interaction of antitumor drugs with human erythrocyte ghost membranes and mastocytoma P815:a spin label study. Biochem. Biophys. Res. Commun. 86:1051, 1979.

83. Zwelling LA, and Kohn, KW: Mechanism of action of *cis*-dichlorodiammineplatinum(II). Cancer Treat. Rep. 63:1439, 1979.

84. Pascoe JM, and Roberts JJ: Interaction between mammalian cell DNA and inorganic platinum compounds. I. DNA interstrand crosslinking and cytotoxic properties of platinum(II) compounds. Biochem. Pharmacol. 23:1345, 1974.

85. Harder HC, and Rosenberg B: Inhibitory effects of antitumor platinum compounds on DNA, RNA and protein synthesis in mammalian cells *in vitro*. Int. J. Cancer 6:207, 1970.

86. Howle JA, and Gale GR: *Cis*-dichlorodiammineplatinum(II). Persistent and selective inhibition of deoxyribonucleic acid synthesis *in vivo*. Biochem. Pharmacol. 19:2757, 1970.

87. Howle JA, Thompson HS, Stone AE, et al.: *Cis*-dichlorodiammineplatinum(II): inhibition of nucleic acid synthesis in lymphocytes stimulated with phytohemagglutinin. Proc. Soc. Exp. Biol. Med. 137:820, 1971.

88. Roberts JJ, and Thomson AJ: The mechanism of action of antitumor platinum compounds. Prog. Nucl. Acid Res. Mol. Biol. 22:71, 1979.

89. Meyn RE, Corry PM, Fletcher SE, et al.: Thermal enhancement of DNA damage in mammalian cells treated with *cis*-diamminedichloroplatinum(II). Cancer Res. 40:1136, 1980.

90. Barlogie B, Corry PM, and Drewinko B: *In vitro* thermochemotherapy of human colon cancer cells with *cis*-dichlorodiammineplatinum(II) and mitomycin C. Cancer Res. 40:1165, 1980.

91. Roberts JJ, and Pascoe JM: Cross-linking of complementary strands of DNA in mammalian cells by antitumour platinum compounds. Nature 235:282, 1972.

92. Kohn KW: DNA as a target in cancer chemotherapy: measurement of macromolecular DNA damage produced in mammalian cells by anticancer agents and carcinogens. Methods Cancer Res. 16:291, 1979.

93. Zwelling LA, Kohn KW, Ross WE, et al.: Kinetics of formation and disappearance of a DNA cross-linking effect in mouse leukemia L1210 cells treated with *cis*- and *trans*-diamminedichloroplatinum(II). Cancer Res. 38:1762, 1978.

94. Burchenal JH, Kalaher K, Dew K, et al.: Studies of cross-resistance, synergistic combination and blocking activity of platinum derivatives. Biochimie 60:961, 1978.

95. Zwelling LA, Filipski J, and Kohn KW: Effects of thiourea on survival and DNA cross-link formation in cells treated with platinum(II) complexes, L-phenylalanine mustard and bis(2-chloroethyl)methylamine. Cancer Res. 39:4989, 1979.

96. Fraval HNA, Rawlings CJ, and Roberts JJ: Increased sensitivity of UV-repair-deficient human cells to DNA bound platinum products which unlike thymine dimers are not recognized by an endonuclease extracted from *Micrococcus luteus*. Mutat. Res. 51:121, 1978.

97. Van Den Berg HW, and Roberts JJ: Investigations into the mechanism of action of anti-tumor platinum compounds: time- and dose-dependent changes in the alkaline sucrose gradient sedimentation profiles of DNA from hamster cells treated with *cis*-platinum(II) diamminedichloride. Chem. Biol. Interact. 11:493, 1975.

98. Van Den Berg HW, and Roberts JJ: Post-replication repair of DNA in Chinese hamster cells treated with *cis*-platinum(II) diamminedichloride. Enhancement of toxicity and chromosome damage by caffeine. Mutat. Res. 33:279, 1975.

99. Van Den Berg HW, and Roberts JJ: Inhibition by caffeine of post-replication repair in Chinese hamster cells treated with *cis*-platinum(II) diamminedichloride: the extent of platinum binding to template DNA in relation to the size of low molecular weight nascent DNA. Chem. Biol. Interact. 12:375, 1976.

100. Zwelling LA, Michaels S, Schwartz H, et al.: DNA cross-linking as an indicator of sensitivity and resistance of mouse L1210 leukemia to *cis*-diamminedichloroplatinum(II) and L-phenylalanine mustard. Cancer Res. 41: 640, 1981.

101. Ducore J, Zwelling L, Kohn K: DNA interstrand crosslinking and cytotoxicity in three Burkitt's lymphoma cell lines treated with cisplatin. Proc. Am. Assoc. Cancer Res. 21:267, 1980.
102. Erickson LC, Zwelling LA, Ducore JM, et al.: Differential cytotoxicity and DNA crosslinking in normal and transformed human fibroblasts treated with *cis*-diamminedichloroplatinum(II). Cancer Res. 41:2791, 1981.
103. Strandberg MC: Studies on the resistance of a murine leukemia L1210 cell line to *cis*-diamminedichloroplatinum(II). Proc. Am. Assoc. Cancer Res. 22:202, 1981.
104. Micetich K, Michaels S, Jude G, et al.: Mechanism of resistance to *cis*-dichlorodiammineplatinum(II) in a line of L1210 cells. Proc. Am. Assoc. Cancer Res. 22:252, 1981.
105. Roberts JJ, and Fraval HNA: The interaction of antitumor platinum compounds with cellular DNA in cultured cells and animal tissues: relationship to DNA cellular repair processes. Biochimie 60:869, 1978.
106. Fraval HNA, and Roberts JJ: G_1 phase Chinese hamster V79-379A cells are inherently more sensitive to platinum bound to their DNA than mid S phase or asynchronously treated cells. Biochem. Pharmacol. 28:1575, 1979.
107. Drewinko B, Brown BW, and Gottlieb JA: The effect of *cis*-diamminedichloroplatinum(II) on cultured human lymphoma cells and its therapeutic implications. Cancer Res. 33:3091, 1973.
108. Fraval HNA, and Roberts JJ: Effects of *cis* platinum(II) diamminedichloride on survival and the rate of DNA synthesis in synchronously growing Chinese hamster V79-379A cells in the absence and presence of caffeine inhibited post-replication repair; evidence for an inducible repair mechanism. Chem. Biol. Interact. 23:99, 1978.
109. Fraval HNA, and Roberts JJ: Excision repair of *cis*-diamminedichloroplatinum(II)-induced damage to DNA of Chinese hamster cells. Cancer Res. 39:1793, 1979.
110. Pera MF, Rawlings CJ, and Roberts JJ: The role of DNA repair in the recovery of human cells from cisplatin toxicity. Proc. Am. Assoc. Cancer Res. 22:206, 1981.
111. Fraval HNA, and Roberts JJ: Effects of *cis*-platinum(II) diamminedichloride on survival and the rate of DNA synthesis in synchronously growing HeLa cells in the absence and presence of caffeine. Chem. Biol. Interact. 23:111, 1978.
112. Bergerat J-P, Barlogie B, and Drewinko B: Effects of *cis*-dichlorodiammineplatinum(II) on human colon carcinoma cells *in vitro*. Cancer Res. 39:1334, 1979.
113. Gerber NL, and Steinberg AD: Clinical use of immunosuppressive drugs: Part I. Drugs 11:14, 1976.
114. Berenbaum MC: Immunosuppression by platinum diamines. Br. J. Cancer 26:208, 1971.
115. Khan A, and Hill JM: Immunosuppression with *cis*-platinum(II)diamminedichloride effect on antibody plaque-forming spleen cells. Infect. Immun. 4:320, 1971.
116. Brambilla G, Cavanna M, and Maura A: Effect of *cis*-diamminedichloroplatinum (NSC-119875) on the allograft reaction in mice. Cancer Chemother. Rep. 58:633, 1974.
117. Khan, A, Albayrak A, and Hill JM: Effect of *cis*-platinum diamminedichloride on graft rejection: prolonged survival of skin grafts against H_2 histocompatibility. Proc. Soc. Exp. Biol. Med. 141:7, 1972.
118. Bowen JR, Gale GR, Gardner WA Jr, et al.: *Cis*-dichlorodiammineplatinum(II): suppression of adjuvant-induced arthritis in rats. Agents Actions 4:108, 1974.
119. Khan A, and Hill JM: Suppression of graft-versus-host reaction by *cis*-platinum(II) diamminedichloride. Transplantation 13:55, 1972.
120. Ohnuma T, Arkin H, Jun M, et al.: Differential chemotherapeutic susceptibility of human T-lymphocytes and B-lymphocytes in culture. J. Natl. Cancer Inst. 60:749, 1978.
121. Mally MB, Taylor RC, and Callewaert DM: Effects of platinum antitumor agents on *in vitro* assays of human antitumor immunity. Chemotherapy 25:117, 1979.
122. Kleinerman ES, Zwelling LA, and Muchmore AV: The enhancement of naturally occurring human spontaneous monocyte-mediated cytotoxicity by *cis*-diamminedichloroplatinum(II). Cancer Res. 40:3099, 1980.
123. Kleinerman ES, Decker JM, and Muchmore AV: *In vitro* cellular regulation of monocyte function: evidence for a radiosensitive suppressor. J. Reticuloendothel. Soc., in press.
124. Mally MB, Taylor RC, and Callewaert DM: Effects of platinum antitumor agents on *in vitro* assays of human antitumor immunity. II. Effects of *cis*-$[Pt(NH_3)_2Cl_2]$ on spontaneous cell-mediated cytotoxicity. Chemotherapy 26:1, 1980.
125. Herberman RB, and Holden HT: Natural cell-mediated immunity. Adv. Cancer Res. 27:305, 1978.
126. Kleinerman E, Zwelling, L, Howser D, et al.: Defective monocyte killing in patients with malignancies and restoration of function during chemotherapy. Lancet 2:1102, 1980.
127. Taylor DM, Jones JD, and Robins AB: Metabolism of platinum [^{14}C]ethylene-diamine dichloride in the rat. Biochem. Pharmacol. 22:833, 1973.
128. DeConti RC, Toftness BR, Lange RC, et al.: Clinical and pharmacological studies with *cis*-diamminedichloroplatinum(II). Cancer Res. 33:1310, 1973.
129. Lange RC, Spencer RP, and Harder MC: The antitumor agent *cis* $Pt(NH_3)_2Cl_2$: distribution studies and dose calculations for ^{193m}Pt and ^{195m}Pt. J. Nucl. Med. 14:191, 1973.
130. Lange RC, Spencer RP, and Harold HC: Synthesis and distribution of a radiolabeled antitumor agent: *cis*-diamminedichloroplatinum(II). J Nucl. Med. 13:328, 1972.
131. Manaka RC, and Wolf W: Distribution of *cis*-platin in blood. Chem. Biol. Interact. 22:353, 1978.
132. Smith PHS, and Taylor DM: Distribution and retention of the antitumor agent ^{195m}Pt-*cis*-dichlorodiammine platinum(II) in man. J. Nucl. Med. 15:349, 1974.
133. LeRoy AF, Wehling ML, Sponseller HL, et al.: Analysis of platinum in biological materials by flameless atomic absorption spectrophotometry. Biochem. Med. 18:184, 1977.
134. Pera MF Jr., and Harder HC: Analysis for platinum in biological material by flameless atomic absorption spectrometry. Clin. Chem. 23:1245, 1977.
135. Bannister SJ, Sternson LA, and Repta AJ: Urine analysis of platinum species derived from *cis*-dichlorodiammineplatinum(II) by high-performance liquid chromatography following derivatization with sodium diethyldithiocarbomate. J. Chromatog. 173:333, 1979.
136. Bannister SJ, Sternson LA, Repta AJ, et al.: Measurement of free-circulating *cis*-dichlorodiammineplatinum(II) in plasma. Clin. Chem. 23:2258, 1977.
137. Seifert W, Caprioli R, Benjamin R, et al.: Energy dispersive x-ray fluorescence determination of platinum in plasma, urine and cerebrospinal fluid of patients administered *cis*-diamminedichloroplatinum(II). Proc. Am. Assoc. Cancer Res. 20:168, 1979.
138. Loo TL, Hall SW, Salem P, et al.: Clinical pharmacological and toxicological studies of *cis*-diamminedichloroplatinum(II) by continuous intravenous infusion. Biochimie 60:957, 1978.
139. Bannister SJ, Chang Y, Sternson LA, et al.: Atomic absorption spectrophotometry of free circulating platinum species in plasma derived from *cis*-dichlorodiammineplatinum(II). Clin. Chem. 24:877, 1978.
140. Crooke SL, and Prestayko AW: The clinical pharmacology of *cis*-diamminedichloroplatinum, a review. *In* Pinedo HM (ed.): Clinical Pharmacology of Anti-Neoplastic Drugs. Elsevier/North Holland Biomedical Press, Amsterdam, 1978, pp. 295–303.
141. Borch RF, Murkovitz JH, and Pleasants ME: A new method of HPLC analysis of Pt(II) in urine. Anal. Lett. 12:917, 1979.
142. Hincal AA, Long DF, and Repta AJ: *Cis*-platin stability in

aqueous parenteral vehicles. J. Parenteral Drug Assoc. 33:107, 1979.

143. Earhart RH: Instability of *cis*-dichlorodiammineplatinum in dextrose solution. Cancer Treat. Rep. 62:1105, 1978.

144. Repta AJ, Long DF, and Hincal AA: *Cis*-dichlorodiammineplatinum(II) stability in aqueous vehicles: an alternative view. Cancer Treat. Rep. 63:229, 1979.

145. LeRoy AF: Some quantitative data on *cis*-dichlorodiammineplatinum(II) species in solution. Cancer Treat. Rep. 63:231, 1979.

146. Bohart R, and Ogawa G: An observation on the stability of *cis*-dichlorodiammineplatinum(II): a caution regarding its administration. Cancer Treat. Rep. 63:2117, 1979.

147. Prestayko AW, Cadiz M, and Crooke ST: Incompatibility of aluminum-containing IV administration equipment with *cis*-dichlorodiammineplatinum(II) administration. Cancer Treat. Rep. 63:2218, 1979.

148. Einhorn LH, and Williams SD: The role of *cis*-platinum in solid-tumor therapy. N. Engl. J. Med. 300:289, 1979.

149. Prestayko AW, D'Aousst JC, Issell BF, et al.: Cisplatin (*cis*-diamminedichloroplatinum II). Cancer Treat. Rev. 6:17, 1979.

150. Rozencweig M, Von Hoff DD, Abele R, et al.: Cisplatin. *In* Cancer Chemotherapy Annuals. Elsevier/North Holland Biomedical Press, Amsterdam, in press.

151. Litterst CL, Gram TE, Dedrick RL, et al.: Distribution and disposition of platinum following intravenous administration of *cis*-diamminedichloroplatinum(II) (NSC-119875) to dogs. Cancer Res. 36:2340, 1976.

152. Gormley PE, Bull JM, LeRoy AF, et al.: Kinetics of *cis*-dichlorodiammineplatinum. Clin. Pharmacol. Ther. 25:351, 1979.

153. Cole WC, and Wolf W: Preparation and metabolism of a cisplatin/serum protein complex. Chem. Biol. Interact. 30:223, 1980.

154. Gullo JJ, Litterst C, Maguire P, Sikic BI, et al.: Pharmacokinetics and protein binding of *cis*-dichlorodiammine-platinum(II) administered as a one-hour or as a twenty-hour infusion. Cancer Chemother. Pharmacol. 5:21, 1980.

155. Gale GR, Morris CR, Atkins LM, et al.: Binding of an antitumor platinum compound to cells as influenced by physical factors and pharmacologically active agents. Cancer Res. 33:813, 1973.

156. Ogawa M, Gale GR, and Keirn SS: Effects of *cis*-diamminedichloroplatinum (NSC 119875) on murine and human hemopoietic precursor cells. Cancer Res. 35:1398, 1975.

157. Gormley P, Poplack D, and Pizzo P: The cerebrospinal fluid (CSF) pharmacokinetics of *cis*-diamminedichloroplatinum(II) (DDP) and several platinum analogues. Proc. Am. Assoc. Cancer Res. 20:279, 1979.

158. Higby DJ, Buchholtz L, Chary K, et al.: Kinetics of *cis*-platinum (DDP) with intensive diversis. Proc. Am. Assoc. Cancer Res. 18:110, 1977.

159. Litterst CL, LeRoy AF, and Guarino AM: The disposition and distribution of platinum following parenteral administration to animals of *cis*-dichlorodiammineplatinum(II). Cancer Treat. Rep. 63:1485, 1979.

160. Patton TF, Himmelstein KJ, Belt R, et al.: Plasma levels and urinary excretion of filterable platinum species following bolus injection and IV infusion of *cis*-dichlorodiammineplatinum (II) in man. Cancer Treat. Rep. 63:1359, 1979.

161. Waldmann TA, and Wochner RD: The use of ^{51}Cr-labeled albumin in the study of protein-losing enteropathy. Protides Biol. Fluids 11:224, 1964.

162. Casper ES, Kelson DP, Alcock NW, et al.: Platinum concentrations in bile and plasma following rapid and six-hour infusion of *cis*-dichlorodiammineplatinum(II). Cancer Treat. Rep. 63:2023, 1979.

163. DeSimone PA, Yancey RS, Coupal JJ, et al.: Effect of a forced diuresis on the distribution and excretion (via urine and bile) of ^{195m}platinum when given as ^{195m}platinum *cis*-dichlorodiammineplatinum. Cancer Treat. Rep. 63:951, 1979.

164. Wolf W, and Manaka RC: Synthesis and distribution of ^{195m}Pt *cis*-dichlorodiammine platinum(II). J. Clin. Hematol. Oncol. 7:79, 1977.

165. Earhart RH, Wheeler RH, and Bull FE: Pharmacokinetic evidence for biotransformation of *cis*-dichlorodiammine platinum(II) in man. Clin. Res. 25:269A, 1977.

166. Belt RJ, Himmelstein KJ, Patton TR, et al.: Pharmacokinetics of non-protein bound platinum species following administration of *cis*-dichlorodiammineplatinum(II). Cancer Treat. Rep. 63:1515, 1979.

167. Taylor DM: The pharmacokinetics of *cis*-diamminodichloro-platinum(II) in animals and man: relation to treatment scheduling. Biochimie 60:949, 1978.

168. Jacobs C, Kalman SM, Tretton M, et al.: Renal handling of *cis*-diamminedichloroplatinum. Cancer Treat. Rep. 64:1223, 1980.

169. Ross DA, and Gale GR: Reduction of the renal toxicity of *cis*-dichlorodiammineplatinum(II) by probenecid. Cancer Treat. Rep. 63:781, 1979.

170. Ettinger LJ, and Freeman AI: The gingival platinum line. A new finding following *cis*-dichlorodiammine platinum(II) treatment. Cancer 44:1882, 1979.

171. Slater TF, Ahmed M, and Ibrahim SA: Studies on the nephrotoxicity of *cis*-dichlorodiammine-platinum 2^+ and related substances. J. Clin. Hematol. Oncol. 7:534, 1977.

172. Madias NE, and Harrington JT: Platinum nephrotoxicity. Am. J. Med. 65:307, 1978.

173. Leonard BJ, Eccleston E, Jones D, et al.: Antileukaemic and nephrotoxic properties of platinum compounds. Nature 234:43, 1971.

174. Ward JM, and Fauvie KA: The nephrotoxic effects of *cis*-dichloroplatinum(II) (NSC-119875) in male F344 rats. Toxicol. Appl. Pharmacol. 38:535, 1976.

175. Kociba RJ, and Sleight SD: Acute toxicologic and pathologic effects of *cis*-diamminedichloroplatinum (NSC-119875) in the male rat. Cancer Chemother. Rep. 55:1, 1971.

176. Carter SK, and Goldsmith M: The development and clinical testing of new anticancer drugs at the National Cancer Institute — example: *cis*-platinum(II) diammine-dichloride (NSC 119875). *In* Connors, TA, and Roberts JJ (eds.): Recent Results in Cancer Research: Platinum Co-ordination Complexes in Cancer Chemotherapy. Springer-Verlag, New York, 1974, p. 137.

177. Dobyan DC, Levi J, Jacobs C, et al.: Mechanism of *cis*-platinum nephrotoxicity. II. Morphologic observations. J. Pharmacol. Exp. Ther. 213:551, 1980.

178. Ward JM, Young DM, Fauvie KA, et al.: Comparative nephrotoxicity of platinum cancer chemotherapeutic agents. Cancer Treat. Rep. 60:1675, 1976.

179. Levi J, Jacobs C, McTigue M, et al.: Effects of *cis*-platinum on renal SH groups. Fed. Proc. 38:852, 1979.

180. Levi J, Jacobs C, Kalman SM, et al.: Mechanism of *cis*-platinum nephrotoxicity. I. Effects of sulfhydryl groups in rat kidneys. J. Pharmacol. Exp. Ther. 213:545, 1980.

181. Dentino M, Luft FL, Yum MN, et al.: Long-term effect of *cis*-diamminedichloride platinum (CDDP) on renal function and structure in man. Cancer 41:1274, 1978.

182. Jones B, Mladek J, Bhalla R, et al.: Enzymuria and β_2 microglobulinuria as a sensitive index of cisplatinum nephrotoxicity. Proc. Am. Soc. Clin. Oncol 20:336, 1979.

183. Kuhn JA, Argy WP, Rakowski TA et al.: Nephrotoxicity of *cis*-diamminedichloroplatinum(II) as measured by urinary beta glucuronidase. Cancer Treat. Rep. 64:1083, 1980.

184. Gonzalez-Vitale JC, Hayes DM, Cvitkovic E, et al.: The renal pathology in clinical trials of *cis*-platinum(II) diamminedichloride. Cancer 39:1362, 1977.

185. Hayes FA, Green AA, Jenzer N, et al.: Tetany: a complication of *cis*-dichlorodiammineplatinum(II) therapy. Cancer Treat. Rep. 63:547, 1979.

186. Nitschke R, Starling KA, Vats T, et al.: *Cis*-diamminedichloroplatinum (NSC-119875) in childhood malignancies: a southwest oncology group study. Med. Pediatr. Oncol. 4:127, 1978.

187. Schilsky RL, and Anderson T: Hypomagnesemia and renal

magnesium wasting in patients receiving cisplatin. Ann. Intern. Med. 90:929, 1979.

188. Carney SL, Wong NLM, Quamme GA, et al.: Effects of magnesium deficiency on renal magnesium and calcium transport in the rat. J. Clin. Invest. 65:180, 1980.

189. Davis S, Kessler W, Haddad BM, et al.: Acute renal tubular dysfunction following *cis*-dichlorodiammineplatinum therapy. J. Med. 11:133, 1980.

190. Chary KK, Higby DJ, Henderson ES, et al.: A phase I study of high-dose *cis*-diamminedichloroplatinum(II) (NSC 119875) with forced diuresis. J. Clin. Hematol. Oncol. 7:633, 1977.

191. Cvitkovic E, Spaulding J, Bethune V, Martin J, Whitmore WF, et al.: Improvement of *cis*-dichlorodiammineplatinum (NSC-119875): therapeutic index in an animal model. Cancer 39:1357, 1977.

192. Ward JM, Grabin ME, Berlin E, et al.: Prevention of renal failure in rats receiving *cis*-diamminedichloroplatinum(II) by administration of furosemide. Cancer Res. 37:1238, 1977.

193. Ward JM, Grabin ME, LeRoy AF, et al.: Modification of the renal toxicity of *cis*-dichlorodiammineplatinum(II) with furosemide in male F344 rats. Cancer Treat. Rep. 61:375, 1977.

194. Earhart RH: Effect of chloride excretion on nephrotoxicity due to *cis*-diamminedichloride platinum(II). Proc. Am. Assoc. Cancer Res. 20:147, 1979.

195. Earhart RH, Martin P, Pruitt B, et al.: Improvement in cisplatin therapeutic index by increased urinary chloride excretion. Fed. Proc. 39:310, 1980.

196. Lehane D, Winston A, Gray R, et al.: The effect of diuretic pre-treatment on clinical, morphological and ultrastructural *cis*-platinum induced nephrotoxicity. Int. J. Radiat. Oncol. Biol. Phys. 5:1393, 1979.

197. Pera MF Jr, Zook BC, and Harder MC: Effects of mannitol or fuorosemide diuresis on the nephrotoxicity and physiological disposition of *cis*-dichlorodiammineplatinum(II) in rats. Cancer Res. 39:1269, 1979.

198. Pera MF Jr, and Harder MC: Effects of mannitol and furosemide diuresis on *cis*-dichlorodiammineplatinum(II) antitumor activity and toxicity to host-renewing cell populations in rats. Cancer Res. 39:1279, 1979.

199. Eshaque M, McKay MJ, and Theophanides T: D-Mannitol platinum complexes. J. Clin. Hematol. Oncol. 7:338, 1977.

200. Chary KK, Higby DJ, Henderson ES, et al.: Phase I study of high-dose *cis*-dichlorodiammineplatinum(II) with forced diuresis. Cancer Treat. Rep. 61:367, 1977.

201. Hayes D, Cvitkovic E, Golbey R, et al.: Amelioration of renal toxicity of high dose *cis*-platinumdiammine dichloride (CPDD) by mannitol induced diuresis. Proc. Am. Assoc. Cancer Res. 17:169, 1976.

202. Merrin C: A new method to prevent toxicity with high doses of *cis*-diammine platinum (therapeutic efficacy in previously treated widespread and recurrent testicular tumors). Proc. Am. Soc. Clin. Oncol. 17:243, 1976.

203. Stark JJ, and Howell SB: Nephrotoxicity of *cis*-platinum(II) dichlorodiammine. Clin. Pharmacol. Ther. 23:461, 1978.

204. Bozzino JM, Prasad V, and Koriech OM: Avoidance of renal toxicity by 24-hour infusion of cisplatin. Cancer Treat. Rep. 65:351, 1981.

205. Borch RF, and Pleasants ME: Inhibition of *cis*-platinum nephrotoxicity by diethyldithiocarbamate rescue in a rat model. Proc. Natl. Acad. Sci. USA 76:6611, 1979.

206. Borch RF, Katz JC, Lieder PH, et al.: Effect of diethyldithiocarbamate rescue on tumor response to *cis*-platinum in a rat model. Proc. Natl. Acad. Sci. USA 77:5441, 1980.

207. Gale GR, and Atkins LM: Cisplatin and diethyldithiocarbamate in treatment of L1210 leukemia. J. Clin. Hematol. Oncol. 11:41, 1981.

208. Gylys JA, Doran KM, and Buyniski JP: Antagonism of cisplatin induced emesis in the dog. Res. Commun. Chem. Pathol. Pharmacol. 23:61, 1979.

209. Kahn T, Elias EG, and Mason GR: A single dose of metoclopramide in the control of vomiting from *cis*-dichlorodiammine(II) in man. Cancer Treat. Rep. 62:1106, 1978.

210. Steele N, Braun D, O'Hehir M, et al.: Double-blind comparison of the antiemetic effects of Nabilone and prochlorperazine on chemotherapy-induced emesis. Proc. Am. Soc. Clin. Oncol. 20:337, 1979.

211. Jacobs, C, Bertino JR, Goffinet DR, et al.: 24-hour infusion of *cis*-platinum in head and neck cancer. Cancer 42:2135, 1978.

212. Ochs JJ, Freeman AI, Douglas HO Jr, et al.: *Cis*-dichlorodiammineplatinum(II) in advanced osteogenic sarcoma. Cancer Treat. Rep. 62:239, 1978.

213. Salem P, Hall SW, Benjamin RS, et al.: Clinical phase I-II study of cis-dichlorodiammine platinum (II) given by continuous IV infusion. Cancer Treat. Rep. 62:1553, 1978.

214. Salem P, Jabboury K, Khalil M, et al.: *Cis*-diamminedichloroplatinum by 5 day-continuous infusion — toxicity pattern. Proc. Am. Assoc. Cancer Res. 20:84, 1979.

215. Lokich JJ: Phase I study *cis*-diamminedichloroplatinum(II) administered as a constant 5-day infusion. Cancer Treat. Rep. 64:905, 1980.

216. Williams CJ, Stevenson KE, and Whitehouse JMA: Pharmacokinetics and toxicity of *cis*-diamminedichloroplatinum (DDP) given by IV bolus 24- or 48-hr. infusion. Proc. Am. Soc. Clin. Oncol. 20:317, 1979.

217. Williams CJ, Stevenson KE, Buchanan RB, et al.: Advanced ovarian carcinoma: a pilot study of *cis*-dichlorodiamminoplatinum(II) in combination in previously untreated patients and as a single agent in previously treated patients. Cancer Treat. Rep. 63:1745, 1979.

218. Corder MP, Elliott TE, and Bell SJ: Dose limiting myelotoxicity in absence of significant nephrotoxicity with a weekly out-patient schedule of *cis*-platinum(II) diamminedichloride. J. Clin. Hematol. Oncol. 7:645, 1977.

219. Wiltshaw E: A review of clinical experience with *cis*-platinum diammine dichloride: 1972–1978. Biochimie 60:925, 1978.

220. Getaz EP, Beckley S, Fitzpatrick J, et al.: Cisplatin-induced hemolysis. N. Engl. J. Med. 302:334, 1980.

221. Kedar A, Cohen ME, and Freeman AI: Peripheral neuropathy as a complication of *cis*-dichlorodiammineplatinum(II) treatment: a case report. Cancer Treat. Rep. 62:819, 1978.

222. Von Hoff DD, Reichert CM, Cuneo R, et al.: Demyelination of peripheral nerves associated with *cis*-diamminedichloroplatinum(II) therapy. Proc. Am. Assoc. Cancer Res. 20:91, 1979.

223. Cowan JD, Kiesms, Roth JL, et al.: Nerve conduction studies in patients treated with *cis*-diamminedichloroplatinum(II). A preliminary report. Cancer Treat. Rep. 64:1119, 1980.

224. Hogenkamp HPC, Kohlmiller NA, and Hausinger R: The interaction of *cis*-diammine diaquo platinum (II) with adenosylcobalamin and alkylcobalamins. Fed. Proc. 38:643, 1979.

225. Stadnicki SW, Fleischman RW, Schaeppi U, et al.: *Cis*-dichlorodiammineplatinum(II) (NSC-119875): hearing loss and other toxic effects in rhesus monkeys. Cancer Chemother. Rep. 59:467, 1975.

226. Helson L, Okonkwo E, Anton L, et al.: *Cis*-platinum ototoxicity. Clin. Toxicol. 13:469, 1978.

227. Piel IJ, Meyer D, Perlia C, et al.: Effects of *cis*-diamminedichloroplatinum (NSC-119875) on hearing function in man. Cancer Chemother. Rep. 58:871, 1974.

228. Khan A, Wakasugi K, Hill B, et al.: Platinum complexes: immunology and allergy. J. Clin. Hematol. Oncol. 7:797, 1977.

229. Khan A, Hill JM, Grater W, et al.: Atopic hypersensitivity to *cis*-dichlorodiammineplatinum(II) and other platinum complexes. Cancer Res. 35:2766, 1975.

230. Von Hoff DD, Slavik M, and Muggia FM: Allergic reactions to *cis*-platinum. Lancet 1:90, 1976.

231. Cleare MJ, Hughes EG, Jacoby B, et al.: Immediate (type I)

allergic responses to platinum compounds. Clin. Allergy 6:183, 1976.
232. Wiesenfeld M, Reinders E, Corder M, et al.: Successful re-treatment with *cis*-DDP after apparent allergic reactions. Cancer Treat. Rep. 63:219, 1979.
233. Ashford RFU, Mclachlan A, Nelson I, et al.: Pyrexia after cisplatin. Lancet 2:691, 1980.
234. Cavalli F, Tschopp L, Sonntag RW, et al.: A case of liver toxicity following *cis*-dichlorodiammineplatinum(II) treatment. Cancer Treat. Rep. 62:2125, 1978.
235. Edwards GS, Lane M, and Smith FE: Long-term treatment with *cis*-dichlorodiammineplatinum(II)-vinblastine-bleomycin: possible association with severe coronary artery disease. Cancer Treat. Rep. 63:551, 1979.

15 NONCLASSICAL ALKYLATING AGENTS

The classical alkylating agents of the nitrogen mustard type incorporate a chloroethyl group as their effector arm, but various other chemical structures have proved capable of forming covalent bonds with biologic macromolecules. These nonclassical alkylators include alkyl, immonium, and sulfonium type structures and epoxide-forming compounds. In this chapter we will consider a group of agents that, though inert as parent compounds, undergo complex metabolic transformation to active alkylating intermediates. Included in this latter group are three drugs that have clinically important action: procarbazine, dacarbazine (DTIC), and hexamethylmelamine.

PROCARBAZINE

Robert J. Weinkam
David A. Shiba

HISTORICAL BACKGROUND

Procarbazine was one of over 200 substituted hydrazine and hydrazide compounds synthesized by Zeller et al.[1] at the Hoffman LaRoche Laboratories in the early 1960s. These analogues were prepared and tested as potential monamine oxidase inhibitors; however, during this process Bollag and Grunberg[2] discovered that 1-methyl-2-benzylhydrazine had significant antitumor activity against several transplantable tumors. This compound proved to be hepatotoxic and to have a low therapeutic index, but approximately 40 other methylhydrazine analogues were found to have antineoplastic activity against rodent tumors. Procarbazine and the N-carbamoyl analogue were chosen for further screening. Procarbazine hydrochloride proved to be the less toxic of these two compounds and is now the only member of this class of cancer chemotherapeutic agents in clinical use.

The first clinical trials were conducted by Martz and co-workers[3] in Switzerland in 1963. Significant response was seen in 16 of 17 patients with malignant lymphoma, but 14 patients with solid tumors failed to respond to treatment. Between 1963 and 1969 procarbazine was used in clinical trials in the United States and found to be effective in the treatment of Hodgkin's disease. A response was observed in 57 per cent of the 480 patients with Hodgkin's disease treated, but only 15 per cent of those with other malignancies showed improved clinical status.[4] Procarbazine is of particular importance in the chemotherapy of Hodgkin's disease because it is not cross-resistant with other chemotherapeutic agents. In 1969 this agent was approved for noninvestigational clinical use in the treatment of Hodgkin's disease and in patients with other malignancies that had become resistant to other forms of therapy. Procarbazine is currently used primarily in combination regimens such as MOPP[5-10] (see Chapter 1, discussion of strategies for clinical Chemotherapy, pp. 8–12).

Procarbazine has been shown to be effective in the treatment of brain tumors. It produces a 50 per cent response rate for a median duration of six months when used as a single agent in the treatment of recurrent brain tumors.[11] A 60 per cent response rate for a median duration of nine months was achieved in patients with recurrent malignant gliomas when procarbazine was used in combination with vincristine and 1-(2-chloroethyl)-2-cyclohexyl-1-nitrosourea (CCNU) (PCV).[12]

CHEMISTRY AND METABOLISM

Procarbazine hydrochloride was developed and brought to clinical use without a clear understanding of its metabolism or mode of action. Procarbazine is chemically stable in acidic solution;[13] however, at neutral pH the hydrazine function (CH_3-*NH-NH*-R) is deprotonated and is rapidly oxidized by molecular oxygen.[13, 14] The rate of this reaction is dependent on the presence of catalysts such as trace metals and metaloporphyrins.[15, 16] In aqueous buffer at physiologic pH and temperature, procarbazine reacts with a half-life of about 15 minutes[17] to give the azo analogue N-isopropyl-α-(2-methyldiazeno)-*p*-toluamide, with hydrogen peroxide formed as a biproduct[15] (Fig. 15–1). The lipophilic azo compound is

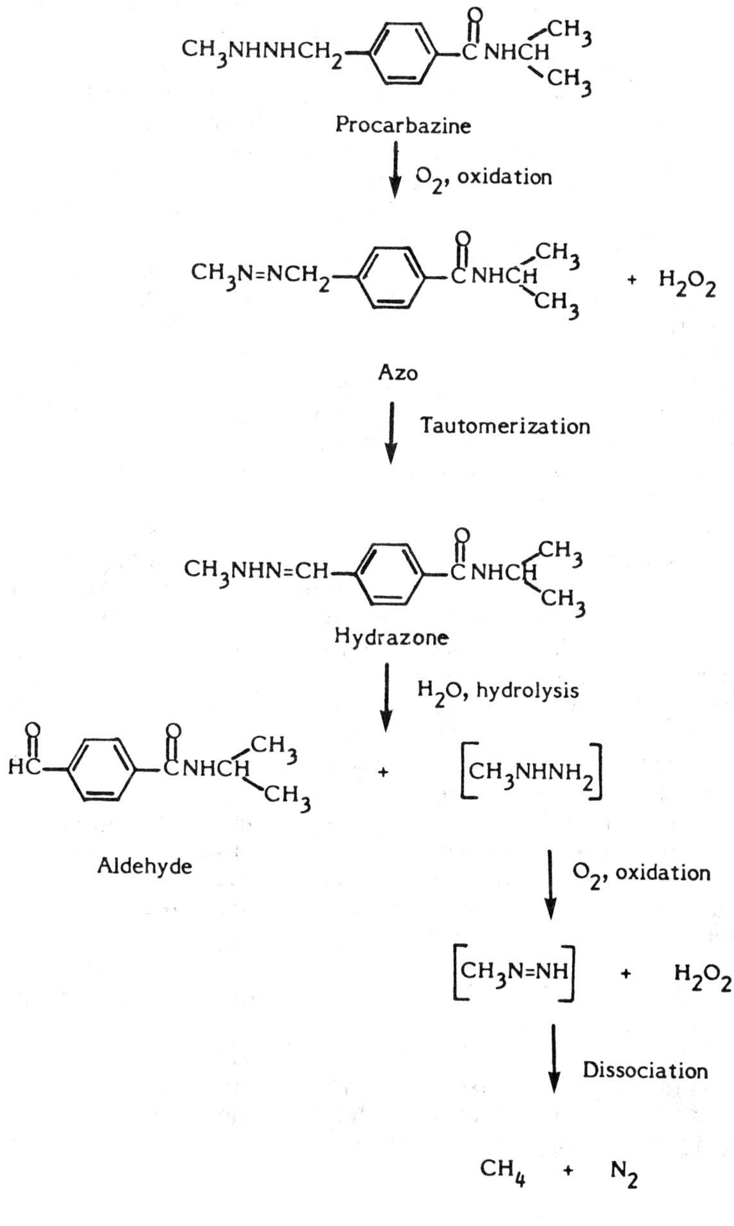

$CH_3NHNHCH_2-C_6H_4-C(=O)NHCH(CH_3)_2$

Procarbazine

↓ O_2, oxidation

$CH_3N{=}NCH_2-C_6H_4-C(=O)NHCH(CH_3)_2$ + H_2O_2

Azo

↓ Tautomerization

$CH_3NHN{=}CH-C_6H_4-C(=O)NHCH(CH_3)_2$

Hydrazone

↓ H_2O, hydrolysis

$HC(=O)-C_6H_4-C(=O)NHCH(CH_3)_2$ + $[CH_3NHNH_2]$

Aldehyde

↓ O_2, oxidation

$[CH_3N{=}NH]$ + H_2O_2

↓ Dissociation

CH_4 + N_2

Figure 15–1. Chemical reactions of procarbazine in aqueous solution in the presence of molecular oxygen at pH 7.4, 37° C. Probable, but thus far unidentified, products are enclosed in brackets.

relatively stable under these conditions, (t½ = 50 min), but slowly isomerizes to the conjugated hydrazone *p*-formyl-N-isopropylbenzamide methylhydrazone. This compound also degrades slowly by hydrolysis to yield the aldehyde *p*-formyl-N-isopropylbenzamide and methylhydrazine, although the latter compound has not been isolated. This monoalkylhydrazine is presumably oxidized to methyldiazene and hydrogen peroxide. Methyldiazenes are known to react rapidly in the presence of molecular oxygen to give methane.[18] The chemical decomposition pathway (Fig. 15–1) leads to the formation of a number of potentially toxic substances that complicate the *in vitro* determination of procarbazine activity.

It is clear that procarbazine itself is not a cytotoxic or mutagenic agent and must undergo chemical or metabolic activation.[19, 20] Recent reports indicate that 9000g rat liver supernatant enzymes can activate procarbazine to produce a cytotoxic intermediate against some L1210 strains[17] and in mutagenesis assays.[21, 22] The first step in the *in vitro* metabolic activation sequence (Fig. 15–2) is the rapid formation of the azo compound.[14, 23-26] This reaction occurs in high yield; the appearance of azo metabolite corresponds to the disappearance of procarbazine.[26] Prough et al. have shown that cytochrome P-450 is the only liver homogenate enzyme catalyzing this oxidation.[23] Procarbazine disappearance may be induced by phenobarbital[23, 27] but not by 3-methylcholanthrene.[23] Carbon monoxide, metyrapone, and microsomal NADPH cytochrome C reductase antibodies inhibit metabolism.[23, 24]

The initial chemical oxidation rate is comparable to the *in vitro* metabolic and *in vivo* plasma clearance rates, and may be a significant factor in the fate of this drug. The subsequent conversions of azo to hydrazone and of hydrazone hydrolysis, however, are slower than the rate of *in vitro* azo metabolism or *in vivo* plasma clearance. Little hydrazone is formed under these conditions, so it is unlikely that the chemical degradation products participate in the *in vivo* cytotoxicity of procarbazine.[14, 24]

The continued metabolism of the azo compound leads to the stereoselective formation of two azoxy isomers[14, 24] (Fig. 15–2). The methylazoxy isomer is formed more rapidly in this rat liver microsome catalyzed reaction. Both azoxy isomers are metabolized, with the benzylazoxy compound consumed at 1.7 times the rate of the methylazoxy isomer. N-isopropyl-*p*-formyl benzamide, N-isopropyl-*p*-hydroxymethylbenzamide, and N-isopropylterephthalamic acid are detected following the microsomal metabolism of procarbazine and of the azo and azoxy isomers.[14, 24] Formaldehyde, formic acid, and carbon dioxide are also generated from the N-methyl group of procarbazine during rat liver microsomal metabolism.[28, 29]

One mechanism for the metabolism of the azoxy isomers that would lead to the formation of cytotoxic alkylating intermediates would be hydroxylation on the methyl and/or benzyl carbons adjacent to the azoxy function. The resulting hydroxy-azoxy metabolites, shown in Figure 15–2, are analogous to methylazoxymethanol, a toxic liver microsomal metabolite of 1,2-dimethylhydrazine.[30] Methylazoxymethanol and, by analogy, the procarbazine hydroxy-azoxy metabolites are chemically unstable substances that react to give alkyldiazonium ion alkylating intermediates and the corresponding aldehyde. An alkylating species formed in an enzyme preparation will alkylate macromolecules, but the predominant product occurs by alkylation of water to give the corresponding alcohol. Both 1,2-dimethylhydrazine[31] and procarbazine[32] are known to be converted to methylating agents that act by transfer of an intact CH_3 group.

The metabolites shown in Figure 15–2 are also observed in rat liver perfusion experiments and as plasma components *in vivo* in rats. Formation of the azo metabolite occurs in high yield in perfused liver, and the rate of azo formation is more rapid than that of N-isopropylterephthalamic acid or CO_2.[26, 28] Procarbazine, azo, both azoxy isomers, N-isopropylterephthalamic acid, and toluamide have been detected in rat plasma following intraperitoneal procarbazine administration[27] (Figs. 15–2 and 15–3). Procarbazine clearance as well as azo and azoxy isomer clearance are increased following phenobarbital pretreatment. The major excreted metabolites from rat are (1) N-isopropylterephthalamic acid, which accounts for 70 per cent of administered CO-^{14}C-procarbazine in rat within 24 hours,[33, 34] with similar findings in man, dog, and mouse;[34, 35] and (2) CO_2, which accounts for 11 to 22 per cent of N-methyl-^{14}C-procarbazine.[36] All these findings are consistent

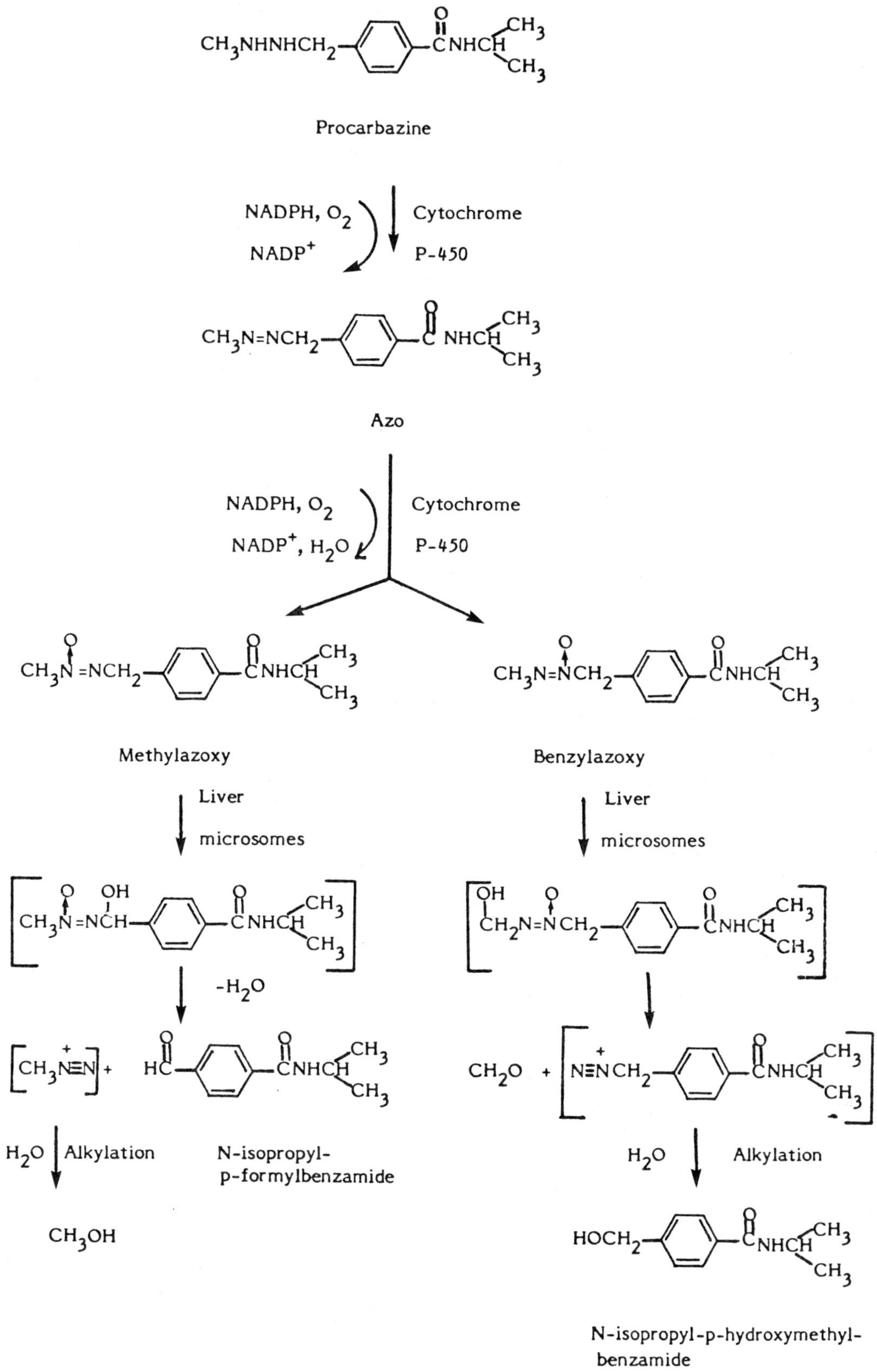

$CH_3NHNHCH_2$–C₆H₄–C(=O)NHCH(CH_3)$_2$

Procarbazine

NADPH, O_2 → $NADP^+$; Cytochrome P-450

$CH_3N{=}NCH_2$–C₆H₄–C(=O)NHCH(CH_3)$_2$

Azo

NADPH, O_2 → $NADP^+$, H_2O ; Cytochrome P-450

$CH_3N(\rightarrow O){=}NCH_2$–C₆H₄–C(=O)NHCH($CH_3$)$_2$

Methylazoxy

$CH_3N{=}N(\rightarrow O)CH_2$–C₆H₄–C(=O)NHCH($CH_3$)$_2$

Benzylazoxy

Liver microsomes

[$CH_3N(\rightarrow O){=}NCH(OH)$–C₆H₄–C(=O)NHCH($CH_3$)$_2$]

$-H_2O$

[$CH_3\overset{+}{N}{\equiv}N$] + HC(=O)–C₆H₄–C(=O)NHCH(CH_3)$_2$

H_2O Alkylation

CH_3OH

N-isopropyl-p-formylbenzamide

Liver microsomes

[$HOCH_2N{=}N(\rightarrow O)CH_2$–C₆H₄–C(=O)NHCH($CH_3$)$_2$]

CH_2O + [$\overset{+}{N}{\equiv}NCH_2$–C₆H₄–C(=O)NHCH($CH_3$)$_2$]

H_2O Alkylation

$HOCH_2$–C₆H₄–C(=O)NHCH(CH_3)$_2$

N-isopropyl-p-hydroxymethyl-benzamide

Figure 15–2. Metabolic activation pathway leading to the generation of alkylating intermediates.

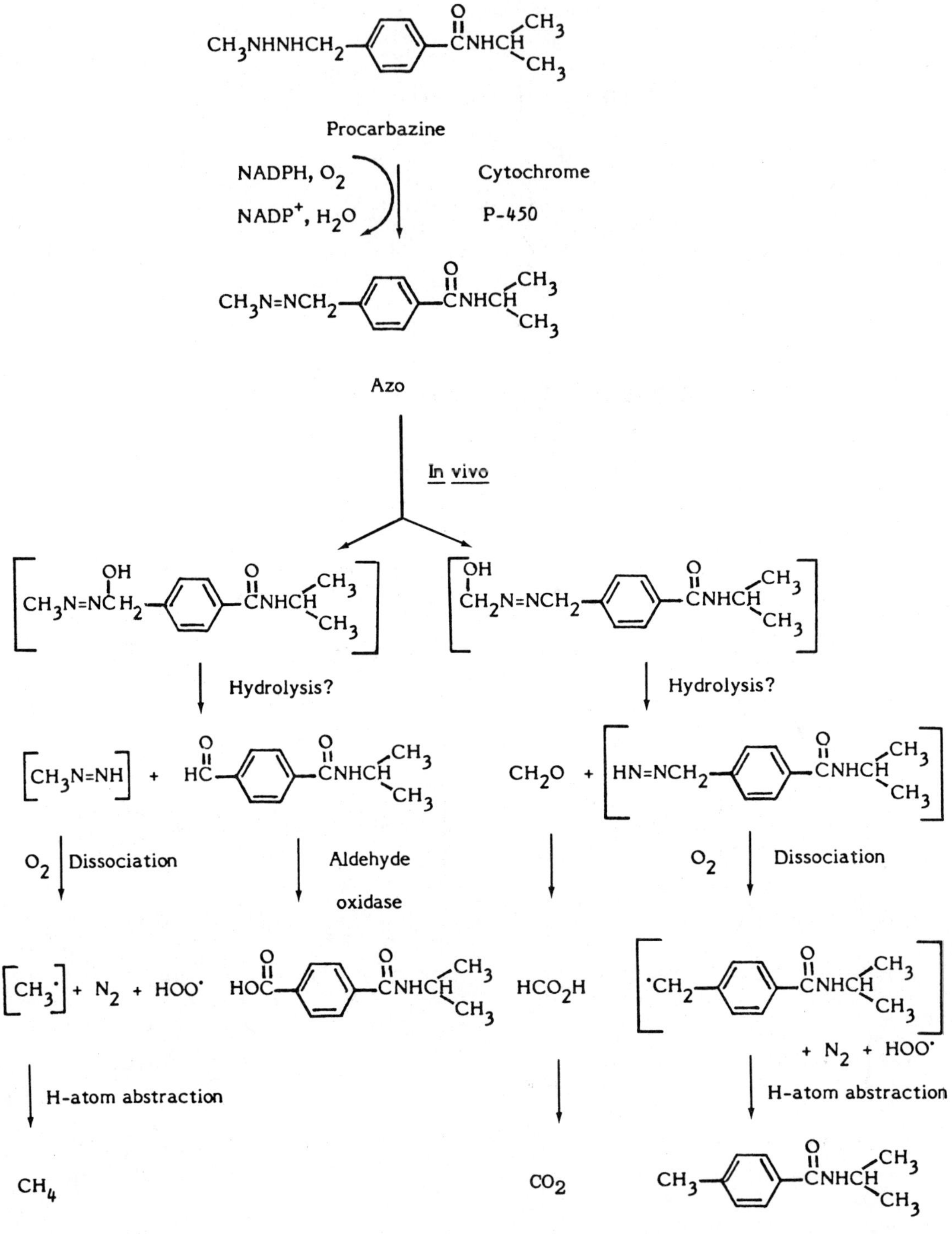

$CH_3NHNHCH_2-C_6H_4-C(=O)NHCH(CH_3)_2$

Procarbazine

NADPH, O_2 / $NADP^+$, H_2O — Cytochrome P-450

$CH_3N{=}NCH_2-C_6H_4-C(=O)NHCH(CH_3)_2$

Azo

In vivo

$[CH_3N{=}NCH(OH)-C_6H_4-C(=O)NHCH(CH_3)_2]$ $[HOCH_2N{=}NCH_2-C_6H_4-C(=O)NHCH(CH_3)_2]$

Hydrolysis? Hydrolysis?

$[CH_3N{=}NH]$ + $HC(=O)-C_6H_4-C(=O)NHCH(CH_3)_2$ CH_2O + $[HN{=}NCH_2-C_6H_4-C(=O)NHCH(CH_3)_2]$

O_2 Dissociation Aldehyde oxidase O_2 Dissociation

$[CH_3^{\cdot}]$ + N_2 + $HOO^{\cdot}$ $HOC(=O)-C_6H_4-C(=O)NHCH(CH_3)_2$ HCO_2H $[{}^{\cdot}CH_2-C_6H_4-C(=O)NHCH(CH_3)_2]$ + N_2 + $HOO^{\cdot}$

H-atom abstraction H-atom abstraction

CH_4 CO_2 $CH_3-C_6H_4-C(=O)NHCH(CH_3)_2$

N-isopropyl-p-toluamide

Figure 15–3. The *in vivo* metabolic pathway proposed for the formation of free radical intermediates from procarbazine.

with the metabolic sequence of Figure 15–2 and indicate that this pathway of activation also occurs *in vivo* in rat. Methylation *in vivo* is indicated by the rapid incorporation of label from N-methyl-^{14}C-procarbazine into P815 leukemia cells implanted in mice.[37] Label was bound to DNA, RNA, phospholipids, and protein. Significant amounts of labeled 7-methylguanine may be detected[38] as the result of transfer of an intact ^{14}C- and ^{3}H-labeled methyl group.[31] Label is also incorporated into nonmethylated purines by *de novo* biosynthesis, using the formate pool enriched by way of N-methyl-^{14}C-procarbazine oxidative demethylation.[31]

In addition to the above pathway, it appears that procarbazine may be metabolized to free radical intermediates *in vivo*. Methane is detected as an expired metabolite of both procarbazine[35] and the azo metabolite[38] following administration to rat. N-isopropyl-*p*-toluamide is present as a metabolite in plasma[14] and brain.[17] There are no other data available to define directly the metabolic pathway leading to these hydrocarbon metabolites. It is reasonable to assume that the methane and N-isopropyl-*p*-toluamide are formed by hydrogen atom abstraction within the organism to give a variety of free radical products. A sequence first proposed by Baggiolini et al.[26] involves oxidation of the azo metabolite (Fig. 15–3). Hydroxylation on the methyl or benzyl carbon adjacent to the azo function would give a product that would rapidly hydrolyze to an aldehyde and diazene. Diazenes, in the presence of molecular oxygen, rapidly decompose to molecular nitrogen and free radicals.[18] Whatever the mechanism of formation, these products appear in relatively low yields. Methane is recovered from rats in 5 to 10 per cent yields after eight hours.[39]

MODE OF ACTION

Procarbazine, even at high concentrations (10^{-2}M), does not alter DNA, RNA, or protein synthesis in Ehrlich ascites cells *in vitro*, although subcutaneous administration of 200 mg per kg to mice bearing this tumor results in increased survival and a 35 to 40 per cent reduction in DNA synthesis.[40] Although these results indicate that the procarbazine molecule is inactive, chemical and metabolic reactions generate a number of potentially toxic products. Hydrogen peroxide and formaldehyde were identified in early studies and proposed as active cytotoxic species. In high concentrations, hydrogen peroxide and formaldehyde do inhibit DNA and RNA polymerase and synthesis of nucleoside triphosphates.[41-43, 60] N-hydroxymethyl compounds formed from formaldehyde also inhibit RNA and DNA polymerase.[33] However, a number of studies[19, 44] have shown that hydrogen peroxide is not responsible for procarbazine activity. The strongest evidence is that azo procarbazine, in the absence of hydrogen peroxide, is an effective cytotoxic agent.[27] Hydrogen peroxide, formaldehyde, and other aldehydes are common metabolic products of compounds that do not possess antitumor activity. Catalase, peroxidase, and alcohol dehydrogenase have the capacity to rapidly detoxify these substances *in vivo*. It is unlikely that toxic amounts will be formed from therapeutic doses of procarbazine.

The antitumor and carcinogenic activity of procarbazine is more probably related to metabolic conversion to alkylating and/or free radical intermediates. Metabolism by way of the alkylation pathway has been related to cytotoxic and mutagenic activity under conditions in which free radical formation does not occur.[21, 22] *In vitro* rat liver homogenate metabolism converts procarbazine to aklylating intermediates by a sequence that is analogous to 1,2-dimethylhydrazine activation. Support for this mechanism of activation comes from the fact that a 2:1 mixture of methyl and benzylazoxy metabolites produces a 140 per cent increased survival in L1210 bearing mice at one half of the dose required of procarbazine or the azo derivative.[27] Both methyl and benzylazoxy isomers have been identified in plasma after procarbazine administration to rat. Because procarbazine is known to be a methylating agent, and other methylating agents such as dimethyltriazenes[45] and 1,2-dimethylhydrazine[46] are known to have antitumor and carcinogenic activity, this appears to be a mechanism by which this drug could exert its toxicity.

Free radical species formed from procarbazine have not been shown to have antitumor activity under conditions during which alkylation does not occur. Nevertheless, free radicals are highly reactive intermediates that are expected to have toxic and possibly antitumor activity. It is not clear that a sufficient number of free radicals are formed during procarbazine metabolism to produce detectable cellular alterations and clinically observable effects.

CELLULAR PHARMACOLOGY

The biochemical basis of procarbazine activity is unclear. This is due, in part, to the fact that several toxic products may be formed from procarbazine by chemical and metabolic reactions. Cellular effects have been observed in culture without evidence that tumor cells can metabolically activate this agent. Cultured cells such as Ehrlich ascites are not affected by freshly prepared procarbazine solutions[19], but do respond to aged solutions[19] or prolonged exposure[47] during which decomposition occurs. The observed effects are presumably due to the activity of aqueous degradation products. *In vivo* metabolic reactions occur at a faster rate than chemical degradation, and lead to the formation of alkylating and/or free radical intermediates. Cytotoxic effects observed *in vivo* are probably caused by different species from those in cell culture. Procarbazine has cytotoxic, mutagenic, carcinogenic, and teratogenic activity.[48, 49] It is possible that these effects are due to DNA damage as a consequence of alkylation and subsequent alterations.[49] However, further studies are required to define the molecular mechanisms by which procarbazine produces biologic effects.

Procarbazine produced chromatid translocations in Ehrlich ascites, 2BF, and L1210 leukemia cells *in vivo* in Therman's study.[50] Maximal inhibition occurred eight hours after procarbazine administration and remained suppressed beyond the period when DNA synthesis was restored. Chromosomal translocations were not observed *in vitro* in Ehrlich ascites or HeLa cells, however, which again suggests that procarbazine requires metabolic activation by mouse tissue enzymes to a compound capable of chromosome breakage.[50] Rutishauser and Bollag reported that a single procarbazine dose decreases the percentage of cells undergoing mitosis from 4.9–9.0 per cent to 0.5 per cent depending on the dose and elapsed time after administration of the drug,[51] suggesting that the drug inhibits progression through a premitotic phase of the cell cycle. Llombart and Minguez[52, 53] found that the interphase of the cell cycle (G_1 phase) is the primary target of procarbazine action during the cell division process. The duration of antimitotic action varies from 12 to 48 hours and coincides with inhibition of a wide range of enzyme activities,[54] including several steps in the tricarboxylic acid cycle. It is uncertain, however, whether there exists a causal relationship between these two events.

Procarbazine, as well as 1-methyl-2-benzylhydrazine, can also produce chromatid breaks.[50, 51] Because no chromosome breaks or damage to pre-existing DNA occur,[44] the breaks probably occur during or after DNA synthesis. The number of breaks is dependent on the dose and elapsed time after treatment.[55]

In addition to chromatid breaks and translocations, procarbazine can inhibit RNA, DNA, and protein synthesis *in vivo* and *in vitro*. A single procarbazine dose decreases tRNA synthesis in implanted P815 ascites tumor cells after two hours; tRNA synthesis recovers after 24 hours.[56, 57] Nuclear RNA synthesis is inhibited by 50 per cent. The inhibition of tRNA synthesis is preceded by inhibition of normal tRNA methylation, and a lack of methylation of tRNA is believed to lead to alteration in its function.[58] Procarbazine also depresses incorporation of orotic acid into RNA uracil by 65 per cent in implanted L5178Y lymphoma.[44, 59]

Procarbazine also inhibits DNA and protein synthesis. A single procarbazine dose given to Ehrlich ascites-bearing mice inhibits its incorporation of thymidine into DNA thymidine.[20] A maximum of 35 to 40 per cent inhibition is reached four to eight hours after procarbazine administration; after eight hours thymidine utilization returns to normal. A similar effect has been observed in L5178Y lymphoma-bearing mice.[50, 59] A maximal inhibition of 70 per cent occurred one to three hours after procarbazine administration. Inhibition was totally absent after 24 hours. The inhibition was dose-related and not due to inhibition of thymidine kinase, monophosphate kinase, or DNA nucleotidyltransferase. Both *de novo* purine and pyrimidine nucleotide synthesis were blocked, although the inhibition of DNA synthesis was not due to the unavailability of one or more deoxynucleotides. Cellular DNA content remained unchanged.[50]

The inhibition of protein synthesis is delayed more than the inhibition of nucleic acid synthesis and does not reach a maximum until 12 to 16 hours after procarbazine administration.[20, 44, 59] Because inhibition of protein synthesis occurs after inhibition of nucleic acid synthesis, it is likely a secondary event. Recovery of inhibition occurs by 24 hours. There is no evidence to indicate that the decrease in protein synthesis is related to a defect in *in vivo* biosynthesis of mRNA or sRNA.[60] The mechanisms for protein synthesis[41, 42] were normal, including the number of polysomes, the ability of the ribosomes to accept polyuridylic acid, the ability of pH 5 enzymes to load sRNA, and the ability of sRNA to accept amino acids. Although the incorporation of labeled leucine into peptides was decreased in polysomes in procarbazine-pretreated animals, the loaded sRNA of pretreated animals could enter normally into the polysomes of untreated animals.

Finally, procarbazine has been reported to affect other cellular processes. Gutterman and co-workers[20] observed no change in oxygen uptake (respiration) or the production of CO_2 from glucose-1-^{14}C or glucose-6-^{14}C in Ehrlich ascites-bearing mice. However, other workers have observed a modest inhibition of oxidative phosphorylation,[61-64] and increases in the intracellular concentration of intermediates in anaerobic glycolysis.[65]

The determinants of procarbazine resistance are not well understood. During the initial testing of procarbazine antineoplastic activity, resistant lines of Walker carcinosarcoma 256 and Ehrlich ascites carcinoma were rapidly induced.[2] Gutterman et al. reported that resistance in Ehrlich ascites cells is possibly related to nucleic acid synthesis.[20] Resistance was induced much more rapidly when procarbazine was administered during periods of normal DNA synthesis than when it was given during a depression in DNA synthesis. In both cases, resistant cells contained two new metacentric chromosomes, the appearance of which coincided with the lack of mitotic inhibition and the presence of resistance to procarbazine.[66] Although the direct relation between this cytologic observation and resistance remains unknown, amplification of a gene coding for a target enzyme is an interesting possibility in light of recent findings of amplified dihydrofolate reductase genes in cells resistant to methotrexate.[67]

No studies have been reported of procarbazine effects upon common mechanisms of cellular resistance toward alkylating agents, such as repair of drug-induced DNA damage, changes in intracellular concentrations of protective sulfhydryl compounds (i.e., glutathione), or changes in cellular transport or permeability.[68] Resistance probably is not related to transport factors, as a recent study by Lam et al. on the *in vitro* mechanism of uptake of procarbazine by L5178Y lymphoblasts showed that transport is likely by simple diffusion.[69]

Assay Methods

The detection and quantitation of procarbazine and its metabolites present difficult problems because of the highly polar nature of the parent compound and the nonpolarity of the primary metabolites, and the chemical instability of these compounds. Initial studies in man were performed with radiolabeled drug, with preliminary identification of metabolites by thin-layer chromatography. High-pressure liquid chromatography (HPLC), using a reverse-phase system, now appears to be the best technique for separation and quantitation of the polar metabolites, including the azo and azoxy derivatives, and *p*-formyl-N-isopropylbenzamide.[14, 24] Procarbazine and N-isopropylterephthalamic acid are not detected in these HPLC systems, but can be measured by mass spectrometry.[14] Neither HPLC analysis nor mass spectrometry has been applied to the study of clinical pharmacokinetics at this time.

Biodistribution and Pharmacokinetics

The biodistribution of procarbazine and biologically active metabolites in humans has not been adequately studied. Raaflaub and Schwartz[35] showed that ^{14}C-procarbazine is cleared from plasma with a seven-minute half-life following intravenous administration of 150 mg. The azo metabolite appeared very rapidly and the inactive N-isopropylterephthalamic acid could be detected after ten minutes. This acid is the major metabolite excreted in urine by humans.[35, 70] Procarbazine and/or unidentified metabolites appeared in the cerebrospinal fluid of dogs 15 minutes after intravenous injection of 100 mg per kg.[70]

The plasma clearance of procarbazine[27] and the appearance of the azo compound, azoxy isomers, and the inactive N-isopropylterephthalamic acid in rats following intraperitoneal administration of 150 mg per kg are shown in Figure 15–4. Procarbazine concentration decreases rapidly and is eliminated by two hours. The azo metabolite peaks within 10 to 20 minutes, followed by the appearance of methyl and benzylazoxy isomers. Liver perfusion studies indicated that procarbazine is converted almost entirely to the azo metabolite.[26, 28] The relatively low azo and azoxy plasma concentrations may reflect the larger volume of distribution of these lipophilic compounds. Both azo and azoxy metabolites appear in brain 10 to 30 minutes after procarbazine administration.[17]

The conversion of procarbazine to an active alkylating intermediate involves liver endoplasmic reticulum enzymes that are subject to induction by agents such as phenobarbital and phenytoin (Dilantin), which are frequently administered along with cancer chemotherapeutic agents. Drug interactions of this type may significantly alter procarbazine activation. Pretreatment of rats with phenobarbital before procarbazine administration results in an increased procarbazine clearance and a slight decrease in peak azo concentrations.[27] Azo and both azoxy metabolites are cleared more rapidly from the phenobarbital-pretreated animal, indicating that azo and azoxy isomers are also subject to microsomal-inducing agents. Microsomal enzyme induction presumably results in the more rapid generation of active alkylating intermediates, because phenobarbital or phenytoin pretreatment increases the survival of procarbazine-treated, tumor-bearing mice. Conversely, procarbazine inhibits the biotransformation of pentobarbital and aminopyrene by rat liver microsomes and prolongs pentobarbital-induced sleeping time.[10, 70, 71] These findings suggest that drug interactions between procarbazine and other agents metabolized by microsomes

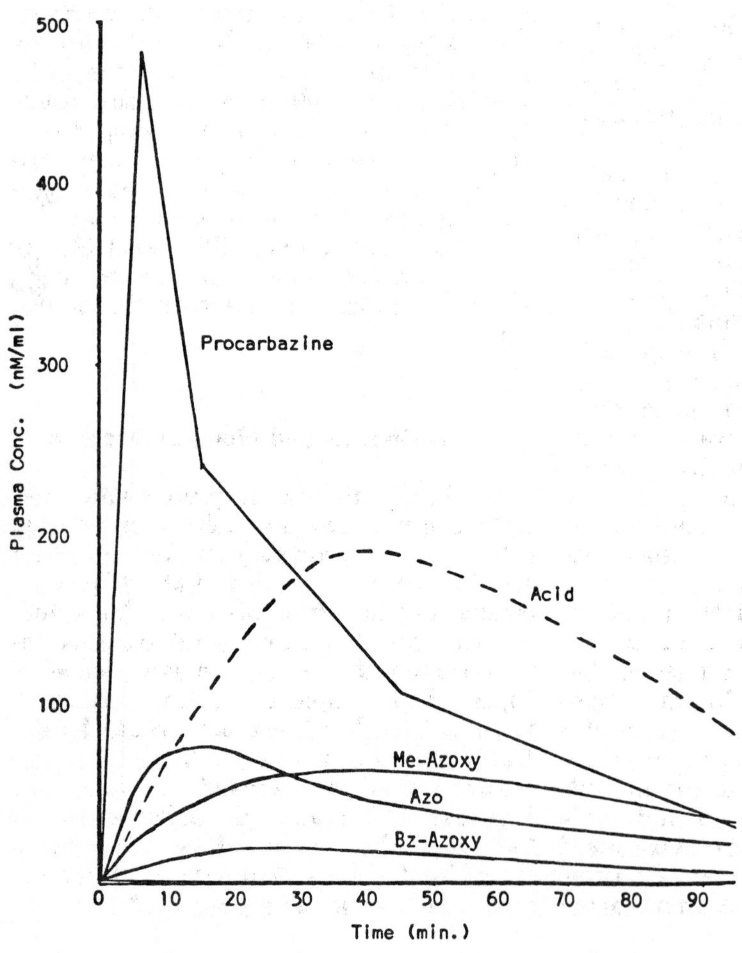

Figure 15–4. Procarbazine plasma clearance and metabolite appearance following the intraperitoneal administration of 150 mg/kg to rat.

may significantly affect the clinical activity and biodistribution of both the anticancer drug and these accessory agents.

Clinical Usage

Procarbazine is used primarily in the combination therapy of Hodgkin's disease and the non-Hodgkin's lymphomas, although it is gaining increased attention in the treatment of brain neoplasms and small cell carcinoma of the lung. It also produces responses in patients with multiple myeloma and malignant melanoma,[9] although the drug is not used in primary treatment protocols in these diseases. Because procarbazine is not cross-resistant with alkylating agents and has relatively mild bone marrow toxicity, it can be used in full therapeutic doses in combination with nitrogen mustard or cyclophosphamide in the highly effective combination therapy of the lymphomas. The MOPP combination widely employed in Hodgkin's disease, a curative regimen in approximately 50 per cent of patients with advanced disease, consists of procarbazine given once daily for 14 days in doses of 100 mg per m^2, plus nitrogen mustard, vincristine (Oncovin), and prednisone. It is commonly used in an identical 14-day schedule with 2-chloroethyl-2-cyclohexyl-1-nitrosourea (CCNU) and vincristine in the treatment of malignant brain tumors.[12] Alternatively, procarbazine may be given as a single agent in daily doses of 4 to 6 mg per kg per day for up to 30 days, with dose adjustment for leukopenia and thrombocytopenia.

Like many other antitumor agents, procarbazine has a broad range of clinical toxicities. Anorexia, nausea, and vomiting are frequent complaints during the initial week of therapy,[5] but usually diminish as treatment continues. The major toxic effect is myelosuppression, which becomes apparent during the second week of treatment and may not completely reverse until two weeks after the end of a course of therapy. The duration and severity of myelosuppression are clearly dose-dependent.

In contrast to the myelosuppressive toxicity of oral procarbazine, its intravenous administration produces primarily neurotoxic symptoms. High single-bolus IV doses (over 1 gm per dose) cause nausea, vomiting, and marked confusion or somnolence. Obtundation may last two to three days.[73] The clinical effectiveness of this route of treatment has not been established; the only apparent advantage is the lack of myelosuppression, but clinical activity may not be equal to the oral route, particularly in view of the possibility that the first pass of drug through the portal circulation may be important in the activation of orally administered procarbazine.

In addition to gastrointestinal toxicity and myelosuppression, orally administered procarbazine produces hemolysis in glucose-6-phosphate dehydrogenase–deficient patients.[74] Occasional patients receiving oral procarbazine may complain of neurotoxic symptoms, including paresthesias and changes in mood or mental status such as depression, somnolence, or agitation. Procarbazine is known to inhibit monamine oxidase activity[75] and to cause depletion of pyridoxal phosphate,[76] probably by interaction of the hydrazine with the aldehyde group of pyridoxal phosphate. Inhibition of monamine oxidase sensitizes patients to foods containing a high content of tyramine, such as wine, bananas, ripe cheeses, and yogurt; ingestion of such foods may cause acute hypertensive reactions. Procarbazine also has a disulfiram-like action that may lead to facial flushing, headache, and sweating in patients who ingest alcohol while receiving the anticancer drug.

Because of its sedative effects and its ability to inhibit the microsomal inactivation of hypnotics, procarbazine-treated patients should not receive barbiturates, phenothiazines, and other hypnotics or sedatives.

Allergic reactions to procarbazine are common and may include urticaria, maculopapular skin rash, pulmonary infiltrates, and eosinophilia.[77, 78] In many patients who develop cutaneous reactions, the drug may be continued in the presence of corticosteroids without exacerbation of the rash.

In addition to its wide range of acute toxicity, procarbazine is profoundly immunosuppressive,[79] highly mutagenic,[21, 22] teratogenic,[80, 81] and potently carcinogenic[82] in animals. The latter toxicity is of particular concern in clinical chemotherapy because of the curative potential of the MOPP combination in Hodgkin's disease, and the small but finite incidence of second malignancies in MOPP-treated patients. The carcinogenicity of procarbazine is discussed in further detail in Chapter 6. Procarbazine also ablates spermatogenesis and may be responsible for the high incidence of infertility in male patients who have been treated with MOPP.

DTIC (DACARBAZINE)

Bruce A. Chabner

The rational synthesis of new antitumor agents presents formidable obstacles. Not only must a key reaction site be identified and understood, but the proposed agent must be able to pass several major hurdles (formulation, bioavailability, intracellular penetration, and metabolism) in order to arrive at its designated site in an active form. In the design of antimetabolites, changes in structure may lead to entirely new and unpredicted cytotoxic mechanisms unrelated to the original intentions of the theorist. One of the best examples of this disparity between hypothesis and practice is provided by 5-methyl-(3,3-dimethyl-1-triazeno)-imidazole-4-carboxamide (DTIC, or dacarbazine). DTIC was conceived as one of several potential analogues of 5-amino-imidazole-4-carboxamide (AIC), an intermediate in synthesis of the purine ring (Fig. 15–5). Montgomery[83] reviewed the development of this series of compounds at the Southern Research Institute in the late 1950s.

The first of these purine analogues synthesized was the nitrous acid addition product 5-diazoimidazole-4-carboxamide, which proved to have significant antitumor activity in experimental testing. The addition of a third nitrogen group created a light-sensitive 5-triazene that spontaneously converted back to the diazo analogue; the latter was found to undergo cyclization to form 2-azahypoxanthine, a compound known to be metabolized to a nucleotide form and potentially an active purine analogue in its own right (Fig. 15–6).[84] Further modification of the triazene analogue was undertaken to form more stable but still light-sensitive derivatives, the most active of which was the dimethyltriazene (DTIC).[85]

MECHANISM OF ACTION

It is now clear that DTIC does not exert its antitumor activity as a purine analogue. The drug is active against various 6-thioguanine- and 6-mercaptopurine-resistant cell lines, and does not show the schedule dependence and cell cycle dependence of other purine

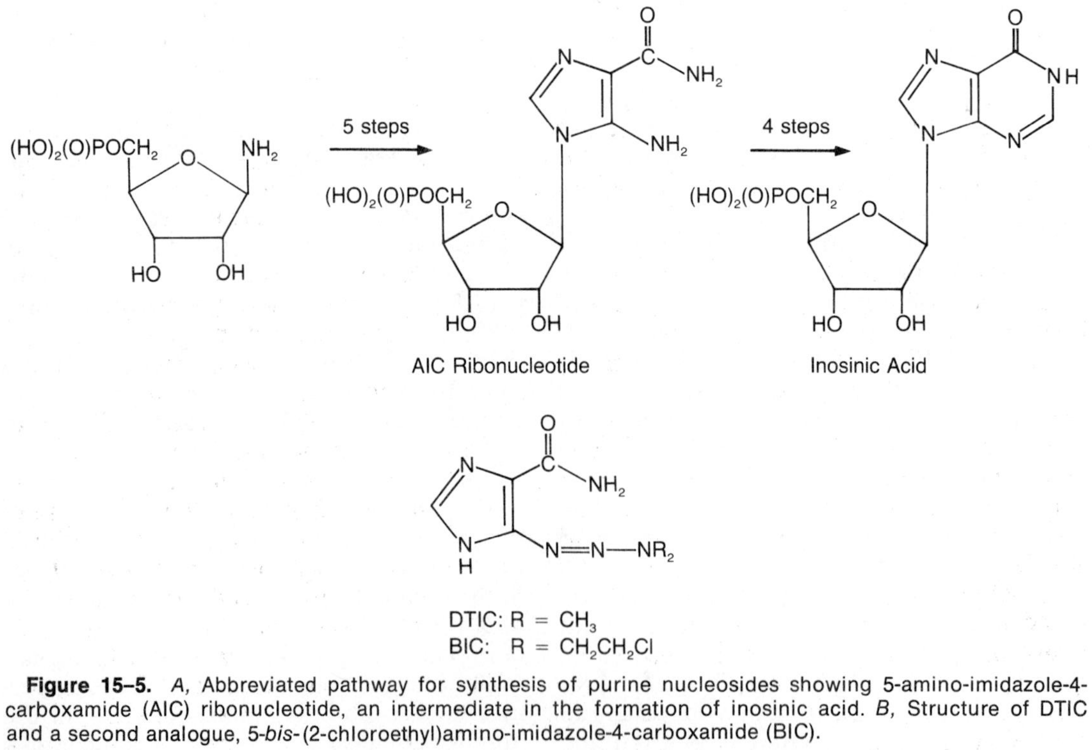

$(HO)_2(O)POCH_2$ — 5 steps → AIC Ribonucleotide — 4 steps → Inosinic Acid

DTIC: R = CH_3
BIC: R = CH_2CH_2Cl

Figure 15–5. *A,* Abbreviated pathway for synthesis of purine nucleosides showing 5-amino-imidazole-4-carboxamide (AIC) ribonucleotide, an intermediate in the formation of inosinic acid. *B,* Structure of DTIC and a second analogue, 5-*bis*-(2-chloroethyl)amino-imidazole-4-carboxamide (BIC).

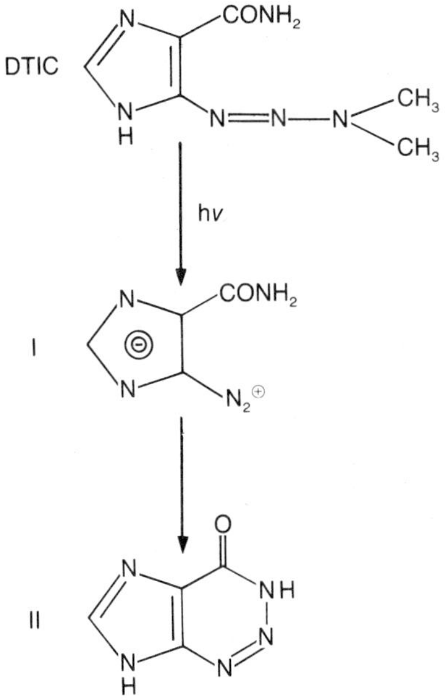

Figure 15–6. Light-induced conversion of DTIC to 5-diazo-imidazole-4-carboxamide (I) and 2-azahypoxanthine (II). (Reproduced with permission from Montgomery JA: Experimental studies at Southern Research Institute with DTIC. Cancer Treat. Rep. 60:141, 1976.)

antimetabolites.[83] The AIC portion of the molecule is not essential for activity and can be replaced by a simple phenylamine substitution.[86] Second, the parent drug has little activity in tissue culture,[86-88] but is believed to undergo metabolic activation to yield a methylating species.[89] The pathway of DTIC activation (Fig. 15–7) requires an initial elimination of one methyl group by a microsomal, NADPH-dependent, mixed-function oxidase to form monomethyl-5-amino-imidazole-4-carboxamide. The latter compound spontaneously tautomerizes and eliminates methyldiazonium ion, $CH_3N^+{\equiv}N$, as the active methylating intermediate. Evidence for methylation of nucleic acids has been obtained in studies of DTIC action in tissue culture[88, 90] and by identification of urinary excretion products in man.[91]

The site of microsomal activation of DTIC in intact animals is not clear. Liver microsomes are known to accomplish this conversion,[89, 92] but Hill was unable to detect enzymatic metabolism of DTIC in homogenates of other mouse tissues or sarcoma 180 cells. However, small amounts of alkylated DNA can be detected after incubation of Chinese hamster ovary cells with DTIC,[88] and the possibility remains that some tumors may possess the necessary microsomal activity.[90] DTIC is active only in high concentrations in tissue culture (see below), indicating that extratumor activation is probably required for this drug.

Further analogues of DTIC have been tested,[83] and several have superior activity in animal systems. One of these, the *bis*-chloroethyl derivative (Fig. 15–5), undergoes very similar metabolism to DTIC to yield an active 2-chloroethyl alkylating group;[94] comparative clinical trials of DTIC and this compound (often referred to as TIC mustard) have shown lesser activity against malignant melanoma for the latter compound.[95]

Dacarbazine retains the light-sensitivity of

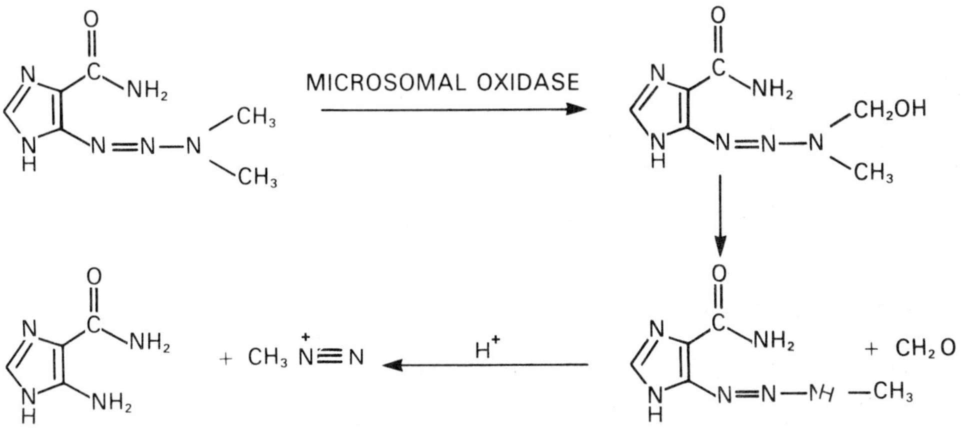

Figure 15–7. Pathway for activation of DTIC to an alkylating intermediate, methyldiazonium ion ($CH_3N^+{\equiv}N$). The initial step is mediated by microsomal mixed function oxidase, but the subsequent reactions are not clearly defined.

its parent triazene and therefore must be protected from light during *in vitro* studies. Interestingly, its photodecomposition (Fig. 15–6) yields 5-diazoimidazole-4-carboxamide, which cyclizes as previously mentioned to form the purine analogue azahypoxanthine. Both azahypoxanthine and 5-diazoimidazole-4-carboxamide are moderately cytotoxic to mammalian cells in tissue culture[87, 96] and could contribute to the cytotoxicity of the parent compound. The light-activation pathway probably accounts for the antitumor effects of DTIC in tissue culture, since in many reported experiments the minimal antitumor activity of DTIC *in vitro* is considerably enhanced by exposure of the culture to light.[88, 92] Although there is no reason to expect that the light-activation pathways are important in the whole animal, a careful study of DTIC metabolism and pharmacokinetics in man is required to determine the relative importance of microsomal metabolism and that of the alternative pathway.

CELLULAR PHARMACOLOGY

The cellular uptake process for DTIC and its potential active intermediates has not been studied. The available information concerning its effect on macromolecular synthesis is also incomplete, since the experiments have been performed in the absence of a microsomal activating system, and many have been conducted in the presence of light. Thus, the results are of uncertain relevance to the antitumor action of DTIC in the whole animal.

When incubated with tumor cells in culture, DTIC inhibits synthesis of DNA, RNA, and protein,[97] but has relatively greater effects on DNA synthesis if experiments are conducted in the presence of light.[90] The effects of DTIC on cell cycle progression are similarly uncertain. The drug appears to kill cells in all phases of the cell cycle[92, 98] and may produce progression delay through the G_2 phase of the cycle.[97]

Experimental Chemotherapy

Dacarbazine is active against a broad spectrum of experimental murine tumors, including L1210, sarcoma 180, adenocarcinoma 755, and the Ehrlich ascites tumor.[83] It shows no cross-resistance with L1210 sublines unresponsive to methotrexate, 5-fluorouracil, and (as previously mentioned) the purine antimetabolites. There is little evidence of schedule-dependency in its effectiveness against L1210; daily doses for 30 days give no better results than single doses on day 1 after tumor implantation. DTIC is active by the oral route in mice, but has not been employed in this manner in clinical trials.

Various combinations employing DTIC have been tested against L1210, but synergism has resulted only for DTIC with melphalan or doxorubicin (Adriamycin). No effect was observed when DTIC was administered with agents that enhance (phenobarbital) or inhibit (SKF-525A) microsomal mixed-function oxidase activity.

Assay Methods

A colorimetric method for DTIC has been the primary assay procedure employed in pharmacokinetic studies in man. The method employs an initial photodecomposition of DTIC to a primary amine; the amine is then coupled to the Bratton-Marshall reagent, and the resulting colored compound may be measured by its ultraviolet absorption.[99, 100] A variation of this assay method, in which protein is precipitated by sulfosalycylic acid rather than trichloroacetic acid, gives lower background values and increased sensitivity.[101] DTIC and its metabolite AIC may also be separated by HPLC, using a μBondapak C_{18} column eluted with heptane sulfonic acid and methanol or with sodium acetate; the compounds are detected by ultraviolet absorption at 300 nm.[102] The HPLC method has significant advantages over the colorimetric method, since the latter measures both parent compound and several of the potential metabolites (the monomethyl derivative and AIC itself). The colorimetric methods have a sensitivity of 0.1 μg per ml in plasma; HPLC appears to be somewhat less sensitive (1 μg/ml) in the preliminary description of its use in clinical studies.

Clinical Pharmacokinetics

Because of the lack of specificity and sensitivity of the available methods for DTIC measurement, the present information on pharmacokinetics of this compound must be regarded as preliminary. The drug appears to be well absorbed by the oral route, as judged by the very similar cumulative urinary excretion of drug administered by the oral versus the intravenous route.[101] Intravenous infusion of 4.5 mg per kg, about 200 mg per m^2, yields peak plasma concentrations of 9 μg per ml, as compared with peak plasma levels of 2 μg per ml for the same dose given by the oral route. About 20 per cent of drug in plasma is loosely bound to protein.[100] The drug distributes into a volume that exceeds total body water, and disappears from the plasma with a half-life of approximately 3.2 hours.[102] Thirty to 40 per cent of an intravenous dose is recovered in the urine within 24 hours, as detected by the colorimetric method; because of the lack of specificity of this method, it is not certain that the drug is excreted unchanged.[100, 101] Urinary clearance of DTIC, calculated on the basis of these data, exceeds inulin clearance and averages 230 ml per minute. However, it is not known whether renal dysfunction has any effect on DTIC pharmacokinetics. As discussed above, it is quite likely that hepatic metabolism (demethylation) of DTIC is a primary feature of its disposition in man, and the ultimate breakdown product, AIC, has been detected in plasma.[102]

DTIC does not penetrate well into the cerebrospinal fluid in dogs. At equilibrium, the ratio between plasma and spinal fluid is 1:7, as judged by the colorimetric method.[108] This poor penetration is consistent with the lack of activity against intracranial L1210 leukemia.[83]

Since DTIC is frequently used in combination with other antineoplastic agents or with immune adjuvants, drug interactions have received attention. *Corynebacterium parvum*, an immune adjuvant frequently used with DTIC in treatment of malignant melanoma, causes a prolongation of the DTIC plasma half-life to 4.8 hours, as opposed to 3.02 for controls,[102] whereas actinomycin D given with *C. parvum* and DTIC reverses this effect and returns the DTIC half-life to 3.0 hours. *C. parvum* treatment has been shown to depress the N-demethylation of other drugs;[103] prolongation of the DTIC half-life by *C. parvum* is consistent with the hypothesis that DTIC undergoes hepatic N-demethylation.

Clinical Chemotherapy

The clinical use of DTIC is confined to the treatment of malignant melanoma, Hodgkin's disease, and soft tissue sarcoma. It is the single most active agent in malignant melanoma,[104] having a response rate of approximately 25 per cent; little, if any, improvement in this response rate has resulted from combination therapy with the few other active drugs in this disease, including BCNU and vincristine.[105] In patients with Hodgkin's disease, DTIC has been combined with doxorubicin, BCNU, and vinblastine (ABVD) to treat patients resistant to the standard MOPP combination, with a high initial response rate of approximately 70 per cent.[106] This combination is now being tested with and without MOPP in previously untreated patients. The value of DTIC in the treatment of soft tissue sarcoma is less well established, although response rates in the order of 20 to 30 per cent have been reported.[107]

A variety of clinical schedules of administration have been used. There appears to be little evidence for schedule-dependency; an equal response rate to single doses of 650 to 1450 mg per m^2 every four to six weeks, as opposed to the more frequently used daily schedule of 150 to 300 mg per m^2 per day for five to ten days, has been reported in studies of malignant melanoma.[108] DTIC in doses of 250 mg per m^2 per day for five days has also been used by intra-arterial infusion to treat malignant melanoma involving the pelvis, soft tissues, or maxillofacial region. Einhorn et al. reported a 41 per cent response rate, with few instances of progression of local disease during therapy.[109] These results are difficult to interpret in view of the likelihood that the drug requires metabolic activation in the liver.

The primary toxicity of DTIC treatment consists of moderate-to-severe nausea and vomiting; these symptoms are usually most severe during the initial days of treatment and may be ameliorated by beginning treatment at a lower dose, with gradual escalation as tolerance develops.[110] Doses of less than 250 mg per m^2 per day for five days produce only modest leukopenia or thrombocytopenia in 10 to 25 per cent of patients, the nadir occurring two to three weeks after completion of treatment. However, escalation above this dose level is prevented by gastrointestinal symptoms. With single, large-bolus doses above 650 mg per m^2, severe nausea and vomiting lasting 24 to 48 hours are observed in most patients.[111] The mild degree of bone marrow suppression has enhanced the attractiveness of DTIC for combination therapy.

Other less frequent toxicities include mild hepatic dysfunction and a flu-like syndrome of fever, myalgias, and malaise lasting through the period of treatment. An enhancement of doxorubicin-induced cardiac toxicity has been suggested on the basis of one report in which four of ten children receiving DTIC, doxorubicin, and vincristine or VP-16 developed congestive heart failure at doxorubicin doses of 300 to 540 mg per m^2.[112] The effects of DTIC on the immune system have received considerable attention,[113-116] but the drug has not been used clinically as an immunosuppressant.

Immunologic Effects

Dacarbazine has been shown to depress both primary antibody responses and allograft rejection in mice.[114, 115] In mice, the depression of antibody response to sheep red blood cells or rejection of an incompatible tumor graft can still be demonstrated 60 days after drug administration.[116] It has no suppressive effect on natural killer-cell activity in mice.[117]

Dacarbazine appears capable of altering the immunogenicity of drug-resistant tumor sublines in mice.[114] Highly immunogenic sublines of L1210 or L5178Y lymphomas have been obtained by repeated passage following DTIC treatment, such that large innoculi of the resistant cell lines are rejected by nonimmunosuppressed mice.[114, 118] The rejection of these tumors correlates with the development of lymphocytes cytotoxic for the challenge cell line.[118] It is not known whether similar enhancement of immunogenicity occurs after clinical use of DTIC.

In man the common clinical schedule of 150 to 250 mg per m^2 per day for five days does not produce consistent suppression of delayed hypersensitivity or antibody production if antigen is given on the first day of drug administration.[119] However, experimental studies indicate that DTIC suppression of delayed hypersensitivity is more effective when the drug is given several days before antigenic challenge.

Delayed Side Effects

Despite having only modest mutagenic activity in the Ames test, DTIC is highly carcinogenic in rodents, producing thymic tumors and mammary carcinoma in female and male buffalo rats when given in either single doses or multiple injections. It is also carcinogenic when given by the oral route.[120, 121] Lung and uterine tumors, and also lymphomas, are produced in mice.[122] Metabolites of DTIC have also been tested for carcinogenicity; of these, 3-methyl-1-triazenoimidazole-4-carboxamide produced a spectrum of tumors resembling that of the parent compound, although in lower frequency.[121]

Dacarbazine has also been found to produce fetal malformations and a high incidence of fetal resorptions when administered to pregnant animals. Specific fetal malformations in rats and rabbits are influenced by the interval of exposure during pregnancy and by the dose of DTIC administered; these abnormalities include malformations of the urogenital system, skeleton, eye, and cardiovascular system in rats, and the urogenital and skeletal systems in rabbits.[123, 124]

HEXAMETHYLMELAMINE

Bruce A. Chabner

The third clinically important agent in this group of biochemically activated alkylating agents is hexamethylmelamine (HMM), a structural analogue of the alkylating agent triethylenemelamine (Fig. 15–8). The synthesis of HMM was first reported in 1951,[125] and its antitumor activity against the Walker 256 sarcoma and the Crocker mouse sarcoma was identified shortly thereafter.[126, 127] Although considerable uncertainty exists as to its mechanism of antitumor action and metabolism, HMM has unmistakable and significant antitumor activity against alkylating agent–resistant tumors in man. These include ovarian cancer (30 per cent response rate),[128] small cell carcinoma of the lung (43 per cent response rate),[129] breast cancer (25 per cent response rate),[130] and the lymphomas,[131] and HMM is currently in use in numerous combination therapy

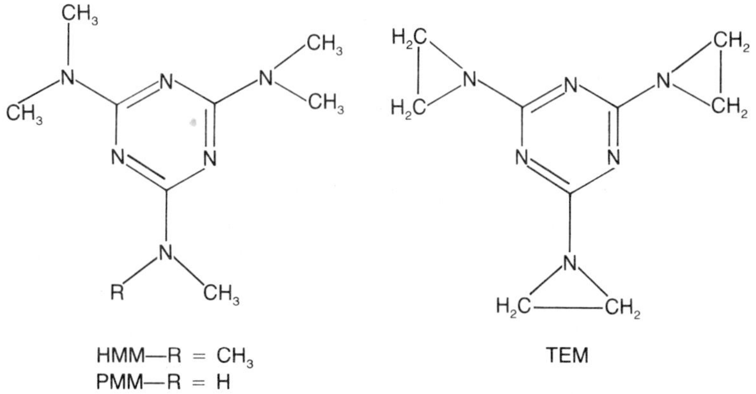

Figure 15–8. Structures of hexamethylmelamine (HMM), pentamethylmelamine (PMM), and triethylenemelamine (TEM).

HMM—R = CH_3
PMM—R = H

TEM

regimens for these diseases. The parent compound does not possess alkylating activity and has cytotoxic effects in tissue culture only in the presence of microsomes,[132, 133] indicating that an active intermediate must be formed *in vivo* by microsomal metabolism. Because of its clinical utility and lack of cross-resistance with conventional alkylating agents, an active search is under way to identify the active intermediate of HMM and to develop new analogues.

STRUCTURE AND MECHANISM OF ACTION

Hexamethylmelamine consists of a symmetric triazine ring system identical to that of the pyrimidine antimetabolite 5-azacytidine; to the ring system are attached three dimethylamine groups (Fig. 15–8). A formulation for intravenous administration has not been possible to date because of the compound's limited aqueous solubility. Thus, the drug is administered exclusively by the oral route. The six methyl groups attached to the amine side chains are unreactive chemically, as indicated by their failure to react with the alkyl-group acceptor, 4-(*p*-nitrobenzyl)pyridine.[134]

Primary attention has been paid to the likelihood that the methyl groups of HMM constitute the reactive site of the compound, but the mechanism whereby a reactive intermediate is formed and the structure of that metabolite have not been elucidated. Rutty and co-workers[135] showed that ring-labeled HMM becomes bound to acid-precipitable material, probably nucleic acids and/or protein, following intravenous administration to mice. No selective uptake by tumor cells was demonstrated, but a high concentration of labeled material was found in the small intestine, an important site of drug toxicity. Methyl-labeled drug also yields covalently bound material in tumor and normal tissues, with somewhat greater binding of the methyl-labeled material than of the ring-labeled compound.[135] This difference in binding of the two parts of the molecule could be explained by N-demethylation of HMM,[134, 136, 137] a process that produces formaldehyde *in vivo*.[135, 138] Formaldehyde could then be reutilized in the one-carbon pool for *de novo* purine or pyrimidine biosynthesis.

Despite this preliminary evidence for alkylation of macromolecules *in vivo*, the identity of the alkylating species remains speculative. Formaldehyde itself is weakly cytotoxic, but the HMM analogue trimethylmelamine, which produces equal plasma levels of formaldehyde, has no antitumor activity.[135] Thus, formaldehyde formation is unlikely to account for HMM cytotoxicity. An alternative candidate for the active intermediate is one of several N-methylol compounds that can be formed by hydroxylation of either the parent compound[139] or pentamethylmelamine (PMM), an *in vivo* metabolite. However, certain differences in the cytotoxic action of HMM and its monomethylol derivative have been noted in tissue culture experiments;[135] in addition, it is uncertain at present whether N-methylol metabolites are formed *in vivo* in significant amounts.

Although HMM is not cross-resistant with the commonly used alkylating agents, either clinically or in experimental systems, this finding does not rule out the possibility of an alkylating mechanism of HMM action. Resistance for specific classic alkylating agents such as nitrogen mustard or phenylalanine mustard may occur at the level of drug transport, and thus would not affect an alkylating agent of an entirely different structure. Mechanisms of HMM action other than alkylation have been proposed, such as antifolate or antimetabolite effects, based on the structural similarity of HMM and other such compounds,[140] but neither proposal has been supported by experimental evidence.

METABOLISM

In rodents,[136, 137] rabbits,[141] and man,[136, 137, 141] HMM undergoes rapid and extensive N-demethylation in a process that can be reproduced *in vitro* by incubation with hepatic microsomes.[142] In man, approximately 10 per cent of ^{14}C-(methyl)-HMM is recovered as respiratory $^{14}CO_2$ within six hours of administration,[136] and 29 per cent is recovered in the urine in the form of various partially demethylated metabolites. The S-triazine ring is not cleaved metabolically, and 90 per cent of ring-labeled material is recovered with the ring intact in the urine.[137] The stability of the triazine ring in compound contrasts with the extreme lability of the triazine ring of 5-azacytidine[142] (see Chapter 8). The primary urinary metabolites are N^2,N^2,N^4,N^6-tetramethylmelamine; N^2,N^4,N^6-trimethylmelamine; N^2,N^4-dimethylmelamine; monomethylmelamine; and melamine (Table 15–1 and Fig. 15–9). None of these metabolites has alkylating activity in solution when tested with 4-(*p*-nitrobenzyl)pyridine.

Analogues

The minor urinary metabolite PMM, along with the tetra-, tri-, di-, and monomethylmelamines, all have *in vivo* antitumor activity against L1210 leukemia.[143] In general, the cytotoxic potency as well as the rate of N-demethylation of these compounds decreases with decreasing numbers of methyl groups.[142,143] Melamine is inactive against L1210.

Of the various possible demethylated analogues, PMM is the only compound to enter clinical trials, being chosen because its aqueous solubility is greater than that of HMM, thus allowing an intravenous formulation for PMM. It was hoped that an intravenous preparation would have less gastrointestinal toxicity than the oral compound, but preliminary trials of PMM have revealed that the new drug causes severe nausea and vomiting, indicating that these side effects are likely the result of an action on the central nervous system. The metabolism of PMM closely resembles that of HMM, in that N-demethylation occurs rapidly; less than 1 per cent of the parent compound is recovered intact in the urine in man.[141]

The chemical synthesis and properties of a number of melamine analogues with antitumor activity have been described by Cumber and Ross.[144] In addition to PMM, a second compound, N^2,N^4,N^6-trimethylolmelamine, has shown activity against a human lung tumor xenograft and may be a candidate for future trials.[145]

Assay Methods

The higher methylated melamine derivatives such as HMM and PMM are readily extracted from plasma with heptane or toluene.[146, 147] Alternatively, in acid solution, PMM and the demethylated metabolites are positively charged and can be concentrated from plasma by absorption on a cation ex-

TABLE 15–1. Percentage of HMM Metabolites in 24-Hour Urine*

	HMM Metabolites (%)		
	PATIENT 1	PATIENT 2	RATS
N^2,N^4,N^6-Trimethylmelamine	6	7	2
N^2,N^4-Dimethylmelamine	23	26	33
Monomethylmelamine	23	19	32
Melamine	5	5	2
Miscellaneous	5	4	5
Total (% of administered dose)	62	61	74

*Reproduced with permission from Worzalla et al.: Metabolism of hexamethylmelamine-ring-C^{14} in rats and man. Cancer Res. 34:2669, 1974.

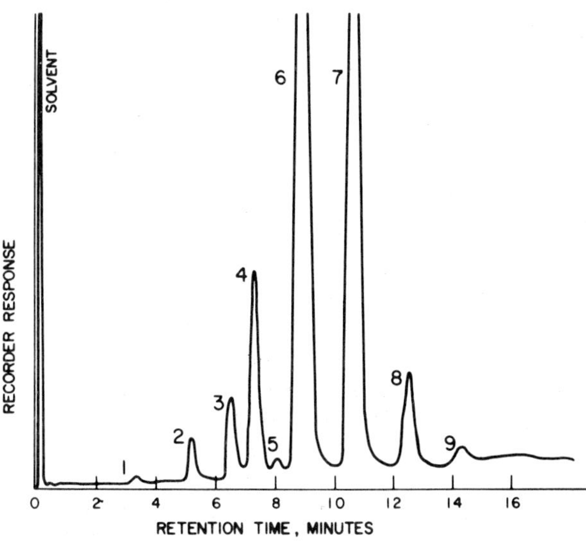

Figure 15–9. Gas chromatogram of 24-hr urine of patient after administration of HMM. The peaks correspond to the following metabolites: *1,* pentamethylmelamine; *2,* N^2,N^2,N^4,N^6-tetramethylmelamine; *3,* N^2,N^2,N^4-trimethylmelamine; *4,* N^2,N^4,N^6-trimethylmelamine; *5,* N^2,N^2-dimethylmelamine; *6,* N^2,N^4-dimethylmelamine; *7,* monomethylmelamine; *8,* melamine; *9,* unknown. (Reproduced with permission from Worzalla et al.: Metabolism of hexamethylmelamine-ring-C^{14} in rats and man. Cancer Res. 34:2669, 1974.)

change minicolumn.[148] These concentration procedures are important because they allow measurement of low concentrations of drug through reduction of background, particularly in work with urine samples; these procedures also allow the application of drug samples concentrated from large volumes of plasma. Initial pharmacologic studies of HMM employed anion and cation exchange resins to separate HMM from metabolites, with ultraviolet spectral detection for quantitation of drug concentration (Table 15–2).[149] These methods were insufficiently sensitive to quantitate HMM or its metabolites in plasma beyond a two-hour time point, and were primarily useful in quantification and identification of urinary excretion products. Measurement sensitivity has been extended to the level of 0.1 to 0.5 μM for both PMM and HMM in plasma, using gas chromatography with a nitrogen detector.[146, 147] This method allows separation of parent compound from the demethylated metabolites, but the metabolites have not been quantitatively determined at this time. An alternative method for measurement of PMM (also adaptable to measurement of HMM) has been described by Dutcher and colleagues,[148] who employed a preliminary cation exchange clean-up procedure, followed by gas chromatography–mass spectrometry. Deuterated parent compound, having a molecular ion of 199 mass units (three more than PMM), was used as an internal standard. Sensitivity for PMM by this method is 0.1 μM in plasma.

TABLE 15–2. Methods for Assay of Melamine Derivatives

Author (ref.)	*Drug*	*Analytical Method*	*Sensitivity*	*Specificity*
Dutcher[148]	PMM HMM	Preliminary cation exchange, then gas chromatography–mass spectrometry	0.1 μM in plasma	Complete
D'Incalci[146]	HMM	Gas chromatography with nitrogen detector	0.1 μM in plasma	Not specified, but probably excellent
Ames[147]	HMM PMM	Gas chromatography with nitrogen detector	0.5 μM HMM 0.05 μM PMM in plasma	Not specified, but probably excellent
Bryan[149]	HMM	Ion-exchange chromatography with ultraviolet detection	Poor	Excellent

Pharmacokinetics

Because of its limited aqueous solubility, HMM is administered by mouth in doses of 4 to 12 mg per kg per day for a course of 14 to 21 days.[150-152] Bioavailability of orally administered drug is highly variable, according to D'Incalci and co-workers,[146] who found a 100-fold variation in peak blood levels ranging from 0.2 to 0.8 μg per ml in a group of 11 patients. This variation could be due to variable absorption or to variable metabolism of the drug in its first pass through the liver via the portal circulation. Peak plasma concentrations are reached within three hours of oral administration, and the primary half-life of drug disappearance from plasma varies from 4.7 to 10.2 hours. Hepatic metabolism constitutes the primary elimination route, a conclusion based on the quantitative excretion of N-demethylated metabolites in the urine and the known ability of hepatic microsomes to accomplish this conversion *in vitro*. Less than 1 per cent of the drug is excreted intact (Table 15–1). Hepatic dysfunction and microsomal enzyme induction would be expected to influence HMM pharmacokinetics, but the necessary studies have not been performed as yet in man.

The pharmacokinetics of PMM have been examined in patients receiving this drug during phase I trials.[141, 148] At an intravenous dose of 80 mg per m^2, a dose considerably below the maximal-tolerated dose of 1000 to 1500 mg per m^2, the peak plasma concentration reaches 4.1 μM, after which a biphasic disappearance curve is observed, with half-lives of 27 and 133 minutes. Less than 0.1 per cent of the administered dose is recovered intact in the urine at doses of 80 mg per m^2.

Little information exists as to the distribution of either HMM or PMM into the central nervous system or into ascites. Preliminary experiments in mice have unexpectedly revealed that the more water-soluble compound, PMM, achieves a higher peak concentration in brain than does a comparable dose of HMM, a finding that may account for the severe nausea and vomiting induced by intravenous PMM.[153]

Schedules of Administration and Toxicity

Although HMM is usually administered in 14- to 21-day courses at doses of 4 to 12 mg per kg, longer periods of continuous administration have been used. These extended courses have led to unacceptable gastrointestinal toxicity, with no improvement in response rate.[128, 130, 154] The most troublesome HMM side effects are nausea and vomiting. Johnson et al. found that daily doses of 8 mg per kg per day led to these symptoms after an average of seven days of therapy and became dose-limiting after approximately six weeks of continuous treatment.[128] Gastrointestinal symptoms are a function of total drug dosage, in that the same total dose of 200 mg per kg is associated with unacceptable toxicity when administered in daily doses of 4 or 8 mg per kg per day. Weight loss frequently accompanies these symptoms, owing to decreased caloric intake. Some clinicians believe that gastrointestinal symptoms can be reduced by taking the drug in divided doses one to two hours after meals and at bedtime.[130]

Hexamethylmelamine also produces myelosuppression in approximately one quarter to one half of patients treated for 21 days or longer. Johnson et al. observed that almost one half of patients receiving 8 mg per kg per day developed leukopenia (WBC less than 3000 cells per mm^3) a median of 41 days after the initiation of treatment.[128] With shorter courses of treatment, such as used in combination chemotherapy, myelosuppression is less severe and frequent, and usually is not dose-limiting.

Neurotoxic symptoms also are produced by HMM in approximately 25 per cent of patients.[130] These side effects include mood changes such as lethargy, depression, or hallucinations, in addition to peripheral neuropathic symptoms such as paresthesias and loss of proprioception. Objective neurologic findings include decreased deep tendon reflexes and an ataxic gait. The neurotoxic side effects usually appear only after extended periods of treatment (one to three months) and abate upon withdrawal of the drug.[128, 155] The etiology of this neurotoxicity is unknown. It has been suggested that pyridoxal phosphate deficiency induced by a chemical reaction between the vitamin and the demethylated amine metabolites of HMM may be responsible, and it is claimed that pyridoxine, 100 mg three times daily, causes partial reversal of neurotoxic symptoms.[130] Rare reports of cutaneous toxicity have described instances of drug-related rash, pruritus, and eczema. The drug has no known renal or hepatic toxicity.

References

Procarbazine

1. Zeller P, Gutmann, H, Hegedus B, et al.: Methylhydrazine derivatives, a new class of cytotoxic agents. Experientia 19:129, 1963.
2. Bollag W, and Grunberg E: Tumor inhibitory effects of a new class of cytotoxic agents: methylhydrazine derivatives. Experientia 19:130, 1963.
3. Martz G: Clinical results with a methylhydrazine derivative. *In* Plattner P (ed.): Proceedings of the International Symposium on Chemotherapy of Cancer, Lugano, Switzerland. Elsevier, New York, 1964, p. 198.
4. Miller E: Development of procarbazine. *In* Carter S (ed.): Proceedings of the Chemotherapy Conference on Procarbazine (Mutalane NSC-77213): Development and Applications, Bethesda, MD. US Government Printing Office, Washington, DC, 1976, p. 3.
5. DeVita J, Serpick A, and Carbone P: Preliminary clinical studies with ibenzmethyzin. Ann. Intern. Med. 73:542, 1970.
6. Mathe G, Berumen L, Schweisguth O, et al.: Methylhydrazine in treatment of Hodgkin's disease. Lancet 2:1077, 1963.
7. Todd I: Experience with ibenzmethyzin. Br. Med. J. 1:628, 1965.
8. Kenis Y, Werli J, Hilbrand J, et al: Action d'un derive de la methylhydrazine. Eur. J. Cancer 1:33, 1965.
9. Jelliffee A, and Marks J (eds.): Natulan (Ibenzmethyzin). John Wright & Sons, Ltd., Bristol, England, 1965, p. 1.
10. Stolinski D, Solomon J, Pugh R, et al.: Clinical experience with procarbazine in Hodgkin's disease, reticulum cell sarcoma, and lymphosarcoma. Cancer 26:984, 1970.
11. Kumar AR, Renaudin J, Wilson CB, et al.: Procarbazine hydrochloride in the treatment of brain tumors. J. Neurosurg. 40:365, 1974.
12. Gutin PH, Wilson CB, Kumar AR, et al.: Phase II study of procarbazine, CCNU, and vincristine combination chemotherapy in the treatment of brain tumors. Cancer 35:1398, 1975.
13. Rucki R: Analytical profile-procarbazine hydrochloride. *In* Florey VK (ed.): Analytical Profiles of Drug Substances. Academic Press, New York, 1976, p. 404.
14. Weinkam RJ, and Shiba DA: Metabolic activation of procarbazine. Life Sci. 22:937, 1978.
15. Aebi H, Dewald B, and Suter H: Autoxydation N^2-substituierter Methylhydrazine Beeinflussung der Cu und Fe Katalyse durch Proteine. Helv. Chim. Acta 48:656, 1965.
16. Aebi H, Dewald B, and Suter H: Peroxidbildung bei der Autoxydation N^2-substituierter Methylhydrazine. Helv. Chim. Acta 48:1380, 1965.
17. Weinkam RJ, and Shiba DA: Unpublished observations.
18. Tsuji T, and Kosower E: Diazenes. VI. Alkyldiazenes. J. Am. Chem. Soc. 93:1992, 1971.
19. Gale GR, Simpson JG, and Smith AB: Studies of the mode of action of N-isopropyl-α-(2-methylhydrazine)-p-toluamide. Cancer Res. 27:1186, 1967.
20. Gutterman J, Huang A, and Hochstein P: Studies on the mode of action of N-isopropyl-α-(2-methylhydrazine)-p-toluamide. Proc. Soc. Exp. Biol. Med. 130:797, 1979.
21. Hansch C: Personal communication.
22. Pueyo C: Natulan induces forward mutations to L-arabinose resistance in *Salmonella typhimurium*. Mutat. Res. 67:189, 1979.
23. Prough RA, Coomes ML, and Dunn DL: Microsomal metabolism of carcinogenic and/or therapeutic hydrazines. *In* Roots I, Ullrich V, Hildebrandt A, et al. (eds): Microsomes and Drug Oxidation. Pergamon Press, New York, 1977, p. 500.
24. Dunn DL, Lubet RA, and Prough RA: Oxidative metabolism of N-isopropyl-alpha-(2-methylhydrazino)-p-toluamide hydrochloride (procarbazine) by rat liver microsomes. Cancer Res. 39:4555, 1979.
25. Prough RA, Wittkop JA, and Reed DJ: Evidence for the hepatic metabolism of some monoalkylhydrazines. Arch. Biochem. Biophys. 131:369, 1969.
26. Baggiolini M, Dewald B, and Aebi H: Oxidation of p-(N^1-methylhydrazinomethyl)-N-isopropylbenzamide to the methylazo derivative and oxidative cleavage of the N^2-C bond in the isolated perfused rat liver. Biochem. Pharmacol. 18:2187, 1969.
27. Shiba DA, and Weinkam RJ: Metabolic activation of procarbazine: activity of the intermediates and the effects of pretreatment. Proc. Am. Assoc. Cancer Res. 20:139, 1979.
28. Baggiolini M, Bickel MM, and Messiha FS: Demethylation *in vivo* of Natulan, a tumor-inhibiting methylhydrazine derivative. Experientia 21:334, 1965.
29. Wittkop J, Prough R, and Rerd D: Oxidative demethylation of N-methylhydrazines by rat liver microsomes. Arch. Biochem. Biophys. 134: 308, 1969.
30. Fiala ES: Investigation into the metabolism and mode of action of the colon carcinogen 1,2-dimethylhydrazine. Cancer 36:2407, 1975.
31. Matsumoto H, and Higa HH: Studies on methylazoxymethanol, the aglycone of cycasin: methylation of nucleic acids in vitro. Biochem. J. 98:20c, 1966.
32. Kreis W: Metabolism of an antineoplastic methylhydrazine derivative in a P815 mouse neoplasm. Cancer Res. 30:82, 1970.
33. Schwartz DE, Bollag W, and Obrecht P: Distribution and excretion studies of procarbazine in animals and man. Arzneimittelforschung 17:1389, 1967.
34. Bollag W: Investigations with methylhydrazine derivatives. *In* Plattner P (ed.): Proceedings of the International Symposium on Chemotherapy of Cancer, Lugano, Switzerland. Elsevier, New York, 1964, p. 191.
35. Raaflaub J, and Schwartz DE: Uber den Metabolismus einer cytostatisch wirksamen Methylhydrazin-Derivates (Natulan). Experientia 21:44, 1965.
36. Reed D, and Dost F: Methane and CO_2 formation by rats during metabolism of a methylhydrazine (Natulan). Proc. Am. Assoc. Cancer Res. 7:57, 1965.
37. Kreis W, and Yen Y: An antineoplastic C^{14}-labeled methylhydrazine derivative in P815 mouse leukemia. A metabolic study. Experientia 21:284, 1965.
38. Brookes P, and Lawley P: Alkylation of *Escherichia coli*: ability of a resistant strain to remove the product of difunctional alkylation of its DNA. British Empire Cancer Campaign for Research, 42nd Annual Report Covering the Year 1964, Part II, 1967, p. 77.
39. Dost F, and Reed D: Methane formation in vivo from N-isopropyl-α-(2-methylhydrazino)-p-toluamide hydrochloride, a tumor-inhibiting methylhydrazine derivative. Biochem. Pharmacol. 16:1741, 1967.
40. Gutterman J, Huang A, and Hochstein P: The mode of action of N-isopropyl-α-(2-methylhydrazine)-p-toluamide. Exp. Biol. Med. 130:797, 1969.
41. Weitzel G, Schneider F, Hirschmann W, et al.: Untersuchungen zum cytostatischen Wirkungsmechanismus der Methylhydrazin. III. Hoppe Seyler Z. Physiol. Chem. 348:443, 1967.
42. Weitzel G, Schneider F, Kummer D, et al.: Cytostatischer Wirkungs-Mechanismus von Natulan. Z. Krebsforsch. 70:354, 1968.
43. Weitzel G, Schneider F, Fretzdorff A, et al: Untersuchungen zum cytostatischen Wirkungsmechanismus der Methylhydrazin. II. Hoppe Seyler Z. Physiol. Chem. 348:433, 1967.
44. Sartorelli A, and Tsunamura S: Studies on the biochemical mode of action of a cytotoxic methylhydrazine derivative, N-isopropyl-α-(2-methylhydrazino)-p-toluamide. Mol. Pharmacol. 2:275, 1966.
45. Mizuno NS, Decker RW, and Zakis B: Effects of 5-(3-methyl-1-triazeno)imidazole-4-carboxamide on alkylating agent derived from 5-(3,3-dimethyl-1-triazeno)-

imidazole-4-carboxamide. Biochem. Pharmacol. 24:615, 1975.
46. Preussmann R, Druckrey H, Ivankovic S, et al.: Chemical structure and carcinogenicity of aliphatic hydrazo, azo, and azoxy compounds of triazenes, potential *in vivo* alkylating agents. Ann. NY Acad. Sc. 163:697, 1969.
47. Lee IP, and Dixon RL: Effects of procarbazine on spermatogenesis determined by velocity sedimentation cell separation. J. Pharmacol. Exp. Ther. 181:219, 1972.
48. Sieber SM, Correa P, Dalgard DW, et al.: Carcinogenic and other adverse effects of procarbazine in nonhuman primates. Cancer Res. 38:2125, 1978.
49. Lee IP, and Dixon RL: Mutagenicity, carcinogenicity and teratogenicity of procarbazine. Mutat. Res. 55:1, 1978.
50. Therman E: Chromosome breakage by 1-methyl-2-benzylhydrazine in mouse cancer cells. Cancer Res. 32:1111, 1972.
51. Rutishauser A, and Bollag W: Cytological investigations with a new class of cytotoxic agent: methylhydrazine derivatives. Experientia 19:131, 1963.
52. Llombart A Jr, and Minguez FP: Antimitotic activity of the methylhydrazine derivative Natulan in the Ehrlich ascites carcinoma. Oncology 23:201, 1969.
53. Llombart A, Llombart A Jr, and Minguez FP: Studies of the effects of an experimental antitumor methylhydrazine. Arch. Camerol. Esp. 5:7, 1966.
54. Llombart A Jr, Peydro A, and Llopia F: Some histochemical alterations induced by the methylhydrazine derivative Natulan on two experimental ascites tumors. Oncology 24:358, 1970.
55. Blijleven W, and Vogel E: The mutational spectrum of procarbazine on *Drosophila melanogaster*. Mutat. Res. 45:47, 1977.
56. Kreis W: Mechanism of action of procarbazine. *In* Carter S (ed.): Proceedings of the Chemotherapy Conference on Procarbazine: Development and Applications. Bethesda, MD. US Government Printing Office, Washington DC, 1970, p. 35.
57. Kreis W: Metabolism and reaction mechanism of a methylhydrazine derivative in DBF P815-leukemic mice. Proc. Am. Cancer Res. 7:39, 1966.
58. Revel M, and Littauer U: The coding properties of methyl-deficient phenylalanine transfer RNA from *Escherichia coli*. J. Mol. Biol. 15:389, 1966.
59. Sartorelli A, and Tsunamura S: Metabolic alteration of L5178Y lymphoma cells induced by procarbazine. Proc. Am. Assoc. Cancer Res. 6:55, 1965.
60. Koblet H, and Diggelmann H: The action of ibenzmethyzin on protein synthesis in the rat liver. Eur. J. Cancer 4:45, 1968.
61. Obrecht P, and Fusenig N: Zur Biochemie der sogenannten cytostatischen Nebenwirkin. Klin. Wochenschr. 44:1339, 1964.
62. Obrecht P, Strickstrock K, and Fusineg N: Die Wirking von Natulan und der Energiestoffwechsel. Z. Krebsforsch. 69:25, 1967.
63. Obrecht P, Strickstrock K, and Woenckhaus J: Zur Froge der biochemeschen Wirkung eines Neuen Zytostatikum und der Klosse der Methylhydrazin Derivate. Chemotherapia 8:106, 1964.
64. Fusenig N, Obrecht P, and Strickstrock K: Zur Biochemie der cytostatischen Nebenwirkungen. Klin. Wochenschr. 44:1335, 1966.
65. Weitzel G, Schneider F, Fritzdorff A, et al.: Untersuchungen zum cytostatischen Wirkungsmechanismus der Methylhydrazine. Z. Physiol. Chem. 336:271, 1964.
66. Huang A, Gutterman J, and Hochstein P: Cytogenetic changes induced by procarbazine in Ehrlich ascites tumor cells. Experientia 25:203, 1969.
67. Biedler J, Albrecht A, and Hutchinson D: Cytogenetics of mouse leukemia L1210. I. Associations of a specific chromosome with dihydrofolate reductase activity in Amethopterin-treated sublines. Cancer Res. 25:246, 1965.
68. Wheeler G: Studies related to mechanisms of resistance to biological alkylating agents. Cancer Res. 23:1334, 1963.
69. Lam H, Begleiter A, Stein W, et al.: On the mechanism of uptake of procarbazine by L5178Y lymphoblasts in vivo. Biochem. Pharmacol. 27:1883, 1978.
70. Oliverio V, Denham C, DeVita V, et al.: Some pharmacologic properties of a new antitumor agent N-isopropyl-α-(2-methylhydrazino)-p-toluamide. Cancer Chemother. Rep. 42:1, 1964.
71. Eade N, MacLeod S, and Renton K: Inhibition of hepatic microsomal drug metabolism by hydrazines. Can. J. Physiol. Pharmacol. 50:721, 1972.
72. Brunnes KW, and Young CW: A methylhydrazine derivative in Hodgkin's disease and other malignant neoplasms. Ann. Intern. Med. 63:69, 1965.
73. Chabner BA, Sponzo R, Hubbard S, et al.: High-dose intermittent intravenous infusion of procarbazine. Cancer Chemother. Rep. 57:361, 1973.
74. Sponzo RW, Arseneau J, and Canellos GP: Procarbazine-induced oxidative haemolysis: relationship to *in vivo* red cell survival. Br. J. Haematol. 27:587, 1974.
75. DeVita V, Hahn M, and Oliverio V: Monoamine oxidase inhibition by a new carcinostatic agent, procarbazine. Proc. Soc. Exp. Biol. Med. 120:561, 1965.
76. Chabner VA, DeVita VT, Considine N, et al: Plasma pyridoxal phosphate depletion by the carcinostatic procarbazine. Proc. Soc. Exp. Biol. Med. 132:1119, 1969.
77. Jones SE, Moore M, Blank N, et al.: Hypersensitivity to procarbazine (Matulane) manifested by fever and pleuropulmonary reaction. Cancer 29:498, 1972.
78. Lokich JJ, and Moloney WC: Allergic reaction to procarbazine. Clin. Pharmacol. Ther. 13:573, 1072.
79. Liske R: A Comparative study of the action of cyclophosphamide and procarbazine on the antibody production in mice. Clin. Exp. Immunol. 15:271, 1973.
80. Chaube S, and Murphy M: The teratogenic effects of 1-methyl-2-p-1-isopropylcarbomoylbenzyl-hydrazine Proc. Am. Assoc. Cancer Res. 5:11, 1964.
81. Chaube S, and Murphy M: Fetal malformations produced in rats by procarbazine. Teratology 2:23, 1969.
82. Sieber SM, Correa P, Dalgard DW, et al: Carcinogenesis and other adverse effects of procarbazine in non-human primates. Cancer Res. 38:2125, 1978.

DTIC

83. Montgomery JA: Experimental studies at Southern Research Institute with DTIC (NSC-45388). Cancer Treat. Rep. 60:125, 1976.
84. Shealy YF, Krauth CA, and Montgomery JA: Imidazoles. I. Coupling reactions of 5-diazoimidazole-4-carboxamide. J. Org. Chem. 27:2150, 1962.
85. Shealy YF, Montgomery JA, and Laster WR Jr: Antitumor activity of triazenoimidazoles. Biochem. Pharmacol. 11:674, 1962.
86. Schmid FA, and Hutchison DJ: Chemotherapeutic, carcinogenic, and cell-regulatory effects of triazenes. Cancer Res. 34:1671, 1974.
87. Beal DD, Skibba, JL, Whitnable KK, et al.: Effects of 5-(3,3-dimethyl-1-triazeno)imidazole-4-carboxamide and its metabolites on Novikoff hepatoma cells. Cancer Res. 36:2827, 1976.
88. Saunders PP, and Chao LY: Fate of the ring moiety of 5-(3,3-dimethyl-1-triazeno)imidazole-4-carboxamide in mammalian cells. Cancer Res. 34:2464, 1974.
89. Skibba JL, Beal DD, Ramirez G, et al.: N-Demethylation of the antineoplastic agent 4(5)--(3,3-dimethyl-1-triazeno)imidazole-5(4)-carboxamide by rats and man. Cancer Res. 30:147, 1970.
90. Loo TL, Housholder GE, Gerulath AH, et al.: Mechanism of action and pharmacology studies with DTIC (NSC-45388). Cancer Treat. Rep. 60:149, 1976.
91. Skibba JL, and Bryan GT: Methylation of nucleic acids and urinary excretion of ^{14}C-labelled 2-methylguanine by rats and man after administration of 4(5)-(3,3 dimethyl-1-triazeno)imidazole-5(4)-carboxamide. Toxic Appl. Pharmacol. 18:707, 1971.
92. Gerulath AH, and Loo TL: Mechanism of action of 5-(3,3-dimethyl-1-triazeno)imidazole-4-carboxamide (NSC-

45388) in mammalian cells in culture. Biochem. Pharmacol. 21:2335, 1972.

93. Hatheway GJ, Hansch C, Kim KH, et al: Antitumor 1-(x-aryl)-3,3-dialkyltriazenes. 1. Quantitative structure activity relationships vs. L1210 leukemia in mice. J. Med. Chem. 21:563, 1978.
94. Shealy YF, Krauth CA, Holum B, et al.: Synthesis and properties of the antileukemic agent 5(or 4)-3,3-bis(2-chlorethyl)-1-triazenoimidazole-4(or 5) carboxamide. J. Pharm. Sci. 57:83, 1969.
95. Costanza ME, Nathanson L, Costello WG, et al.: Results of a randomized study comparing DTIC with TIC mustard in malignant melanoma. Cancer 37:1654, 1976.
96. Montgomery JA, Laseter AG, Shortnacy AT, et al.: Nucleosides of 2-azapurines. 7H-Imidazo[4-5-*d*]-1,2,3-triazines. J. Med. Chem. 18:564, 1975.
97. Shirakawa S, and Frei E III: Comparative effects of antitumor agents 5-(dimethyltriazeno)-imidazole-4-carboxamide and 1,3-bis(2-chloroethyl)-1-nitrosourea on cell cycle of L1210 leukemia cells *in vivo*. Cancer Res. 30:2173, 1970.
98. Wodinsky I, Swiniarski J, and Kensler CJ: Spleen colony studies of leukemia L1210. IV. Sensitivities of L1210 and L1210/6-MP to triazenoimidazole carboxamides — a preliminary report. Cancer Chemother. Rep. 52:393, 1968.
99. Loo TL, and Stasswender EA: Colorimetric determination of dialkyltriazenoimidazoles. J. Pharm. Sci. 56:1016, 1967.
100. Loo TL, Luce JK, Jardine H, et al.: Pharmacologic studies of the antitumor agent 5-(dimethyltriazeno)imidazole-4-carboxamide. Cancer Res. 28:2448, 1968.
101. Skibba JL, Ramirez G, Beal DD, et al.: Preliminary clinical trial and the physiologic disposition of 4(5)-(3,3-dimethyl-1-triazeno)imidazole-5(4)-carboxamide in man. Cancer Res. 29:1944, 1969.
102. Benvenuto JA, Hall SW, Farquhar D, et al.: High-pressure liquid chromatography in pharmacological studies of anticancer drugs. Chromatog. Sci. 10:377, 1979.
103. Lipton A, Hepner GW, White DS, et al.: Decreased hepatic drug demethylation in patients receiving chemoimmunotherapy. Cancer 41:1680, 1978.
104. Comis RL: DTIC (NSC-45388) in malignant melanoma: a retrospective. Cancer Treat. Rep. 60:165, 1976.
105. Einhorn LH, and Furnas B: Combination chemotherapy for disseminated melanoma with DTIC, vincristine, and methyl-CCNU. Cancer Treat. Rep. 61:881, 1977.
106. Bonadonna G, Zucali R, Manfardini S, et al.: Combination chemotherapy of Hodgkin's disease with Adriamycin, bleomycin, vinblastine, and imidazole carboxamide versus MOPP. Cancer 36:252, 1975.
107. Gottlieb JA, Benjamin RS, Baker LH, et al.: Role of DTIC (NSC-45388) in the chemotherapy of sarcoma. Cancer Treat. Rep. 60:199, 1976.
108. Cowan DH, and Bergsagel DE: Intermittent treatment of metastatic malignant melanoma with high dose 5-(3, 3-dimethyl-1-triazeno)imidazole-4-carboxamide (NSC-45388). Cancer Chemother. Rep. 55:175, 1971.
109. Einhorn LH, McBride CM, Luce JK, et al.: Intra-arterial infusion therapy with 5-(3,3-dimethyl-1-triazeno)-imidazole-4-carboxamide (NSC 45388) for malignant melanoma. Cancer 32:749, 1973.
110. Moore GE, and Meiselbaugh D: DTIC (NSC 45388) toxicity. Cancer Treat. Rep. 60:219, 1976.
111. Smith PJ, Ekert H, Waters KD, et al.: High incidence of cardiomyopathy in children treated with Adriamycin and DTIC in combination chemotherapy. Cancer Treat. Rep. 61:1736, 1977.
112. Samson MK, Baker LH, Talley RW, et al.: Phase I–II Study of intermittent bolus administration of DTIC and actinomycin D in metastatic malignant melanoma. Cancer Treat. Rep. 62:1223, 1978.
113. Fioretti MC: Immunopharmacology of 5-(3,3-dimethyl-1-triazeno)-imidazole-4-carboxamide (DTIC). Pharmacol. Res. Commun. 7:481, 1975.
114. Bonmassar E, Bonmassar A, Vadlamudi S, et al.: Immunological alteration of leukemic cells *in vitro* after treatment with an antitumor drug. Proc. Natl. Acad. Sci. USA 66:1089, 1970.
115. Spreafico F, Mantovani A, Menconi E, et al.: Immunodepressive activity of dimethyl-triazeno-imidazole-carboxamide (DTIC) in mice. Fed. Proc. 33:572, 1974.
116. Puccetti P, Giampietri A, and Fioretti MC: Long-term depression of two primary immune responses induced by a single dose of 5-(3,3-dimethyl-1-triazeno)-imidazole-4-carboxamide (DTIC). Experientia 34:799, 1978.
117. Mantovani A, Luini W, Peri G, et al.: Effect of chemotherapeutic agents on natural cell-mediated cytotoxicity in mice. J. Natl. Cancer Inst. 61:1255, 1978.
118. Nicolin A, Bini A, Coronetti E, et al.: Cellular immune responses to a drug-treated L51784 lymphoma subline. Nature 251:654, 1974.
119. Bruckner HW, Mokyr MB, and Mitchell MS: Effect of imidazole-4-carboxamide, 5-(3,3-dimethyl-1-triazeno) on immunity in patients with malignant melanoma. Cancer Res. 34:181, 1974.
120. Skibba JL, Erturk E, and Bryan GT: Induction of thymic lymphosarcomas and mammary adenocarcinomas in rats by oral administration of the antitumor agent 4(5)-3,3-dimethyl-1-triazeno)imidazole-5(4)-carboxamide. Cancer 26:1000, 1970.
121. Beal DD, Skibba JL, Croft WA, et al.: Carcinogenicity of the antineoplastic agent, 5-(3,3-dimethyl-1-triazeno)-imidazole-4-carboxamide, and its metabolites in rats. J. Natl. Cancer Inst. 54:951, 1975.
122. Weisburger JH, Griswold DP, Prejean JD, et al.: The carcinogenic properties of some of the principal drugs used in clinical cancer chemotherapy. Recent Results Cancer Res. 52:1, 1975.
123. Chaube S, and Swinyard CA: Urogenital anomalies in fetal rats produced by the anticancer agent 4(5)-(3,3-dimethyl-1-triazeno)-imidazole-4-carboxamide. Anat. Record. 186:461, 1976.
124. Thompson DJ, Molello JA, Strebing RJ, et al: Reprodution and teratology studies with oncolytic agents in the rat and rabbits. II. 5-(3,3-Dimethyl-1-triazeno)imidazole-4-carboxamide (DTIC). Toxicol. Appl. Pharmacol. 33:281, 1975.

Hexamethylmelamine

125. Kaiser DW, Thurston IT, Dudley JR, et al.: Cyanuric chloride derivatives. II. Substituted melamines. J. Am. Chem. Soc. 73:2984, 1951.
126. Hendry JA, Rose FL, and Walpole AL: Cytotoxic agents. III. Derivatives of ethylenimines. Br. J. Pharmacol. 6:357, 1951.
127. Buckley SM, Stock CC, Crossley ML, et al.: Inhibition of the Crocker mouse sarcoma 180 by certain ethylenimine derivatives and related compounds. Cancer 5:144, 1952.
128. Johnson BL, Fisher RI, Bender RA, et al.: Hexamethylmelamine in alkylating agent-resistant ovarian carcinoma. Cancer 42:2157, 1978.
129. Takita H, and Didolkar MS: Effect of hexamethylmelamine (NSC-13875) on small cell carcinoma of the lung (phase II study). Cancer Chemother. Rep. 58:371, 1974.
130. Legha SS, Slavik M, and Carter SK: Hexamethylmelamine. An evaluation of its role in the therapy of cancer. Cancer 38:27, 1976.
131. Borden EC, Larson P, Ansfield FJ, et al.: Hexamethylmelamine treatment of sarcomas and lymphomas. Med. Pediatr. Oncol. 3:401, 1977.
132. Rutty CJ, and Connors TA: *In vitro* studies with hexamethylmelamine. Biochem. Pharmacol. 26:2385, 1972.
133. Worzalla JF, Lee DM, Johnson RO, et al.: Effect of microsomal enzyme-inducing chemicals on the metabolism of hexamethylmelamine (NSC-13875) in rats. Proc. Am. Assoc. Cancer Res. 12:41, 1972.
134. Worzalla JF, Kaima BD, Johnson BM, et al.: N-Demethylation of the antineoplastic agent hexamethylmelamine by rats and man. Cancer Res. 33:2810, 1973.

135. Rutty CJ, Connors TA, Nguyen HN, et al.: *In vivo* studies with hexamethylmelamine. Eur. J. Cancer 14:713, 1978.
136. Chang SC, DeMilo AB, Woods CW, et al.: Metabolism of C^{14}-labeled hemel in male house flies. J. Econ. Entomol. 61:1357, 1968.
137. Worzalla JF, Kaima BD, Johnson BM, et al.: Metabolism of hexamethylmelamine-ring-C^{14} in rats and man. Cancer Res. 34:2669, 1974.
138. Borkovec AB, and DeMilo AB: Insect chemosterilants. V. Derivatives of melamine. J. Med. Chem. 10:457, 1967.
139. Mitchley BCV, Clarke SA, Connors TA, et al.: The assessment of antitumor activity of chemotherapeutic agents using human xenografts. Cancer Treat. Rep. 61:3, 1977.
140. Baker BR, and Ashton WT: Irreversible enzyme inhibitors. 196. Active-site-directed irreversible inhibitors of dihydrofolate reductase derived from 1-(4-benzyloxy-3-chlorophenyl)-4,6-diamino-1,2-dihydro-2,2-dimethyl-s-triazine and bearing a terminal phenyl sulfonate group. J. Med. Chem. 15:945, 1972.
141. Ames M, Powis G, Kovach JS, et al.: Disposition and metabolism of pentamethylmelamine and hexamethylmelamine in rabbits and humans. Cancer Res. 39:5016, 1979.
142. Beisler J: Isolation, characterization, and properties of a labile hydrolysis product of the antitumor nucleoside, 5-azacytidine. J. Med. Chem. 21:204, 1978.
143. Lake LM, Grunden EE, and Johnson BM: Toxicity and antitumor activity of hexamethylmelamine and its N demthylated metabolites in mice with transplantable tumors. Cancer Res. 35:2858, 1975.
144. Cumber AJ, and Ross WCJ: Analogues of hexamethylmelamine: the antineoplastic activity of derivatives with enhanced water solubility. Chem. Biol. Interact. 17:349, 1977.
145. Connors TA, Cumber AJ, Ross WCJ, et al.: Regression of human lung tumor xenographs induced by water-soluble analogues of hexamethylmelamine. Cancer Treat. Rep. 61:927, 1977.
146. D'Incalci M, Bolis G, Mangioni C, et al.: Variable absorption of hexamethylmelamine in man. Cancer Treat. Rep. 62:2117, 1978.
147. Ames MM, and Powis G: Determination of pentamethylmelamine and hexamethylmelamine in plasma and urine by nitrogen-phosphorus gas-liquid chromatography. J. Chromatog. 174:245, 1979.
148. Dutcher JS, Jones RB, and Boyd MR: A sensitive and specific assay for pentamethylmelamine in plasma; applicability to clinical studies. Cancer Treat. Rep. 65:755, 1981.
149. Bryan GT, and Gorske AL: Use of ion-exchange chromatography in the spectrophotometric assay for the antineoplastic agent, hexamethylmelamine, in biological fluids. J. Chromatog. 34:67, 1968.
150. Bryan GT, Worzalla JF, Gorske AL, et al.: Plasma levels and urinary excretion of hexamethylmelamine following oral administration to human subjects with cancer. Clin. Pharmacol. Ther. 9:777, 1968.
151. Wilson WL, Schroeder JM, Bisel HF, et al.: Phase II study of hexamethylmelamine (NSC-13875). Cancer 23:132, 1969.
152. Louis J, Louis NB, Linman JB, et al.: The clinical pharmacology of hexamethylmelamine: phase I study. Clin. Pharmacol. Ther. 8:55, 1967.
153. Morimoto M, Schein PS, and Engle R: Comparative pharmacology of pentamethylmelamine (PMM) and hexamethylmelamine (HMM) in mice. Proc. Am. Assoc. Cancer Res. 20:980, 1979.
154. Wilson WL, Bisel HF, Cole D, et al.: Prolonged low-dose administration of hexamethylmelamine (NSC-13875). Cancer 25:568, 1970.
155. Bergevin PR, Tormey DC, and Blom J: Clinical evaluation of hexamethylmelamine (NSC-13875). Cancer Chemother. Rep. 57:51, 1973.

ALLOPURINOL

Kenneth R. Hande

16

Allopurinol, unlike other drugs described in this book, has little or no antineoplastic activity. However, it is frequently used in patients with malignant disease to prevent hyperuricemia and uric acid nephropathy. Thus, the optimal clinical use of allopurinol by itself, and its potential interactions with various antitumor agents, are of both theoretical and practice importance in cancer chemotherapy.

HISTORY

The development of allopurinol as a clinically useful drug for the treatment of hyperuricemia is an example of the rational clinical application of a new agent based on a knowledge of its biochemical mechanism of action and its likely effects on nucleic acid metabolism. In the late 1940s, Hitchings and Elion began a series of experiments investigating the relationship of the chemical structure of various purine analogues to their ability to modify nucleic acid synthesis.[1] Allopurinol, or 4-hydroxypyrazolo(3,4-d)pyrimidine, was found to be a potent inhibitor of the enzyme xanthine oxidase, but showed no antitumor activity upon *in vitro* testing.[2] Other purine analogues tested, including 6-mercaptopurine (6-MP) and 6-thioguanine (6-TG), did demonstrate significant antitumor activity *in vitro.*[3] In subsequent clinical trials, 6-MP was found to be effective in reducing the major leukemic manifestations of chronic granulocytic leukemia. However, not all patients remained responsive to the action of 6-MP. Pharmacologic studies in these patients showed that a significant portion of 6-MP was inactivated by xanthine oxidase[4] and excreted in the urine as the inactive metabolite 6-thiouric acid. In an attempt to decrease the rate of drug inactivation and increase the therapeutic effectiveness of 6-MP, Rundles et al.[5] combined allopurinol with 6-MP in the treatment of chronic granulocytic leukemia. This combination increased both the antileukemic effect of 6-MP and the toxicity, but did not improve the overall therapeutic effectiveness as compared with that of 6-MP alone. However, the hyperuricemia and uricosuria commonly seen in patients with chronic granulocytic leukemia was notably reduced in patients treated with allopurinol. The effectiveness of allopurinol in preventing the formation of uric acid was soon verified in other clinical studies, and by the mid-1960s it was being widely used for the treatment of hyperuricemia, both the hyperuricemia found secondary to the presence of malignant disease[6, 7] and that arising as a consequence of primary gout.[8, 9]

STRUCTURE AND MECHANISM OF ACTION

Allopurinol is an analogue of hypoxanthine in which the 7-nitrogen and the 8-carbon of the purine ring are found in reversed position as compared with the naturally occurring purines. Allopurinol inhibits the enzyme xanthine oxidase and thereby blocks the conversion of hypoxanthine and xanthine to uric acid (Fig. 16–1). Allopurinol is an alternate substrate of xanthine oxidase, being converted to oxipurinol [4,6-dihydroxypyrazolo(3,4-*d*)pyrimidine], a structural analogue of xanthine (Fig. 16–1); oxipurinol acts as a tight-binding inhibitor of xanthine oxidase.

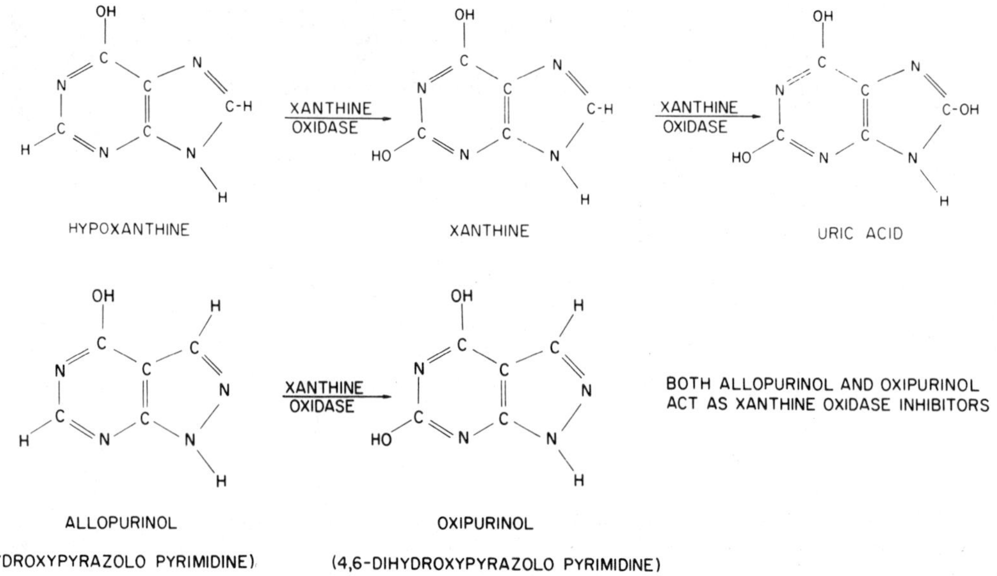

HYPOXANTHINE → XANTHINE OXIDASE → XANTHINE → XANTHINE OXIDASE → URIC ACID

ALLOPURINOL (4-HYDROXYPYRAZOLO PYRIMIDINE) → XANTHINE OXIDASE → OXIPURINOL (4,6-DIHYDROXYPYRAZOLO PYRIMIDINE)

BOTH ALLOPURINOL AND OXIPURINOL ACT AS XANTHINE OXIDASE INHIBITORS

Figure 16–1. Metabolic pathway for the conversion of hypoxanthine and xanthine to uric acid and of allopurinol to oxipurinol.

Mechanism of Inhibition of Xanthine Oxidase by Allopurinol and Oxipurinol

The initial biochemical studies of Elion[10] demonstrated that the interactions of both allopurinol and oxipurinol with xanthine oxidase were complex, the inhibition kinetics being dependent on the conditions under which the reaction was studied. The complex mechanism of xanthine oxidase inhibition by allopurinol and oxipurinol has been clarified by the subsequent studies of Massey et al.[11] and Spector and Johns.[12] These investigators have shown that as xanthine is converted to uric acid, xanthine oxidase accepts electrons and becomes reduced. These electrons are passed through the electron transport chain of xanthine oxidase and are eventually transferred to molecular oxygen, returning the enzyme to its oxidized state. Allopurinol as an alternate substrate binds to xanthine oxidase and undergoes oxidation to oxipurinol, simultaneously reducing xanthine oxidase (Fig. 16–2). Oxipurinol produced in this reaction then binds tightly to reduce xanthine oxidase, preventing further electron transfer and freezing the enzyme in its inactive reduced state. Oxipurinol appears to attach at the active site of xanthine oxidase in what is thought to be a stoichiometric fashion, i.e., one molecule of oxipurinol for each functionally active site of xanthine oxidase. The enzyme may undergo reoxidation under specific conditions *in vitro*, with gradual dissociation of oxipurinol, but the reversibility of this reaction *in vivo* is uncertain. The active inhibitor of xanthine oxidase is thought to be oxipurinol, whether this agent is given initially or is internally generated through conversion from allopurinol. The tight-binding interaction of oxipurinol with reduced xanthine oxidase has an estimated binding constant of 5.4×10^{-10}M.[12] A more detailed discussion of the interaction of allopurinol with xanthine oxidase may be found in a review article by Spector.[13]

Effects on Purine Metabolism

Administration of allopurinol to patients with primary gout lowers serum uric acid concentrations and results in a concomitant rise in serum xanthine and hypoxanthine concentrations, as would be expected with inhibition of xanthine oxidase. A similar decline in urinary uric acid excretion and a rise in urinary xanthine and hypoxanthine excretion are also noted. However, the quantitative rise in excretion of xanthine and hypoxanthine usually does not account for the accompanying decline in urinary uric acid excretion. In several studies[8,9] the total purine excretion (xanthine plus hypoxanthine plus uric acid) has been found to

$[K_I = 5 \times 10^{-10} M]$

Figure 16–2. Proposed mechanism of tight-binding inhibition of reduced xanthine oxidase. Xanthine oxidase is reduced as allopurinol is converted to oxipurinol or as xanthine is converted to urate. Oxipurinol binds tightly to reduced xanthine oxidase inhibiting enzyme activity. (Reproduced from Spector T: Inhibition of urate production by allopurinol. Biochem. Pharmacol. 26:355–358, 1977. By permission of the author and Pergamon Press.Inc.)

decrease by 30 to 40 per cent following initiation of allopurinol therapy. These studies suggest that allopurinol lowers serum uric acid levels in primary gout not only by inhibiting xanthine oxidase, but also by decreasing the rate of *de novo* purine biosynthesis in these patients. Inhibition of purine biosynthesis probably occurs at the level of the initial and rate-limiting step of *de novo* purine formation catalyzed by phos-

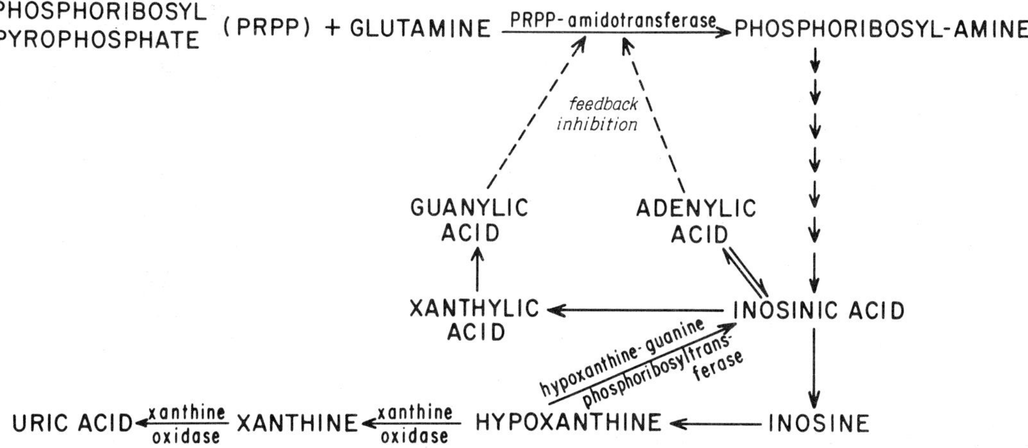

Figure 16–3. Feedback inhibition of *de novo* purine biosynthesis. Inhibition of xanthine oxidase by allopurinol causes an increase in serum hypoxanthine concentration, which in turn results in elevated intracellular concentrations of inosinic, xanthylic, adenylic, and guanylic acids. Guanylic and adenylic acids are inhibitors of phosphoribosylpyrophosphate amidotransferase (PRPP-amidotransferase).

phoribosylpyrophosphate amidotransferase (PRPP-amidotransferase). By blocking the conversion of hypoxanthine and xanthine to uric acid, allopurinol results in an increased conversion of hypoxanthine to inosinic acid via the enzyme hypoxanthine-guanine phosphoribosyltransferase (HG-PRTase) (Fig. 16–3). Inosinic acid, in turn, can be converted to adenylic and guanylic acid, which are allosteric inhibitors of PRPP-amidotransferase.[14, 15]

In addition to adenylic and guanylic acid, certain allopurinol metabolites are also potential inhibitors of PRPP-amidotransferase. Some of the ribonucleotide metabolites of allopurinol and oxipurinol (shown in Fig. 16–4 and described later in this chapter) have been found to inhibit PRPP-amidotransferase under *in vitro* conditions.[16] However, under most circumstances these allopurinol metabolites are found in 100- to 1000-fold lower concentrations than needed for *in vitro* inhibition of PRPP-amidotransferase.[17] The conversion of allopurinol and oxipurinol to their respective ribonucleotides does lead to decreased intracellular concen-

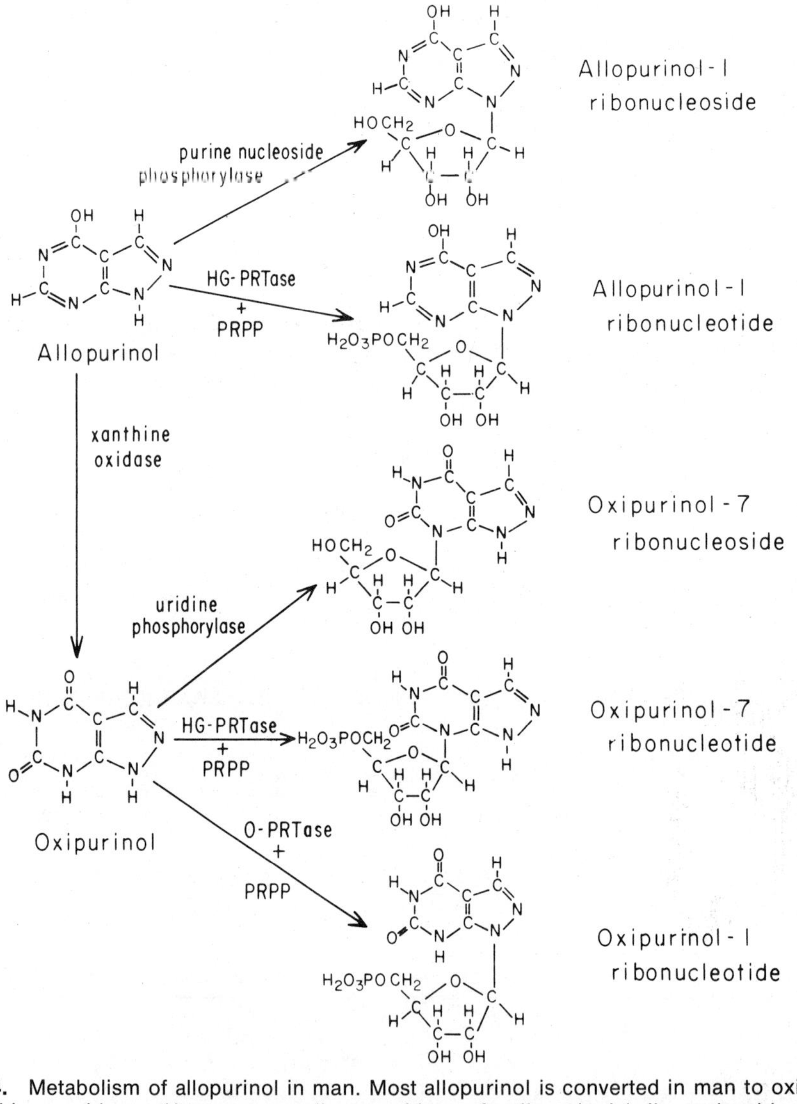

Figure 16–4. Metabolism of allopurinol in man. Most allopurinol is converted in man to oxipurinol via the enzyme xanthine oxidase. However, small quantities of allopurinol-1-ribonucleoside, allopurinol-1-ribonucleotide, oxipurinol-7-ribonucleoside, oxipurinol-7-ribonucleotide, and oxipurinol-1-ribonucleotide have also been found in mammalian tissues or serum. Abbreviations used are: HG-PRTase, hypoxanthine-guanine phosphoribosyltransferase; PRPP, phosphoribosylpyrophosphate; O-PRTase, orotidylic phosphoribosyltransferase.

trations of PRPP following allopurinol administration in man (Fig. 16–4).[18] PRPP plays an important and rate-limiting role in *de novo* purine biosynthesis and may be important in several other steps of intermediary metabolism.[19] Depletion of PRPP by allopurinol metabolite formation, therefore, may be a major reason for the decreased rate of *de novo* purine biosynthesis.

Not all gouty patients treated with allopurinol have a deficit in total purine excretion following allopurinol therapy.[15, 20] Those patients who do not demonstrate an overall decrease in *de novo* purine synthesis following allopurinol therapy have been shown to have a deficiency of the enzyme HG-PRTase.[15] With a deficiency in this enzyme, conversion of hypoxanthine to inosinic acid does not occur, and concentrations of adenylic and guanylic acid sufficient for inhibition of PRPP-amidotransferase are not formed. Lack of HG-PRTase may, therefore, afford partial resistance to allopurinol therapy.

EFFECTS ON PYRIMIDINE BIOSYNTHESIS

In addition to the previously described effects on *de novo* purine biosynthesis, allopurinol interferes with *de novo* pyrimidine synthesis. Allopurinol administration leads to a marked increase in the urinary excretion of both orotic acid and orotidine in man.[21, 22] Orotic acid is the immediate precursor of orotidylic acid (OMP) in the *de novo* pyrimidine synthetic pathway, and orotidine arises from the catabolism of orotidylic acid (Fig. 16–5). The conversion of OMP to uridylic acid (UMP) is catalyzed by the enzyme orotidylic acid decarboxylase. OMP-decarboxylase is inhibited both by xanthylic acid (XMP) and by certain allopurinol and oxipurinol ribonucleotide metabolites of allopurinol.[22] Inibition of xanthine oxidase by allopurinol results in increased formation of XMP (Fig. 16–3). Both 1-oxipurinol-5-monophosphate and 7-oxipurinol-5-monophosphate have been shown to be present in sufficient tissue concentrations to inhibit OMP-decarboxylase *in vitro.*[17]

CLINICAL PHARMACOLOGY AND PHARMACOKINETICS

Allopurinol can be administered intravenously or orally. The oral preparation is commercially available as 100- or 300-mg scored tablets (Zyloprim, Burroughs Wellcome Co.). The intravenous preparation is available only for investigational use. Following intravenous administration of 100 to 300 mg (1 to 5 mg/kg) of allopurinol to man, plasma allopurinol concentrations of 0.5 to 2.0×10^{-5}M (0.7–2.7 mg/l) are attained.[23] The plasma half-life of allopurinol is short (30 to 100 minutes),[23, 24] with rapid conversion of allopurinol to oxipurinol. The volumes of distribution of both allopurinol and oxipurinol are roughtly equal to total body water, with little binding of either drug to plasma proteins.[24] A small amount of allopurinol is excreted directly in the urine (clearance rate 13 to 19 ml/min),[23] but most of an administered dose of allopurinol is excreted as oxipurinol. Allopurinol is well absorbed orally (80 per cent of an administered dose);[24] by contrast, the oral absorption of oxipurinol is incomplete (40 per cent of an administered dose).[25] Therefore, higher oxipurinol dosages are necessary to achieve a comparable therapeutic effect.[26] Following oral administration of 300 mg of allopurinol, plasma oxipurinol concentrations of roughly 1×10^{-5}M (1.5 mg/L) are attained within one to two hours (Fig. 16–6).[21] Patients with normal renal function receiving 300 mg oral allopurinol per day maintain plasma oxipurinol concentrations of 3 to 6×10^{-5}M.[23]

The bulk of administered allopurinol is

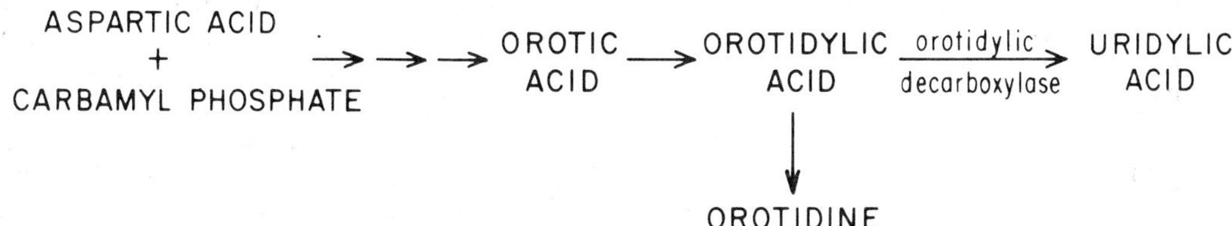

Figure 16–5. Schematic representation of *de novo* pyrimidine biosynthesis. Xanthylic acid and ribonucleotide metabolites of allopurinol are inhibitors of orotidylic decarboxylase.

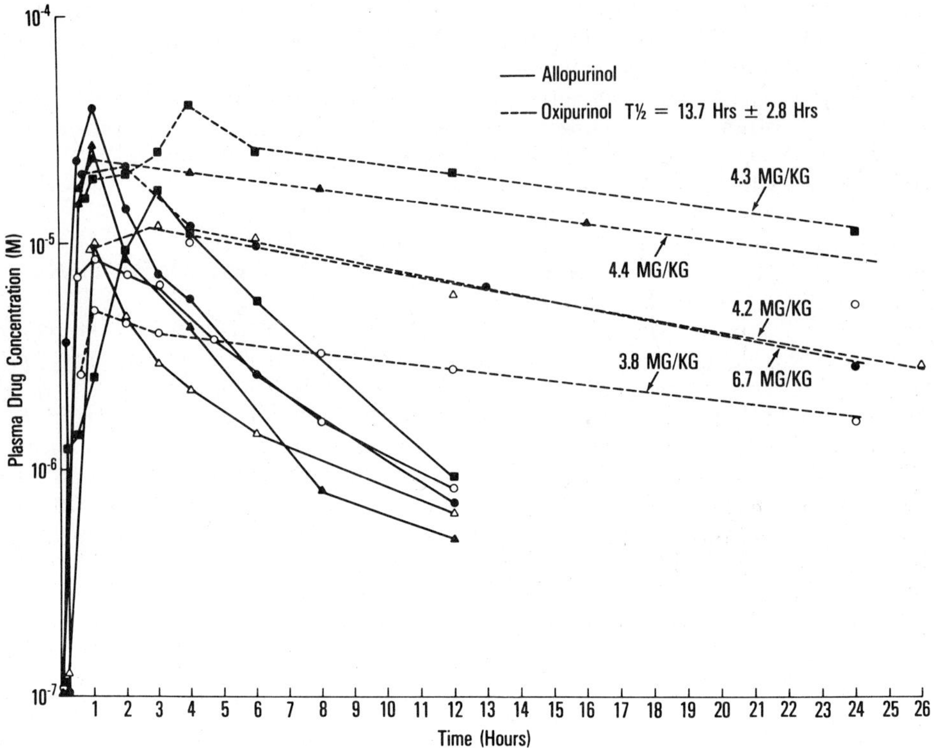

Figure 16–6. Kinetics of oral allopurinol. Serum drug levels (in molar concentrations) following oral administration of 300 mg allopurinol are plotted on a log scale against time. Doses of allopurinol in mg/kg are indicated for each patient. (Reproduced from Hande KR, Reed E, and Chabner BA: Allopurinol kinetics. Clin. Pharmacol. Ther. 23:598–605, 1978. By permission of C.V. Mosby Co.)

excreted through the kidneys as intact oxipurinol. In patients with normal renal function (normal serum creatinine and BUN), the renal clearance of oxipurinol is 12 to 35 ml per min.[23, 25] This relatively slow renal clearance leads to a prolonged plasma half-life for oxipurinol of 14 to 28 hours.[23, 24] The clearance of oxipurinol by the kidney is similar to that of urate.[25] Patients with renal failure have delayed oxipurinol excretion and may require a dose reduction to prevent drug accumulation in plasma. Preliminary studies in patients with chronic renal failure suggest that doses of allopurinol should be reduced by 30 to 75 per cent in those with serum creatinine of 1.5 to 3.0 mg/dl, and by 60 to 90 per cent in those with serum creatinine of greater than 3.0 mg/dl, to maintain serum oxipurinol levels comparable with those found in patients with normal renal function.[27] The clearance of oxipurinol by hemodialysis has been incompletely investigated, but preliminary studies by Hayes et al. on two patients found the clearance of oxipurinol to be roughly 78 ml per minute.[28]

Estimated renal clearance rates of allopurinol (13 to 19 ml/min)[23] indicate that the short half-life of allopurinol is due primarily to enzymatic conversion of allopurinol to oxipurinol, and not to rapid renal clearance of the drug. If allopurinol is converted to oxipurinol via xanthine oxidase in a manner similar to the conversion of xanthine to uric acid, a delayed rate of conversion of allopurinol to oxipurinol would be expected in patients with high plasma oxipurinol concentrations. However, the rapid conversion of allopurinol to oxipurinol is not significantly altered by chronic allopurinol therapy.[23] This is consistent with either a relatively weak inhibition of xanthine oxidase *in vivo* or an alternative (non-xanthine oxidase) pathway for the conversion of allopurinol to oxipurinol. A separate flavoprotein enzyme distinct from xanthine oxidase can convert allopurinol to oxipurinol, but is unable to convert xanthine or hypoxanthine to uric acid.[29] This enzyme, hepatic aldehyde oxidase, is able to convert allopurinol to oxipurinol, but does so only at extremely slow rates *in vitro*. The role of this enzyme in the pharmacology of allopurinol *in vivo* has not been determined. The presence of an enzyme other than xanthine oxidase that is able to convert allopurinol to oxipurinol is also suggested by the findings of Chalmers et al.,[30] who demonstrated the production of oxipurinol from allopurinol in a patient with congenital xanthine oxidase deficiency.

Although the major metabolite of allopurinol in man is oxipurinol, several other allopurinol metabolites have been identified in both *in vitro* and *in vivo* investigations. As mentioned above, some metabolites may play an important role in certain metabolic effects of allopurinol. Both allopurinol and oxipurinol can be converted to their respective nucleosides *in vitro* in a reaction catalyzed by purine nucleoside phosphorylase.[31] However, allopurinol is a much better substrate for purine nucleoside phosphorylase than is oxipurinol, so that only allopurinol-1-ribonucleoside, and not oxipurinol-1-ribonucleoside, is found in the urine of allopurinol-treated patients (Fig. 16–4). Oxipurinol-7-ribonucleoside has been found in the urine of patients receiving allopurinol and is presumably formed *in vitro* through a reaction mediated by uridine phosphorylase.[31] Neither allopurinol nor oxipurinol ribonucleosides can be phosphorylated to ribonucleotides in man because of the lack of the appropriate phosphorylating enzyme. The importance of ribonucleoside metabolites of allopurinol or oxipurinol on intermediary metabolism in man is unknown.

There is evidence for formation of allopurinol-derived ribonucleotides by mammalian tissues both *in vitro* and *in vivo*. Allopurinol can be converted to allopurinol-1-ribonucleotide *in vitro* by the addition of PRPP and the enzyme HG-PRTase.[17] Oxipurinol is also converted by HG-PRTase to oxipurinol-1-ribonucleotide, but is a much poorer substrate for this enzyme than is allopurinol. Oxipurinol is metabolized to oxipurinol-7-ribonucleotide by the addition of PRPP and the enzyme orotidylic phosphoribosyltransferase (O-PRTase).[17] Studies by Nelson[17] have shown that plasma concentrations of allopurinol and oxipurinol ribonucleosides account for 5 to 10 per cent of total radioactive drug in plasma following administration of a dose of 4.6 mg per kg of ^{14}C-allopurinol to rats; following administration of higher doses of ^{14}C-allopurinol (50 mg/kg), more drug (10 to 30 per cent) is converted to allopurinol or oxipurinol ribonucleosides. In Nelson's studies, neither allopurinol nor oxipurinol ribonucleotides were identified in tissue of rats given doses of 4.6 mg per kg of radioactive allopurinol, but were found following doses of 50 mg per kg allopurinol. Formation of even small quantities of allopurinol and oxipurinol ribonucleotides is probably important in interfering with *de novo* pyrimidine biosynthesis by inhibition of OMP-decarboxylase, since both oxipurinol ribonucleotides are potent inhibitors of this enzyme.[17] Allopurinol and oxipurinol ribonucleotide are also inhibitors of PRPP-amidotransferase.[16] However, as previously mentioned, the concentrations of allopurinol and oxipurinol ribonucleotides found *in vivo* are probably inadequate to inhibit PRPP-amidotransferase and block *de novo* purine synthesis significantly.[17]

Although both allopurinol and oxipurinol ribonucleoside monophosphates are formed following allopurinol therapy, nucleoside monophosphate kinases capable of phosphorylating these compounds to nucleoside di- and triphosphates are not present in man. The ribonucleoside monophosphates of allopurinol and oxipurinol are also poor substrates for the enzymes that would catalyze their amination to produce analogues of guanosine monophosphate and adenosine monophosphate.[32, 33] Therefore, incorporation of allopurinol into RNA and DNA does not occur.[34]

CLINICAL USES

Gout

Primary gout is a metabolic disease in which there is either an overproduction or an underexcretion of uric acid. The clinical use of allopurinol and its effects on urate metabolism have been investigated most extensively in primary gout. Primary gout is generally characterized by chronic steady elevations of uric acid, in contrast to some forms of secondary hyperuricemia that are characterized by intermittent increases in uric acid formation. In the treatment of primary gout, allopurinol generally produces a fall in serum uric acid concentration and a fall in urinary uric acid excretion starting within one to two days following initiation of therapy, and produces a maximal reduction in serum urate levels within four to 14 days.[8, 9] In addition to lowering serum and urinary uric acid concentrations, allopurinol therapy produces a decrease in the frequency of urate stone formation and a shrinkage in size of gouty tophi. An empiric dose of 300 mg allopurinol per day is effective therapy in a majority of patients with primary gout, but occasional patients require higher drug doses. In those who do not respond to 300 mg allopurinol per day, dosages of 600 to 1000 mg per day are usually effective in lowering serum uric acid concentrations. Normal serum urate values are 2.2 to 7.5 mg/dl in males and 2.2 to 6.6 mg/dl in females, as determined by automated colorimetric methods.* The normal daily rate of uric acid production is roughly 750 mg per day, with 60 to 80 per cent of that quantity being excreted in the urine each day.[36] In gout patients treated with allopurinol, urinary urate excretion falls from more than 1 gm per day down to normal levels of 300 to 700 mg per day. Studies by Rodnan et al.[37] have demonstrated that a once daily dose of 300 mg allopurinol is clinically as effective as three equally divided doses of 100 mg, probably because of the long plasma half-life of oxipurinol.

Lowering of serum uric acid concentrations by allopurinol will lead to the gradual resolution of gouty tophi and improvement in destructive arthritis. Slow improvement in renal insufficiency due to uric acid nephropathy may also occur.[36] Although allopurinol administration generally improves the clinical symptoms in patients with primary gout, an acute arthritic flare may occasionally occur following initiation of allopurinol therapy and may require temporary treatment with colchicine.

*Two major automated methods for determining serum uric acid values are generally available. One is a colorimetric assay based on the reduction by uric acid of a phosphotungstate complex (Sequential Multiple Analyzer Computer, or SMAC, Technicon Instrument Corp., Tarrytown, NY). The other uric acid assay is based on the decreased light absorption at 293 nm when uric acid is converted to allantoin by the action of the enzyme uricase (Automated Clinical Analyzer, DuPont Co., Wilmington, DE). The change in absorption at 293 nm is directly proportional to the concentration of uric acid in the serum. The phosphotungstate determination for uric acid generally exceeds the value obtained by the uricase method by 0.5–1.0 mg/dl.[35]

Treatment of Hyperuricemia Secondary to Tumor Lysis

Hyperuricemia may occur in patients with primary gout or as a consequence of several conditions, including hemolytic anemias, polycythemia vera, lead ingestion, renal failure, hypertension, and various malignant diseases. Secondary hyperuricemia following rapid tumor lysis contrasts with primary gout in that there is a sudden, temporary rise in uric acid production that is due not to increased *de novo* synthesis but to cell destruction with release of preformed purines. Uric acid is sparingly soluble in both water and urine (Table 16–1). The rapid release of uric acid following sudden tumor destruction from chemotherapy may lead to a marked increase in urinary excretion of uric acid, with renal failure due to the precipitation of urate crystals in the distal renal tubules where concentration and acidification are maximal.[38]

The use of allopurinol in preventing secondary hyperuricemia due to tumor lysis has been empiric. DeConti and Calabresi[7] and Krakoff and Meyer[6] have used daily doses of 200 to 800 mg allopurinol before initiation of chemotherapy and have demonstrated these doses to be effective in preventing elevations of serum uric acid in most cases. The incidence of urate stones as a complication of untreated chronic myeloproliferative disease has been established at 40 per cent.[38] However, the incidence of uric acid nephropathy and complications of tumor lysis in various other neoplastic diseases and situ-

TABLE 16–1. Solubility of Purine Analogues and Physiologic Purines

pH	*Uric Acid**	*Xanthine**	*Hypoxanthine**	*Allopurinol†*	*Oxipurinol†*
5	150 mg/L (8.9×10^{-4}M)	50 mg/L (3.2×10^{-4}M)	1400 mg/L (1.0×10^{-2}M)	650 mg/L (4.8×10^{-3}M)	130 mg/L (8.2×10^{-4}M)
7	200 mg/L (1.2×10^{-3}M)	130 mg/L (8.5×10^{-4}M)	1500 mg/L (1.1×10^{-3}M)	710 mg/L (5.2×10^{-3}M)	210 mg/L (1.4×10^{-3}M)

*Solubility in urine (from Klinenberg et al.[20]).
†Solubility in 0.05 M phosphate buffer (Hande, unpublished studies).

ations has not been extensively investigated. The development of hyperuricemia following chemotherapy of certain malignancies such as lymphoma or leukemia has been recognized as a significant problem for several years. The exact incidence of hyperuricemia following treatment of lymphoma or leukemia is unknown, but is sufficiently common that hydration and allopurinol therapy are recommended treatments prior to the initiation of chemotherapy for these diseases.

With recent advances in combination chemotherapy, rapid tumor shrinkage has been described with testicular carcinoma[39] and small cell carcinoma of the lung.[40] The development of more effective chemotherapeutic regimens may lead to the "tumor lysis syndromes" in association with other common malignancies.[41] The optimal dose of allopurinol and the necessity for its use in different types of malignant disease are not known. However, the objective of therapy in this situation, establishment of a block in xanthine oxidase activity, is somewhat different from the need to lower the existing plasma concentration of uric acid. Thus, the four- to eight-day period required to lower serum uric acid is less important in cancer treatment and, if rapid antineoplastic treatment is required, significant oxipurinol blood levels can be achieved within 30 minutes of an intravenous allopurinol infusion and within two to four hours of oral allopurinol administration.[23]

Recent Trials in Experimental Settings

In vitro studies have suggested that allopurinol may be effective as an antiparasitic agent for the treatment of leishmaniasis and trypanosomiasis.[42] The toxic effect of allopurinol in these parasites appears to occur as a result of a different metabolism of allopurinol in these organisms from that in man.[42] Oxipurinol is the major metabolite of allopurinol in man, but *T. cruzi* lacks xanthine oxidase and instead converts allopurinol to a ribonucleotide metabolite not found in man. This metabolite, 4-aminopyrazolopyrimidine monophosphate, is then phosphorylated further and incorporated into RNA to cause cell death. Further clinical studies on the effects of allopurinol in the treatment of leishmaniasis or Chagas' disease will undoubtedly be completed in the next few years.

Allopurinol has also been used as an experimental agent for the treatment of Duchenne muscular dystrophy. Some studies have indicated that this dystrophy is associated with depleted concentrations of certain purine nucleotides in affected muscle cells. Thompson and Smith[43] have used allopurinol in these patients in hopes of blocking purine excretion and repleting purine pools. Clinical improvement has been noted in a significant number of patients following allopurinol therapy. Further investigations into this area are needed.

TOXICITY

Allopurinol therapy is well tolerated in most patients, producing few side effects, but occasional toxicity from its administration can occur. Development of xanthine or hypoxanthine nephropathy has long been considered a potential complication of allopurinol therapy. Hypoxanthine is considerably more soluble than uric acid, and precipitation nephropathy should not be a clinical problem with this compound. Xanthine, on the other hand, is less soluble than uric acid (Table 16–1) and therefore has the potential for causing precipitation nephropathy in selected patients. In addition, the pKa's of uric acid are at 5.4 and 10.4 whereas those of xanthine are at 7.4 and 11. Therefore, increasing urinary pH above 5.4 will greatly improve the solubility of uric acid, but the solubility of xanthine will not improve significantly until the urine is alkalinized to a pH above 7.4. It is difficult to raise the urinary pH above 7.5 and efforts in this direction may cause significant systemic alkalosis. Therefore increasing the solubility of xanthine by adjusting the pH may not be clinically feasible.

Xanthine nephropathy, although a potential problem, is a rare complication of allopurinol therapy and has not been seen in the treatment of primary gout. Normal urinary excretion of either xanthine or hypoxanthine is less than 30 mg per day.[44] Following administration of allopurinol to patients with primary gout, the renal excretion of total oxipurines (xanthine plus hypoxanthine) increases to 40 to 500 mg per day with 55 to 70 per cent of the total excretion being xanthine.[8, 9] Plasma oxipurine concentrations rarely rise higher than 1 to 2 mg/dl[44, 45] following allopurinol therapy of primary gout owing to (1) a decreased rate of *de novo* purine synthesis, as described earlier in this chapter; and (2) a tenfold greater rate of renal clearance of xanthine than that of uric acid.

Development of xanthine nephropathy has occurred in patients receiving allopurinol who have had rapid tumor lysis[46-48] and in occasional patients with Lesch-Nyhan syndrome.[49] *De novo* purine biosynthesis does not contribute in a significant manner to the acute purine load seen following rapid tumor lysis. Therefore, the fall in uric acid excretion in this situation should be accompanied by a near-equal rise in the excretion of xanthine and hypoxanthine. The formation of xanthine nephropathy following treatment of lymphoma patients on allopurinol has been reported in three cases.[46-48] In the two cases in which serum xanthine concentrations have been measured,[47, 48] these concentrations have reached levels of 6 to 14 mg/dl following chemotherapy; such levels are over 200-fold higher than normal plasma xanthine concentrations. These high xanthine concentrations may lead to concomitantly high urinary xanthine concentrations, resulting in xanthine precipitation in the renal tubule in a manner similar to uric acid deposition. In addition, xanthine concentrations in excess of 5 mg/dl may cause a falsely low uric acid measurement as determined by the uricase method.[48] In one patient, serum xanthine concentrations of 14 mg/dl caused a 50 per cent underestimation of serum uric acid concentrations. Elevated xanthine concentrations do not affect uric acid measurements determined by the phosphotungstate colorimetric assay.

The problem of marked hyperxanthinuria following chemotherapy of sensitive tumors may be more frequent than is recognized based on the total of three cases reported in the medical literature. Unexplained renal failure following chemotherapy in patients with Burkitt's lymphoma and other lymphomas sensitive to chemotherapy is not an uncommon problem. In a preliminary study,[50] six of 11 lymphoma patients on allopurinol had postchemotherapy urinary xanthine concentrations exceeding the solubility of xanthine (150 mg/L). Three of these six patients developed transient renal failure, suggesting that xanthine nephropathy may be a cause of unexplained renal failure following chemotherapy treatment of lymphoma patients on allopurinol. Although xanthine precipitation is a potential complication of allopurinol therapy in patients who have massive tumor lysis, allopurinol treatment is beneficial to such patients in that it enables them to excrete a larger total purine load. Since the solubility of a single purine such as xanthine, hypoxanthine, or uric acid is independent of the others, dividing the purine load among these three purines by the use of allopurinol increases the total amount of purine that can be excreted in the urine.

Not only can elevated concentrations of xanthine and uric acid lead to precipitation nephropathy, but overdoses of allopurinol potentially can lead to precipitation of oxipurinol in muscle tissue and in the renal tubules. Standard oral doses of 300 mg per day of allopurinol given on a chronic basis produce plasma oxipurinol levels of 3 to 5 $\times 10^{-5}$M and urinary oxipurinol levels roughly tenfold higher (3 to 5 $\times 10^{-4}$M).[23] As shown in Table 16–1, the maximal solubility of oxipurinol in buffer at pH 5 is 8.2 $\times 10^{-4}$M. Doses of allopurinol exceeding 1 gm per day potentially could achieve urine oxipurinol concentrations of greater than 1 $\times 10^{-3}$M and exceed the solubility of oxipurinol in the urine. Watts et al.[51] have demonstrated the presence of oxipurinol crystals in the muscle biopsies of patients with primary gout following treatment with allopurinol. Oxipurinol stones have also been identified in the urine of a patient being treated with oxipurinol.[52]

Many other side effects of allopurinol therapy have been reported. Fortunately, most of these are mild and self-limiting with cessation of drug therapy. The most common toxicity associated with allopurinol therapy is skin rash, which often occurs in patients taking concomitant ampicillin.[53] The Boston Collaborative Drug Surveillance Program found a 2 per cent incidence of skin rash in patients on allopurinol alone and a 7 per cent incidence in those on ampicillin alone, but a 22 per cent incidence in those on allopurinol plus ampicillin. In patients allergic to allopurinol, oxipurinol may be tried as an alternative therapy for xanthine oxidase inhibition. However, cross-sensitivity between allopurinol and oxipurinol has been noted.[54] Gastrointestinal intolerance, fever, and alopecia[55] are other relatively mild complications of allopurinol therapy.

Significant, life-threatening toxicities following allopurinol administration have also been described, including bone marrow suppression with agranulocytosis,[56, 57] jaundice,[58] granulomatous hepatitis,[59] and hepatic necrosis.[60] Several cases of a severe, potentially life-threatening hypersensitivity syndrome resulting from allopurinol have been reported.[61-64] These patients have illnesses characterized by fever, eosinophilia, skin rash including toxic epidermal necrolysis, renal dysfunction, and hepatic failure. This hypersensitivity syndrome usually appears four to six weeks after initiation of allopurinol therapy and occurs most commonly in patients with underlying renal failure. The overall incidence of allopurinol toxicity of all kinds appears to be about 20 per cent, most of these toxicities being mild. However, significant and life-threatening toxic side effects appear to occur more frequently in the presence of renal insufficiency, suggesting that elevated plasma allopurinol or oxipurinol concentrations may play a role in their development.

ASSAYS FOR ALLOPURINOL OR OXIPURINOL

In most clinical situations, dosages of allopurinol in man can be adjusted by increasing the amount of drug administered until a decrease in the serum uric acid concentration is noted. However, in some circumstances, such as in the prevention of hyperuricemia secondary to tumor lysis, a reduction in serum uric acid concentrations prior to antineoplastic therapy cannot be used as an accurate guide to the effectiveness of allopurinol therapy. In addition, monitoring serum uric acid concentrations does not necessarily prevent the use of excessive amounts of allopurinol, particularly in patients with compromised renal function. In these clinical situations, a sensitive, specific assay for allopurinol and oxipurinol would be useful as a guide to allopurinol therapy.

Several analytical assay systems for allopurinol and oxipurinol have been described, but each has limitations for routine analysis of these purines in biologic fluids. Previously described methods include isotope dilution techniques,[22] cation exchange chromatography,[65] and high-pressure liquid chromatography.[66] Recently, a competitive protein binding assay for allopurinol and oxipurinol (which employs reduced xanthine oxidase as the binding protein) has been developed, with little interference from other common purines such as uric acid, xanthine, hypoxanthine, or 6-MP.[67] With this assay, from one to 30 samples may be analyzed within a two- to three-hour period. This assay is rapid and sensitive enough (lower level of sensitivity is 0.1 μM) to be used for routine pharmacologic monitoring, and may prove to be clinically useful for monitoring both allopurinol and oxipurinol levels.

DRUG INTERACTIONS

Interactions between allopurinol and several other drugs, including antineoplastic agents, have been described, and it is important to recognize these in order to minimize the toxic side effects and maximize the therapeutic effectiveness of these agents. The recognition of the potential interaction between allopurinol and 6-MP or azathioprine was one of the major developments leading to the clinical use of allopurinol.[5] Xanthine oxidase catalyzes the conversion of both azathioprine and 6-MP to the inactive metabolite 6-thiouric acid. Concomitant administration of allopurinol with either of these two agents results in decreased urinary excretion of 6-thiouric acid and increased toxicity.[5, 68] The concomitant administration of allopurinol with 6-MP does not appear to prolong the plasma half-life of 6-MP;[69] however, levels of 6-thioinosinic acid (the active metabolite of 6-MP) may be increased in this setting and may account for the increased toxicity. Doses of 6-MP or azathioprine should be reduced by one half to two thirds when allopurinol is used concomitantly, and white blood cell counts should be monitored frequently. Inactivation of 6-thioguanine occurs through the enzyme guanase and not via xanthine oxidase, so that no dose reduction is needed when allopurinol and 6-thioguanine are used in combination.

Both allopurinol and oxipurinol appear to be reabsorbed in the renal tubules.[25] The concomitant use of the uricosuric agent probenecid with allopurinol results in a shorter oxipurinol plasma half-life, owing to more rapid renal excretion of the drug. Conversely, allopurinol lengthens the biologic half-life of probenecid and potentiates its uricosuric effect.[70] In addition to probenecid, the thiazide diuretics may also interfere with the renal handling of allopurinol and oxipurinol. When thiazides are used with allopurinol, an increase in the rate of orotic acid excretion is noted[71] and the risk of allopurinol hypersensitivity reactions also appears to increase.[62] These effects suggest that the thiazides may delay the renal excretion of oxipurinol, but specific pharmacologic studies have not been performed.

Allopurinol reduces the activity of the hepatic microsomal enzyme system through unknown mechanisms.[72] Therefore, drugs such as bishydroxycoumarin or barbiturates that are inactivated by the hepatic microsomal enzyme system may have a more prolonged drug half-life when used in combination with allopurinol. Patients receiving allopurinol with drugs metabolized by the hepatic microsomal enzyme system should be monitored closely for increased risk of drug toxicity. Allopurinol also appears to enhance the activity of cyclophosphamide. In a retrospective study, the Boston Collaborative Drug Surveillance Program[70] demonstrated an increase in cyclophosphamide toxicity when allopurinol was used in combination with this alkylating agent, compared with the toxicity of cyclophosphamide alone. Cyclophosphamide is activated through the hepatic microsomal enzyme system, and the effects of allopurinol may be related to its ability to slow activation and prolong the duration of exposure of cells to active cyclophosphamide intermediates. However, Alberts[74] could find no change in the pharmacokinetics of cyclophosphamide when combined with allopurinol. In Albert's study, doses of allopurinol five- to tenfold greater than those normally used in man were needed in order to find increased cyclophosphamide activity in mice, suggesting that the increased toxicity in man may be of marginal significance.

In addition to its effects on the antitumor drugs already mentioned (6-MP, azathioprine, and cyclophosphamide), allopurinol alters the toxicity of several other antineoplastic agents. Grindey[75] has demonstrated that the antitumor effects of methotrexate can be partially reversed by allopurinol in an *in vitro* cell culture system. Methotrexate is a folic acid antagonist that inhibits the formation of tetrahydrofolates needed for the synthesis of both thymidylate and purines (see Chapter 10 for a more complete review). Allopurinol increases plasma and tissue concentrations of hypoxanthine and xanthine, and thus potentially can rescue cells from the antipurine effects of methotrexate, thereby decreasing toxicity.

Studies by Schwartz and Handschumacher[76] have demonstrated that allopurinol can antagonize the antitumor effect of 5-fluorouracil (5-FU) in both *in vitro* and *in vivo* settings. As mentioned earlier in this chapter, allopurinol causes an increase in plasma concentrations of orotic acid. 5-Fluorouracil is converted to its active metabolite, 5-fluorouridine monophosphate (5-FUMP), through the action of the enzyme orotate phosphoribosyltransferase. This enzyme is inhibited by the high levels of orotic acid that result from allopurinol administration. However, certain tumor cell lines appear to activate 5-FU through a different enzymatic pathway. Schwartz[76] has suggested that the combination of allopurinol and 5-FU may offer a therapeutic advantage in the therapy of such tumors by decreasing 5-FU activation in normal bone marrow while maintaining toxicity in tumor cells.

References

1. Hitchings GH, and Elion, GB: Studies on analogs of purines and pyrimidines. Ann. N.Y. Acad. Sci. 52:1318–1335, 1950.
2. Lorz DC, and Hitchings GH: Specificity of xanthine oxidase. Am. Chem. Soc. 30C, 1956 (abstr.).
3. Elion GB, Singer S, and Hitchings GH: Microbiological effects of 6-mercaptopurine. Ann. N.Y. Acad. Sc. 60:235–243, 1954.
4. Elion GB, Callahan SW, Hitchings GH, et al.: Experimental, clinical and metabolic studies of thiopurines. Cancer Chemother. Rep. 16:197–202, 1962.
5. Rundles RW, Wyngaarden JB, Hitchings GH, et al.: Effects of a xanthine oxidase inhibitor on thiopurine metabolism, hyperuricemia and gout. Trans. Assoc. Am. Physicians 76:126–140, 1963.
6. Krakoff IH, and Meyer RL: Prevention of hyperuricemia in leukemia and lymphoma: use of allopurinol, a xanthine oxidase inhibitor. J.A.M.A. 193:1–6, 1965.
7. DeConti RC, and Calabresi P: Use of allopurinol for prevention and control of hyperuricemia in patients with neoplastic disease. N. Engl. J. Med. 274:481–486, 1966.
8. Yu TF, and Gutman AB: Effect of allopurinol on serum uric acid in primary and secondary gout. Am. J. Med. 37:885–898, 1964.
9. Rundles RW, Metz EM, and Silberman HR: Allopurinol in the treatment of gout. Ann. Intern. Med. 64:229–258, 1966.
10. Elion GB: Enzymatic and metabolic studies with allopurinol. Ann. Rheum. Dis. 25:608–680, 1966.
11. Massey V, Komai H, Palmer G, et al.: Mechanism of inactivation of xanthine oxidase by allopurinol and other (3,4-*d*) pyrimidines. J. Biol. Chem. 245:2837–2844, 1970.
12. Spector T, and Johns DG: Stoichiometric inhibition of reduced xanthine oxidase by hydroxypyrazolo (3,4-*d*) pyrimidines. J. Biol. Chem. 245:5079–5085, 1970.
13. Spector T: Inhibition of urate production by allopurinol. Biochem. Pharmacol. 26:355–358, 19
14. Caskey CT, Ashton, DM, and Wyngaarden JB: The enzymology of feedback inhibition of glutamine phosphoribosylpyrosphosphate amidotransferase by purine ribonucleotides. J. Biol. Chem. 239:2570–2579, 1964.
15. Kelley WN, Rosenbloom FM, Miller J, et al.: An enzymatic basis for variation in response to allopurinol. N. Engl. J. Med. 278:287–293, 1968.

16. McCollister RJ, Gilbert WR, Ashton DM, et al.: Pseudofeedback inhibition of purine synthesis by 6-mercaptopurine ribonucleotide and other purine analogs. J. Biol. Chem. 239:1560–1563, 1964.
17. Nelson DJ, Bugge C, Krasny HC, et al.: Formation of nucleotides of 6-^{14}C allopurinol and 6-^{14}C oxipurinol in rat tissue and effects on uridine nucleotide pools. Biochem. Pharmacol. 22:2003–2022, 1973.
18. Fox IH, Wyngaarden JB, and Kelley WN: Depletion of erythrocyte phosphoribosylpyrophosphate in man: a newly observed effect of allopurinol. N. Engl. J. Med. 283:1172–1182, 1970.
19. Fox IH, and Kelley WN: Phosphoribosylpyrophosphate in man: biochemical and clinical significance. Ann. Intern. Med. 74:424–433, 1971.
20. Klinenberg JR, Goldfinger SE, and Seegmiller JE: The effectiveness of the xanthine oxidase inhibitor allopurinol in the treatment of gout. Ann. Intern. Med. 62:639–647, 1965.
21. Fox RM, Royse-Smith MD, and O'Sullivan WJ: Orotidinuria induced by allopurinol. Science 169:861–862, 1970.
22. Kelley W, and Beardmore T: Allopurinol: alteration in pyrimidine metabolism in man. Science 169:388–390, 1970.
23. Hande KR, Reed E, and Chabner BA: Allopurinol kinetics. Clin. Pharmacol. Ther. 23:598–605, 1978.
24. Elion GB, Kovensky A, Hitchings GH, et al.: Metabolic studies of allopurinol, an inhibitor of xanthine oxidase. Biochem. Pharmacol. 15:863–880, 1966.
25. Elion GB, Yu TF, Gutman AB, et al.: Renal clearnace of oxipurinol, the chief metabolite of allopurinol. Am. J. Med. 45:69–77, 1968.
26. Chalmers RA, Kromer H, Scott JT, et al.: A comparative study of the xanthine oxidase inhibitors allopurinol and oxipurinol in man. Clin. Sci. 35:353–362, 1968.
27. Hande KR, and Stone W: Plasma oxipurinol levels following allopurinol therapy in patients with renal failure. Clin. Res. 27:738A, 1979 (abstr.).
28. Hayes CP, Metz EN, Robinson RR, et al.: The use of allopurinol to control hyperuricemia in patients on chronic intermittent hemodialysis. Trans. Am. Soc. Artif. Intern. Organs 11:247–251, 1965.
29. Johns DG, Spector T, and Robins RK: Studies on the mode of oxidation of pyrazolo (3,4-*d*) pyrimidine by aldehyde oxidase and xanthine oxidase. Biochem. Pharmacol. 18:2371–2383.
30. Chalmers RA, Parker R, Simmonds HA, et al.: The conversion of 4-hydroxypyrazolo (3,4-*d*) pyrimidine (allopurinol) into 4,6-dihydroxypyrazolo (3,4-*d*) pyrimidine (oxipurinol) *in vivo* in the absence of xanthine-oxygen oxidoreductase. Biochem. J. 112:527–532, 1968.
31. Krenitsky TA, Elion GB, Strelity RA, et al.: Ribonucleosides of allopurinol and oxipurinol. J. Biol. Chem. 242:2675–2682, 1967.
32. Spector T: Studies with GMP synthetase from Ehrlich ascites cells. J. Biol. Chem. 250:7372–7376, 1973.
33. Spector T, and Miller R: Mammalian adenosyl succinate synthetase: nucleotide monophosphate substrates and inhibitors. Biochim. Biophys. Acta 445:509–517, 1976.
34. Nelson DJ, and Elion GB: Metabolism of 6-^{14}C allopurinol: lack of incorporation of allopurinol into nucleic acids. Biochem. Pharmacol. 24:1235–1237, 1975.
35. Lum G, and Gambino SR: Comparison of four methods for measuring uric acid: copper-chelate, phosphotungstate. Manual uricase and automated kinetic uricase. Clin. Chem. 19:1184–1186, 1973.
36. Wyngaarden JB, and Kelley WN: Gout and Hyperuricemia. Grune & Stratton, New York, 1976.
37. Rodnan GP, Robin JA, Tolchin SF, et al.: Allopurinol and gouty hyperuricemia. J.A.M.A. 231:1143–1147, 1975.
38. Rieselbach RE, Bentzel CJ, Cotlove E, et al.: Uric acid excretion and renal function in the acute hyperuricemia of leukemia. Am. J. Med. 37:872–884, 1964.
39. Einhorn L, and Donohue J: *cis*-Diamminedichloroplatinum, vinblastine, and bleomycin combination chemotherapy in disseminated testicular cancer. Ann. Intern. Med. 87:293–298, 1977.
40. Greco FA, Richardson RL, Snell JD, et al.: Small cell lung cancer: complete remission and improved survival. Am. J. Med. 66:625–630, 1979.
41. Murinson DS, and Arseneau JC: The tumor lysis syndrome: a consequence of successful chemotherapy. Proc. Am. Assoc. Clin. Oncol. 18:356, 1977 (abstr.).
42. Marr JJ, Berens RL, and Nelson DJ: Antitrypanosomal effect of allopurinol: conversion *in vivo* to aminopyrazolopyrimidine nucleotides by *Trypanosoma cruzi*. Science 201:1918–1920, 1978.
43. Thompson WH, and Smith I: X-linked recessive (Duchenne) muscular dystrophy (DMD) and purine metabolism: effects of oral allopurinol and adenylate. Metabolism 27:151–163, 1978.
44. Goldfinger S, Klinenberg JR, and Seegmiller JE: The renal excretion of oxipurines. J. Clin. Invest. 44:623–628, 1965.
45. Klinenberg JR, Goldfinger S, Bradley KH, et al.: An enzymatic spectrophotometer method for the determination of xanthine and hypoxanthine. Clin. Chem. 13:834–848, 1967.
46. Band PR, Silverberg DS, Henderson JF, et al.: Xanthine nephropathy in a patient with lymphosarcoma treated with allopurinol. N. Engl. J. Med. 283:354–357, 1970.
47. Ablin A, Stephens B, Hirata T, et al.: Nephropathy, xanthinuria and orotic aciduria complicating Burkitt's lymphoma treated with chemotherapy and allopurinol. Metabolism 21:771–778, 1972.
48. Hande KR, Perini F, Putterman G, et al.: Hyperxanthinemia causes interference with serum uric determinations by the uricase method. Clin. Chem. 25:1492–1497, 1979.
49. Green ML, Fujimoto WY, and Seegmiller JE: Urinary xanthine stones — a rare complication of allopurinol therapy. N. Engl. J. Med. 280:426–427, 1969.
50. Hande KR, Hixson CU, and Chabner BA: Post-chemotherapy purine excretion in lymphoma patients receiving allopurinol. Cancer Res. 41:2273–2279, 1981.
51. Watts WE, Scott JR, Chalmers RA, et al.: Microscopic studies on skeletal muscle in gout patients treated with allopurinol. Q. J. Med. 40:1–14, 1971.
52. Landgrebe AR, Nyhan WL, and Coleman M: Urinary tract stones resulting from the excretion of oxipurinol. N. Engl. J. Med. 292:626–627, 1975.
53. Boston Collaborative Drug Surveillance Program: Excess of ampicillin rashes associated with allopurinol or hyperuricemia. N. Engl. J. Med. 286:505–507, 1972.
54. Lockard O, Harmon C, Nolph K, et al.: Allergic reaction to allopurinol with cross-reactivity to oxypurinol. Ann. Intern. Med. 85:333–335, 1978.
55. Auerbach R, and Orentrich N: Alopecia and ichthyosis secondary to allopurinol therapy. J.A.M.A. 211:478–489, 1970.
56. Greenberg MS, and Zambrino SS: Aplastic agranulocytosis after allopurinol therapy. Arthritis Rheum. 15:413–416, 1972.
57. Wilkinson DS: Allopurinol and agranulocytosis. Lancet 2:1282–1283, 1977.
58. Mills RM: Severe hypersensitivity reactions associated with allopurinol. J.A.M.A. 216:799–802, 1971.
59. Chawla SK, Patel HD, Parrino GR, et al.: Allopurinol hepatotoxicity. Arthritis Rheum. 20:146–154, 1977.
60. Butler RC, Shah SM, Grunow WA, et al.: Massive hepatic necrosis in a patient receiving allopurinol. J.A.M.A. 237:473–474, 1977.
61. Kantor GL: Toxic epidermal necrolysis, azotemia, and death after allopurinol therapy. J.A.M.A. 211:478–489, 1970.
62. Young JL, Boswell RB, and Nies AS: Severe allopurinol hypersensitivity. Arch. Intern. Med. 14:553–558, 1974.
63. Lindsey SW, and Evans EF: Allopurinol hypersensitivity syndrome: effects and treatment. Va. Med. 105:297–299, 1978.
64. Chan HL, Hu G, and Khoo OT: Allopurinol associated hypersensitivity reactions: cutaneous and renal manifestations. Aust. N.Z. J. Med. 7:518–522, 1977.
65. Sweetman L, and Nyhan W: Quantitation of oxypurines and allopurinol metabolites in biological fluids by cation-exchange chromatography. Anal. Biochem. 31:358–365, 1969.
66. Brown M, and Bye A: The determination of allopurinol and

oxipurinol in human plasma and urine. J. Chromatogr. 99:587–595, 1974.
67. Hande KR, and Chabner BA: A competitive protein binding assay for allopurinol and oxipurinol. Anal. Biochem. 101:26–33, 1980.
68. Ragab AH, Gilkerson E, and Myers M: The effect of 6-mercaptopurine and allopurinol on granulopoiesis. Cancer Res. 34:2246–2249, 1974.
69. Coffey JJ, White CA, Lesk AB et al.: Effect of allopurinol on the pharmacokinetics of 6-mercaptopurine in cancer patients. Cancer Res. 32:1283–1289, 1972.
70. Tjandramaga TB, Cucinell SA, Israili ZH, et al.: Observations on the disposition of probenecid in patients receiving allopurinol. Pharmacology 8:259–272, 1972.
71. Wood MH, Sebel E, and O'Sullivan WJ: Allopurinol and thiazides. Lancet 1:751 (letter), 1972.
72. Vessel ES, Passanti GT, and Green F: Impairment of drug metabolism in man by allopurinol and nortriptyline. N. Engl. J. Med. 283:1484–1488, 1970.
73. Boston Collaborative Drug Surveillance Program: Allopurinol and cytotoxic drugs. J.A.M.A. 227:1036–1040, 1974.
74. Alberts DS, and Van Doalen Weters T: The effect of allopurinol on cyclophosphamide antitumor activity. Cancer Res. 36:2790–2794, 1976.
75. Grindey GB, and Moran RG: The effects of allopurinol on the therapeutic efficacy of methotrexate. Cancer Res. 35:1702–1705, 1975.
76. Schwartz PM, and Handschumacher RE: Selective antagonism of 5-fluorouracil cytotoxicity by 4-hydroxyprazolopyrimidine (allopurinol) *in vitro*. Cancer Res. 39:3095–3101, 1979.

17 BLEOMYCIN

Bruce A. Chabner

In a search for new antimicrobial and antineoplastic agents, Umezawa and colleagues isolated a number of small glycopeptides from culture broths of the fungus *Streptomyces verticillis*.[1] The most active antitumor agent found in these broths was a mixture of peptides now known in clinical usage as bleomycin, a drug that has important activity against Hodgkin's disease, non-Hodgkin's lymphoma, testicular cancer, and head and neck cancer. Bleomycin used in combination with vinblastine and *cis*-dichlorodiammineplatinum has produced a high rate of complete remissions and probable cures in patients with germinal neoplasms of the testis,[2] and has attracted great interest because of the unique features of its biochemical action and its virtual lack of toxicity for normal hematopoietic tissue.

STRUCTURE AND MECHANISM OF ACTION

The bleomycins are a family of peptides with a molecular weight of approximately 1500 (Fig. 17–1). All contain a unique structural component, bleomycinic acid, and differ only in their terminal alkylamine group. Because of their unusual structure, catalytic properties, and important antitumor activity, the bleomycin antibiotics have been the subject of intensive basic and clinical investigation. Additional bleomycin-like antitumor antibiotics have been isolated and are likely to enter clinical trial. Pepleomycin differs from bleomycin in its terminal amino acid and has lesser pulmonary toxicity in rodents.[3] Tallysomycin A, an isolate from actinomycetes, differs both in amino acid

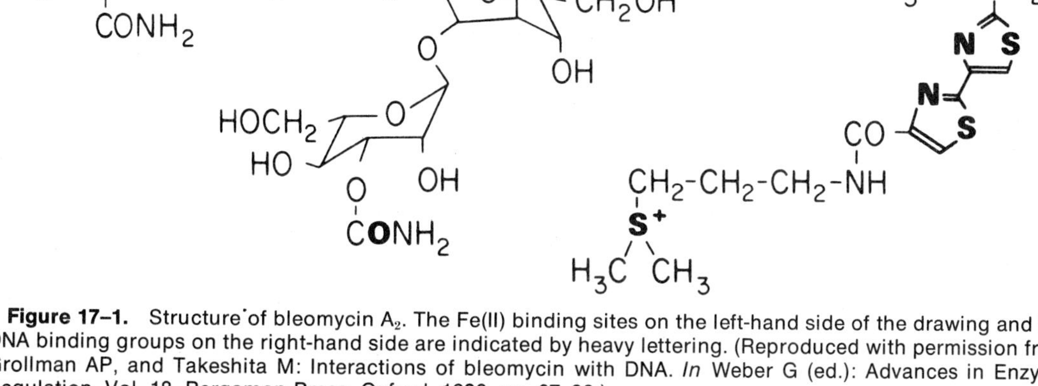

Figure 17–1. Structure of bleomycin A_2. The Fe(II) binding sites on the left-hand side of the drawing and the DNA binding groups on the right-hand side are indicated by heavy lettering. (Reproduced with permission from Grollman AP, and Takeshita M: Interactions of bleomycin with DNA. *In* Weber G (ed.): Advances in Enzyme Regulation, Vol. 18. Pergamon Press, Oxford, 1980, pp. 67–83.)

composition and in the presence of an additional sugar, and has greater affinity for DNA.[4]

The clinical mixture of bleomycin peptides is formulated as a sulfate salt, and its potency is measured in units of antimicrobial activity. Each unit contains between 1.2 and 1.7 mg of polypeptide protein. The clinical mixture is stable for at least one year at room temperature, and for four weeks following reconstitution in aqueous solution if stored at 4°C.

The multiple glycopeptides found in the clinical preparation of bleomycin have been separated and purified by paper and column chromatography;[5] the predominant active component is the A_2 peptide shown in Figure 17–1. The native compound isolated from S. *verticillus* contains copper bound in a coordinate complex. The bleomcyin–Cu(II) complex has been studied spectroscopically[6] and by x ray crystallography,[7] but has no antitumor activity in tissue culture. Active forms of bleomycin contain Fe(II) rather than Cu(II) in complex with the antibiotic.[8,9] As indicated in Figure 17–1, six distinct nitrogens are thought to participate in metal binding,[10] including: (1) β-aminoalanine; (2) proprionamide; (3) pyrimidinylmethyl; (4) β-hydroxyhistidine; (5) mannose 3′; and (6) methylvalerate.

The primary biochemical action of the A_2 peptide is to produce single- and double-strand breaks in DNA, both in cultured cells exposed to the drug and in isolated DNA incubated with bleomycin in solution. This breakage is reflected in the chromosomal gaps, deletions, and fragments seen in cytogenetic studies of whole cells. The drug is ineffective in producing strand breakage of native RNA or synthetic ribonucleotide polymers. The mechanism of DNA breakage has been clarified by investigation of the action of bleomycin on both viral and mammalian DNA, and appears to result from the production of free radicals by an Fe(II)–bleomycin complex intercalated between opposing strands of DNA. The initial step in this reaction sequence is the binding of bleomycin to DNA, which occurs with a dissociation constant of 8.3×10^{-6}M.[11] At saturating concentrations of bleomycin, one molecule of drug is bound per 4 to 5 base pairs of DNA. Binding to DNA occurs principally through the aminoterminal tripeptide of bleomycin (called the S tripeptide) to guanine bases on DNA.[11] Chien and co-workers[11] have shown that the bithiazole rings of the S tripeptide intercalate between guanine-cytosine base pairs.[12] The terminal dimethyl sulfonium group also participates in DNA binding, as indicated by the broadening of proton magnetic resonance of the sulfonium group in the presence of DNA.[11] Evidence for intercalation (insertion between base pairs) comes from the observation that the mixing of either bleomycin or its S tripeptide with DNA results in a lengthening of linear DNA and a relaxation of supercoiled circular DNA; both effects are indicative of unwinding of the double helical structure as the result of intercalation.[13]

The second step in the action of bleomycin is the induction of DNA breaks, mediated by free radicals produced by the bleomycin–Fe(II) complex. Although other metals are capable of binding to bleomycin, including Cu(II), Co(II), and Zn(II), only Fe(II) produces a complex capable of causing DNA breaks *in vitro*.[8,9] The importance of Fe(II) is further indicated by the observation that iron chelating agents inhibit the DNA scission reaction.[8] The bleomycin–Fe(II) complex functions as a ferrous oxidase,[14] catalyzing the reduction of molecular oxygen to superoxide or hydroxyl radicals. In the process, Fe(II) undergoes oxidation to Fe(III); regeneration of the active ferrous iron oxidation state requires the presence of a reducing agent such as mercaptoethanol *in vitro*. Caspary and co-workers[14] have calculated that the reaction, as monitored by measurement of oxygen consumption, has a maximal velocity of 27 moles of oxygen consumed per minute per mole bleomycin; the K_m for Fe(II) is 1.8 mM.

Oxidation of bleomycin–Fe(II) can be monitored by rapid optical spectrum shifts. The initial bleomycin–Fe(II) complex can be detected by optical absorption at 475 nm.[15] Addition of oxygen leads to the appearance of a short-lived intermediate with the spectral characteristics of bleomycin–Fe(II)–0_2, followed immediately by transition to an optical spectrum consistent with bleomycin–Fe(III). In the absence of oxygen, the bleomycin–Fe(II) complex is stable. As might be expected from its properties as an oxygenase, the bleomycin–Fe(II) complex is also capable of binding carbon monoxide or isocyanide in place of oxygen.[16] The carbon monoxide complex has been useful in defining the ligand sites on bleomycin that participate in metal binding,[16] as indicated in Figure 17–1.

The actual toxic products generated by the redox reaction involving bleomycin–Fe(II)–O_2 are conjectural. Hydroxyl and superoxide radicals have been identified by electron spin resonance,[17] and could result from the transfer of a single electron from Fe(II) to O_2, producing $\cdot O_2^-$, which in turn can generate the very toxic hydroxyl radical • OH through the so-called Haber-Weiss reaction. Other possible reaction sequences generating free radicals have been reviewed by Giloni and colleagues.[18]

DNA Cleavage

The hypothesis that oxygen radicals participate in the DNA cleavage mediated by bleomycin is based on the following observations: (1) strand breakage requires the presence of O_2 and ceases in an anaerobic environment;[19, 20] (2) coincident with the oxidation of bleomycin–Fe(II), oxygen is consumed[14] and superoxide and hydroxyl radicals are generated;[17] (3) free radical scavengers and superoxide dismutase (which inactivates $\cdot O_2^-$) inhibit DNA strand breakage;[21] and (4) peroxidation products of DNA deoxyribose have been identifed.[18, 22]

Incubation of DNA with bleomycin results in the release of all four bases (thymine, cytosine, adenine, guanine),[23] as well as lesser amounts of partially degraded nucleosides of the same four bases.[24] These latter products have now been identified as base-propenal compounds, the result of cleavage of the deoxyribose ring at the 3′-4′ bond.[18] A reaction sequence leading to the propenal base configuration (compound 7) is given in Figure 17–2. A second product of the reaction, the glycolic ester (compound 8),

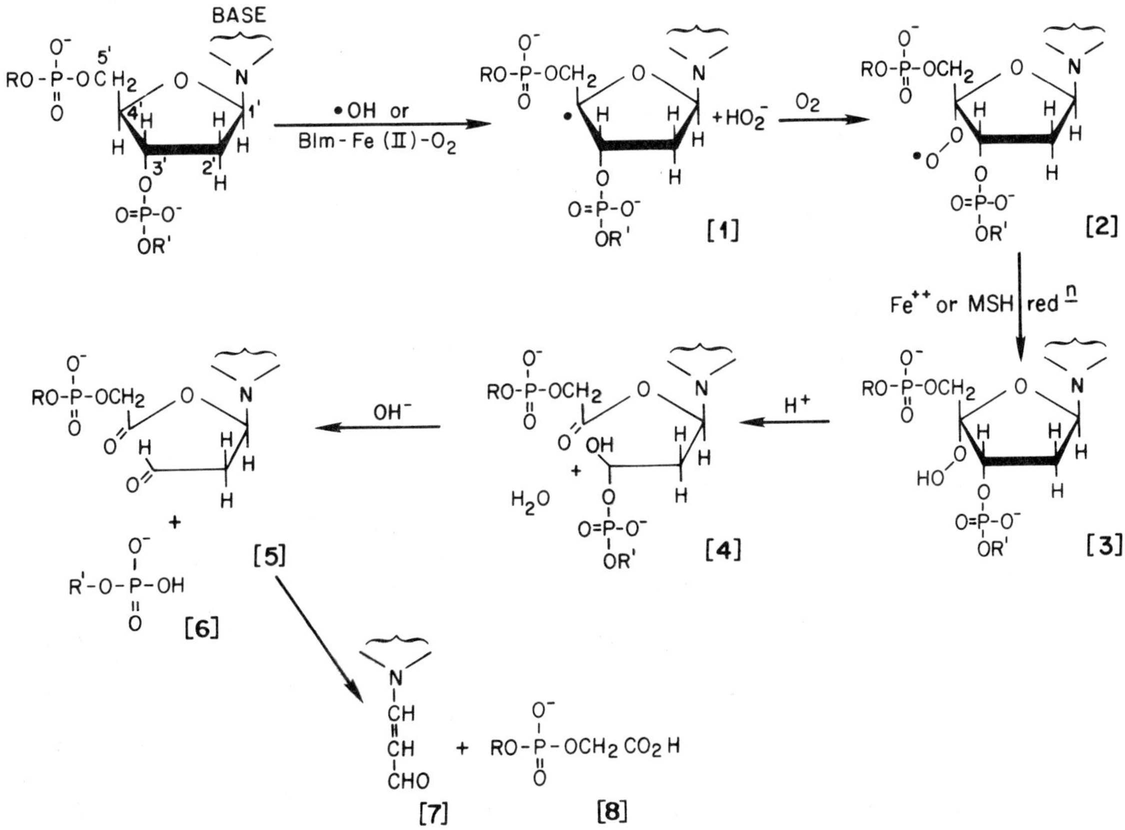

Figure 17–2. Reaction sequence for cleavage of the C-3′-C-4′ deoxyribose bond, as postulated by Grollman and Takeshita.[24] Reaction products are a base-propenal [7], a glycolic acid ester [8], free base, and the degradation product of [7] — malondialdehyde. (Reproduced with permission from Grollman AP, and Takeshita M: Interactions of bleomycin with DNA. *In* Weber G (ed.): Advances in Enzyme Regulation, Vol. 18. Pergamon Press, Oxford, 1980, pp. 67–83.)

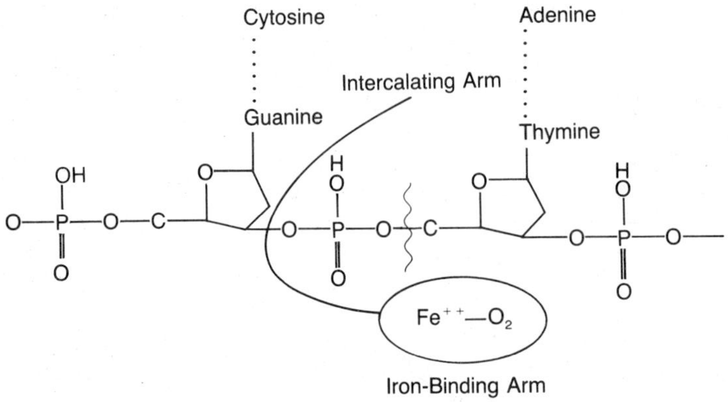

Figure 17–3. Intercalation of the bithiazole groups between DNA base pairs, at least one of which contains the GpT of GpC sequence. Also shown is the apposition of the Fe(II) binding portion of bleomycin to the deoxyribose group, which is cleaved in the subsequent release of free radicals. (Reproduced with permission from Grollman AP, and Takeshita M: Interactions of bleomycin with DNA. *In* Weber G (ed.): Advances in Enzyme Regulation, Vol. 18. Pergamon Press, Oxford, 1980, pp. 67–83.)

has also been identified and is thought to represent the C-4′ and C-5′ fragment and its phosphate group attached to the C-3′ carbon of the neighboring bases. The malondialdehyde repeatedly observed in the reaction solution resulting from bleomycin action on DNA is likely generated from the base-propenal adduct during distillation or assay of the reaction mixture,[18] and is not a direct product of the reaction.

Analysis of the products of DNA cleavage, using either viral or mammalian DNA, has consistently shown a preferential release of thymine[22] or thymine-propenal,[18] with lesser amounts of the other three bases or their propenal adducts. The propensity for attack at thymine bases likely results from the previously mentioned preference for intercalation of bleomycin between base pairs in which at least one strand contains the sequence GpT. The specificity for cleavage of DNA at a residue located at the 3′ side of G appears to be absolute.[25] A schematic representation of the intercalation and cleavage processes as conceived by Grollman and Takeshita[24] is given in Figure 17–3, and summarizes the structural specificities and reaction mechanisms discussed in this chapter.

CELLULAR PHARMACOLOGY

The cellular uptake of bleomycin has not been examined in detail. Autoradiographic studies with ^{14}C-bleomycin have demonstrated early accumulation of labeled material at the cell membrane of murine tumor cells, with gradual appearance of labeling at the nuclear membrane only after four hours of exposure.[26] The fate of intracellular bleomycin is similarly unclear; a bleomycin-inactivating enzyme has been described in samples of normal and malignant cells,[27] and has been partially purified from liver. Interestingly, this enzyme was not found in lung and skin, the two normal tissues most susceptible to bleomycin damage.[28] Bleomycin degrading activity was increased in two resistant rat hepatomas studied by Mayaki et al.,[29] but this change does not appear to account for resistance in all cell lines. Brabbs and Warr[30] isolated three stably resistant CHO cell lines after mutagenesis with ethylmethane sulfonate. Bleomycin inactivating enzyme activity was not increased in any of these lines. One line was cross-resistant to vinblastine and puromycin, and showed increased sensitivity to bleomycin in the presence of the detergent polysorbate 80 (Tween 80). Both observations suggest that an alteration in membrane permeability was responsible for bleomycin resistance in this cell line.

Cells exposed to bleomycin in culture appear to be most susceptible in mitosis or in the G_2, or intermitotic, phase of the cell cycle;[31, 32] in addition, progression of cells through G_2 into mitosis is blocked by the drug.[33] In mouse L cells, S phase is also lengthened, prior to G_2 blockade.[34] However, Barlogie et al. observed that, although cell killing was maximal in G_2, cell death also occurred in cells exposed during G_1.[35] Despite the apparent increased toxicity for cells in G_2, there is no agreement regarding preferential kill of logarithmically growing cells as compared with plateau-phase cells; indeed, some workers have observed greater fractional cell kill for plateau-phase cells.[36, 37] However, the possibility of enhancing cell kill by exposure during G_2 has led to the clinical use of bleomycin by continuous infusion in order to maximize the chances of tumor cell exposure during the most sensitive phase of the cell cycle.

The intracellular lesions caused by bleomycin include chromosomal breaks and deletions, and both single- and (less frequently) double-strand breaks. In nonmitotic cells, DNA is organized into nucleosomes, or small beads, which are joined by long strands, or linker regions. The primary point of attack appears to be in the linker regions of DNA, between nucleosomes.[38] The technique of alkaline elution has been used by Iqbal and coworkers, who observed a biphasic survival curve for cell survival or DNA single-strand breaks versus dose.[39] The reason for the biphasic characteristics of this curve is unclear, but may be related to the differing susceptibility of cells during different phases of the cell cycle. It is clear, however, that cell kill and DNA strand breakage increase in proportion to the duration of drug exposure for at least six hours; this finding implies a greater effectiveness for bleomycin when given by prolonged infusion than when administered via intravenous bolus.

Little is known about the potential of cells to repair bleomycin-induced DNA breaks. A delay in plating cells after bleomycin exposure has been shown to increase plating efficiency substantially, presumably by allowing time for repair of so-called potentially lethal damage.[40] Indirect evidence suggests that repair processes similar to those required for repair of lesions induced by *ionizing radiation* play a role in limiting damage due to bleomycin,[41,42] while cells deficient in repair mechanisms for *ultraviolet radiation* damage have no increased sensitivity to bleomycin.

CLINICAL PHARMACOKINETICS

A variety of techniques have been developed for assay of bleomycin in biologic fluids, including microbiologic,[43] high-pressure liquid chromatographic (HPLC),[44] biochemical (degradation of DNA),[45] and radioimmunoassay methods.[46] The most rapid and simplest for clinical studies is the radioimmunoassay, which, utilizing ^{125}I or ^{57}Co-labeled bleomycin, has provided insight into the disposition of bleomycin in man and has superseded the less sensitive and less specific microbiologic assay techniques. The antibodies described by Broughton and Strong react quantitatively with the component peptides of the clinically used bleomycin formulation.[46] The primary component peptides A_2 and B_2 give 75 to 100 per cent reactivity as compared with the mixture in standard curve determinations. HPLC, using the ion-pairing technique, allows resolution of the component peptides, but is more time-consuming and of unproved value in clinical studies.

The hallmark of bleomycin pharmacokinetics in patients with normal serum creatinine is a rapid, two-phase drug disappearance from plasma with 45[52] to 70 per cent[53] of the dose excreted in the urine within 24 hours. For intravenous bolus doses, the half-lives for plasma disappearance have varied somewhat among the published studies. Alberts et al.[47] reported half-lives α and β of 24 minutes and four hours, respectively, whereas Crooke[48] estimated half-life β to be approximately two hours. Peak plasma concentrations reach 1 to 10 milliunits per ml for intravenous bolus doses of 15 units per m^2.

For patients receiving bleomycin by continuous intravenous infusion, the postinfusion half-life is approximately three hours. Intramuscular injection of bleomycin (2 to 10 units per m^2) gave peak plasma levels of 0.13 to 0.6 milliunits per ml, or approximately one tenth the peak level achieved by the intravenous bolus doses.[49] The mean half-life after intramuscular injection was 2.5 hours, or about the same as that following intravenous injection. Peak serum concentrations were reached approximately one hour after injection (Fig. 17–4). Bleomycin pharmacokinetics have also been studied in patients receiving intrapleural or intraperitoneal injections. These routes have proved effective in controlling malignant effusions due to breast, lung, and ovarian cancer.[50] Intracavitary bleomycin, in doses of 60 mg per m^2, gives peak plasma levels of 0.4 to 5.0 milliunits per ml, with a plasma half-life of 3.4 hours after intrapleural doses and 5.3 hours after intraperitoneal injection.[51] Corresponding intracavitary levels are tenfold higher than simultaneous plasma concentrations. Approximately 45 per cent of an intracavitary dose is absorbed into the systemic circulation.

As might be expected, bleomycin pharmacokinetics are markedly altered in patients with abnormal renal function, particularly those with creatinine clearance of less than 35 ml per minute. Alberts et al.[47] noted a terminal half-life of approximately ten hours

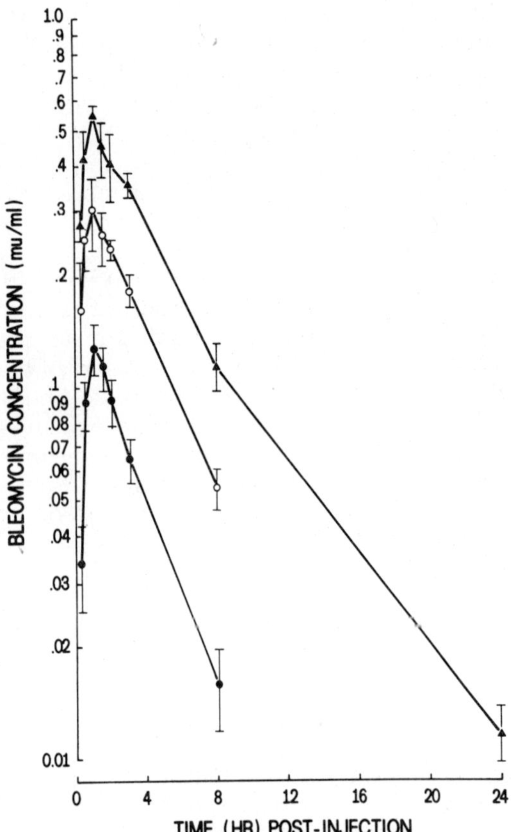

Figure 17–4. Pharmacokinetics of bleomycin following intramuscular administration of 2 (•—•—•), 5 (○–○–○), and 10 (▲-▲-▲) mg/m² bleomycin. (Reproduced with permission from Oken et al.: Pharmacokinetics of bleomycin after IM administration in man. Cancer Treat. Rep. 64:485–489, 1981.)

in a patient with a slightly elevated creatinine clearance of 1.5 mg per dl, and Crooke[52] reported a patient with a creatinine clearance of 10.7 ml per minute and a half-life β of 21 hours. However, the available data are too limited to provide accurate guidelines for dosage adjustment in patients with renal failure. It would appear prudent to decrease doses in proportion to the decrease in creatinine clearance for patients with clearances below 25 ml per minute per m². Fatal bleomycin pulmonary toxicity has been observed in a patient with *cis*-platinum–induced renal failure who received a six-day course of bleomycin (total dose 185 units).[53]

CLINICAL TOXICITY AND SIDE EFFECTS

The most important toxic actions of bleomycin affect the lungs and skin; there is usually little evidence of myelosuppression except in patients with severely compromised bone marrow function due to extensive previous chemotherapy.[54] In such patients, myelosuppression is usually mild and is seen primarily with high-dose therapy. Fever occurs in the 48 hours following drug administration in one quarter of patients.[55] Some investigators advocate using a 1-unit test dose of bleomycin in patients receiving their initial dose.[55A]

Pulmonary toxicity is manifest as a subacute or chronic interstitial pneumonitis complicated in its later stages by progressive interstitial fibrosis, hypoxia, and death. Evidence of pulmonary toxicity, usually in the form of bibasilar pulmonary infiltrates on chest x-ray and cough and dyspnea clinically, occurs in 3 to 5 per cent of patients receiving a total dose of less than 450 mg bleomycin, increasing significantly to a 10 per cent incidence in those treated with greater cumulative doses.[55] Toxicity is also more frequent in patients older than 70 years, in those with underlying emphysema, and in those receiving single doses greater than 25 mg per m².[54] There is also growing evidence that previous radiotherapy to the chest predisposes to bleomycin pulmonary toxicity.[56] It should be remembered that, although the risk of lung toxicity increases with doses greater than 450 mg, severe pulmonary sequelae have been observed at total doses below 100 mg.

Raisfeld has considered the possibility that bleomycin lung toxicity is caused by the terminal amine substituent linked to the bithiazole group of the various bleomycins.[56A] She has examined the ability of the various terminal amines of bleomycin A_2, A_5, A_6, and B_2 to cause pulmonary fibrosis and epithelial metaplasia when instilled into the trachea of mice. Her findings indicate that these amines can reproduce the lung toxicity caused by their corresponding bleomycins. The A_2 substituent diaminopropane and the A_5 end-group spermidine both were potent inducers of pulmonary fibrosis, whereas the B_2 terminal amine, agmatine, resembled its parent compound in that it produced much milder changes. These findings raise the possibility that by chemical modification of the terminal amine it may be possible to select an analogue lacking pulmonary toxicity.

The pathogenesis of the pulmonary toxicity is poorly understood. Animal models indicate that the initial lesion occurs in pulmonary arterioles and veins.[57] The progression of changes thereafter, as revealed by studies in mice[58] and baboons,[59] consists of edema and an inflammatory intra-alveolar infiltrate, proliferation of Type II alveolar macrophages, and interstitial fibrosis. In the later stages of development, pulmonary function becomes abnormal, as reflected by a decrease in total lung capacity, increased lung stiffness (a shift in pressure-volume relationships), and finally a decrease in carbon monoxide diffusion capacity. In mice, hydroxyproline content (a convenient measure of collagen content) increases in parallel with pulmonary fibrosis and can be used as a quantitative assay for the progression of bleomycin-related toxicity.[58]

The process of evolution of pulmonary fibrosis can be observed in organ culture. Following endotracheal instillation of bleomycin in rats, lung explants placed in organ culture synthesize up to threefold increased quantities of collagen from the fourth to the 15th day after drug exposure.[60] It is not clear whether increased collagen synthesis is due to an increased synthetic rate by individual cells or a recruitment of new cells into collagen synthesis. The process of collagen deposition can be prevented in rats by administration of dehydroproline, an inhibitor of prolylhydroxylase, which is required for synthesis of hydroxyproline, a required constituent of collagen. Dehydroproline, as might be expected, prevents bleomycin-induced changes in pulmonary function and compliance in rats.[61] It has not yet been tested in man. There is preliminary evidence from studies of bleomycin toxicity in rats that the anti-inflammatory agent indomethacin may prevent or reduce bleomycin-induced pulmonary fibrosis.[62] It should be emphasized that the pathologic changes observed in the late stages of bleomycin toxicity are not unique to this drug, since similar findings are seen in a variety of toxic lung lesions, including those due to paraquat, oxygen, radiation, idiopathic pulmonary fibrosis, and other antineoplastic agents such as cyclophosphamide, BCNU, and busulfan. These changes appear to be common sequelae of primary injury to the alveolar epithelium or small vessels.[63]

In animal toxicology studies, single high doses of bleomycin produced greater pulmonary collagen deposition and poorer therapeutic results than did small daily doses or continuous infusion schedules of administration.[64] These results constitute strong evidence for more extensive testing of continuous infusions of bleomycin in clinical trials, as has been done in patients with testicular cancer.[65]

Clinical symptoms of bleomycin pulmonary injury include a nonproductive cough, dyspnea, and occasionally fever and pleuritic pain. Physical examination usually reveals little auscultatory evidence of pulmonary alveolar infiltrates, and initial chest films are often negative or may reveal an increase in interstitial markings, especially in the lower lobes, with a predilection for subpleural areas. Gallium-67 lung scans may show the presence of a diffuse lung lesion at a time of minimal radiologic abnormality, but this finding does not differentiate bleomycin lung toxicity from other forms of interstitial lung disease,[66] and particularly from *Pneumocystis carinii* pneumonia. Arterial oxygen desaturation and an abnormal carbon monoxide diffusion capacity are present in symptomatic patients with bleomycin toxicity, as is also the case in patients with other forms of interstitial pulmonary disease. Thus, open lung biopsy is usually required to distinguish between the primary differential diagnostic considerations, specifically a drug-induced pulmonary lesion, an infectious interstitial pneumonitis, and neoplastic pulmonary infiltration. The findings on histologic examination of human lung following bleomycin treatment closely resemble those previously described in the experimental animal, and include an acute inflammatory infiltrate in the alveoli, interstitial and intra-alveolar edema, pulmonary hyaline membrane formation, and intra-alveolar and interstitial fibrosis. In addition, squamous metaplasia of the alveolar lining cells has been described as a characteristic finding.[67]

Pulmonary function tests, particularly of the carbon monoxide diffusing capacity, are of possible value in predicting a high risk of pulmonary toxicity. Patients treated with bleomycin show a general trend of progressive deterioration in diffusion capacity with increasing total dose, and a marked increase in changes above a 240-mg total dose. It is not clear, however, whether the diffusion capacity test can be used to predict which patients will subsequently develop pulmonary toxicity.[68] As mentioned above, at advanced stages in the evolution of bleomycin pulmonary toxicity the diffusion capacity, as well as arterial O_2 saturation and total lung capacity, becomes markedly abnormal.

Patients who have received bleomycin appear to be at greater risk of respiratory failure in the postoperative recovery period following surgery.[69] In one study five of five patients treated with 200 mg per m^2 bleomycin (cumulative dose) for testicular cancer died of postoperative respiratory failure; a reduction in inspired O_2 to an FiO_2 of 0.24 and a decrease in fluids administered during surgery prevented mortality in subsequent patients.[69] The sensitivity of bleomycin-treated patients to high concentrations of inspired O_2 is intriguing in view of the molecular action of bleomycin, which is dependent on, and mediated by, the formation of oxygen-derived free radicals. Current safeguards for anesthesia of bleomycin-treated patients include the use of the minimal tolerated concentration of inspired oxygen, and modest fluid replacement to prevent pulmonary edema.

There is no specific therapy for patients with bleomycin lung toxicity. Discontinuation of the drug may be followed by a period of continued progression of the pulmonary findings, with partial reversal of the abnormalities in pulmonary function only after several months. The inflammatory component of the pathologic process does resolve in experimental models[59] and interstitial infiltrates resolve clinically, but the reversibility of pulmonary fibrosis has not been documented. The value of corticosteroids in promoting recovery from bleomycin lung toxicity remains in doubt, although beneficial effects have been described in isolated case studies.[70]

A more common but less serious toxicity of bleomycin is its effect on skin. Approximately 50 per cent of patients treated with conventional once- or twice-daily doses of this agent develop erythema, induration, and hyperkeratosis and peeling of skin that may progress to frank ulceration.[55] These changes predominantly affect digits, hands, and joints and areas of previous irradiation. Hyperpigmentation, alopecia, and nail changes do not necessitate discontinuation of therapy, particularly if clear benefit is being derived from the drug. Rarely, patients may develop Raynaud's phenomenon while receiving bleomycin.[71]

Because of the greater effect of bleomycin on cells in the mitotic and G_2 phases of the cell cycle, this drug has been used in continuous infusion schedules to produce a prolonged period of toxic concentrations. Doses of 25 mg per day for five days, as employed for the treatment of testicular cancer, have produced the expected incidence of pulmonary toxicity, particularly in patients with previous chest irradiation,[56, 72] but additionally have caused hypertensive episodes in 17 per cent of patients and hyperbilirubinemia in 30 per cent.[56] These latter toxicities are rarely seen with conventional bolus doses.

Continuous intra-arterial infusion has also been employed for patients with carcinoma of the cervix[73] and of the head and neck.[74] The former study noted a disappointing 12 per cent response rate to infusion of 20 mg per m^2 per week for courses of up to three weeks. Pulmonary toxicity was observed in 20 per cent of patients.

Other toxic reactions to bleomycin include hypersensitivity reactions, with urticaria, periorbital edema, and bronchospasm.[55]

Bleomycin has also been applied topically as a 3.5 per cent ointment in a xipamide (Aquaphor) base. Two-week courses of treatment produced complete regression of Paget's disease of the vulva in four of seven patients,[75] with no serious local toxicity.

Bleomycin has been instilled into the urinary bladder in doses of 60 units in 30 ml of sterile water.[76] Seven of 26 patients with superficial transitional cell carcinomas had a complete disappearance of disease after seven to eight weekly treatments, but all had relatively small lesions. The primary toxicity was cystitis. Plasma drug level monitoring revealed little evidence of systemic absorption.

RADIATION AND DRUG INTERACTION

Bleomycin is used frequently in combination therapy regimens for treatment of lymphomas and squamous carcinomas of the esophagus and head and neck, primarily because of its lack of myelosuppressive toxicity. The pharmacologic basis of synergism between bleomycin and various agents has received considerable attention,[77, 78] but is only poorly understood. Bleomycin given within three hours of irradiation, either before or after, produces greater than additive effects,[79] possibly owing to the production of free radical damage to DNA by both agents. As mentioned earlier, synergistic pulmonary toxicity has been reported in patients receiving bleomycin following previous chest irradiation.

References

1. Umezawa H, Meada K, Takeuchi T, et al.: New antibiotics, bleomycin A and B. J. Antibiot. Ser. A 19:200, 1966.
2. Einhorn L, and Donohue J: *cis*-Diamminedichloroplatinum, vinblastine, and bleomycin combination chemotherapy in disseminated testicular cancer. Ann. Intern. Med. 87:293, 1977.
3. Sikic BI, Siddik ZH, and Gram TE: Relative pulmonary toxicity and antitumor effects of two new bleomycin analogs, pepleomycin and tallysomycin A. Cancer Treat. Rep. 64:659–667, 1980.
4. Lown JW, and Joshua AV: Intervention of the glycopeptide antitumor antibiotics bleomycin and tallysomycin with deoxyribonucleotide *in vitro*. Biochem. Pharmacol. 29:521–532, 1980.
5. Umezawa H, Suhara Y, Takita T, et al.: Purification of bleomycin. J. Antibiot. Ser. A 19:210, 1966.
6. Dabrowiak JC, Greenaway FT, Santillo FS, et al.: The iron complexes of bleomycin and tallysomycin. Biochem. Biophys. Res. Commun. 91:721, 1979.
7. Takita T, Muraoka Y, Nakatani T, et al.: Chemistry of bleomycin. XXI. Metal-complex and its implication for the mechanism of bleomycin action. J. Antibiot. (Tokyo) 31:1073–1077, 1978.
8. Sausville EA, Peisach J, and Horwitz SB: Effects of chelating agents and metal ions on the degradation of DNA by bleomycin. Biochemistry 17:2740, 1978.
9. Sausville EA, Peisach J, and Horwitz SB: A role for ferrous ion and oxygen in the degradation of DNA by bleomycin. Biochem. Biophys. Res. Commun. 73:814, 1976.
10. Oppenheimer NJ, Rodriquez LO, and Hecht SM: Proton magnetic resonance study of the structure of bleomycin and the zinc-bleomycin complex. Biochemistry 18:3439–3445, 1979.
11. Chien M, Grollman AP, and Horwitz SB: Bleomycin-DNA interactions: fluorescence and proton magnetic resonance studies. Biochemistry 16:3641, 1977.
12. Kasai H, Naganawa H, Takita T, et al.: Chemistry of bleomycin. XXII. Interaction of bleomycin with nucleic acids, preferential binding to guanine base and electrostatic effect of the terminal amine. J. Antibiot. (Tokyo) 31:1316, 1978.
13. Povirk LF, Hogan M, and Dattagupta N: Binding of bleomycin to DNA: intercalation of the bithiazole rings. Biochemistry 18:96, 1979.
14. Caspary WJ, Niziak C, Lanzo DA, et al.: Bleomycin A_2: a ferrous oxidase. Mol. Pharmacol. 16:256–260, 1979.
15. Burger RM, Horwitz SB, Peisach J, et al.: Oxygenated iron bleomycin. A short-lived intermediate in the reaction of ferrous bleomycin with O_2. J. Biol. Chem. 254:12299–12302, 1979.
16. Burger RM, Peisach J, Blumberg WE, et al.: Iron-bleomycin interactions with oxygen and oxygen analogues. Effects on spectra and drug activity. J. Biol. Chem. 254:10906–10912, 1979.
17. Sugiura Y, and Kikuchi TK: Formation of superoxide and hydroxy radicals by bleomycin and iron (II). J. Antibiot. (Tokyo) 31:1310–1312, 1978.
18. Giloni L, Takeshita M, Johnson F, et al.: Bleomycin-induced strand-scission of DNA: mechanism of deoxyribose cleavage. J. Biol. Chem. 256:8608–8615, 1981.
19. Onishi T, Iwata H, and Takagi Y: Effects of reducing or oxidizing agents on the action of bleomycin. J. Biochem. 77:745–752, 1975.
20. Horwitz SB, Sausville EA, and Peisach J: Role for iron in the degradation of DNA by bleomycin. *In* Hecht S (ed.): Bleomycin: Chemical, Biochemical and Biological Aspects. Springer, New York, 1979, pp. 170–183.
21. Lown JW, and Sim S: The mechanism of the bleomycin-induced cleavage of DNA. Biochem. Biophys. Res. Commun. 77:1150–1157, 1977.
22. Burger RM, Berkowitz AR, Peisach J, et al.: Origin of malondialdehyde from DNA degraded by Fe(II)-bleomycin. J. Biol. Chem. 255:11832–11838, 1980.
23. Sausville E, Stein R, Peisach J, et al.: Properties and products of the degradation of DNA by bleomycin. Biochemistry 17:2746, 1978.
24. Grollman AP, and Takeshita M: Interactions of bleomycin with DNA. *In* Weber G (ed.): Advances in Enzyme Regulation, Vol. 18. Pergamon Press, Oxford, 1980, pp. 67–83.
25. Takeshita M, Grollman AP, Ohtsubo E, et al.: Interaction of bleomycin with DNA. Proc. Natl. Acad. Sci. USA 75:5983, 1978.
26. Fugimito J, Higashi H, and Kosaki G: Intracellular distribution of [^{14}C] bleomycin and the cytokinetic effects of bleomycin in the mouse tumor. Cancer Res. 36:2248, 1976.
27. Muller WEG, and Zahn RK: Bleomycin: mode of action on DNA. *In* Carter SK, Ichikawa T, Mathe G, et al. (eds.): Fundamental and Clinical Studies of Bleomycin (Gann Monograph on Cancer Research No. 19). University Park, Baltimore–London–New York, 1976, pp. 51–62.
28. Umezawa H, Hori S, Sawa T, et al.: A bleomycin-inactivating enzyme in mouse liver. J. Antibiot. Ser. A 27:419, 1974.
29. Mayaki M, Ono T, Hori S, et al.: Binding of bleomycin to DNA in bleomycin-sensitive and -resistant rat ascites hepatoma cells. Cancer Res. 35:2015, 1975.
30. Brabbs S, and Warr JR: Isolation and characterization of bleomycin-resistant clones of OHO cells. Genet. Res. 34:269–279, 1979.
31. Kunimoto TM, Hori M, and Umezawa H: Modes of action of phleomycin, bleomycin, and formycin on HeLa 53 cells in synchronized culture. J. Antibiot. Ser. A 20:277, 1967.
32. Barranco SC, and Humphrey RM: The effects of bleomycin on survival and cell progression in Chinese hamster cells *in vitro*. Cancer Res. 31:1218, 1971.
33. Tobey RA: Arrest of Chinese hamster cells in G_2 following treatment with the antitumor drug bleomycin. J. Cell. Physiol. 79:259, 1972.
34. Wanatabe M, Takabe Y, Katsumata T, et al.: Effects of bleomycin on progression through the cell cycle of mouse L cells. Cancer Res. 34:2726–2732, 1974.
35. Barlogie B, Drewinko B, Schumann J, et al: Pulse cytophotometric analysis of cell cycle perturbation with bleomycin *in vitro*. Cancer Res. 36:1182, 1976.
36. Twentyman PR, and Bleehen NM: The sensitivity to bleomycin in spleen colony forming units in the mouse. Br. J. Cancer 28:66, 1973.
37. Barranco SC, Novak JK, and Humphrey RM: Response of mammalian cells following treatment with bleomycin and 1,3-bis(2-chloroethyl)1-nitrosourea. Cancer Res. 33:691, 1973.
38. Kuo MT, and Hsu TC: Bleomycin causes release of nucleosomes from chromatin and chromosomes. Nature 271:83, 1978.
39. Iqbal ZM, Kohn KW, Ewig RAG, et al.: Single-strand scission and repair of DNA in mammalian cells by bleomycin. Cancer Res. 36:3834, 1976.
40. Barranco SC, Novak JK, and Humphrey RM: Studies on recovery from chemically induced damage in mammalian cells. Cancer Res. 35:1194, 1975.
41. Onishi T, Shimada K, and Takagi Y: Effects of bleomycin on *Escherichia coli* strains with various sensitivities to radiation. Biochem. Biophys. Acta 312:248, 1973.
42. Cramer P, and Printer RB: Bleomycin-resistant DNA synthesis in ataxia telangiectasia cells. Nature 291:671–672, 1981.
43. Umezawa H, Takeuchi T, Hori S, et al.: Studies on the mechanism of antitumor effect of bleomycin on squamous cell carcinoma. J. Antibiot. (Tokyo) 25:409–420, 1972.
44. Shiu GK, and Goehl TJ: High performance liquid chromatographic determination of bleomycin A_2 in urine. J. Chromatogr. 181:127–131, 1980.

45. Galvan L, Strong JE, and Crooke ST: Use of PM-2 DNA degradation as a pharmacokinetic assay for bleomycin. Cancer Res. 39:3948–3951, 1979.
46. Broughton A, and Strong JE: Radioimmunoassay of bleomycin. Cancer Res. 36:1418, 1976.
47. Alberts DS, Chen HSG, Liu R, et al.: Bleomycin pharmacokinetics in man. I. Intravenous administration. Cancer Chemother. Pharmacol. 1:177, 1978.
48. Crooke ST, Comis RL, Einhorn LH, et al.: Effects of variations in renal function on the clinical pharmacology of bleomycin administered as an IV bolus. Cancer Treat. Rep. 61:1631, 1977.
49. Oken MM, Crooke ST, Elson MK, et al.: Pharmacokinetics of bleomycin after IM administration in man. Cancer Treat. Rep. 65:485–489, 1981.
50. Paladine W, Cunningham TJ, Sponzo R, et al.: Intracavitary bleomycin in the management of malignant effusions. Cancer 38:1903, 1976.
51. Alberts DS, Chen HSG, Mayersohn M, et al.: Bleomycin pharmacokinetics in man. II. Intracavitary administration. Cancer Chemother. Pharmacol. 2:127, 1979.
52. Crooke ST, Luft F, Broughton A, et al.: Bleomycin serum pharmacokinetics as determined by a radioimmunoassay and a microbiologic assay in a patient with compromised renal function. Cancer 39:1430, 1977.
53. Bennett WM, Pastore L, and Houghton DC: Fatal pulmonary bleomycin toxicity in *cis*-platin–induced acute renal failure. Cancer Treat. Rep. 64:921–924, 1980.
54. Hubbard SP, Chabner BA, Canellos GP, et al.: High-dose intravenous bleomycin in treatment of advanced lymphomas. Eur. J. Cancer 11:623, 1975.
55. Blum RH, Carter SK, and Agre K: A clinical review of bleomycin — a new antineoplastic agent. Cancer 31:903, 1973.
55A. Levy RL, and Chiarillo S: Hyperpyrexia, allergic-type response, and death occurring with bleomycin administration. Oncology 37:316, 1980.
56. Samuels ML, Johnson DE, Holoye PH, et al.: Large-dose bleomycin therapy and pulmonary toxicity. A possible role of prior radiotherapy. J.A.M.A. 235:1117, 1976.
56A. Raisfeld IH: Role of terminal substituents in the pulmonary toxicity of bleomycins. Toxicol. Appl. Pharmacol. 57:355, 1981.
57. Adamson IY, and Bowden DH: The pathogenesis of bleomycin-induced pulmonary fibrosis in mice. Am. J. Pathol. 77:185, 1974.
58. Sikic BI, Young DM, Mimnaugh EG, et al.: Quantification of bleomycin pulmonary toxicity in mice by changes in lung hydroxyproline content and morphometric histopathology. Cancer Res. 38:787, 1978.
59. McCullough B, Collins JF, Johanson WG Jr, et al.: Bleomycin-induced diffuse interstitial pulmonary fibrosis in baboons. J. Clin. Invest. 61:79, 1978.
60. Phan SH, Thrall RS, and Ward PA: Bleomycin-induced pulmonary fibrosis in rats: biochemical demonstration of increased rates of collagen synthesis. Am. Rev. Respir. Dis. 121:501–506, 1980.
61. Kelley J, Newman RA, and Evans JN: Bleomycin-induced pulmonary fibrosis in the rat. Prevention with an inhibitor of collagen synthesis. J. Lab. Clin. Med. 96:954–964, 1980.
62. Thrau RS, McCormick JR, Jack RM, et al.: Bleomycin-induced pulmonary fibrosis in the rat. Inhibition by indomethacin. Am. J. Pathol. 95:117, 1979.
63. Witschi H: Exploitable biochemical approaches for the evaluation of toxic lung damage. Essays Toxicol. 6:125, 1975.
64. Sikic BI, Collins JM, Mimnaugh EG, et al.: Improved therapeutic index of bleomycin when administered by continuous infusion in mice. Cancer Treat. Rep. 62:2011, 1978.
65. Samuels ML, Johnson DE, and Holoye PY: Continuous intravenous bleomycin (NSC-125066) therapy with vinblastine (NSC-49842) in Stage III testicular neoplasia. Cancer Chemother. Rep. 59:563, 1975.
66. Richman SD, Levenson SM, Bunn PA, et al.: 67-Ga-accumulation in pulmonary lesions associated with bleomycin toxicity. Cancer 36:1975.
67. Burkhardt A, Gebbers JO, and Holtje WJ: Die Bleomycin-Lunge. Deutsch. Med. Wochenschr. 102:281, 1977.
68. Comis RL, Kuppinger MS, Ginsberg SJ, et al.: Role of single-breath carbon monoxide-diffusing capacity in monitoring the pulmonary effects of bleomycin in germ-free tumor patients. Cancer Res. 39:5076, 1979.
69. Goldiner PL, Carlon GC, Critkovic E, et al.: Factors influencing post-operative morbidity and mortality in patients treated with bleomycin. Br. Med. J. 1:1664–1667, 1978.
70. Yagoda A, Etcubanas E, and Tan CTC: Bleomycin, an antitumor antibiotic. Clinical experience in 274 patients. Ann. Intern. Med. 77:861, 1972.
71. See Cancer Treatment Reports 62(4), 1978, for a series of Letters to the Editors on this subject.
72. Einhorn L, Krause M, Hornbach N, et al.: Enhanced pulmonary toxicity with bleomycin and radiotherapy in oat cell lung cancer. Cancer 37:2414, 1976.
73. Morrow CP, DiSaia PJ, Mangan CF, et al.: Continuous pelvic arterial infusion with bleomycin for squamous carcinoma of the cervix recurrent after irradiation therapy. Cancer Treat. Rep. 61:1403, 1977.
74. Bitter K: Pharmacokinetic behaviour of bleomycin-cobalt-57 with special regard to intra-arterial perfusion of the maxillofacial region. J. Maxillofac. Surg. 4:226, 1976.
75. Watring WG, Roberts JA, Lagasse LD, et al.: Treatment of recurrent Paget's disease of the vulva with topical bleomycin. Cancer 41:10, 1978.
76. Bracken RB, Johnson DE, Rodriquez L, et al.: Treatment of multiple superficial tumors of bladder with intravesical bleomycin. Urology 9:161, 1977.
77. Crooke ST, and Bradner WT: Bleomycin, a review. J. Med. 7:333, 1976.
78. Blehan NM, Gillies NE, and Twentyman PR: The effect of bleomycin and radiation in combination on bacteria and mammalian cells in culture. Br. J. Radiol. 47:346, 1974.
79. Takabe Y, Miyamoto T, Watanabe M, et al.: Synergism of x-ray and bleomycin on Ehrlich ascites tumour cells. Br. J. Cancer 36:391, 1977.

CYTOSINE ARABINOSIDE 18

Bruce A. Chabner

Arabinose nucleosides are a unique class of compounds, first isolated from the sponge *Cryptothethya crypta*,[1] that differ from the physiologic nucleosides found in animal tissues by the presence of a β-OH group in the 2′ position of the sugar (Fig. 18–1). Several arabinose nucleosides have useful antitumor and antiviral activity. The most active cytotoxic agent is the chemically synthesized cytosine arabinoside (ara-C),[2] the most potent antileukemic agent in man. Arabinosyl adenine (ara-A), a purine arabinosyl nucleoside, has antitumor and antiviral action, and is considered in detail in Chapter 9.[3,4]

Ara-C is used primarily in combination with doxorubicin (Adriamycin) or daunomycin for remission induction in acute myeloblastic leukemia.[5] It is also employed in combination therapy for histiocytic lymphoma and as secondary therapy for childhood acute lymphocytic leukemia,[7] but has little activity in solid tumors. The reasons for this limited spectrum of activity relate to the unique tumor cell metabolism of this agent and its restricted activity against rapidly dividing cells.

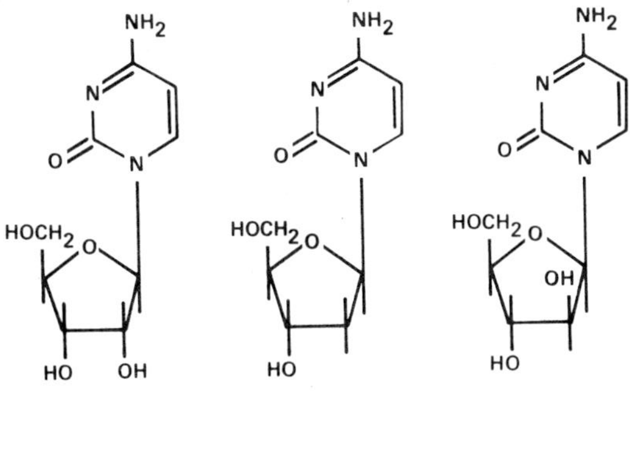

Figure 18–1. Structure of cytidine, deoxycytidine, and the analogue, cytosine arabinoside.

MECHANISM OF ACTION

In human cells, ara-C acts as an analogue of the physiologic nucleoside deoxycytidine and has multiple effects on DNA synthesis (Table 18–1). Ara-C undergoes phosphorylation to form ara-CTP, which competitively inhibits DNA polymerase in opposition to the normal substrate dCTP.[8] This competitive inhibition has been demonstrated with crude DNA polymerase from calf thymus[8] and from human leukemic cells,[9] as well as with enzyme from a variety of murine tumors.[10,11] Ara-CTP and dCTP have relatively equal affinities for DNA polymerase α in the range of 1×10^{-5}M, and the inhibition is reversible in cell-free systems by addition of dCTP, or in intact cells by addition of deoxycytidine, the precursor of dCTP.[12] The DNA polymerase responsible for repair is weakly inhibited by ara-C. The K_i for inhibition of the repair enzyme is 26 μM, as compared with the fivefold greater affinity for the natural substrate dCTP.[13] Thus, repair of single-strand breaks in DNA induced by ultraviolet irradiation is inhibited by the presence of 0.1 mM ara-C only if dCTP pools are depleted by additional pharmacologic manipulation.[14,15] In addition to its effects on eukaryotic DNA polymerases, ara-CTP is an extremely potent inhibitor of viral RNA–directed DNA polymerase (K_i = 0.1 μM).[13]

The effects of ara-C on DNA synthesis are compounded by its incorporation into DNA, the degree of which correlates closely with cytotoxicity to L1210 cells in culture.[16] A

TABLE 18–1. Mechanisms of Cytosine Arabinoside Cytotoxicity

Effects on DNA Synthesis
1. Inhibition of *de novo* synthesis (DNA polymerase α)
2. Inhibition of DNA repair (DNA polymerase β)
3. Incorporation into DNA
   a. Reiteration of DNA sequence
   b. Failure to ligate small pieces of nascent DNA
   c. Termination of chain elongation

Other Actions
1. Inhibition of ribonucleotide reductase
2. Inhibition of glycolipid and glycoprotein synthesis

linear relationship exists between pmoles of ara-C incorporated and the log of cell survival for a wide range of drug concentrations and durations of exposure. In addition, a given level of ara-C incorporation can be achieved by various combinations of concentrations (C) and times (T) of exposure that yield a specific C × T product. Thus, drug toxicity is a direct function of incorporation into DNA, and the latter varies directly with the C × T product. These experiments support the hypothesis that ara-C incorporation into DNA is a prerequisite for drug action and is responsible for cytotoxicity.

The reasons for cell death following drug incorporation into DNA are unclear. DNA containing ara-C is susceptible to degradation under alkaline conditions normally nondestructive to the nucleic acids.[16] Other explanations have been offered for the lethality of ara-C incorporation. In several experimental systems, ara-C incorporation blocks initiation and elongation of the growing DNA strand.[17] In cell-free systems for studying DNA synthesis, ara-C incorporation leads to premature termination of DNA chains[18] through incorporation into DNA in terminal positions. However, analysis of DNA from whole cells has not disclosed the presence of ara-C in terminal position;[19] thus, chain termination does not appear to explain ara-C cytotoxicity in intact cells. In intact cell systems, ara-C causes accumulation of small pieces of DNA, suggesting either defective ligation or incomplete synthesis of the DNA fragments; these fragments (also called Okazaki pieces) are rapidly joined to form complete strands when ara-C is removed from the medium,[20] a further indication that ara-C incorporation does not cause irreversible termination of DNA synthesis.

Ara-C also causes an unusual reiteration of DNA segments.[21] Human lymphocytes exposed to ara-C in culture synthesize small reduplicated segments of DNA, resulting in multiple copies of limited portions of DNA. These reduplicated segments increase the possibility of recombination and cross-over, and may explain the gaps and breaks observed in karyotype preparations following ara-C treatment. These findings may also have bearing on the process of gene reduplication induced by other antimetabolites such as methotrexate and other pyrimidine antagonists (see Chapters 8 and 10).

In summary, although ara-C has multiple effects on DNA synthesis, it is unclear which of these actions is responsible for its cytotoxicity.

Other biochemical actions of ara-C have been described and include inhibition of ribonucleotide reductase, incorporation into RNA,[12] and interference with the synthesis of membrane glycolipids and glycoproteins.[22] Very little drug is incorporated into RNA in comparison with that incorporated into DNA.[16] The drug also induces terminal differentiation of erythroleukemia cells in culture.[23] These actions are of unproved significance in the antitumor action of ara-C[24] and are probably less important than incorporation into DNA.

CELLULAR PHARMACOLOGY AND METABOLISM

Ara-C penetrates cells by a carrier-mediated process that is shared by deoxycytidine.[25] The characteristics of this process have been difficult to define since it occurs with extreme rapidity, and equilibrium between the cytoplasm and extracellular fluid occurs within 90 seconds at 37°C. Because the transported drug quickly undergoes phosphorylation in the cells, and thus is effectively removed from the equilibrium, one must separate unchanged intracellular drug from metabolites in studying the transport process. Preliminary estimates of the affinity of the transport carrier, based on studies in cells lacking deoxycytidine kinase, indicate an affinity of about 0.4 mM, but this result may have been influenced by deamination of ara-C and efflux of the product ara-U. Indeed, if one extrapolates from studies of the transport of another pyrimidine nucleoside, 5-fluorodeoxyuridine,[26] a higher affinity and more rapid achievement

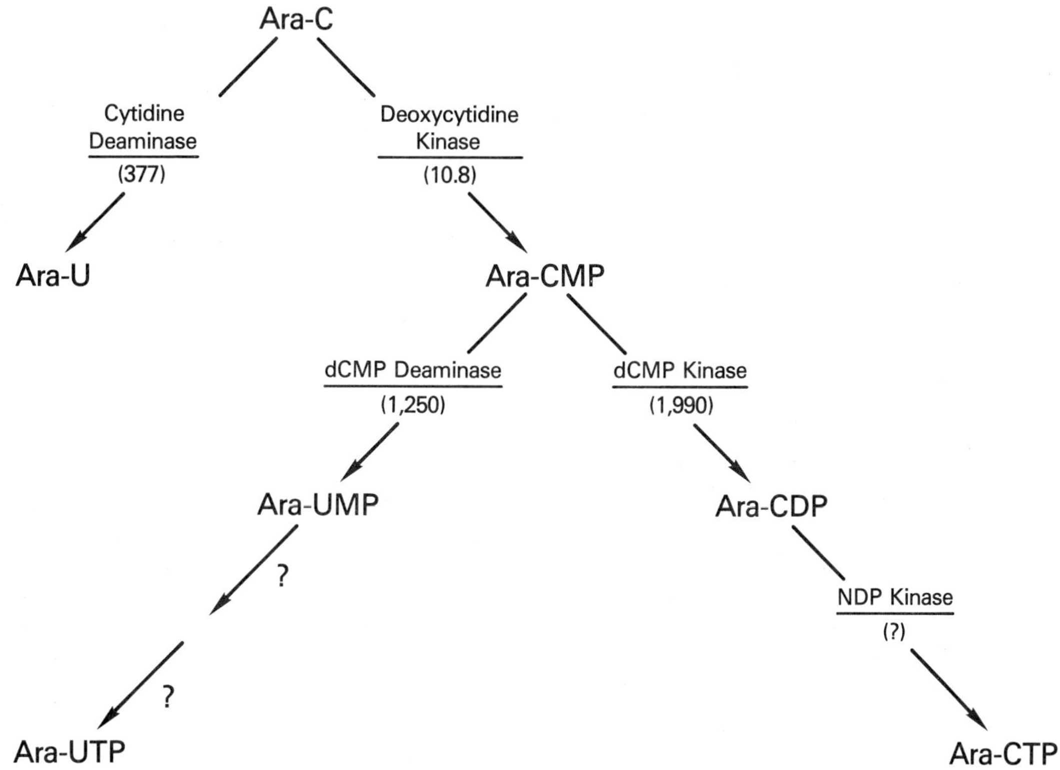

Figure 18–2. Sequential biochemical reactions that lead to activation (ara-CTP formation) or degradation of cytosine arabinoside (ara-C). Enzyme activities, expressed in *n* moles per hour per mg protein, are given in parentheses for each enzyme as found in human AML cells. NDP kinase: nucleoside diphosphate kinase.

of equilibrium may be expected. Although the process of ara-C transport is incompletely understood, there is no evidence to suggest that transport plays a limiting role in the action of this agent, either in sensitive or in resistant cells.

As shown in Figure 18–2, ara-C must be converted to its active form, ara-CTP, through the sequential action of three enzymes: (1) deoxycytidine (CdR) kinase, (2) deoxycytidylate (dCMP) kinase, and (3) nucleoside diphosphate (NDP) kinase. Ara-C is subject to degradation by cytidine deaminase, forming the inactive product ara-U; ara-CMP is likewise degraded by a second enzyme, dCMP deaminase, to the inactive ara-UMP. Each of these enzymes, with the possible exception of NDP kinase, has been examined in detail because of its possible relevance to ara-C resistance.

The first activating enzyme, CdR kinase, is found in lowest concentration (Table 18–2) and is believed to be rate-limiting in the process of ara-CTP formation. The K_m, or affinity constant, for ara-C is 20 μM, as compared with the higher affinity, 7.8 μM, for the physiologic substrate CdR.[27] However, this enzyme is strongly inhibited by dCTP, but weakly inhibited by ara-CTP, thus allowing accumulation of the ara-C nucleotide to higher concentrations. The second activating enzyme, dCMP kinase,[28] is found in several hundredfold higher concentration than CdR kinase. Its affinity for ara-CMP is low ($K_m = 6.8 \times 10^{-4}$M), but greater than the affinity for the competitive physiologic substrate dCMP. Because of its relatively poor affinity for ara-CMP, this enzyme could become rate-limiting at low ara-C concentrations.

The third activating enzyme, the diphosphate kinase, has received less attention than the two preceding enzymes, but appears not to be rate-limiting since the intra-

TABLE 18–2. Kinetic Parameters of ara-C Metabolizing Enzymes

Enzyme	*Substrate*	$K_m(M)$	*Activity in AML Cells (nmoles/hr/mg protein at 37°)*
CdR kinase	ara-C CdR	2.6×10^{-5} 7.8×10^{-6}	15.4 ± 16
dCMP kinase	ara-CMP dCMP	6.8×10^{-4} 1.9×10^{-3}	1990 ± 1500
dCDP kinase	ara-CDP other NDP's	? ?	not known
CR deaminase	ara-C CdR	$8.8 \quad 10^{-5}$ 1.1×10^{-5}	372 ± 614
dCMP deaminase	ara-CMP dCMP	1×10^{-3} 3×10^{-3}	1250 (5 patients)

cellular pool of diphosphate (ara-CDP) is only a fraction of the ara-CTP pool in the few cell lines studied.[29]

Opposing the activation pathway are two deaminases, which are found in high concentration in some tumor cells as well as normal tissues. Cytidine deaminase is widely distributed in mammalian tissues, including intestinal mucosa, liver, and granulocytes.[30-33] It is also found in leukemic myeloblasts in varying concentrations, but usually in excess of the concentration of CdR kinase, the initial activating enzyme.[27, 32] The second degradative enzyme, dCMP deaminase (Fig. 18–2), regulates the flow of nucleotides from the dCMP pool into the dUMP pool, and ultimately to dTMP via thymidylate synthetase.[34] It is strongly activated by intracellular dCTP ($K_m = 0.2\ \mu M$) and strongly inhibited by dTTP in concentrations of 0.2 μM or greater. Ara-CTP weakly activates this enzyme ($K_m = 40\ \mu M$),[35] and thus would not promote degradation of its own precursor nucleotide, ara-CMP. The affinity of dCMP deaminase for ara-CMP is somewhat higher than that of dCMP kinase for the same substrate, but depends greatly on the degree of activation or inhibition by triphosphates. dCMP deaminase concentration in leukemic myeloblasts is slightly less than that of dCMP kinase, about 1250 units per mg protein (see Table 18–2).[36]

The balance between activating and degrading enzymes thus appears to be crucial in determining the quantity of drug converted to the active intermediate, ara-CTP. This balance varies greatly among cell types[27] and within specific disease groups such as acute myeloblastic leukemia. Thus, AML cells in general have higher cytidine deaminase activity and lower deoxycytidine kinase activity than do lymphoblastic leukemia cells. Enzyme activities vary also with cell maturation; deaminase increases dramatically with maturation of granulocyte precursors, while kinase activity decreases correspondingly.[32] Thus, admixture of normal granulocyte precursors with leukemic cells in human bone marrow samples will complicate the interpretation of enzyme measurements unless cells are separated by density centrifugation. In general, cytidine deaminase activity greatly exceeds kinase (the so-called K/D ratio averages 0.03) in human acute myeloblastic leukemia, whereas the enzyme activities are approximately equal in acute lymphoblastic leukemia and Burkitt's lymphoma. Thus, the biochemical setting would appear to favor drug activation by lymphoblastic leukemia cells, if these initial enzymes play a rate-limiting role.

In fact, this may not be the case. Chou et al.[29] found that human acute myeloblastic leukemia cells formed 12.8 ng ara-CTP per 10^6 cells after 45 minutes incubation with 1×10^{-5}M ara-C. Acute lymphoblastic leukemia cells formed less ara-CTP, 6.3 ng per 10^6 cells, and as expected the more mature chronic myelocytic and chronic lymphocytic leukemia cells formed lesser amounts of ara-CTP (4.7 to 5.2 ng per 10^6 cells). From this study, and other evidence to be discussed below, it appears likely that the complex regulation of CdR kinase and dCMP deaminase by dCTP, as well as the activity of enzymes further in the metabolic pathway, plays an important but poorly understood role in drug activation.

In addition to the above metabolic pathways, ara-C is converted intracellularly to ara-CDP choline,[37] an analogue of the physiologic CDP-choline lipid precursor. However, ara-C does not inhibit incorporation of choline into phospholipids of normal or transformed hamster embryo fibroblasts.[38] Ara-CMP does inhibit the transfer of galactose, N-acetylglucosamine, and sialic acid to cell surface glycoproteins. Further, ara-CTP inhibits the synthesis of CMP-acetylneuraminic acid, an essential substrate in sialylation of glycoproteins, although high ara-CTP concentrations (0.1 to 1 mM) are needed to produce this effect.[39] Thus, ara-C treatment could have important effects on membrane structure, antigenicity, and function.

ara-C Resistance

A number of different mechanisms for resistance to ara-C have been identified in experimental tumors and cultured cells. Deletion of the initial activating enzyme, CdR kinase, has been the most frequently reported finding in resistant murine tumor cell lines,[17, 40, 41] but other mechanisms have been identified, such as increased intracellular pools of dCTP[42] and decreased ability to retain intracellular ara-CTP following elimination of extracellular drug.[43] However, increase or decrease in the activity of any one of the several enzymes in the pathway could lead to resistance, and such changes have not been systematically examined in animal systems.

In vitro systems can be used to examine mutational events responsible for ara-C resistance.[44, 45] Chinese hamster fibroblasts exposed to a mutagen (EMS) and to low concentrations of ara-C develop a single-step resistance to the antimetabolite with a frequency of about 1×10^{-5}M. Resistant clones occur in several phenotypes: (1) deficiency in CdR kinase, a change that confers a high level of resistance; and (2) a markedly expanded dCTP pool, presumably due to increased CTP synthetase activity with or without an additional deficiency of dCMP deaminase.[46] These latter cells have a markedly depleted intracellular pool of dUMP and, consequently, dTTP.* Cells with expanded pools of dCTP are quite resistant to high concentrations of thymidine, which is unable to deplete intracellular dCTP pools in these cells.

Studies with *human tumors* have confirmed the idea that formation and retention of ara-CTP are determinants of response, but have not identified the responsible biochemical lesion. Rustum and Priesler[47] found a clear relationship between the duration of complete remission in patients with acute myeloblastic leukemia and the ability of the tumor cells to form and retain ara-CTP (Fig. 18–3). In earlier work, Chou et al. observed greater ara-CTP formation *in vitro* by leukemic cells from patients achieving complete remission than in nonresponders.[29] From these studies, however, it is not clear whether formation or retention of ara-CTP is the more important factor.

*These cells should be collaterally sensitive to inhibitors of thymidylate synthesis, such as the fluoropyrimidines and methotrexate, but this possibility has not been investigated.

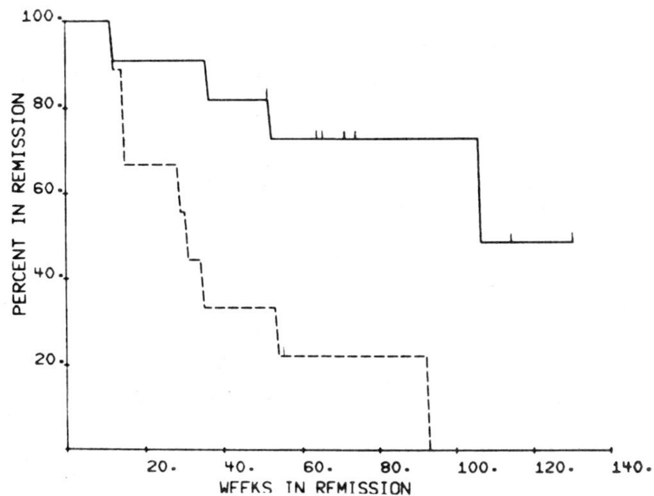

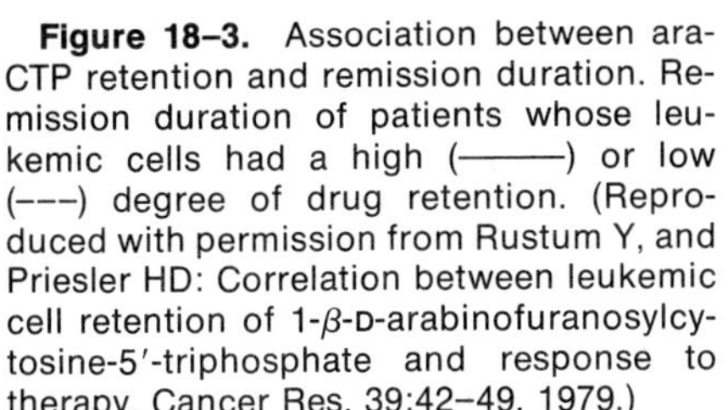
Figure 18–3. Association between ara-CTP retention and remission duration. Remission duration of patients whose leukemic cells had a high (———) or low (---) degree of drug retention. (Reproduced with permission from Rustum Y, and Priesler HD: Correlation between leukemic cell retention of 1-β-D-arabinofuranosylcytosine-5′-triphosphate and response to therapy. Cancer Res. 39:42–49, 1979.)

Specific biochemical lesions responsible for decreased formation or retention of ara-CTP have not been pinpointed in human acute myeloblastic leukemia (AML), the most frequently studied disease. However, it is clear that the concentrations of cytidine deaminase and deoxycytidine kinase in AML cells are extremely variable from one patient to the next (Fig. 18–4).[48-51] One group has reported high cytidine deaminase levels in patients with myeloblastic and lymphoblastic leukemia who were resistant *de novo* or who had become resistant after initial remission induction with ara-C.[48] Subsequent workers have been unable to confirm that deamination correlates with resistance.[49-51] A decrease in CdR kinase activity was reported by Tattersall et al.[49] in patients resistant to ara-C, but Chang and colleagues were unable to correlate activity of this enzyme, or the ratio of kinase to deaminase activities, with either remission induction or the duration of complete remission.[51]

These clinical studies of ara-C resistance are complicated by the fact that ara-C is almost always given in combination with other drugs. Thus, response (remission induction) does not necessarily imply sensitivity to ara-C. A lack of response does imply resistance to each agent in the combination except for the frequent cases in which failure can be attributed to infection or advanced patient age and poor performance status. The duration of complete response may be a more appropriate yardstick of drug sensitivity, as it reflects the fractional cell kill during induction therapy. However, other factors, such as the efficacy of maintenance therapy and the presence of sublines of resistant cells at the time of induction treatment, may well affect the duration of complete response.

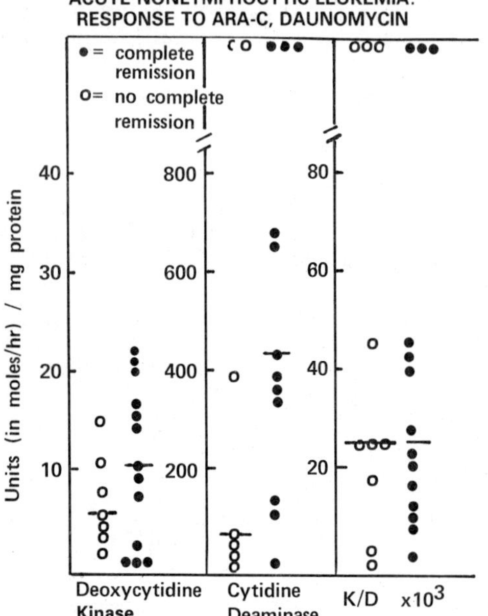

Figure 18–4. Response as a function of deoxycytidine kinase and cytidine deaminase activities, and their ratio, in patients with acute myelogenous leukemia. (Reproduced with permission from Chang P et al.: Prediction of response to cytosine arabinoside and daunorubicin in acute nonlymphocytic leukemia. *In* Mandelli F (ed.): Therapy of Acute Leukemias, Proc. 2nd International Symposium, Rome, 1977. Lombardo Editore, Rome, 1979, pp. 148–156.)

In addition to biochemical factors that determine response, cell kinetic properties have been shown to exert an important effect on the results of treatment. As an inhibitor of DNA synthesis, ara-C has its greatest cytotoxic effects during the S phase of the cell cycle.[52] The cytotoxic action of ara-C is not only cell cycle phase–dependent, but also dependent on the rate of DNA synthesis.[53] That is, cell kill in tissue culture is greatest if cells are exposed during periods of maximal rates of DNA synthesis, as in the recovery period following exposure to a cytotoxic agent. In experimental situations it has been possible to schedule sequential doses of ara-C to coincide with the peak in recovery of DNA synthesis, and thus to improve the therapeutic results.[54]

The cell cycle–specificity of ara-C has been exploited in the experimental treatment of acute myeloid leukemia in the Norway brown rat. This tumor has a high nonproliferative (G_0) fraction of cells (approximately 50 per cent) in its advanced stages two weeks after inoculation of recipient animals, and in this respect resembles human AML. An initial dose of ara-C produces a block in DNA synthesis and a modest kill of the proliferating fraction of cells, followed in 12 to 15 hours by a marked increase in DNA synthetic activity by recruited cells. Retreatment with ara-C at this time produces optimal cell kill and maximal increased survival, as compared with second doses administered either before or after this vulnerable period.[55] Burke and co-workers have exploited kinetic effects that occur at a later time after ara-C treatment. They have found that, following initial cytoreductive chemotherapy, patients with AML develop a circulating humoral factor that stimulates the DNA synthetic rate of leukemic cells.[56] Thus, retreatment eight to ten days after an initial dose of ara-C has yielded a promising improvement in the duration of unmaintained remission in adult leukemic patients in uncontrolled studies.[57] From both experimental and clinical work, it appears likely that optimal treatment with ara-C depends on a precise timing of second doses of chemotherapy to take advantage of recruitment.

In man there is additional evidence that kinetic features of AML, irrespective of the timing of chemotherapy, play a role in determining response. The complete remission rate appears to be higher in patients with tumors that have a high percentage of cells in S phase.[58]

Assay Methods

A variety of assay methods have been used to measure ara-C concentration in plasma, but none have proved entirely satisfactory because of limitations in sensitivity, rapidity, and simplicity. The initial pharmacokinetic studies of this agent employed ^{3}H-ara-C,[59, 60] and the parent drug was separated from its primary metabolite, ara-U, by thin-layer chromatography. However, this method required the use of radioactive drug, and thus was not applicable to general clinical studies. An alternative method employed an ara-C–sensitive strain of *Streptococcus faecalis* and had requisite sensitivity (less than 0.4 μM), but suffered the major disadvantages of a long incubation time, potential interference by other chemotherapeutic agents, and the requirement for maintaining the resistant organism.[61] A second bioassay was developed by van Prooijen et al.,[62] based on the inhibition of DNA synthesis in mouse bone marrow cells by ara-C. Again, this method suffers from lack of specificity, and would be unable to distinguish between ara-C and other antimetabolites used in combination with ara-C.

For routine monitoring, more sensitive, rapid, and specific methods are required. A highly sensitive radioimmunoassay based on antibody raised to ara-C–ovalbumin conjugate has provided the necessary features;[63] it is able to measure concentrations of 4 nM in plasma in a process requiring only three hours. The antibody cross-reacts quantitatively with ara-CMP and ara-CTP, but these products are not found in plasma. There is little reactivity with cytidine.

An equally rapid and specific method utilizes cation-exchange high-pressure liquid chromatography. However, the sensitivity of this method, performed without the benefit of sample clean-up, is only 0.1 μM.[64] An alternative method employing gas chromatography–mass spectroscopy combines the features of high specificity and sensitivity (4 nM), but suffers from the need for derivatization of samples, and thus prolonged performance time.[65]

Because of the presence of cytidine deaminase in plasma, it is necessary to add the deaminase inhibitor tetrahydrouridine to plasma samples immediately after blood samples are obtained.

PHARMACOKINETICS

As a nucleoside, ara-C readily passes into the intracellular compartment and has a volume of distribution that approximates total body water in its initial pharmacokinetic phase.[66, 67] It crosses into the central nervous system less rapidly, reaching 50 per cent of corresponding plasma levels after two hours of continuous intravenous administration.[60] However, ara-C is not deaminated in spinal fluid; therefore, the ratio of ara-C to ara-U lies in favor of the parent drug in the cerebrospinal fluid.

The pharmacokinetics of ara-C are characterized by rapid disappearance[12] from plasma owing to deamination, but marked variability in the clearance rate is seen among individual patients.[60, 62, 65, 67] Peak plasma concentrations of ara-C reach 1×10^{-4}M following intravenous doses of 100 mg and are proportional to dose over the clinical dose range.[60, 66] Thereafter, the plasma concentration declines with a half-life of seven to 20 minutes (Fig. 18–5). A final late phase of drug disappearance has been detected with a terminal half-life of 0.5 to 2.6 hours.[60, 65, 67] Plasma clearance rates vary from approximately 4 to 18 liters per minute. Seventy to 80 per cent of the dose is excreted in 36 hours, primarily in the form of ara-U.[60] Within minutes after injection, ara-U becomes the predominant form of drug found in the plasma, presumably through enzymatic conversion of ara-C to ara-U in liver, plasma, and other sites. The primary half-life of ara-C in plasma appears to be independent

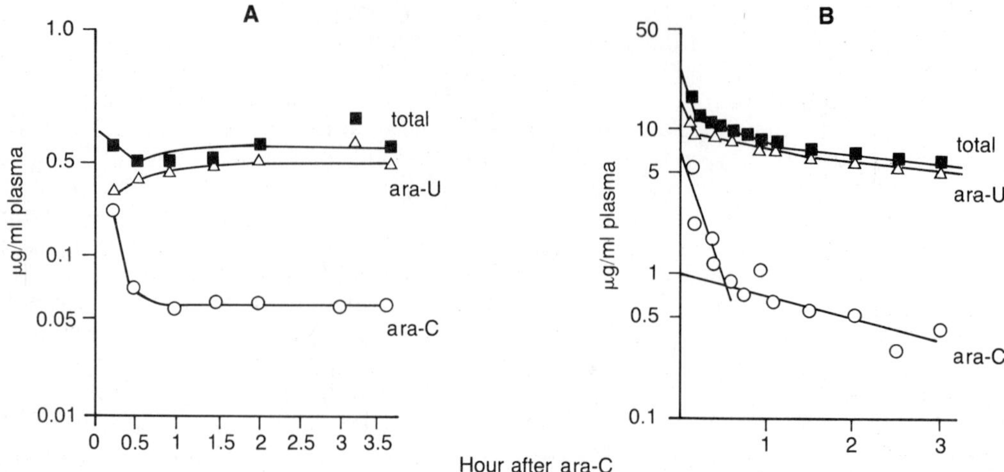

Figure 18–5. Plasma pharmacokinetics of ara-C. *A*, Patient received 30 mg/m² as an intravenous loading dose, and 112 mg/m²/day as a continuous intravenous infusion thereafter. *B*, Patient received a single intravenous bolus of 200 mg/m². Both *A* and *B* demonstrate the rapid conversion of ara-C to ara-U. *B* illustrates the biphasic disappearance curve of ara-C. (Reproduced with permission from Ho DHW, and Frei E III: Clinical pharmacology of 1-β-D-arabinofuranosylcytosine. Clin. Pharmacol. Ther. 12:944–954, 1971.)

of dose over the therapeutic range of 50 to 200 mg per m².[60]

Pharmacokinetic studies have also been performed in patients receiving ara-C by continuous intravenous infusion; an infusion rate of 5 to 10 mg per hour provides plasma levels of about 3×10^{-7}M after four hours,[60, 67] but the steady-state concentration varied over a broad range for a group of 14 patients studied by Harris et al.[65] and could not be predicted on the basis of dose for individual patients. Drug clearance during intravenous infusion was 0.35 to 5.25 liters per minute, or less than 25 per cent of the clearance of bolus doses of ara-C. Because of the slow rate of achieving a steady-state concentration, it is recommended that a loading dose of three times the hourly infusion rate be given prior to infusion.[67]

Owing to the presence of high concentrations of cytidine deaminase in the gastrointestinal mucosa and liver, orally administered ara-C provides proportionately lower plasma levels than does direct intravenous administration. Three- to tenfold higher doses must be given in animals to achieve an equal biologic effect. The oral route, therefore, is not routinely used in man.

Ara-C is effective when administered intrathecally for treatment of metastatic neoplasms. Direct administration of ara-C (50 mg/m²) yields peak levels of 1 mM, which decline slowly with a half-life of approximately two hours.[60] Concentrations presumed to be cytotoxic (0.1 μg/ml or 0.4 μM) on the basis of tissue culture experiments are maintained in the cerebrospinal fluid for 24 hours, following a 50 mg per m² intrathecal injection. Although ara-C is not rapidly deaminated in the spinal fluid, its disappearance from this compartment is delayed by concurrent systemic or intrathecal administration of the deaminase inhibitor tetrahydrouridine.

TOXICITY

The primary determinants of ara-C toxicity are drug concentration and duration of exposure. As a cell cycle phase–specific drug, the duration of cell exposure to the drug is critical in determining the number of cells exposed during the vulnerable phase of the cell cycle. This point was strikingly revealed in experiments with murine L1210 by Skipper and colleagues, who demonstrated the curative potential of schedules employing small doses of drug administered every eight hours and repeated every fourth day, in contrast to lesser therapeutic effects of larger daily doses of drug.[68] In man, bolus doses of ara-C as large as 4.2 gm per m² are well tolerated owing to the rapid inactivation of the parent compound and the brief period of exposure, whereas constant infusion of drug for 48 hours utilizing total doses of 1 gm per m² produces severe myelosuppression.[69]

In the treatment of acute myeloblastic leukemia, schedules that employ either continuous intravenous administration for five days or bolus doses every eight hours for 15 doses yield therapeutic results superior to those achieved with five daily intravenous injections.[69, 70] Two clinical studies have demonstrated a correlation between remission induction and the plasma half-life of ara-C,[66, 71, 72] further evidence that concentration and duration of exposure are important in clinical chemotherapy. In the most comprehensive study to date, van Prooijen et al.[72] found that, of a group of 14 patients with acute myeloblastic leukemia, two patients with the briefest ara-C half-life failed to achieve remission and had the least inhibition of DNA synthesis in leukemic bone marrow cells, as compared with the 12 patients with longer half-lives, eight of whom achieved complete remission. The remaining four died during the aplastic phase of treatment. Harris et al., using a more sensitive and specific assay system, were unable to confirm this association between pharmacokinetics and response in a small series of 13 patients.[65]

Myelosuppression and gastrointestinal epithelial injury are the primary toxic side effects of ara-C. With the conventional five- to seven-day courses of treatment, the period of maximal toxicity begins during the first week of treatment and lasts seven to 14 days. The primary target of ara-C is granulopoiesis, although anemia also occurs. There is little acute effect on the lymphocyte count, although a depression of cell-mediated immunity is found in patients receiving ara-C.[73] Megaloblastic changes consistent with suppression of DNA synthesis are observed in both the white and red cell precursors.[74]

Gastrointestinal symptoms including nausea, vomiting, and diarrhea are frequent during the period of drug administration, but subside quickly after treatment. Severe gastrointestinal lesions occur in patients treated with ara-C as part of complex chemotherapy regimens, and the specific contribution of ara-C is difficult to ascertain in these cases. Clinical symptoms of diarrhea, ileus, and abdominal pain may be accompanied by gastrointestinal bleeding, electrolyte abnormalities, and protein-losing enteropathy. Pathologic findings not specific for ara-C toxicity include denudation of the epithelial surface and loss of crypt cell mitotic activity. Oral mucositis also occurs, and may be severe and prolonged in patients receiving more than five days of continuous treatment. Reversible hepatic dysfunction occurs frequently in patients receiving ara-C for induction therapy, but requires cessation of therapy in less than 25 per cent of patients;[75, 76] it is manifested primarily as an increase in hepatic enzymes in the serum, together with mild jaundice, and rapidly reverses with discontinuation of treatment. The contribution of transfusion-related hepatitis to these early reports of treatment-induced hepatitis is unclear.

Ara-C given intrathecally is infrequently associated with seizures occurring within 24 hours of administration.[77] At least some of the children in this study had drug-related fever at the time of the seizure, a factor that may have contributed to the neurologic toxicity. Intrathecal ara-C should be used with caution in patients who have evidence of methotrexate neurotoxicity.

Although ara-C causes chromosomal breaks in cultured cells and in bone marrow of patients receiving therapy,[78] it is not an established carcinogen in man. The drug is teratogenic in animals.[79]

DRUG INTERACTIONS

Synergistic activity between ara-C and a number of other antitumor agents has been described in animal tumor systems; these other agents include alkylating compounds such as cyclophosphamide[80] and BCNU,[81] 6-thiopurines,[82] 3-deazauridine,[83] and various inhibitors of *de novo* pyrimidine synthesis. The basis for synergism with irradiation and alkylating agents is felt to be ara-C inhibition of the repair of DNA strand breaks.[17]

The synergistic interaction of ara-C with 6-thioguanine is not well understood; the latter compound is thought to exert its cytotoxic action through its incorporation into DNA, an action that is inhibited by simultaneous treatment with ara-C. The combination of ara-C and 6-thioguanine given 12 hours apart does lead to augmented 6-thioguanine incorporation into DNA.[84] 6-Mercaptopurine monophosphate, a metabolite of 6-mercaptopurine, increases incorporation of arabinose nucleotides into DNA by inhibiting the repair exonuclease activity inherent in DNA polymerase. It is possible that 6-thioguanine monophosphate aug-

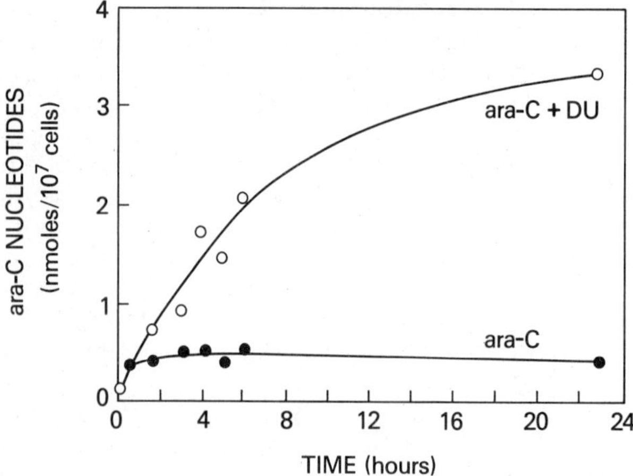

Figure 18–6. Enhanced ara-C nucleotide formation by 6410 cells in the presence of 3-deazauridine. To duplicate cultures of 3.5 × 10^5 cells/ml were added to 3-deazauridine (final concentration 23 μM) or control medium; 50 min later 5 μM ara-C was added, and ara-C nucleotide formation was measured by paper chromatography. (Reproduced with permission from Mills-Yamamoto C, Lauzon GJ, and Paterson ARP: Toxicity of combinations of arabinosyl cytosine and 3-deazauridine toward neoplastic cells in culture. Biochem. Pharmacol. 27:181–186, 1978.)

ments ara-C incorporation in a similar manner.[85] The combination, given simultaneously in man, has improved the complete remission rate in acute myeloblastic leukemia to 50 per cent or greater, as compared with the less favorable results achieved by either drug alone.

A striking enhancement of ara-C conversion to its active product, ara-CTP, has been observed in selected cell lines in the presence of 3-deazauridine[83] (Fig. 18–6). This enhancement of ara-CTP formation is associated with synergistic killing of the human myeloblastic cell line RPMI 1640 in tissue culture. However, a number of other human acute leukemia cell samples do not show enhancement of ara-CTP formation.[86] In addition, a striking increase in ara-C toxicity to bone marrow and gastrointestinal epithelium was noted when this agent was given in combination with 3-deazauridine.[87] The basis for ara-C interaction with 3-deazauridine is not known, but could occur on several levels. 3-Deazauridine is known to inhibit CTP synthetase[88] (Fig. 18–7), and therefore decreases the concentration of dCTP, the natural substrate with which ara-CTP competes. Second, 3-deazauridine, by lowering dCTP concentrations, would tend to decrease the feedback inhibition of dCTP on deoxycytidine kinase, and thus would augment ara-C phosphorylation. Finally, 3-deazauridine is a moderately strong inhibitor of cytidine deaminase ($K_i = 1 \times 10^{-5}$M), and thus would retard the inactivation of ara-C in both normal and malignant tissues that contain this enzyme.[89] An alteration in ara-C pharmacokinetics might be anticipated in patients treated with this combination.

Tetrahydrouridine, a potent inhibitor of

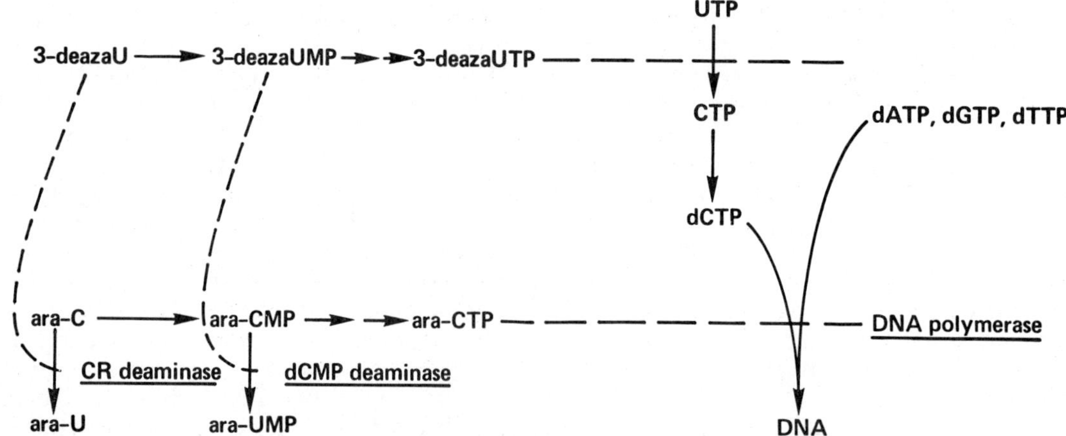

Figure 18–7. Sites of possible interaction of 3-deazauridine and ara-C. Key enzymes inhibited by 3-deazauridine or ara-C nucleotides are indicated by dashed lines.

cytidine deaminase ($K_i = 3 \times 10^{-8}$M),[90] also enhances ara-CTP formation in AML cells *in vitro*,[29, 91] but not in chronic lymphocytic leukemia cells, which lack the deaminase.[91] Tetrahydrouridine enhances the growth-inhibitory effects of sublethal concentrations of ara-C in experiments with the sarcoma 180 cell line, which contains high amounts of cytidine deaminase.[92] Initial clinical evaluation of the combination indicates that tetrahydrouridine in intravenous doses of 50 mg per m^2 markedly prolongs the plasma half-life of ara-C from approximately 10 to 120 minutes, and causes a corresponding enhancement of toxicity to bone marrow.[93, 94] In combination with tetrahydrouridine, the tolerable dosage of ara-C is reduced 30-fold to 0.1 mg per kg per day for five days. It is unclear whether the combination will have greater therapeutic effects, and an improved therapeutic ratio, as compared with ara-C alone.

The combination of ara-C and thymidine has a strong rational basis and is supported by experimental evidence. Thymidine (TdR) is converted to thymidine triphosphate (TTP), and the latter, in concentrations above 0.1 mM, inhibits tumor growth by blocking the reduction of CDP to dCDP, thus depleting the intracellular pool of dCTP. A decrease in dCTP should have at least two beneficial effects on ara-C activity. CdR kinase, the enzyme that converts ara-C to ara-CMP (Fig. 18–2), is inhibited by dCTP; a decrease in dCTP pools should thus increase ara-C nucleotide formation. Second, since ara-CTP and dCTP compete for the same active site on DNA polymerase, a decrease in dCTP pools should lead to greater inhibition of DNA polymerase and to a relative increase in the amount of ara-C incorporated into DNA. These effects of TdR on ara-C metabolism are summarized in Figure 18–8.

Experimental studies have confirmed that these interventions occur in some but not all tumor cell lines. Harris et al.[42] found a strong correlation between dCTP pool size and sensitivity to ara-C in a series of 13 murine tumor cell lines (Fig. 18–9). TdR reduced the dCTP pool and increased sensitivity to ara-C in four lymphoma and plasma cell lines, but not in two myeloid cell lines in culture. The TdR-insensitive lines contained high concentrations of the enzyme TdR phosphorylase, which degrades thymidine. In additional studies, TdR pretreatment led to decreased dCTP pools and increased ara-CTP formation in the L1210 lymphoma and in the Novikoff hepatoma lines; these perturbations resulted in increased incorporation of ara-C into DNA[25] and increased cell kill.[94] The combination of ara-C and TdR has received only limited testing in intact animals. In rats bearing a carcinogen-induced colon carcinoma, pretreatment with TdR (7 gm/kg/day for 24 hours, followed by combined TdR and ara-C) resulted in greatly augmented ara-C toxicity (necessitating a 35-fold reduction in ara-C dosage), but no improvement in therapeutic result.[95] The combination of ara-C and TdR is now entering clinical trial. It should be remembered that tumor cells may develop resistance to both agents by a single-step mutation related

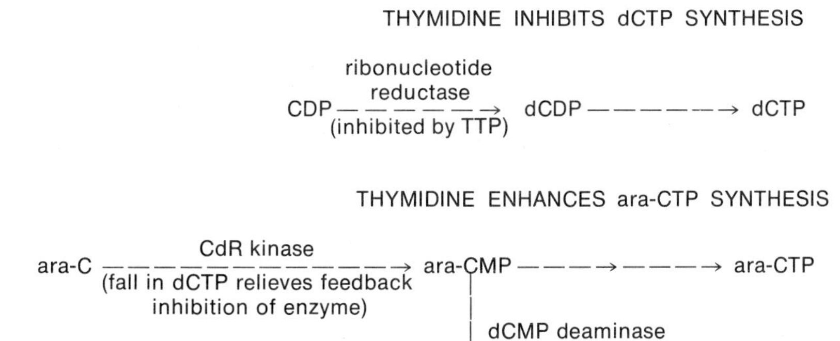

Figure 18–8. Thymidine (TdR) effect on formation of dCTP and ara-CTP. Inhibition of ribonucleotide reductase by TTP and release of inhibition of CdR kinase are indicated.

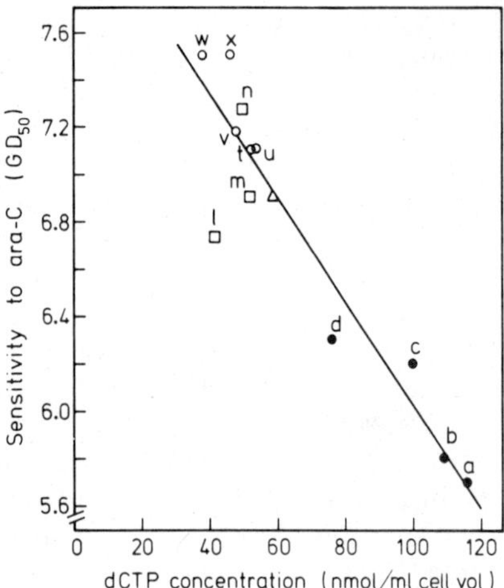

Figure 18–9. Correlation of sensitivity to growth inhibition by ara-C with intracellular dCTP concentration. •, myeloma cell lines: *a,* HPC-108.1; *b,* MPC-11.45.6.2.4; *c,* C1.18; *d,* HPC10. □, myeloid tumor lines: *1,* WEHI-274; *m,* WEHI-265.1; *n,* RAW 8.2. ○, lymphoma cell lines; *t,* WEHI 7.1; *u,* S49.1; *v,* WEHI-112.1.G; *w,* EL-4.1; *x,* ABLS-8.1. △, mastocytoma cell line: P-815 X-2.1. (Reproduced with permission from Harris AW, Reynolds EC, and Finch LR: Effects of thymidine on the sensitivity of cultured mouse tumor cells to 1-β-D-arabinofuranosylcytosine. Cancer Res. 39:538–541, 1979.)

to expansion of the dCTP pool, as a result of either deletion of dCMP deaminase or increased *de novo* synthesis of pyrimidines.[44]

The conversion of ara-C to its active form, ara-CTP, is also augmented by pretreatment with methotrexate, according to studies of the murine lymphoma cell lines L1210 and L5178Y.[96, 97] Simultaneous administration of ara-C and methotrexate is associated with greater retention of ara-CTP in tumor cells and improved therapeutic results, as compared with schedules employing ara-C alone or ara-C and methotrexate separated by 24 hours.[98] The biochemical basis for this interaction is unclear.

NEW CYTIDINE ANALOGUES

The primary objective of analogue development in the general area of cytidine antimetabolites has been to find compounds that preserve the inhibitory activity of ara-C, but which are resistant to deamination. This rationale is primarily based on the assumption that the rapid metabolism of ara-C and its short half-life in plasma not only constitute an inconvenience — requiring continuous infusion of drug rather than intermittent bolus administration — but also may play a role in tumor cell resistance. As reviewed earlier in this chapter, the evidence that nucleoside deamination is responsible for resistance is limited to the study of Steuart and Burke,[48] and has not been confirmed by subsequent work. Nonetheless, a number of deaminase-resistant analogues have been developed, and at least one, cyclocytidine (O^2,2′-cyclocytidine),[100] has undergone limited clinical trial. Representative compounds are listed in Table 18–3. Cyclocytidine proved to have undesirable side effects, including hypotension and parotid pain, and did not have superior activity to ara-C in its initial clinical trials. None of the other compounds is based on a firm biochemical rationale. For example, there is no evidence that membrane transport limits ara-C uptake

TABLE 18–3. Alternative Forms of Cytidine Antimetabolite Chemotherapy

	Rationale	*Effect*	*Ref.*
1. Entrapment of ara-C in liposomes	Prevents deamination; preferential uptake by tumor cells	Acts as depot form of ara-C with slow release	103
2. N^4-acyl ara-C (e.g., N^4-palmitoyl-ara-C)	Resistant to deaminase, highly lipid-soluble	Greater ara-C nucleotide formation *in vitro,* longer $t_{1/2}$	104
3. 2′azido-2′-deoxy-ara-C	Resistant to deaminase	Has antitumor activity	105
4. 5′-(cortisone-21-phosphoryl) ester of ara-C	Resistant to deaminase, combines two active drugs, targets to steroid receptor + cells	Less active than ara-C *in vivo*	106
5. 5′-acyl esters of ara-C (e.g., 5′-palmitate ester)	Lipid-soluble, depot form, resistant to deamination	Prolonged $t_{1/2}$, has antitumor activity, but clinical formulation difficult owing to poor aqueous solubility	107

by tumor cells; thus, the lipid-soluble conjugates, such as ara-CDP–dipalmitoylphosphatidic acid, will likely have no advantage with respect to uptake. It may, however, have novel effects as an analogue of the physiologic lipid conjugate ribo-CDP–L-palmitin, a precursor of membrane lipids.

The unique C nucleoside 5-(β-D-ribofuranosyl) isocytosine, or isocytidine, competes with cytidine for incorporation into RNA and DNA. It is activated by cytidine kinase, but, because of its poor affinity for this enzyme, high doses are required to express antitumor activity.[101] This agent is highly active against some ara-C–resistant tumors, probably on the basis of increased utilization of ribonucleotide pathways for maintaining cellular dCTP pools in these cells. An initial Phase I trial of this agent failed to disclose antitumor activity. The dose-limiting toxicity was hepatic necrosis at doses above 120 mg per m^2 daily for five days.[102]

References

1. Bergmann W, and Feeney R: Contributions to the study of marine products. XXXII. The nucleosides of sponges. J. Org. Chem. 16:981–987, 1951.
2. Walwick ER, Robert WK, and Dekker CA: Cyclisation during the phosphorylation of uridine and cytidine by polyphosphoric acid: a new route to the O²-2′-cyclonucleoside. Proc. Chem. Soc., 84, 1959.
3. Lee WW, Benitez A, Goodman L, et al.: Potential anticancer agents. XL. Synthesis of the beta-anomer of 9-(D-arabinofuranosyl) adenine. J. Am. Chem. Soc. 82:2648–2649, 1960.
4. Cohen SS: The lethality of ara nucleotides. Med. Biol. 54:299–326, 1976.
5. Ellison RR, Holland JF, Weil M, et al.: Arabinosyl cytosine: a useful agent in the treatment of acute leukemia in adults. Blood 32:507–523, 1968.
6. Cadman E, Farber L, Berd D, et al.: Combination therapy for diffuse leukocytic lymphoma that includes antimetabolites. Cancer Treat. Rep. 61:1109–1116, 1977.
7. Bryan JH, Henderson ES, and Leventhal BG: Cytosine arabinoside and 6-thioguanine in refractory acute lymphocytic leukemia. Cancer 33:539–544, 1974.
8. Furth JJ, and Cohen SS: Inhibition of mammalian DNA polymerase by the 5′-triphosphate of 9-β-D-arabinofuranosylcytosine and the 5′-triphosphate of 9-β-D-arabinofuranosyladenine. Cancer Res. 28:2061–2067, 1968.
9. Inagati A, Nakamera T, and Wakinsoka G: Studies on the mechanism of action of 1-beta-D-arabinofuranosylcytosine as an inhibitor of DNA synthesis in human leukemic leukocytes. Cancer Res. 29:2169–2176, 1969.
10. Kimball AP, and Wilson MJ: Inhibition of DNA polymerase by β-D-arabinosylcytosine and reversal of inhibition by deoxycytidine-5′-triphosphate. Proc. Soc. Exp. Biol. 127:429–432, 1968.
11. Graham FL, and Whitmore GF: Studies in mouse L-cells on the incorporation of 1-β-D-arabinofuranosylcytosine into DNA and on inhibition of DNA polymerase by 1-β-D-arabinofuranosylcytosine-5′-triphosphate. Cancer Res. 30:2636–2644, 1970.
12. Chu MY, and Fischer GA: A proposed mechanism of action of 1-β-D-arabinofuranosylcytosine as an inhibitor of the growth of leukemic cells. Biochem. Pharmacol. 11:423–430, 1962.
13. Muller WEG: Rational design of arabinosyl nucleosides as antitumor and antiviral agents. J. Antibiot. (Tokyo) 30 (Suppl.): 104–120, 1977.
14. Hiss EA, and Preston RJ: The effect of cytosine arabinoside on the pregnancy of single strand breaks in DNA of mammalian cells following irradiation or chemical treatment. Biochim. Biophys. Acta 478:1–8, 1978.
15. Dunn WC, and Regan JD: Inhibition of DNA excision repair in human cells by arabinofuranosyl cytosine: effect on normal and xeroderma pigmentosa cells. Mol. Pharmacol. 15:367–374, 1979.
16. Kufe WE, Major PP, Egan EM, et al.: Correlation of cytotoxicity with incorporation of ara-C into DNA. J. Biol. Chem. 255:8997–9000, 1980.
17. Chu MY, and Fischer GA: Comparative studies of leukemic cells sensitive and resistant to cytosine arabinoside. Biochem. Pharmacol. 14:333–341, 1965.
18. Atkinson MR, Deutscher M, Kornberg A, et al.: Enzymatic synthesis of deoxyribonucleic acid. XXXIV. Termination of chain growth by a 2′-3′-dideoxyribonucleotide. Biochemistry 8:4897–4904, 1969.
19. Mantenil S, Kopecka H, Curaux J, et al.: *In vivo* incorporation of cytosine arabinoside into simian virus 40 DNA. J. Mol. Biol. 90:751–756, 1974.
20. Dijkwel PA, and Wanka F: Enhanced release of nascent single strands from DNA synthesized in the presence of arabinosylcytosine. Biochim. Biophys. Acta 520:461–471, 1978.
21. Woodcock DM, Fox RM, and Cooper IA: Evidence for a new mechanism of cytotoxicity of 1-β-D-arabinofuranosylcytosine. Cancer Res. 39:1418–1424, 1979.
22. Hawtrey AO, Scott-Burden T, and Robertson G: Inhibition of glycoprotein and glycolipid synthesis in hamster embryo cells by cytosine arabinoside and hydroxyurea. Nature 252:58–60, 1974.
23. Scher W, and Friend C: Breakage of DNA and alterations in folded genomes by inducers of differentiation in Friend erythroleukemic cells. Cancer Res. 38:841–849, 1978.
24. Moore EC, and Cohen SS: Effects of arabinonucleotides on ribonucleotide reduction by an enzyme system from rat tumor. J. Biol. Chem. 242:2116–2118, 1967.
25. Plagemann PGW, Marz R, and Wolhueter RM: Transport and metabolism of deoxycytidine and 1-β-D-arabinofuranosylcytosine into cultured Novikoff rat hepatoma cells, relationship to phosphorylation, and regulation of triphosphate synthesis. Cancer Res. 38:978–989, 1978.
26. Bowen D, Diasio RB, and Goldman ID: Distinguishing between membrane transport and intracellular metabolism of fluorodeoxyuridine in Ehrlich ascites tumor cells by application of kinetic and high-performance liquid chromatographic techniques. J. Biol. Chem. 254:5333–5339, 1979.
27. Coleman CN, Stoller RG, Drake JC, et al.: Deoxycytidine kinase: properties of the enzyme from human leukemic granulocytes. Blood 46:791–803, 1975.
28. Hande KR, and Chabner BA: Pyrimidine nucleoside monophosphate kinase from human leukemic blast cells. Cancer Res. 38:579–585, 1978.
29. Chou T-C, Arlin Z, Clarkson BD, et al.: Metabolism of 1-β-D-arabinofuranosylcytosine in human leukemic cells. Cancer Res. 37:3561–3570, 1977.
30. Chou T-C, Hutchison DJ, Schmid FA, et al.: Metabolism and selective effects of 1-β-D-arabinofuranosylcytosine in L1210 and host tissues *in vivo*. Cancer Res. 35:225–236, 1975.
31. Camiener GW, and Smith CG: Studies of the enzymatic deamination of cytosine arabinoside. I. Enzyme distribution and species specificity. Biochem. Pharmacol. 14:1405–1416, 1965.
32. Chabner B, Johns D, Coleman C, et al.: Purification and properties of cytidine deaminase from normal and leukemic granulocytes. J. Clin. Invest. 53:922–931, 1974.
33. Stoller RG, Myers CE, and Chabner BA: Analysis of cytidine deaminase and tetrahydrouridine interaction by

use of ligand techniques. Biochem. Pharmacol. 27:53–59, 1978.

34. Jackson RC: The regulation of thymidylate biosynthesis in Novikoff hepatoma cells and the effects of Amethopterin, 5-fluorodeoxyuridine, and 3-deazauridine. J. Biol. Chem. 253:7440–7446, 1978.
35. Ellims P, Kao AH, and Chabner BA: Deoxycytidylate deaminase: purification and kinetic properties of the enzyme isolated from human spleen. J. Biol. Chem. 256:6335–6340, 1981.
36. Stoller RG, Coleman CN, Chang P, et al.: Biochemical pharmacology of cytidine analog metabolism in human leukemic cells. Bibl. Haematol. 43:531–533, 1976.
37. Lauzon GJ, Paran JH, and Paterson ARP: Formation of 1-β-D-arabinofuranosylcytosine diphosphate choline in cultured human leukemic RPMI 6410 cells. Cancer Res. 38:1723–1729, 1978.
38. Hawtrey AO, Scott-Burden T, and Robertson G: Inhibition of glycoprotein and glycolipid synthesis in hamster embryo cells by cytosine arabinoside and hydroxyurea. Nature 252:58–60, 1974.
39. Myers-Robfogel MW, and Spatato AC: 1-β-D-arabinofuranosylcytosine nucleotide inhibition of sialic acid metabolism in WI-38 cells. Cancer Res. 40:1940–1943, 1980.
40. Schrecker AW, and Urshel MJ: Metabolism of 1-β-D-arabinofuranosylcytosine in leukemia L1210: studies with intact cells. Cancer Res. 28:793–810, 1968.
41. Drahovsky D, and Kreis W: Studies on drug resistance. II. Kinase patterns in P815 neoplasms sensitive and resistant to 1-β-D-arabinofuranosylcytosine. Biochem. Pharmacol. 19:940–944, 1970.
42. Harris AW, Reynolds EC, and Finch LR: Effects of thymidine on the sensitivity of cultured mouse tumor cells to 1-β-D-arabinofuranosylcytosine. Cancer Res. 39:538–541, 1979.
43. Rustum YM, and Preisler H: Metabolism and intracellular retention of ^{3}H-arabinosylcytosine as predictors of response of animal tumors. Cancer Res. 38:543–549, 1978.
44. de Saint Vincent BR, Dechamps M, and Buttin G: The modulation of the thymidine triphosphate pool of Chinese hamster cells by dCMP deaminase and UDP reductase. J. Biol. Chem. 255:162–167, 1980.
45. de Saint Vincent BR, and Buttin G: Studies on 1-beta-D-arabinofuranosyl cytosine–resistant mutants of Chinese hamster fibroblasts. III. Joint resistance to arabinofuranosyl cytosine and to excess thymidine — a semidominant manifestation of deoxycytidine triphosphate pool expansion. Somatic Cell Genet. 5:67–82, 1979.
46. de Saint Vincent BR, and Buttin G: Studies on 1-beta-D-arabinofuranosyl cytosine–resistant mutants of Chinese hamster fibroblasts. IV. Altered regulation of CTP synthetase generates arabinosylcytosine and thymidine resistance. Biochim. Biophys. Acta 610:352–359, 1980.
47. Rustum Y, and Priesler HD: Correlation between leukemic cell retention of 1-β-D-arabinofuranosylcytosine-5′-triphosphate and response to therapy. Cancer Res. 39:42–49, 1979.
48. Steuart CD, and Burke PJ: Cytidine deaminase and the development of resistance to arabinosylcytosine. Nature New Biol. 233:109–110, 1971.
49. Tattersall MNH, Ganeshaguru K, and Hoffbrand AV: Mechanisms of resistance of human acute leukaemia cells to cytosine arabinosine. Br. J. Haematol. 27:39–46, 1974.
50. Smyth JF, Robins AB, and Leese CL: The metabolism of cytosine arabinoside as a predictive test for clinical response to the drug in acute myeloid leukaemia. Eur. J. Cancer 12:567–573, 1976.
51. Chang P, Wiernik PH, Reich SD, et al.: Prediction of response to cytosine arabinoside and daunorubicin in acute nonlymphocytic leukemia. *In* Mandelli F (ed.): Therapy of Acute Leukemias, Proc. 2nd International Symposium, Rome, 1977. Lombardo Editore, Rome, 1979, pp. 148–156.
52. Karon M, and Chirakawa S: The locus of action of 1-β-D-arabinofuranosylcytosine in the cell cycle. Cancer Res. 29:687–696, 1970.
53. Shackney SE, Ericson CE, and Lengel CE: Schedule optimization of cytosine arabinoside (CA) and hydroxyurea (HU) and sarcoma 180 *in vitro*. Proc. Am. Assoc. Cancer Res. 19:225, 1978.
54. Young RC, and Schein PS: Enhanced antitumor effect of cytosine arabinoside given in a schedule dictated by kinetic studies *in vivo*. Biochem. Pharmacol. 22:277–280, 1973.
55. Aglietta M, and Colly L: Relevance of recruitment-synchronization in the scheduling of 1-β-D-arabinofuranosylcytosine in a slow-growing acute myeloid leukemia of the rat. Cancer Res. 39:2727–2732, 1979.
56. Karp JE, and Burke PJ: Enhancement of drug cytotoxicity by recruitment of malignant myeloblasts with humoral stimulation. Cancer Res. 36:3600–3603, 1976.
57. Vaughan WP, Kark JE, and Burke PJ: Long chemotherapy-free remission after single cycle timed sequential chemotherapy of acute myelocytic leukemia. Cancer 45:859–865, 1980.
58. Hillen H, Wessels J, and Haanen C: Bone marrow proliferation patterns in acute myeloblastic leukaemia determined by pulse cytophotometry. Lancet 1:609–611, 1975.
59. Creasey WA, Papac RJ, Markiso ME, et al.: Biochemical and pharmacological studies with 1-β-D-arabinofuranosylcytosine in man. Biochem. Pharmacol. 15:1417–1428, 1966.
60. Ho DHW, and Frei E III: Clinical pharmacology of 1 β D arabinofuranosylcytosine. Clin. Pharmacol. Ther. 12:944–954, 1971.
61. Mehta BM, Meyers MB, and Hutchison DJ: Microbiologic assay for cytosine arabinoside (NSC-63878): the use of a mutant of *streptococcus faecium* var. *durans* resistant to methotrexate (NSC-740) and 6-mercaptopurine (NSC-755). Cancer Chemother. Rep. 59:515–522, 1975.
62. van Prooijen HC, Vierwinden G, van Egmond J, et al.: A sensitive bioassay for pharmacokinetic studies of cytosine arabinoside in man. Eur. J. Cancer 12:899–905, 1976.
63. Piall EM, Aherne GW, and Marks VM: A radioimmunoassay for cytosine arabinoside. Br. J. Cancer 40:548–556, 1979.
64. Boutagy J, and Harvey DJ: Determination of cytosine arabinoside in human plasma by gas chromatography with a nitrogen-sensitive detector and by gas chromatography–mass spectrometry. J. Chromatogr. 146:283–296, 1978.
65. Harris AL, Potter C, Bunch C, et al.: Pharmacokinetics of cytosine arabinoside in patients with acute myeloid leukaemia. Br. J. Clin. Pharmacol. 8:219–227, 1979.
66. van Prooijen R, van der Kleijn E, and Haanen C: Pharmacokinetics of cytosine arabinoside in acute leukemia. Clin. Pharmacol. Ther. 21:744–750, 1977.
67. Wau SH, Huffman DH, Azarnoff DL, et al.: Pharmacokinetics of 1-β-D-arabinofuranosylcytosine in humans. Cancer Res. 34:392–397, 1974.
68. Skipper HE, Schabel FM Jr, and Wilcox WS: Experimental evaluation of potential anticancer agents. XXI. Scheduling of arabinosyl cytosine to take advantage of its S-phase specificity against leukemia cells. Cancer Chemother. Rep. 51:125–141, 1967.
69. Frei E III, Bickers JN, Hewlett JS, et al.: Dose schedule and antitumor studies of arabinosyl cytosine (NSC 63878). Cancer Res. 29:1325–1332, 1969.
70. Freireich EJ, Bodey GP, Hart JS, et al.: Current status of therapy for acute leukemia. Recent Results Cancer Res. 36:119–125, 1971.
71. Baguley BC, and Faulkenhaug EM: Plasma half-life of cytosine arabinoside in patients with leukaemia — the effect of uridine. Eur. J. Cancer 11:43–49, 1975.
72. van Prooijen HC: Clinical pharmacology of cytosine arabinoside in acute myeloid leukemia. *In* Pinedo HM (ed.): Clinical Pharmacology of Antineoplastic Drugs. Elsevier/North Holland Biomedical Press, Amsterdam, 1978, pp. 177–191.
73. Mitchell MS, Wade ME, DeConti RC, et al.: Immunosuppressive effects of cytosine arabinoside and methotrexate in man. Ann. Intern. Med. 70:535–547, 1969.

74. Talley RW, and Vaitkevicius VK: Megaloblastosis produced by a cytosine antagonist, 1-β-D-arabinofuranosyl cytosine. Blood 21:352–362, 1963.
75. Slavin RE, Dias MA, and Saral R: Cytosine arabinoside-induced gastrointestinal toxic alterations in sequential chemotherapeutic protocols. Cancer 42:1747–1759, 1978.
76. Goode UB, Leventhal B, and Henderson E: Cytosine arabinoside in acute granulocytic leukemia. Clin. Pharmacol. Ther. 12:599–606, 1971.
77. Eden OB, Goldie W, Wood T, et al.: Seizures following intrathecal cytosine arabinoside in young children with acute lymphoblastic leukemia. Cancer 42:53–58, 1978.
78. Bell WR, Whang JJ, Carbone PP, et al.: Cytogenetic and morphologic abnormalities in human bone marrow cells during cytosine arabinoside therapy. Blood 27:771–781, 1966.
79. Dixon RL, and Adamson RH: Antitumor activity and pharmacologic disposition of cytosine arabinoside (NSC 63878). Cancer Chemother. Rep. 48:11–16, 1965.
80. Schabel FM Jr: *In vivo* leukemic cell kill kinetics and curability in experimental systems. *In* The Proliferation and Spread of Neoplastic Cells. Williams & Wilkins Co., Baltimore, 1968, p. 379.
81. Tyrer DD, Kline I, Vendetti JM, et al.: Separate and sequential chemotherapy of mouse leukemia L1210 with 1-β-D-arabinofuranosylcytosine hydrochloride and 1,3-*bis*-(2-chloroethyl)-1-nitrosourea. Cancer Res. 27:873–879, 1968.
82. Burchenal JH, and Dollinger MR: Cytosine arabinoside in combination with 6-mercaptopurine, methotrexate, or fluorouracil in L1210 mouse leukemia. Cancer Chemother. Rep. 51:435–438, 1967.
83. Mills-Yamamoto C, Lauzon GJ, and Paterson ARP: Toxicity of combinations of arabinosyl cytosine and 3-deazauridine toward neoplastic cells in culture. Biochem. Pharmacol. 27:181–186, 1978.
84. LePage GA, and White SC: Scheduling of arabinosylcytosine (ara-C) and 6-thioguanine (TG). Proc. Am. Assoc. Cancer Res. 13:11, 1972.
85. Lee MYW, Byrnes JJ, Downey KM, et al.: Mechanism of inhibition of deoxyribonucleic acid synthesis by 1-β-D-arabinofuranosyladenosine triphosphate and its potentiation by 6-mercaptopurine ribonucleoside 5′monophosphate. Biochemistry 19:213–219, 1980.
86. Lauzon GJ, Paterson ARP, and Belch AW: Formation of 1-β-D-arabinofuranosylcytosine diphosphate choline in neoplastic and normal cells. Cancer Res. 38:1730–1733, 1978.
87. Paterson ARP, Jakobs ES, Lauzon GJ, et al.: Drug sequence–dependent toxicity and small bowel mucosal injury in mice treated with low doses of 3-deazauridine and 1-beta-D-arabinofuranosylcytosine. Cancer Res. 39:2216–2219, 1979.
88. McPartland RP, Wang MC, Block A, et al.: Cytidine 5′-triphosphate synthetase as a target for inhibition of the antitumor agent 3-deazauridine. Cancer Res. 34:3107–3111, 1974.
89. Drake JC, Hande KR, Fuller RW, and Chabner BA: Cytidine and deoxycytidylate deaminase inhibition by uridine analogs. Biochem. Pharmacol. 29:807–811, 1980.
90. Stoller RG, Myers CE, and Chabner BA: Analysis of cytidine deaminase and tetrahydrouridine interaction by use of ligand techniques. Biochem. Pharmacol. 27:53–59, 1978.
91. Ho DHW, Carter CJ, Brown NS, et al.: Effects of tetrahydrouridine on the uptake and metabolism of 1-β-D-arabinofuranosylcytosine in human normal and leukemic cells. Cancer Res. 40:2441–2446, 1980.
92. Chabner BA, Hande KR, and Drake JC: Ara-C metabolism: implications for drug resistance and drug interactions. Bull. Cancer (Paris) 66:89–92, 1979.
93. Kreis W, Woodcock TM, and Gordon CS: Tetrahydrouridine: physiologic disposition and effect upon deamination of cytosine arabinoside in man. Cancer Treat. Rep. 61:1347–1353, 1977.
94. Wong PP, Currie VE, Mackey RW, et al.: Phase I evaluation of tetrahydrouridine combined with cytosine arabinoside. Cancer Treat. Rep. 63:1245–1249, 1979.
95. Grant S, Lehman C, and Cadman E: Enhancement of 1-β-D-arabinofuranosylcytosine accumulation with L1210 cells and increased cytotoxicity following thymidine exposure. Cancer Res. 40:1525–1531, 1980.
96. Danhauser LL, and Rustum YM: Effect of thymidine on the toxicity, antitumor activity and metabolism of 1-β-D-arabinofuranosylcytosine in rats bearing a chemically induced colon carcinoma. Cancer Res. 40:1274–1280, 1980.
97. Cadman E, and Eiferman F: Mechanism of synergistic cell killing when methotrexate precedes cytosine arabinoside. J. Clin. Invest. 64:788–797, 1979.
98. Hoovis ML, and Chu MY: Enhancement of the antiproliferative action of 1-β-D-arabinofuranosylcytosine by methotrexate in murine leukemic cells (L5178Y). Cancer Res. 33:521–525, 1973.
99. Roberts D, Peck C, Hillard S, et al.: Methotrexate-induced changes in the level of 1-β-D-arabinofuranosylcytosine triphosphate in L1210 cells. Cancer Res. 39:4048–4054, 1979.
100. Ho DHW: Biochemical studies of a new antitumor agent, O^2, 2′-cyclocytidine. Biochem. Pharmacol. 23:1235–1244, 1974.
101. Chow T-C, Burchenal JH, Fox JJ, et al.: Metabolism and effects of 5-(β-D-ribofuranosyl) isocytosine in P815 cells. Cancer Res. 39:721–728, 1979.
102. Woodcock TM, Chou T-C, Tan CTC, et al.: Biochemical, pharmacological, and phase I clinical evaluation of pseudoisocytidine. Cancer Res. 40:4243–4249, 1980.
103. Rustum YM, Dave C, Mayhew E, et al.: Role of liposome type and route of administration in the antitumor activity of liposome-entrapped 1-β-D-arabinofuranosylcytosine against mouse L1210 leukemia. Cancer Res. 39: 1390–1395, 1979.
104. Tsurou T, Iida H, Tsukagoshi S, et al.: Comparison of cytotoxic effect and cellular uptake of 1-beta-D-arabinofuranosylcytosine and its N^4-acyl derivatives using cultured KB cells. Cancer Res. 39:1063–1070, 1979.
105. Bobeck M, Chen Y-C, and Bloch A: Novel arabinofuranosyl derivatives of cytosine resistant to enzymatic deamination and possessing potent antitumor activity. J. Med. Chem. 21:597–598, 1978.
106. Hong CI, Nechaev A, and West CR: Synthesis and antitumor activity of 1-beta-D-arabinofuranosylcytosine conjugates of cortisol and cortisone. Biochem. Biophys. Res. Commun. 88:1223–1229, 1979.
107. Ho DHW, and Neil GL: Pharmacology of 5′ esters of 1-β-D-arabinofuranosylcytosine. Cancer Res. 37:1640–1643, 1977.

19 ANTITUMOR ANTIBIOTICS

Daniel Glaubiger
Avner Ramu

In contrast to the meager results of plant extract screening, similar examination of microbial broths has yielded an impressive variety of clinically important drugs. In other chapters we deal with a number of microbial products, including purine and pyrimidine antimetabolites (cytosine arabinoside, 5-azacytidine, 2′-deoxycoformycin), the anthracyclines, and bleomycin. In this chapter we will consider the remaining fermentation products in common use, three drugs of diverse structure and mechanism of action, each of which plays an important role in cancer treatment. Actinomycin D, mitomycin C, and mithramycin have narrowly defined but significant activity in specific clinical settings. Actinomycin D is one of the most valuable drugs in the treatment of pediatric solid tumors such as Wilms' tumor, Ewing's sarcoma, and others. Mitomycin C is primarily employed in adult gastrointestinal carcinomas. Mithramycin, although it has efficacy against testicular carcinoma, is rarely used for this purpose because of its unusual and potent toxicity for the kidneys and clotting mechanisms; its primary use is for the control of hypercalcemia.

Because of their unique chemical structures, these agents have been the subject of considerable research into their mechanisms of action. Less is known about their pharmacokinetics, transmembrane transport, metabolism, and interaction with other classes of antineoplastic drugs.

ACTINOMYCIN D

Actinomycin D is one of a family of antibiotic substances synthesized by *Streptomyces* species, and initially discovered in 1940.[1] A yellow chromophore purified from the fungal broth, actinomycin D, was introduced as an oncolytic agent in 1954.[2] This drug has significant clinical activity against gestational choriocarcinoma,[3] Wilms' tumor,[4,5] neuroblastoma,[5] rhabdomyosarcoma,[6] and Ewing's sarcoma.[7] Activity has also been noted in Hodgkin's disease and in non-Hodgkin's lymphomas, but actinomycin D is rarely used to treat these diseases, because numerous other, more effective agents are available.

STRUCTURE AND MECHANISM OF ACTION

The structures of the actinomycins have been elucidated by Brockmann and coworkers.[8-10] All the active, naturally occurring compounds are related to actinomycin D (Fig. 19–1) and consist of two symmetric polypeptide chains attached to a central phenoxazone ring. Changes have been found in the peptide chains in naturally occurring actinomycins,[8,11] but not in the phenoxazone ring system. Derivatives with altered substituents on the ring system[8] have been synthesized and some of these may have a different spectrum of antitumor activity from that of the parent compound,[12] but none have completed clinical evaluation at this writing. The ring system itself can be formed by enzymatic condensation[13] of 3-hydroxy-4-methylanthranilic acid with a mixture of *o*-aminophenols, a mechanism that may account for the biosynthesis of the active compound. The naturally occurring actinomycins, which differ in the structures of the peptide side chains, are not synthesized in fixed proportions by *Streptomyces* sp. The

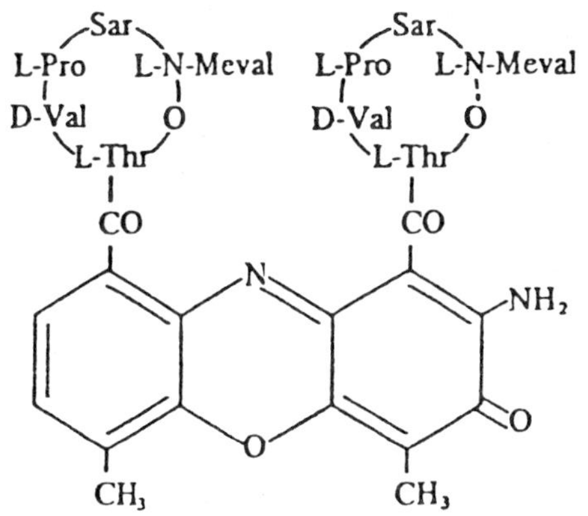

Figure 19–1. Structure of actinomycin-D. Sar = sarcosine; L-N-Meval = methylvaline; L-Thr = L-threonine; D-Val = D-valine; L-Pro = L-proline.

relative amounts of the antibiotic compounds produced depend, at least in part, on the amino acid composition of the medium.[14]

The interaction of actinomycin with DNA is a complex story that provides important insights into the interactions of drug molecules, particularly intercalating compounds, with nucleic acids. The reader is referred to an extensive review of the interaction of intercalating drugs with nucleic acids for a more detailed discussion of this process.[14A] The functional consequences of these interactions in terms of inhibition of RNA and protein synthesis and of cytotoxic effects are not yet completely understood. The fact that actinomycin D interacts with native DNA was established by several investigators who observed inhibition of DNA and RNA syntheses after exposure to actinomycin. Actual binding to DNA was first suspected because of a shift in the actinomycin u.v. spectrum on incubation with DNA. Further, actinomycin co-migrates with DNA in electrophoretic fields after *in vitro* mixing.[15-17] It was later established that actinomycin interacts preferentially with guanine residues.

Spectral studies indicated that (1) actinomycin binds to guanosine; (2) purine nucleosides reverse the biochemical effects of actinomycin (inhibition of DNA synthesis); and (3) actinomycin does not bind to apurinic DNA, or to DNA homologues lacking guanine residues.[18, 19] Subsequently, it became apparent that this preference is relative, and that binding could also occur to polynucleotides composed of other bases, although the binding is less firm.[20] An initial model for the DNA–actinomycin complex was proposed in which the chromophore lies entirely in the minor groove of DNA.[21] This model is in agreement with some of the data obtained subsequently, but another model proposed by Muller and Crothers[22] seems to be more attractive. In this model, the phenoxazone ring lies intercalated between base pairs perpendicular to the long axis of DNA, while the peptide chains lie in the DNA minor groove (Fig. 19–2A and B). The cyclic pentapeptide rings completely prevent rotation of the phenoxazone ring, and form a hydrophobic shield that prevents solvent access to the bonds formed between the ring and DNA. Hydrodynamic measurements made using sonicated, low-molecular-weight DNA are consistent with this model. The intrinsic viscosity of the actinomycin–DNA complex is increased compared with that of DNA alone, and the sedimentation constant is decreased compared with that of DNA alone. Both changes resemble previous results obtained for intercalating dyes, such as acridines.[23]

Further refinement of this intercalating model resulted from structural information obtained by x-ray crystallographic studies of complexes of actinomycin D and deoxyguanosine[24, 25] and the analysis of molecular models of the actinomycin–DNA complex based on the crystallographic data.[26] The tight-binding complex of actinomycin with DNA is formed by interaction of the drug with the sequence dGpdC on one DNA strand and the complementary sequence on the strand. The chromophore intercalates between base pairs (Fig. 19–2), as noted above, but possibly with some tilt relative to the base planes, while the peptide chains lie in the DNA minor groove. There are hydrogen bonds between the 2-amino and N3 ring nitrogens of the guanine residues and the carbonyl and amide groups of the threonine residues. Although this appears to be the structure of the most stable complex, there is kinetic evidence for several classes of binding sites other than this one based on rapid mixing experiments,[22] and actinomycin D may bind to other base sequences on DNA.[20]

An x-ray crystallographic determination of a complex between actinomycin D and the presumed receptor sequence deoxyguanylyl-3′,5′-deoxycytidine (dGpdC) reveals a "pseudo"-intercalated structure[25A] (Fig. 19–3).

Rather than stacking between bases of a single duplex, as would be expected in the intercalation model, the drug was discovered to stack between the dG of one duplex and the dC of an adjacent duplex to form infinite chains. These and other findings[25B] imply that the preferred binding configuration may not be the simple intercalation of a planar ring between adjacent bases.

The functional consequences of actinomycin D binding to DNA, in terms of cellular biochemistry, are the inhibition of RNA and protein synthesis. The predominant effect is the inhibition of DNA-directed RNA synthesis. All classes of nuclear RNA are affected, and the inhibition is such that both DNA and protein synthesis can continue for some time after RNA synthesis ceases,[27] although at diminished rates. RNA is synthesized from DNA templates by a process called "transcription" in which RNA chains are initiated, elongated, and then terminated and released from the template. Antinomycin D appears to affect primarily chain elongation, rather than initiation.[28] Subsequent inhibition of protein synthesis and DNA synthesis is thought to result from inhibition of RNA-dependent steps rather than from a direct drug effect on these processes.[29, 30] This differential sensitivity to actinomycin D exposure, with RNA synthesis being most affected, has been widely used in molecular biology studies to probe the dependence of various cellular functions on RNA synthesis, as well as to measure degradation half-lives and transport properties of various RNA fractions. Studies of the latter type are done by prelabeling RNA with radioactive tracers, then stopping subsequent RNA synthesis by exposing cells to actinomycin D, and following the distribution and transformation of the labeled material.

CELLULAR PHARMACOLOGY

Transport of actinomycin D into cells from the surrounding medium is temperature- but not energy-dependent,[31, 32] and is not affect-

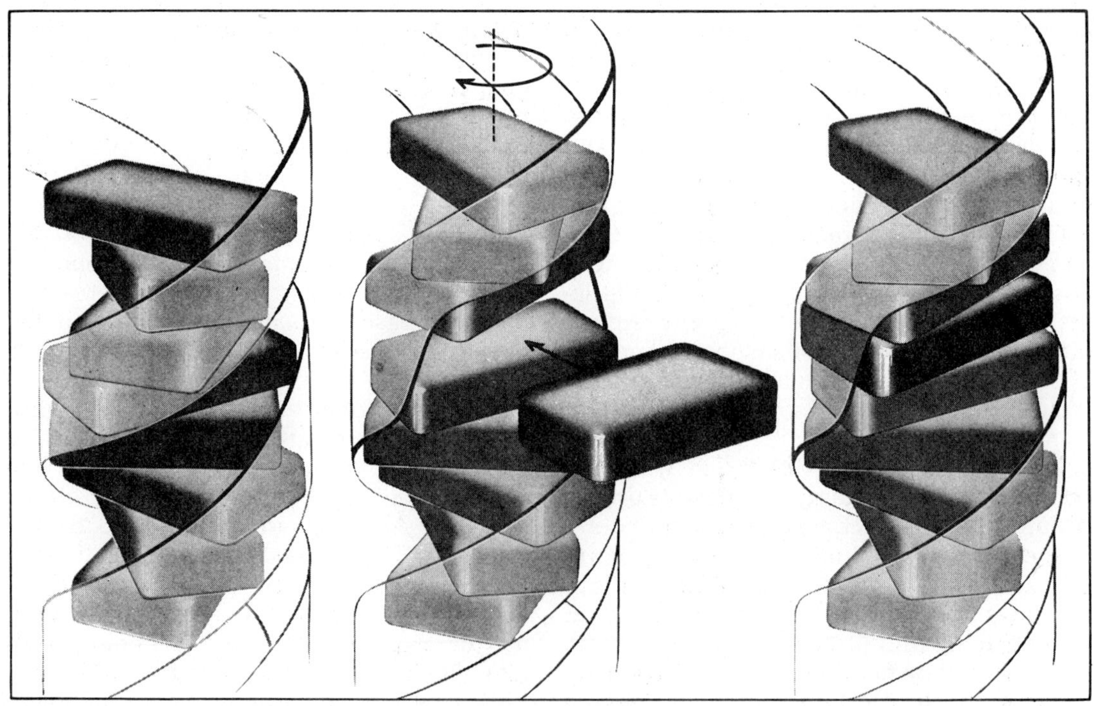

A

Figure 19–2. *A.* Intercalation model of actinomycin D–DNA complex. The phenoxazone ring, which is the chromophore of actinomycin D that gives it the characteristic yellow color, lies intercalated between adjacent base pairs ot DNA. Not shown are the cyclic pentapeptide rings. (Reproduced with permission from Sobell HM: How actinomycin binds to DNA. Sci. Am. 231:86, 1974. Copyright © 1974 by Scientific American, Inc. All rights reserved.)

Illustration continued on opposite page

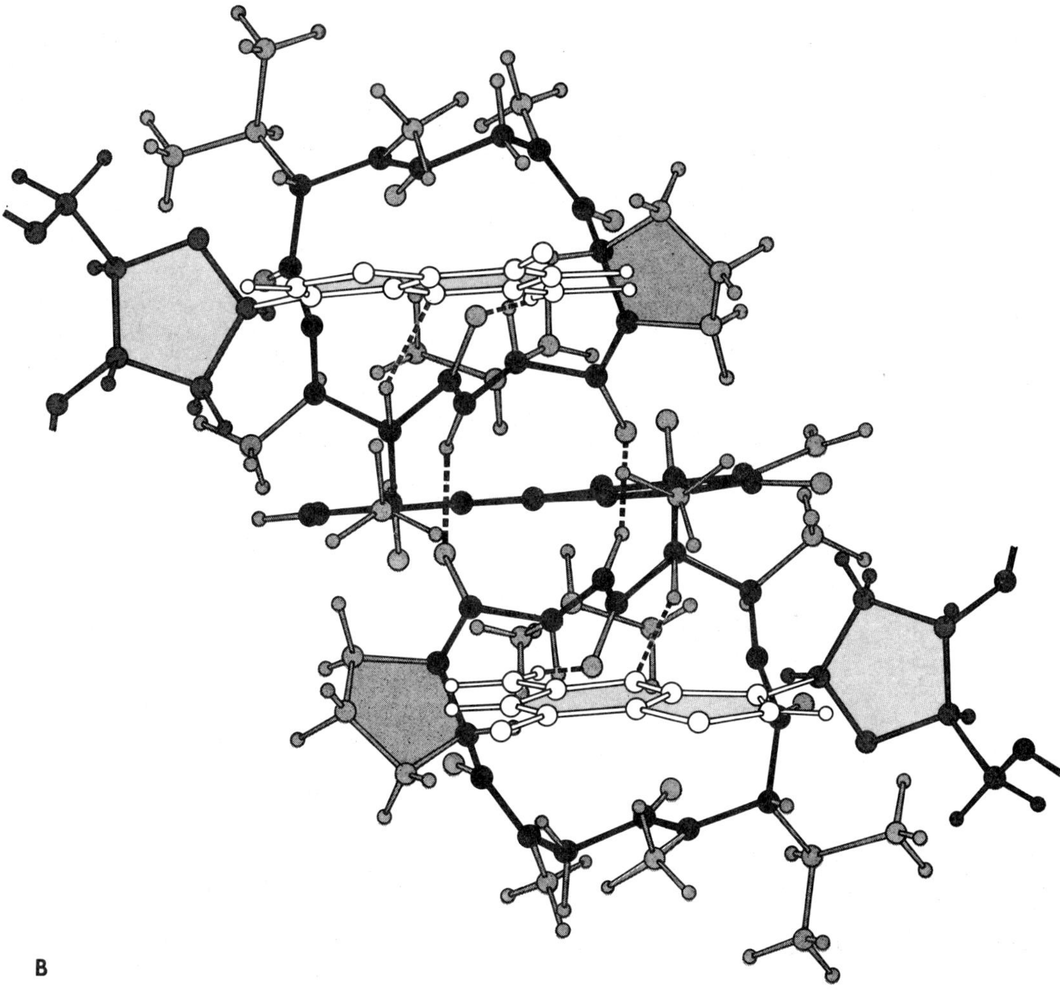

Figure 19–2 *Continued.* *B.* Structure of actinomycin D–deoxyguanosine complex showing the polypeptide chains of actinomycin D (represented by black figures) lying perpendicular to the planar phenoxazone ring. In the proposed complex with DNA the polypeptide chains would lie in the DNA minor groove. (Reproduced with permission from Sobell HM: How actinomycin binds to DNA. Sci. Am. 231:89, 1974. Copyright © 1974 by Scientific American, Inc. All rights reserved.)

ed by metabolic inhibitors.[31] It is thought to be a passive diffusion process, with subsequent binding to several classes (by binding constant) of intracellular sites. The composition and structure of the cell membrane may determine the rate and amount of drug intake. In L5178Y mouse leukemia cells resistant to actinomycin, altered membrane glycoprotein composition is found, compared with the parent line, as well as different membrane-associated enzyme activities.[33] Cells derived from different sources (Chinese hamster, human amnion, human lymphocytes) have different rates of actinomycin uptake.[32] All cell types showed markedly increased uptake when treated with ethanol/acetone (1:1 mixture) to remove the membrane barrier to transport.[32] Drugs that alter the structure of the membrane, such as detergents (e.g., polysorbate 80 [Tween 80][35] or amphotericin B[36]), which tend to make the membrane more permeable, also enhance drug uptake. The implication of data obtained on a variety of mammalian cell lines is that resistance to actinomycin treatment is associated with decreased cell membrane permeability to the drug.[34, 35] Detergents such as polysorbate 80, which increase membrane permeability, can overcome resistance. Nontoxic (by trypan blue exclusion) concentrations of amphotericin B (30 μg/ml) also result in a significantly increased intracellular uptake of actinomycin (five- to sevenfold) and increase cytotoxicity to actinomycin-resistant HeLa cells.[36]

Treatment of an actinomycin-resistant

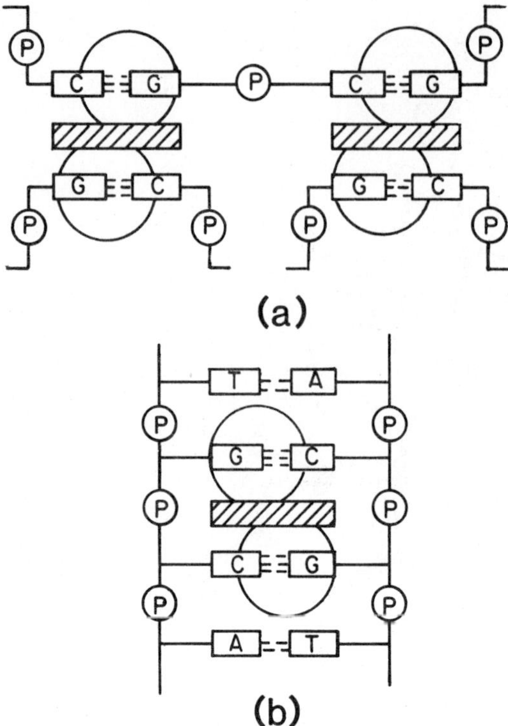

Figure 19–3. Models of actinomycin-D binding to DNA. (*a*), Schematic view of the crystal structure of the 2:1 complex of dGpC-actinomycin D.[25A] In the figure, the phenoxazone rings are striped and the cyclic pentapeptide rings schematically illustrated as circles. G-P-C indicates a dGpC molecule. The Watson Crick base pair hydrogen bonds are shown by dashed lines. This model illustrates a "pseudo"-intercalated structure in which the drug stacks between a base from one strand and a second base from an adjacent strand. (*b*), Schematic view of an intercalated duplex model in which the drug stacks between bases of the same DNA strand. (Figure kindly furnished by Dr. Helen Berman, Institute for Cancer Research, Fox Chase, Philadelphia, Pa.)

subline of Chinese hamster cells with actinomycin contained in unilamellar lipid vesicles, which are themselves nontoxic, also resulted in enhanced incorporation of ^{3}H-actinomycin into the cells and increased cytotoxicity when compared with exposure to free actinomycin at the same concentration.[37] These techniques for increasing transport have not yet been tested clinicallly.

CLINICAL PHARMACOLOGY

Pharmacokinetics of actinomycin D have been studied, both in animals and man, following bolus intravenous administration of ^{3}H-actinomycin D (200 μCi given in 10 to 15 μg/kg in man). Metabolites were isolated and measured using two-dimensional thin-layer chromatography and electrophoresis.[38, 39] The pharmacokinetics of actinomycin D in both animals and man show rapid initial decay of drug concentration in the plasma and a concomitant increase in tissue concentration. The subsequent biologic excretion is slow, with half-disappearance times of 36 hours in man[38] and 47 hours in animals.[40] In three patients with malignant melanoma, 20 per cent of the administered dose was excreted in the urine over the subsequent eight days and 14 per cent in the feces over the same period. Metabolism of the labeled material was minimal; less than 4 per cent of the material in the urine was identified as monolactones.

Based on both animal and human pharmacokinetic data, as well as the schedule-dependency of actinomycin D in tumor-bearing mice,[41] several investigators have suggested that intermittent higher-dose therapy with actinomycin D might be more effective than the usual schedule of 10 to 15 μg/kg/day × 5. A single-dose intermittent schedule of 50 μg/kg every three weeks has been employed at several centers without compromising antitumor activity[42, 44] and without significantly increased toxicity.[43]

TOXICITY

The toxic effects of actinomycin D include nausea, vomiting, diarrhea, and mucosal ulcerations of the oropharynx and gastrointestinal tract. The dose-limiting toxicity is depression of peripheral granulocyte and platelet counts, the nadir occurring eight to 14 days after the drug is given. Alopecia is a common effect and acneiform skin eruptions also can occur particularly at higher dose levels. Actinomycin D is highly toxic to tissues; extravasation may result in necrosis and ulceration of the involved tissue. Actinomycin D acts as a radiation sensitizer when given concomitantly with radiation therapy,[45–47] and may also cause radiation recall phenomena, in which patients experience inflammatory reactions in previously irradiated sites after receiving actinomycin D.[46] The latter effect can be observed up to two years after irradiation. Although there have been attempts to quantitate the radiosensitizing effects of actinomycin D on various tissues,[48] there is at present no satisfactory biochemical explanation of this effect. The clinical consequences of such reactions can be severe, particularly when vital structures such as the lungs are involved. The inflammatory reaction is ameliorated by the administration of systemic steroids, but may be exacerbated when steroids are discontinued.

MITOMYCIN C

Mitomycin C is one of several potent antineoplastic compounds produced by the actinomycete *Streptomyces caespitosus.*[49] Other products of the same microbe, labeled A and B, have both antibiotic and antineoplastic action, but mitomycin C has a broader spectrum of action against animal tumors and has undergone intensive pharmacologic and clinical investigation.[50] Its broad range of activity has been confirmed in man, and encompasses breast,[51] gastrointestinal,[52-53] lung, and head and neck carcinomas;[51] osteogenic sarcoma;[54] and soft tissue sarcomas.[54, 55] This agent has also produced responses in gynecologic malignancies, bladder cancer, and malignant melanoma.[56, 57] Further interest in mitomycin C has been evoked by its synergy with 5-fluorouracil and 6-thioguanine in experimental tumors,[58] leading to its use in combination regimens with 5-fluorouracil against breast cancer[59] and gastrointestinal neoplasms.[60, 61] Despite its broad range of experimental and clinical activity, clinical results with mitomycin C have been disappointing, not only because of its consistently severe bone marrow toxicity, but also because combination therapy regimens, with few exceptions,[61] have produced no improvement over the use of single agents.

STRUCTURE AND MECHANISM OF ACTION

The structure of mitomycin C, shown in Figure 19–4, was first defined by Webb and co-workers.[62, 63] It consists of quinone (A) ring linked to an indole (B) group, and two labile side groups, the first a methoxyformamide side chain and the second an aziridine (C) ring. Mitomycin C has a molecular weight of 334 and is readily soluble in both aqueous and organic solvents. It is formulated for intravenous use in a water solution. A number of derivatives have been synthesized and tested in attempts to enhance antitumor activity and diminish toxicity,[64-66] but the parent compound remains the most potent experimentally and the only drug of this general structure in clinical use.

The mechanism of action of mitomycin C is not defined with certainty, but its cytotoxicity likely results from its activation to a reactive species that alkylates, and possibly crosslinks, DNA.[67] Mitomycin C is not reactive with DNA *in vitro*, but becomes so when mixed with cell lysates, probably through reduction of the quinone ring, as shown in Figure 19–5A. Chemical reducing agents such as sodium borohydride, molecular hydrogen (with a palladium catalyst), and sodium hydrosulfite also activate mitomycin C and promote its alkylation of DNA. As seen in Figure 19–5A, reduction of the quinone ring produces three potential active sites on the molecule, labeled X, Y, and Z. Both the carbamate side chain (Y) and the aziridine C-1 carbon (X) are highly reactive,[68] but opening of the aziridine ring leads to a loss of reactivity of the other two sites and a loss of bifunctional alkylation. The actual site(s) of attachment of mitomycin C to DNA have not been identified.

An alternative mechanism for mitomycin C cytotoxicity has been proposed,[69] based on studies of chemical reduction products of the parent compound[70] (Fig. 19–5B). It is proposed that a free radical semiquinone intermediate may be formed; electron spin resonance studies have confirmed the presence of a free radical form of the drug *in vitro*. Additional evidence for free radical formation has come from the observation that mitomycin C may generate superoxide and hydroxyl radicals in solution.[71] Whether free radical formation occurs spontaneously, or is enzyme-mediated, is still unclear.[72]

The ultimate effects of mitomycin C on DNA are alkylation and single-strand scission. Alkylation takes place preferentially at the O-6 residue of guanine; adducts formed at the N-7 position of guanine are less stable

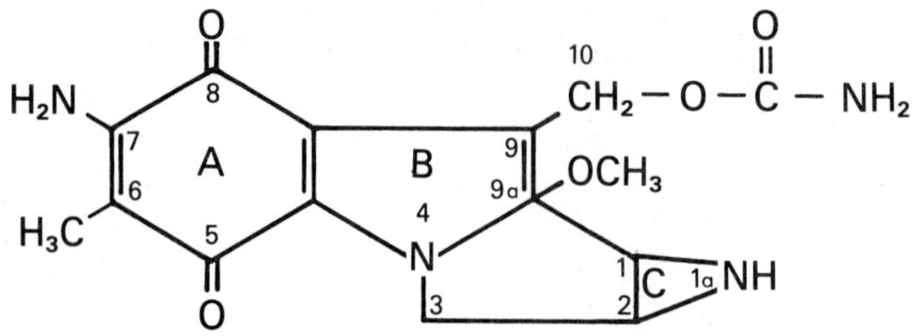

Figure 19–4. Structure of mitomycin C.

thermally. The preference for guanine has been confirmed by studies of alkylation of synthetic polynucleotides and of DNAs of varying base composition.[73]

The induction of single-strand breaks may occur either through the action of free radical intermediates such as superoxide or hydroxyl radicals, which produce breaks in the phosphodiester backbone of DNA, or through attempts to repair alkylated sites on DNA. The induction of breaks by reduced mitomycin C has been studied using closed supercoiled viral (PM2) DNA;[74] binding of a fluorescent compound, ethidium bromide, to DNA increases in the presence of single-strand breaks caused by mitomycin C. Strand breakage induced by reduced mitomycin C can be prevented by free radical scavengers such as mannitol as well as by protective enzymes such as superoxide dismutase or catalase, confirming the importance of the reactive oxygen intermediates.

In summary, mitomycin C is activated *in vivo* by reduction to one of several potentially cytotoxic species that alkylate DNA and cause single-strand breaks. Alkylation occurs predominantly at the O-6 position of guanine, and crosslinkage of DNA may result from the presence of multiple reactive sites on the drug. The relative importance of the three potentially alkylating sites on the drug is unclear, although an intact aziridine ring is required for bifunctional crosslinkage. Single-strand breaks, produced either by attempts to repair alkylation or by free radical intermediates, are also found following mitomycin C treatment of cells.

In addition to its aklylation and scission of DNA, mitomycin C causes an inhibition of DNA synthesis (as measured by ^{3}H-thymidine incorporation into DNA), as well as inhibition of RNA and protein synthesis.[73] The drug produces chromosomal breaks and the appearance of short fragments of DNA.[75,76] Lymphocytes incubated *in vitro* with mitomycin C become unresponsive to immunologic stimuli, and thus can be used in so-called "one-way" mixed lymphocyte cultures[77,78] as the non-effector cell.

CLINICAL PHARMACOLOGY AND PHARMACOKINETICS

Mitomycin C is usually administered by intravenous bolus infusion at doses of 10 to 20 mg per m^2 It is erratically absorbed after oral administration in both animals[79] and man.[80] Intravesicular instillation of mitomycin C in doses of 20 mg has resulted in regression of bladder tumors without significant systemic toxicity. The drug has also been employed intrapleurally and intra-arterially,[81] but its efficacy by these routes is unproved.

Relatively few pharmacokinetic studies have been performed with mitomycin C in animals or in man because of the difficulty in assaying the compound. The assay system most widely used is based on growth inhibition of the bacterium, *Bacillus subtilis*.[82] The method is sensitive to about 0.1 g/ml, but can be increased in sensitivity depending on the bacterial strain used. Its specificity is unproved.

Mitomycin C pharmacokinetics in man are dose-dependent, with prolongation of the plasma disappearance curve at higher doses, possibly owing to saturation of drug metabolism. At conventional doses of mitomycin C, 10 to 20 mg per m^2, the plasma half-lives are two to seven and 30 to 45 minutes.[83] The metabolites of mitomycin C in man have not been identified.

The drug distributes rapidly into the intracellular compartment, and high concentrations are found in muscle, heart, lung, and kidney.[84] Little drug crosses into the central nervous system. Peripheral tissues such as brain, heart, kidney, liver, and spleen are able to inactivate the drug,[82] although the product of this inactivation reaction has not been defined.

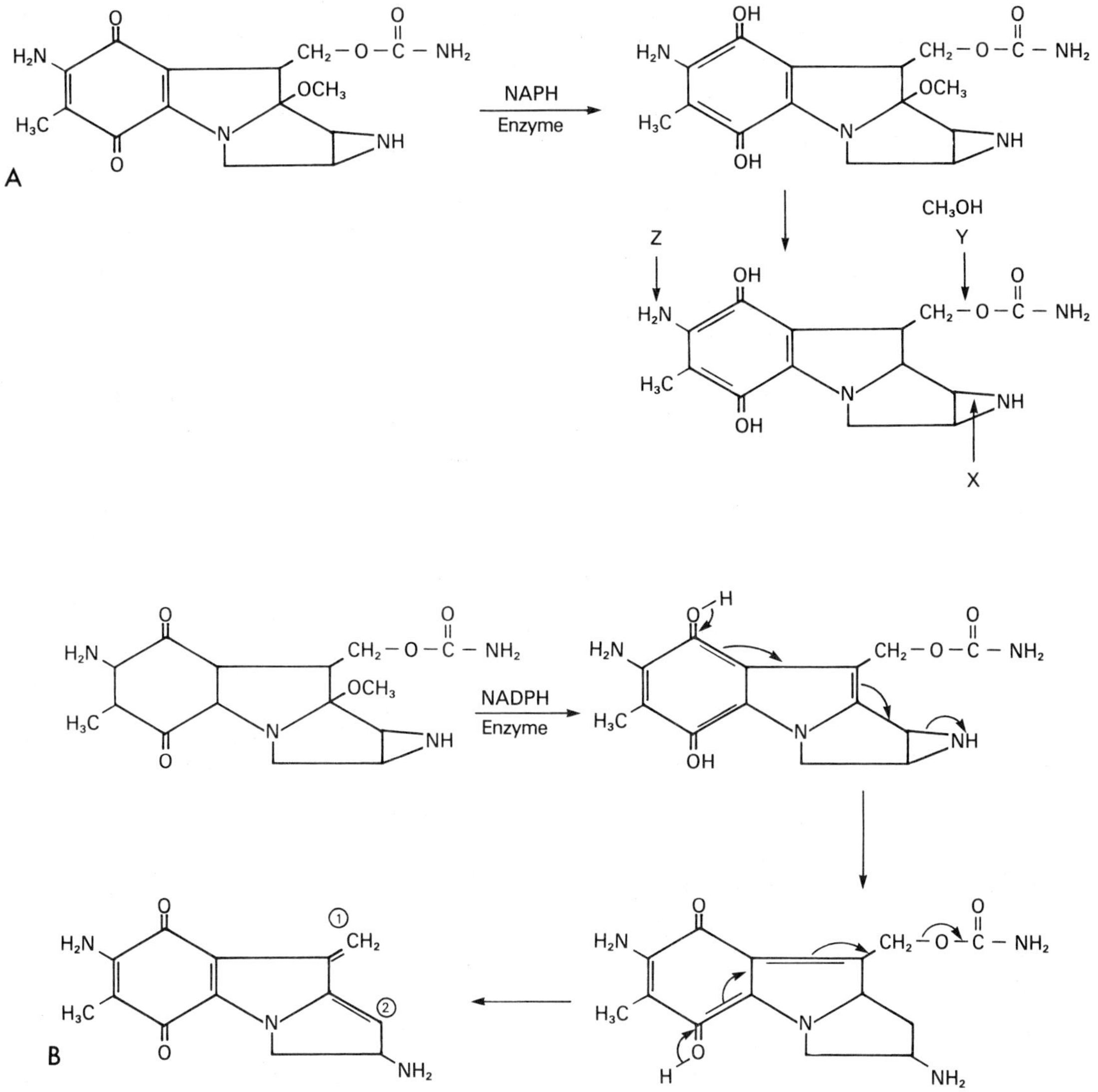

Figure 19–5. *A*, Mechanism of activation of mitomycin C proposed by Iyer and Szybalski.[68] *B*, Mechanism of activation of mitomycin C proposed by Moore.[69] Sites denoted (1) and (2) represent sites of reactivity with DNA.

TOXICITY

The dose-limiting toxicity of mitomycin is delayed myelosuppression. A daily dose of 50 μg per kg per day (15 mg/m^2 for six days) produces thrombocytopenia and leukopenia in most patients, the nadir of these toxicities occurring five to eight weeks after administration.[51] It is unclear whether myelosuppression is cumulative with successive courses of treatment. The drug also causes nausea and vomiting in about 25 per cent of patients, diarrhea in 10 per cent, and, following extravasation at the site of injection, local tissue necrosis and ulceration. Other, less frequent toxicities include fever, alopecia, a maculopapular rash, and stomatitis.

Mitomycin C is suspected of being the cause of renal failure in up to 20 per cent of patients receiving total doses of 100 mg or more. The renal failure appears to be reversible in most cases, although one patient has been reported with chronic renal insufficiency following mitomycin C treatment.[85] Occasional patients may develop diffuse pulmonary infiltrates with underlying pulmonary fibrosis during treatment with as few as two courses of mitomycin.[80, 86] This toxicity is not clearly related to the total dose or duration of treatment. Finally, mitomycin C is believed to increase the incidence of cardiotoxicity in patients receiving this antibiotic in combination with the known cardiotoxin doxorubicin (Adriamycin);[87] this potentiation of doxorubicin cardiac toxicity may be explained by the documented ability of both drugs to cause free radical formation in cells.

MITHRAMYCIN

Mithramycin (NSC-24559), also known as aureolic acid, aurelic acid, Mithracin, and mitramycin, is an antitumor antibiotic substance isolated from a fermentation broth of *Streptomyces plicatus*.[88] Initial clinical trials showed that mithramycin has modest activity against a variety of human tumors, but causes severe hemorrhagic complications when used at optimal antitumor doses.[89] Its clinical antineoplastic use is now limited to secondary treatment of disseminated testicular cancer. The most frequent use of mithramycin is for control of hypercalcemia secondary to malignant disease, as well as in the treatment of Paget's disease of bone.[90-92] There is also a report indicating that mithramycin may be helpful in the control of hypoglycemia associated with malignant insulinoma.[93]

STRUCTURE AND MECHANISM OF ACTION

The structure of mithramycin consists of the aglycone chromomycinone attached to three sugar moieties, olivose, oliose, and mycarose (Fig. 19–6). The drug is a yellow crystalline material with a molecular weight of 1085.2 daltons. It is soluble in short-chain alcohols, acetone, ethyl acetate, and water, but not in diethyl ether or benzene. The drug is relatively more bactericidal to gram-positive than to gram-negative bacteria.[94, 95] The replication of DNA viruses is inhibited by mithramycin; however, replication of RNA viruses is not inhibited.[96] In cell-free systems, mithramycin, like chromomycin A_3, inhibits DNA-directed RNA synthesis.[97]

The antitumor action of mithramycin is thought to result from the binding of this agent to DNA, although the nature of this binding is uncertain. Spectroscopic studies on *in vitro* binding of mithramycin to DNA have shown an alteration in the spectrum of mithramycin only in the presence of divalent cations such as Mg^{++}. The maximal bathychromic shift occurs at equimolar concentrations of drug and divalent cation. No spectral shift is noted in the absence of divalent cations. The spectrum of the drug is likewise unchanged in the presence of RNA, with or without divalent cations being present. The binding of mithramycin to DNA does not appear to alter the sedimentation constant or intrinsic viscosity of the DNA, in contrast to the binding of anthracyclines and acridine dyes.[97] Alterations in sedimentation and viscosity properties of nucleic acids may result from intercalation of drug molecules between adjacent base pairs.[95, 98] Circular dichroism spectra of drug–DNA complexes are not amenable to simple interpretation, but likewise do not appear to indicate intercalation of drug molecules.[99] However, more recent studies show that mithramycin can form a complex with DNA that has some hydrodynamic characteristics of drug intercalation into the DNA structure.[100]

Mithramycin binds preferentially to guanine-cytosine base pairs, and fluorescence enhancement of mithramycin on bind-

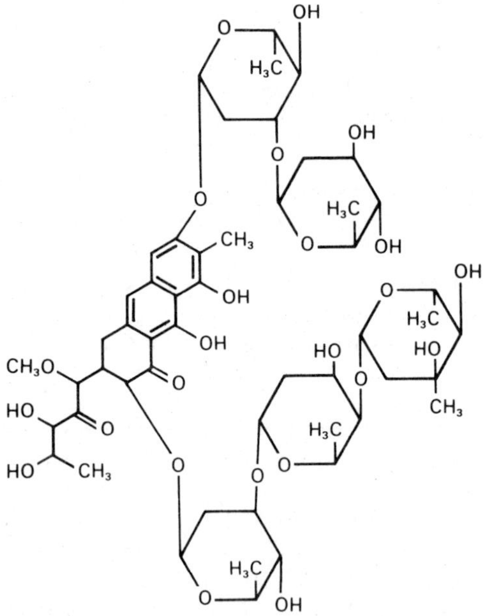

Figure 19–6. Structure of mithramycin.

ing DNA is correlated with increasing guanine-cytosine content in DNA.[101] This finding correlates with the fact that mithramycin inhibits transcription of poly(dG)-poly(dC),[102] but does not affect the transcription of poly[d(A-T)].[97] The fact that mithramycin and actinomycin D compete for binding sites on DNA is also consistent with the preference of mithramycin for guanine binding sites.[103]

In vitro studies on mithramycin, using HeLa cells, have shown decreased growth rates of the cells subsequent to exposure to mithramycin to approximately one half the control value, at mithramycin concentration of 10^{-8}M, and exposure times of 24 hours. When the drug concentration was increased to 5×10^{-8}M, total inhibition of growth was observed. This higher concentration of mithramycin also inhibits incorporation of labeled phosphate into DNA and RNA, to an equal extent.[104] In another cell line, BHK-21, mithramycin incubation for four hours showed relatively more inhibition of RNA synthesis than of DNA or protein synthesis. The preferential inhibition of RNA synthesis became more obvious at higher concentrations of mithramycin.[105] Similar findings have also been noted with the murine ascites tumor line, 6C3HED.[106] Mithramycin causes a significant reduction in the 6C3HED tumor within 24 hours after intraperitoneal treatment with 500 μg/kg (0.2 of LD50). Incorporation of labeled phosphate into tumor cell RNA was inhibited by 60 per cent within three hours of drug administration. No inhibition of labeled phosphate incorporation into DNA of tumor cells was demonstrable at this time point. This inhibitory effect on RNA synthesis lasted less than 24 hours. RNA synthesis in normal cells (liver cells) was inhibited to a comparable degree by mithramycin.[106] Morphologic changes in liver cell nucleoli were also noted, which correlated with the time course of inhibition of RNA synthesis.[107] Similar observations have been made in another murine ascites tumor (Yoshida ascites sarcoma) at similar concentrations of mithramycin. The concentration of mithramycin had to be increased 100-fold to inhibit RNA synthesis in isolated nuclei derived from the same tumor, implying that the binding of the drug to cellular DNA is not the sole mechanism by which transcription and tumor growth are inhibited.[108] At higher concentrations (10^{-4}M), which inhibit DNA synthesis rates by 60 per cent in Morris hepatoma cells, mithramycin also causes extensive single-strand breaks in DNA. Single-strand breaks and inhibition of DNA synthesis also occur in isolated liver nuclei incubated with mithramycin synthesis.[109]

Another effect of mithramycin is the inhibition of adenosine deaminase. Mithramycin appears to be a noncompetitive inhibitor of adenosine deaminase of lymphocytic origin, with a K_i of 6.4×10^{-5}M.[110]

In summary, it is clear that mithramycin binds to DNA and, at appropriate concentrations, can inhibit RNA, DNA, and protein synthesis, with RNA synthesis being most sensitive. It is not clear whether the cytostatic and cytotoxic effects of the drug are related to its binding to DNA and to its inhibition of nucleic acid and DNA synthesis, since these macromolecular effects were demonstrated only at drug concentrations significantly higher than those required to inhibit tumor cell growth.

PHARMACOKINETICS

There is at present no convenient, sensitive assay for mithramycin, and therefore very few studies on pharmacokinetics have been done. The only kinetic study in man was performed in a patient with glioblastoma who was injected with tritium-labeled mithramycin (147 μCi/mg). One mg of drug was given intravenously, and blood, urine, and CSF samples were collected subsequently over 15 hours. Plasma radioactivity declined by a factor of 10 in the first three hours (half-life about one hour) and more slowly over the next 12 hours. Twenty-seven per cent of the total administered radioactivity was excreted in the urine within the first two hours and 15 per cent more over the next 13 hours. The CSF radioactivity was equilibrated with plasma levels after about four hours. Drug concentration in the cystic fluid of the glioblastoma sampled after four hours was equal to that of the CSF. No attempt was made to separate the drug from its metabolites in this study.[111]

Relative tissue distributions in mice have been measured using a microbiologic assay with a sensitivity limit of approximately 10^{-7}M. Inhibitory material concentrated primarily in the kidneys, liver, and lungs.[112] Absorption of drug through the gastrointestinal tract is poor; oral doses 100-fold higher than the intravenous LD50 are not lethal to mice.[113] Nothing is known of the metabolic fate of mithramycin in these animals.[114] The recent development of a GLC–mass spectrometry technique allowing the determination of small quantities of mithramycin and its metabolites may permit better studies of both tissue distribution and kinetics.[115]

Mithramycin is administered in two basic dose regimens. In the first regimen, doses of 25 to 30 μg per kg per day for eight to ten days are given in four- to six-hour infusions in order to minimize nausea and vomiting. The second is an alternate-day administration of 50 μg per kg per day given for three to eight doses per course. Courses are repeated every four weeks for up to six courses. Clinical responses usually occur within two to four weeks after the start of treatment. In the absence of response, treatments are usually stopped after two courses.[116] Although there are no clinical data to suggest increased therapeutic efficacy for either of the two regimens, a comparison of their relative toxicity shows a markedly decreased incidence of severe toxic effects (particularly hemorrhagic diathesis) with the alternate-day schedule.[116]

TOXICITY

Clinical toxicity and side effects of mithramycin have been carefully documented in a report of 1060 patients receiving 1709 treatment courses with mithramycin.[117] The most serious toxic effect recorded is a diffuse hemorrhagic syndrome, which occurs in about 5 per cent of patients treated with mithramycin doses of up to 30 μg per kg per day in courses of less than ten days' duration. The incidence of this syndrome increases to above 10 per cent if higher doses or longer courses are used. Findings associated with this syndrome include thrombocytopenia, swelling of the capillary endothelial cells, and perivascular infiltration with leukocytes.[118] Platelets from patients treated with mithramycin fail to aggregate normally and have reduced ADP content.[119-122] Studies of coagulation factors have indicated reductions in Factors II, V, VII, and X, with prolonged clotting and prothrombin times.[118] Increased fibrinolytic activity has also been reported.[118, 123] The reports delineating the abnormalities of coagulation associated with mithramycin administration were made before the recognition of the syndrome of disseminated intravascular coagulation (DIC). It appears from the observations that the DIC syndrome may be caused by mithramycin in addition to depletion of liver-dependent clotting factors.

Other side effects commonly associated with mithramycin include nausea, vomiting, and anorexia; occasional patients experience diarrhea and stomatitis. Fever occurs in approximately 15 per cent of courses. Dermatologic side effects include skin rash, facial flushing, and (rarely) toxic epidermal necrolysis.[124] Neurologic symptoms such as drowsiness, headache, depression, or weakness are reported by occasional patients. Hepatotoxicity is common with elevated liver enzymes, serum bilirubin, and increased BSP retention.[89, 116, 117] Mithramycin also commonly causes serious renal toxicity with elevated BUN and creatinine levels, proteinuria, hypophosphatemia, hypokalemia, and hypocalcemia.[89] Renal toxicity is not clearly dose-related, but occurs less frequently in patients treated on an alternate-day schedule.[116]

Fatal complications following mithramycin administration have mainly been related to the hemorrhagic syndrome or to renal toxicity. Alternate-day treatment with mithramycin is associated with markedly diminished toxicity.[116]

Mithramycin also has a potent and clinically useful inhibitory effect on bone resorption, and is commonly used to treat hypercalcemia with malignancy.[123] The hypocalcemic effect occurs at doses lower then those required for antitumor activity. A single injection of 10 μg per kg produces a fall in serum Ca^{++} in hypercalcemic (and normocalcemic) patients within 24 hours. The duration of this action is variable, usually lasting several days to one week, and must be supplemented by diuresis and treatment of the underlying malignancy. The mechanism of mithramycin-induced hypocalcemia appears to be inhibition of bone resorption, as documented by *in vitro* studies and by evaluation of bone turnover.[125-128] Mithramycin inhibits resorption of bone caused by a variety of factors, including parathyroid hormone,[128] prostaglandin E_2,[129] or serum factors from patients with multiple myeloma.[129]

References

Actinomycin D

1. Waksman SA, and Woodruff HB: Bacteriostatic and bactericidal substances produced by a soil *Actinomyces*. Proc. Soc. Exp. Biol. Med. 45:609, 1940.
2. Farber S, Tock R, Sears EM, et al.: Advances in chemotherapy of cancer in man. Adv. Cancer Res. 4:1, 1956.
3. Lewis JL: Chemotherapy of gestational choriocarcinoma. Cancer 30:1517, 1972.
4. Farber S: Chemotherapy in the treatment of leukemia with Wilms' tumor. J.A.M.A. 198:826, 1966.
5. Tan, CTC, Dargeon HW, and Burchenal JH: The effect of actinomycin D on cancer in childhood. Pediatrics 24:544, 1959.
6. Pinkel D: Actinomycin D in childhood cancer. A preliminary report. Pediatrics 23:242, 1959.
7. Senyszyn JJ, Johnson RE, and Curran RE: Treatment of metastatic Ewing's sarcoma with actinomycin D (NSC–3053). Cancer Chemother. Rep. 54:103, 1970.
8. Brockmann H: Structural differences of the actinomycins and their derivatives. Ann. N.Y. Acad. Sci. 89:323, 1960.
9. Brockmann H, and Lackner H: Totalsynthese von Actinomycin C[1] (D). Naturwissenschaften 51:384, 1964.
10. Brockmann H, and Lackner H: Totalsynthese von Actinomycin C[2]. Tetrahedron Letters 47:3517, 1964.
11. Katz, E: Biogenesis of actinomycins. Ann. N.Y. Acad. Sci. 89:304, 1960.
12. Sengupta SK, Trites DH, Madhavarao MS, et al.: Actinomycin D oxazinones as improved antitumor agents. J. Med. Chem. 22:797, 1979.
13. Weissbach H, and Katz E: Studies on the biosynthesis of actinomycin: enzymic synthesis of the phenoxazone chromophore. J. Biol. Chem. 236:PC16, 1961.
14. Katz E: Biogenesis of actinomycins. Ann. N.Y. Acad. Sci. 89:304, 1960.

14A. Berman HM, and Young PR: The interaction of intercalating drugs with nucleic acids. Annu. Rev. Biophys. Bioeng. 10:87, 1981.

15. Kersten W, Kersten H, and Rauen HM: Action of nucleic acids on the inhibition of growth by actinomycin of *Neurospora crassa*. Nature 187:60, 1960.
16. Kirk JM: The mode of action of actinomycin D. Biochim. Biophys. Acta 42:167, 1960.
17. Kamawata J, and Imanishi M: Interaction of actinomycin with DNA. Nature 187:1112, 1960.
18. Kersten W: Interaction of actinomycin C with constituents of nucleic acid. Biochim. Biophys. Acta 47:610, 1962.
19. Goldberg IH, Rabinowitz M, and Reich E: Basis of actinomycin action. I. DNA binding and inhibition of RNA-polymerase synthetic reactions by actinomycin. Proc. Natl. Acad. Sci. USA 48:2094, 1962.
20. Wells RD, and Larson JE: Studies on the binding of actinomycin D to DNA and DNA model polymers. J. Mol. Biol. 49:319, 1970.
21. Hamilton LD, Fuller W, and Reich E: X-ray diffraction and molecular model building studies of the interaction of actinomycin with nucleic acids. Nature 198:538, 1963.
22. Muller W, and Crothers D: Studies of the binding of actinomycin and related compounds to DNA. J. Mol. Biol. 35:251, 1968.
23. Lerman LS: Structural considerations in the interaction of DNA and acridines. J. Mol. Biol. 3:18, 1961.
24. Sobell HM, Jam SC, Sakore TD, et al.: Concerning the stereochemistry of actinomycin binding to DNA: an actinomycin-deoxyguanosine crystalline complex. Cold Spring Harbor Symp. Quant. Biol. 36:263, 1971.
25. Sobell HM, Jam SC, Sakore TD, et al.: Stereochemistry of actinomycin D binding to DNA through formation of a crystalline complex. Nature New Biol. 231:200, 1971.

25A. Takusagawa F, Berman H, Neidle S, and Dabrow M: 12th Congress of the IUCR Associated Meeting on Molecular Structure and Biological Activity, Buffalo, N.Y. Aug. 26–28, 1981, p. 55.

25B. Sengupta SK, Anderson JE, and Kogan Y: N^2- and C-7-substituted actinomycin d analogues: synthesis, DNA-binding affinity, and biochemical and biological properties. Structure-activity relationship. J. Med. Chem. 24:9, 1052, 1981.

26. Sobell HM, and Jam SC: Stereochemistry of actinomycin D binding to DNA. II. Detailed molecular model of actinomycin-DNA complex and its implications. J. Mol. Biol. 68:21, 1972.
27. Reich E, Franklin RM, Shatkin AJ, et al.: Action of actinomycin D on animal cells and viruses. Proc. Natl. Acad. Sci. USA 48:1238, 1962.
28. Maitra U, Nakata Y, and Hurwitz J: The role of deoxyribonucleic acid in ribonucleic acid synthesis. XIV. A study of the initiation of ribonucleic acid syntheses. J. Biol. Chem. 242:4908, 1967.
29. Guy AL, and Taylor JH: Actinomycin D inhibits initiation of DNA replication in mammalian cells. Proc. Natl. Acad. Sci. USA 75:6088, 1978.
30. Cooper HL, and Braverman R: The mechanism by which actinomycin D inhibits protein synthesis in animal cells. Nature 269:527, 1977.
31. Bowen, D, and Goldman ID: The relationship among transport, intracellular binding, and inhibition of RNA synthesis by actinomycin D in Ehrlich ascites tumor cells *in vitro*. Cancer Res. 35:3054, 1975.
32. Polet H: Role of the cell membrane in the uptake of ^{3}H-actinomycin D by mammalian cells *in vitro*. J. Pharmacol. Exp. Ther. 192:270, 1975.
33. Kessel D, and Bosmann HB: On the characteristics of actinomycin D resistance in L5178Y cells. Cancer Res. 30:2695, 1970.
34. Bosmann H: Mechanism of cellular drug resistance. Nature 233:566, 1971.
35. Riehm H, and Biedler JL: Potentiation of drug effect by Tween 80 in Chinese hamster cells resistant to actinomycin D and daunomycin. Cancer Res. 32:1195, 1972.
36. Medoff J, Medoff G, Goldstein MN, et al.: Amphotericin B-induced sensitivity to actinomycin D in drug-resistant HeLa cells. Cancer Res. 35:2548, 1976.
37. Papahadjopoulos D, Poste G, Vail WJ, et al.: Use of lipid vesicles as carriers to introduce actinomycin D into resistant tumor cells. Cancer Res. 36:2988, 1976.
38. Tattersall MHN, Sodergren JE, Sengupta SK, et al.: Pharmacokinetics of actinomycin D in patients with malignant melanoma. Clin. Pharmacol. Ther. 17:701, 1975.
39. Perlman D, Mauger AB, and Weissbach H: Microbial transformation of peptide antibiotics. I. Degradation of actinomycins by Actinoplanes species. Antimicrob. Agents Chemother. 6:581, 1966.
40. Galbraith WM, and Mellett LB: Tissue disposition of ^{3}H-actinomycin D (NSC-3053) in the rat, monkey, and dog. Cancer Chemother. Rep. 59:1061, 1975.
41. Galbraith WM, and Mellett LB: Disposition of ^{3}H-actinomycin D in tumor-bearing mice. Cancer Res. 36:1242, 1976.
42. Benjamin RS, Hall, SW, and Burgess MA: A pharmacokinetically based I-II study of single dose actinomycin D (NSC-3053). Cancer Treat. Rep. 60:289, 1976.
43. Blatt J, Trigg, ME, Pizzo PA, et al.: Single dose actinomycin D in childhood solid tumors. Cancer Treat. Rep. 65:145, 1981.
44. Hayes, A.: Personal communication.
45. D'Angio GJ, Farber S, and Maddock CI: Potentiation of x-ray effects by actinomycin D. Radiology 73:175, 1959.
46. D'Angio GJ: Clinical and biologic studies of actinomycin D and roentgen irradiation. Am. J. Roentgenol. 87:106, 1962.
47. Phillips TL, Wharan MD, and Margolis LW: Modification of radiation injury to normal tissues by chemotherapeutic agents. Cancer 35:1678, 1975.
48. Phillips TL, and Fu KK: Quantification of combined radia-

tion therapy and chemotherapy effects on critical normal tissues. Cancer 37:1186, 1976.

Mitomycin C

49. Hata T, Sano Y, Sugawara R, et al.: Mitomycin, a new antibiotic from *Streptomyces*. J. Antibiot. (Tokyo) 9:141, 1956.
50. Sugura K: Studies in a tumor spectrum. VIII: The effect of mitomycin C on the growth of a variety of mouse, rat and hamster tumors. Cancer Res. 19:438, 1959.
51. Moore GE, Bross IDJ, Ausman R, et al.: Effects of mitomycin C (NSC-26980) in 346 patients with advanced cancer. Cancer Chemother. Rep. 52:675, 1968.
52. Woolley PV III, MacDonald JS, and Schein PS: Chemotherapy of colorectal carcinoma. Semin. Oncol. 3:415, 1976.
53. Frank W, and Osterberg AE: Mitomycin C (NSC-26980), an evaluation of the Japanese reports. Cancer Chemother. Rep. 9:114, 1960.
54. Evans AE: Mitomycin C. Cancer Chemother. Rep. 14:1, 1961.
55. Sutow WW, Wilbur JR, Vietti TJ, et al.: Evaluation of dosage schedules of mitomycin C (NSC-26980) in children. Cancer Chemother. Rep. 55:285, 1971.
56. Carter SK: Mitomycin — clinical brochure. Cancer Chemother. Rep. 1:99, 1968.
57. Crooke ST, and Bradner WT: Mitomycin C — a review. Cancer Treat. Rev. 3:121, 1976.
58. Sartorelli AC, and Booth BA: The synergistic antineoplastic activity of combinations of mitomycins with either 6-thioguanine or 5-fluorouracil. Cancer Res. 25:1393, 1965.
59. Godfrey TE: Mitomycin C in breast cancer. *In* Carter SK, and Crooke ST (eds.): Mitomycin C: Current Status and New Developments. Academic Press, New York, 1979, p. 91.
60. Bunn PA, Jr, Nugent JL, Ihde DC, et al.: 5-Fluorouracil, methyl CCNU, Adriamycin, and mitomycin C in the treatment of advanced gastric cancer. Cancer Treat. Rep. 62:1287, 1978.
61. MacDonald JS, Woolley PV III, Smaythe T, et al.: 5-Fluorouracil, Adriamycin, and mitomycin C (FAM): combination chemotherapy in the treatment of advanced gastric cancer. Cancer 44:42, 1979.
62. Webb JS, Cosulich DB, Mowat JH, et al.: The structures of mitomycin A, B and C and porfiromycin. Part I. J. Am. Chem. Soc. 84:3185, 1962.
63. Webb, JS, Cosulich DB, Mowat JH, et al.: The structures of mitomycins A, B and C and porfiromycin. Part II. J. Am. Chem. Soc. 84:3187, 1962.
64. Usubuchi I, Sobajima Y, Hongo T, et al.: Antitumor studies on mitomycin derivatives. I. Effect on Hirosaki ascites sarcoma. Gann 58:307, 1967.
65. Oboshi S, Matsui M, Ishii S, et al.: Antitumor studies on mitomycin derivatives. II. Effect on solid tumor of sarcoma 180. Gann 58:315, 1967.
66. Remers WA, and Schepman CS: Structure activity relationships of the mitomycins and certain synthetic analogs. J. Med. Chem. 17:729, 1974.
67. Iyer VN, and Szybalski W: A molecular mechanism of mitomycin action: linking of complementary DNA strands. Proc. Natl. Acad. Sci., USA 50:355, 1963.
68. Iyer VN, and Szybalski W: Mitomycin and porfiromycin: chemical mechanism of activation and cross-linking of DNA. Science 145:55, 1964.
69. Moore HW: Bioactivation as a model for drug design. Bioreductive alkylation. Science 197:527, 1977.
70. Tomasz M, Mercado CM, Olson J, et al.: The mode of interaction of mitomycin C with deoxyribonucleic acid and other polynucleotides *in vitro*. Biochemistry 13:4878, 1974.
71. Lown JW, Sim SK, and Chen HH: Hydroxyl radical production by free and DNA-bound aminoquinone antibiotics and its role in DNA degradation. Electron spin resonance detection of hydroxyl radicals by spin trapping. Can. J. Biochem. 56:1042, 1978.
72. Bachur NR, Gordon SL, and Gee MV: Anthracycline antibiotic augmentation of microsomal electron transport and free radical formation. Mol. Pharmacol. 13:901, 1977.
73. Lerman MI, and Benyumovich MS: Effect of mitomycin C on protein synthesis in human neoplastic cell lines. Nature 206:1231, 1965.
74. Lown JW, Begleiter A, Johnson D, et al.: Studies related to antitumor antibiotics. Part V. Reactions of mitomycin C with DNA examined by ethidium fluorescence assay. Can. J. Biochem. 54:110, 1976.
75. Makino F, and Okada S: Comparative studies of the effects of carcinogenic and antitumor agents on the DNA replication of cultured mammalian cells. Mutat. Res. 23:387, 1974.
76. Cook PR, and Brazell IA: Detection and repair of single-strand breaks in nuclear DNA. Nature 263:679, 1976.
77. Elves MW: Comparison of mitomycin C and x-rays for the production of one-way stimulation in mixed leucocyte cultures. Nature 223:90, 1969.
78. Etheridge EE, Shons AR, Hohenthanes KL, et al.: Mitomycin C inactivation of leukocytes in the mixed leukocyte culture. Transplantation 15:331, 1973.
79. Bradner WT: Oral activity of mitomycin (NSC-26980) on Walker 256 (intramuscular) tumor. Cancer Chemother. Rep. 52:389, 1968.
80. Martino S, Baker LH, Pollard RJ, et al.: Pulmonary toxicity of mitomycin. *In* Carter SK, and Crooke ST (eds.): Mitomycin C: Current Status and New Developments. Academic Press, New York, 1979, p. 231.
81. Theologides H, and Kennedy BJ: Hepatic arterial infusion for liver metastases from colon cancer. Comparison of mitomycin C (NSC-26980) and 5-fluorouracil (NSC-19893). Cancer Chemother. Rep. 59:401, 1975.
82. Schwartz HS, and Philips FS: Pharmacology of mitomycin C. II. Renal excretion and metabolism by tissue homogenates. J. Pharmacol. Exp. Ther. 133:335, 1961.
83. Reich SD: Clinical pharmacology of mitomycin C. *In* Carter SK, and Crooke ST (eds.): Mitomycin C: Current Status and New Developments. Academic Press, New York, 1979, p. 243.
84. Philips FS, Schwartz HS, and Sternberg SS: Pharmacology of mitomycin C. I. Toxicity and pathologic effects. Cancer Res. 20:1354, 1960.
85. Liu K, Mittelman A, Sproul EE, et al: Renal toxicity in man treated with mitomycin C. Cancer 28:1314, 1971.
86. Arwoll, ES, Kressling PJ, and Patterson JR: Interstitial pneumonia from mitomycin. Ann. Intern. Med. 89:352, 1978.
87. Buzdar, AU, Legha SS, Tashima CK, et al.: Adriamycin and mitomycin C: possible synergistic cardiotoxicity. Cancer Treat. Rep. 62:1005, 1978.

Mithramycin

88. Rao KV, Cullen WP, and Sobin BA: Mithramycin: an antibiotic with antitumor properties. Proc. Am. Assoc. Cancer Res. 3:143, 1960.
89. Slavik M, and Carter SK: Chromomycin A_3, mithramycin, and olivomycin: antitumor antibiotics of related structure. Adv. Pharmacol. Ther. 12:1, 1975.
90. Hadjipavlou AG, Tsoukas GM, Siller TN, et al.: Combination drug therapy in treatment of Paget's disease of bone. J. Bone Joint Surg. 59:1045, 1977.
91. Davies J, Trask C, and Souhami RL: Effect of mithramycin on widespread painful bone metastases in cancer of the breast. Cancer Treat. Rep. 63:1835, 1979.
92. Ryan WG, Schwartz TB, and Fordham EW: Mithramycin and long remission of Paget's disease of bone. Ann. Intern. Med. 92:129, 1980.
93. Kiang DT, Frenning DH, and Bauer GE: Mithramycin for hypoglycemia in malignant insulinoma. N. Engl. J. Med. 299:134, 1978.
94. Kiseleva OA, Volkova NG, Stukacheve EA, et al.: Relationship between the structure and activity of antibiotics of the group of aureolic acid. Formation of complexes with DNA and suppression of RNA synthesis. Mol. Biol. 7:741, 1974.
95. Kersten W, Kersten H, and Szybalski W: Physicochemical properties of complexes between deoxyribonucleic acid

and antibiotics which affect ribonucleic acid synthesis (actinomycin, daunomycin, mithramycin and olivomycin). Biochemistry 5:236, 1966.

96. Smith RD, Henson D, Gehrke J, et al.: Reversible inhibition of DNA virus replication with mithramycin. Proc. Soc. Exp. Biol. Med. 121:209, 1966.

97. Ward DC, Reich E, and Goldberg IH: Base specificity in the interaction of polynucleotides with antibiotic drugs. Science 149:1259, 1965.

98. Waring MJ: Variation of the supercoils in closed circular DNA by binding of antibiotics and drugs: evidence for molecular models involving intercalation. J. Mol. Biol. 54:247, 1970.

99. Dalgleish DG, Fey G, and Kersten W: Circular dichroism studies of complexes of the antibiotics daunomycin, nogalamycin, chromomycin, and mithramycin with DNA. Biopolymers 13:1757, 1974.

100. Dasgupta D, Shashiprabha BK, and Podder SK: Mode of action of antitumor antibiotic. Part II — Evidence for intercalation of mithramycin between DNA bases in the presence of Mg^{2+}. Indian J. Biochem. Biophys. 16:18, 1979.

101. Van De Sande JH, Lin CC, and Jorgenson KF: Reverse binding on chromosomes produced by a guanosine-cytosine specific DNA binding antibiotic: olivomycin. Science 195:400, 1977.

102. Behr W, Honikel K, and Hartmann G: Interaction of the RNA polymerase inhibitor chromomycin with DNA. Eur. J. Biochem. 9:82, 1969.

103. Blau L, and Bittman R: Equilibrium and kinetic measurements of actinomycin binding to deoxyribonucleic acid in the presence of competing drugs. Mol. Pharmacol. 11:716, 1975.

104. Sandberg-Wollheim M, Yarbro JW, and Kennedy BJ: Effect of mithramycin on HeLa cells. Cancer 21:22, 1968.

105. Northrop G, Taylor SG III, and Northrop RL: Biochemical effects of mithramycin on cultured cells. Cancer Res. 29:1916, 1969.

106. Yarbro JW, Kennedy BJ, and Barnum CP: Mithramycin inhibition of ribonucleic acid synthesis. Cancer Res. 26:36, 1966.

107. Kume F, Maruyama S, D'Agostino AN, et al.: Nuclear change produced by mithramycin in rat hepatic cell. Exp. Mol. Pathol. 6:254, 1967.

108. Prasad KS, Nayak R, Sirsi M, et al.: Mechanism of action of antitumor antibiotic mithramycin. Indian J. Cancer 13:371, 1976.

109. Coetzee ML, Sartiano GP, Klein K, et al.: The effect of several antitumor agents on ^{3}H-TTP incorporation in host liver and hepatoma nuclei. Oncology 34:68, 1977.

110. Evans JT, Tritsch GL, and Mittelman A: Mithramycin inhibition of adenosine deaminase activity. Proc. Am. Assoc. Ca. 20:85, 1979.

111. Ransohoff J, Martin BF, Medrek TJ, et al.: Preliminary clinical study of mithramycin (NSC-24559) in primary tumors of the central nervous system. Cancer Chemother. Rep. 49:51, 1965.

112. Woolley C, and Pittillo RF: Microbiological assay and tissue distribution of mithramycin (NSC-24559) in mice. Cancer Chemother. Rep. 58:311, 1974.

113. Morrison RK, Brown DE, and Oleson JJ: A toxicologic study of mithramycin. Toxicol. Appl. Pharmacol. 11:468, 1967.

114. Kennedy BJ, Sandberg-Wollheim M, Loken M, et al.: Studies with tritiated mithramycin in C3H mice. Cancer Res. 27:1534, 1967.

115. Watson E, and Chan KK: GLC-mass spectrometry of several important anti-cancer drugs. I: Petri-methylsilylation and O-methoxime formation. J. Pharm. Sci. 67:1243, 1978.

116. Kennedy BJ: Mithramycin therapy in advanced testicular neoplasms. Cancer 26:755, 1970.

117. Pitts N: *In* Carter SK, and Friedman MA (eds.): Proceedings of the Chemotherapy Conference on Mithramycin: Development and Application. Cancer Therapy Evaluation Branch, National Cancer Institute, Bethesda, MD, 1970, p. 33.

118. Monto RW, Talley RW, Caldwell MJ, et al.: Observations on the mechanism of hemorrhagic toxicity in mithramycin (NSC-24559) therapy. Cancer Res. 29:697, 1969.

119. Ream NW, Perlia CP, Wolter J, et al.: Mithramycin therapy in disseminated germinal testicular cancer. J.A.M.A. 204:96, 1968.

120. Koons CR, Sensenbrenner LL, and Owens AH Jr: Clinical studies of mithramycin in patients with embryonal cancer. Bull. Johns Hopkins Hosp. 118:462, 1966.

121. Ahr DJ, Scialla SJ, and Kimball DB Jr: Acquired platelet dysfunction following mithramycin therapy. Cancer 41:448, 1978.

122. Kubisz P, Klener P, and Cronberg S: Influence of mithramycin on some platelet functions in vitro. Acta Haematol. 63:101, 1980.

123. Brown JH, and Kennedy BJ: Mithramycin in the treatment of disseminated testicular neoplasms. N. Engl. J. Med. 272:111, 1965.

124. Purpora D, Ahern MJ, and Shverman N: Toxic epidermal necrolysis after mithramycin. N. Engl. J. Med. 299:1412, 1978.

125. Kiang DT, Loken MK, and Kennedy BJ: Mechanism of the hypocalcemic effect of mithramycin. J. Clin. Endocrinol. Metab. 48:341, 1979.

126. Kiang DT, and Kennedy BJ: Effect of mithramycin on the bone metabolism. Clin. Res. 19:493, 1971.

127. Cortes EP, Holland JF, Moskowitz R, et al.: Effects of mithramycin on bone resorption *in vitro*. Cancer Res. 32:74, 1972.

128. Minkin C: Inhibition of parathyroid hormone stimulated bone resorption *in vitro* by the antibiotic mithramycin. Calcif. Tiss. Res. 13:249, 1973.

129. Rubenstein M: The use of mithramycin to impair release from bone of ^{45}Ca induced by prostaglandin E_2 and multiple myeloma sera. Proc. Am. Soc. Clin. Oncol. 21: 17, 1980.

20 ANTHRACYCLINES

Charles E. Myers

Doxorubicin (Adriamycin) and daunorubicin (daunomycin), the anthracyclines currently in widespread and routine clinical use, are among the most active anticancer drugs. Doxorubicin is employed in the treatment of such common tumors as small cell carcinoma of the lung and breast cancer, and less common tumors such as soft tissue sarcoma and anaplastic carcinoma of the thyroid. Daunorubicin, on the other hand, is primarily used in the treatment of acute lymphocytic and myelocytic leukemias.

ORIGIN AND STRUCTURE

The anthracyclines are members of a large group of antibiotics, the rhodomycins, that are produced by various *Streptomyces* species.[1] Anthracyclines in general are composed of tetracyclic chromophores, usually red, orange, or yellow in color, linked to a sugar. These antibiotics are classified by the structure of the chromophore or aglycone. Figure 20–1 shows the general structure and major specific aglycone classes. Note that the B ring quinone functionality is a constant feature. In the case of doxorubicin and daunorubicin, the A ring possesses a methoxy group and the B ring hydroquinone functionalities. The sugar most commonly attached to the chromophore is daunosamine (Fig. 20–2); however, other sugars may be involved and can be linked together in carbohydrate chains of up to three sugars in length. Other sugars found include 2-deoxy-L-fucose, L-cinerulose A, L-cinerulose B, D-cinerulose A, L-rhodosamine, L-rhodinose, L-amicetose, and L-aculose.[2] Although the two commonly used anthracyclines, daunorubicin and doxorubicin, belong to the daunomycinone group and possess a single sugar, daunosamine, several anthracyclines of markedly different structure appear to be of some clinical interest. Aclacinomycin A, for example, is composed of the aglycone aklavinone and the sugars L-rhodosamine, 2-deoxy-L-fucose, and L-cinerulose A. Musettamycin is composed of the aglycone pyrromycinone linked to L-rhodosamine and 2-deoxy-L-fucose. Some, such as 7-con-O-methylnogarol, are active as aglycones. The foregoing are but a small sample of the large spectrum of structural variations possible in this drug class; over 500 different anthracyclines have been described or synthesized. The study of the structure-activity relationships and the clinical utility of this large class of drugs is far from complete.

It is important to realize that the anthracyclines are not unique structures with unique chemistry. The tetracyclic chromophore that characterizes this antibiotic class shares many distinguishing features with the hydroxyanthraquinones, a class of compounds ubiquitous in nature. Figure 20–3 illustrates some of these compounds, which include substances such as rhein, alizarin, aloe emodin, and purpurin. These compounds are often intensely colored and are present in large quantities in rhubarb, aloe, and *Cassia* species. Many of the biochemical effects attributed to the anthracyclines are also characteristic of these compounds. Thus, various anthraquinones produce emesis and diarrhea, bind to and cleave DNA, and are mutagenic and carcinogenic. As might be expected, some, such as mitoxantrone and the closely related bisantrene, also exhibit antitumor activity. In addition, rhein (4,5-dihydroxyanthraquinone 2-carboxylic acid) is known to inhibit NAD^+-linked mitochondrial oxidation.[2A]

The parallelism between hydroxyanthraquinones and anthracyclines becomes espe-

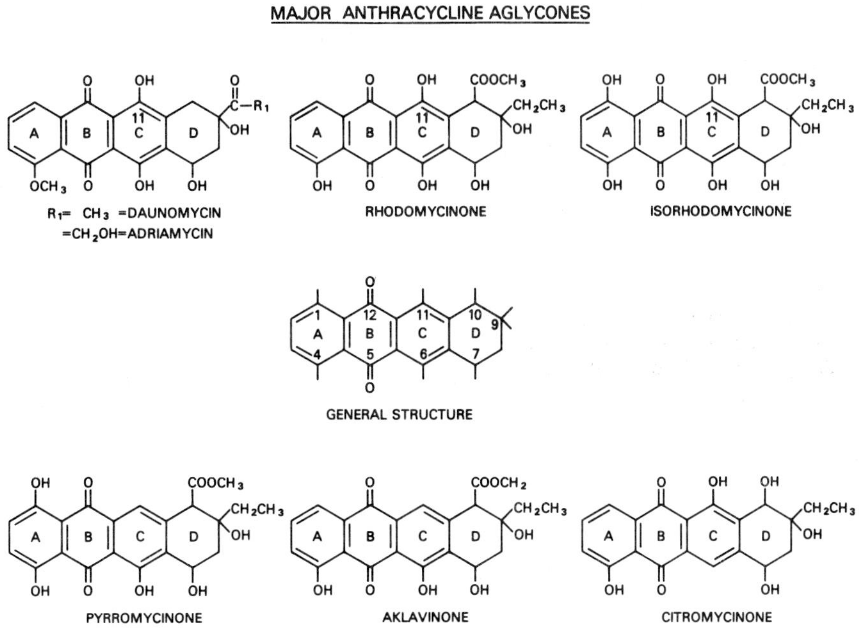

MAJOR ANTHRACYCLINE AGLYCONES

R_1 = CH_3 = DAUNOMYCIN
= CH_2OH = ADRIAMYCIN

RHODOMYCINONE

ISORHODOMYCINONE

GENERAL STRUCTURE

PYRROMYCINONE

AKLAVINONE

CITROMYCINONE

Figure 20–1. Structure of important anthracyclines. The general structure and numbering system for the ring carbons is shown in the central figure.

cially apparent when one compares the spectral characteristics of doxorubicin with the known properties of 1,4-dihydroxyanthraquinone. Thus, the characteristic absorption peak of doxorubicin at 479 nm is similar to the intense change transfer band of the above quinone in the same spectral region. As with the anthraquinones, this may be attributed to an intramolecular hydrogen bond between the phenolic proton and the oxygen of the adjacent quinone.[3] The dramatic blue shift of this peak at basic pH is consistent with

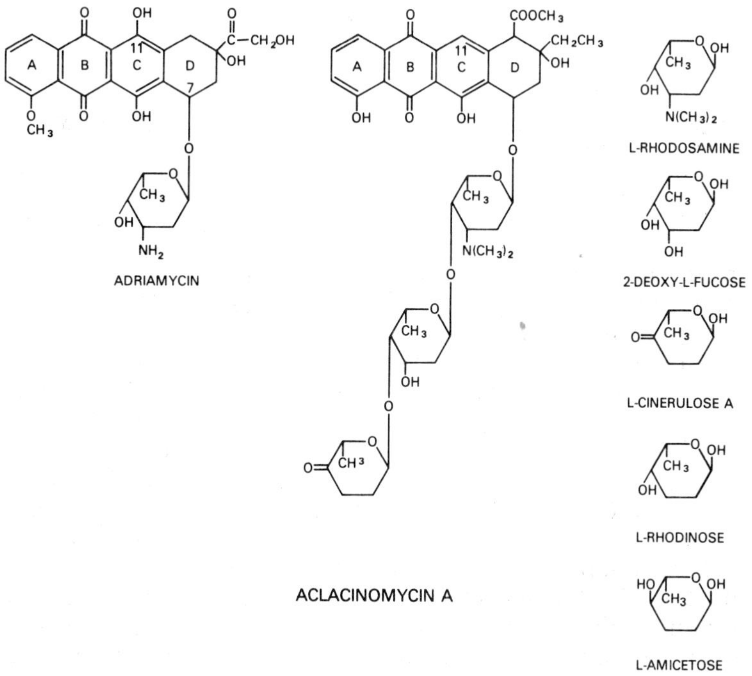

ADRIAMYCIN

ACLACINOMYCIN A

L-RHODOSAMINE

2-DEOXY-L-FUCOSE

L-CINERULOSE A

L-RHODINOSE

L-AMICETOSE

Figure 20–2. Doxorubicin (Adriamycin), aclacinomycin A, and various sugars found on other naturally occurring anthracyclines.

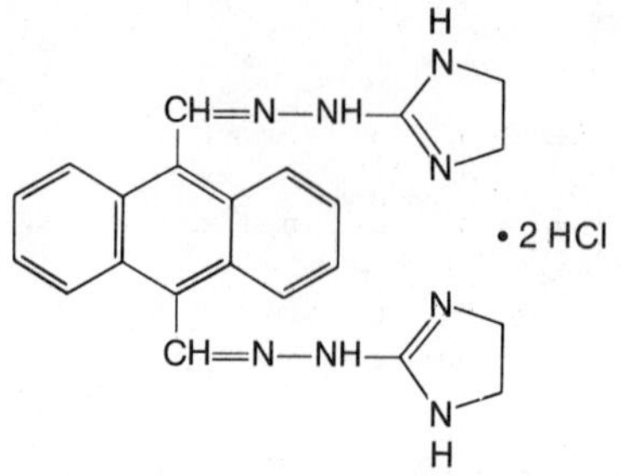

Bisantrene (Orange Crush):
9,10-Anthracenedicarboxaldehyde, bis[(4,5-dihydro-1*H*-imidazol-2-yl)hydrazone] dihydrochloride

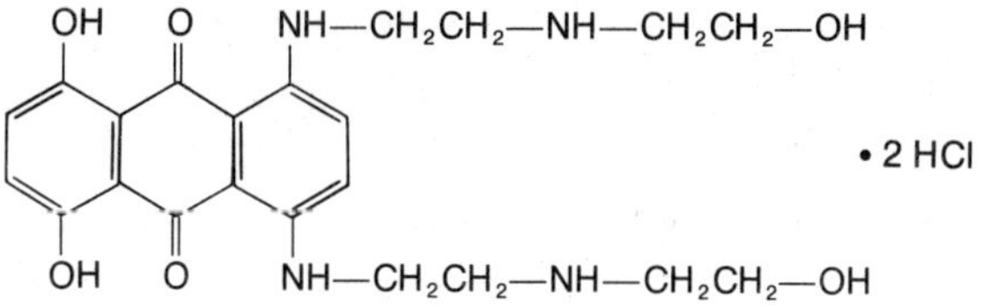

Mitoxantrone
(Dihydroxyanthracenedione dihydrochloride)
1,4-dihydroxy-5,8-bis[(2-hydroxyethyl)-amino]-9,10-anthracenedione dihydrochloride

Naturally Occurring Anthraquinone Dyes

Alizarin

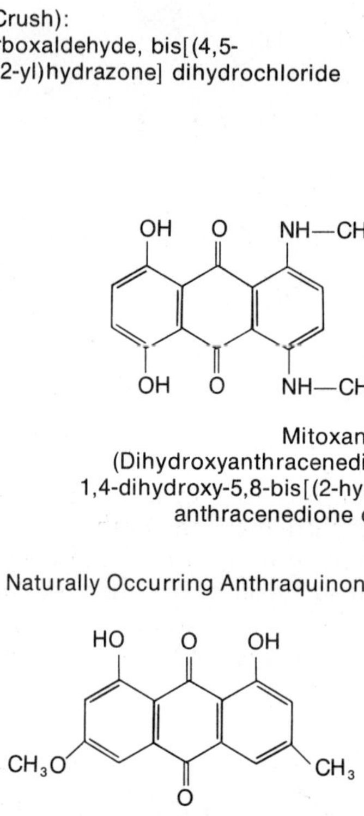

Emodin

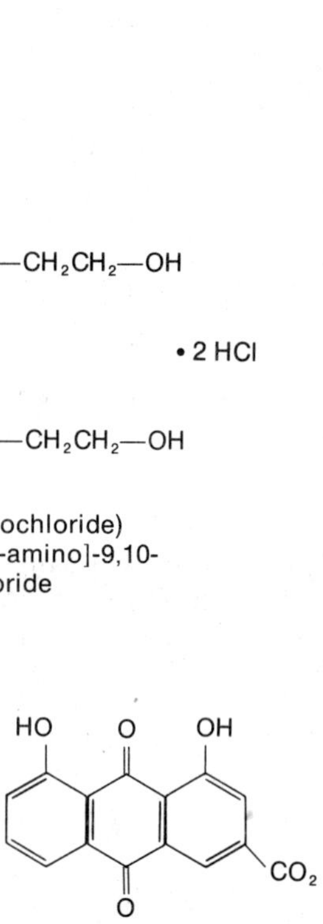

Rhein

Figure 20–3. Naturally occurring dihydroxyanthraquinones, and two related anticancer drugs, bisantrene and mitoxantrone.

ionization of this phenolic proton. In a similar fashion, both the absorption of 1,4-dihydroxyanthraquinone at 252 nm and of doxorubicin in the same region is almost certainly due to a benzonoid π–π^* transition.

MECHANISMS OF ACTION

Doxorubicin and daunorubicin have a number of biochemical actions that may be of clinical relevance to either the antitumor action or the toxicity of the drugs.

DNA Binding

The ability of both these drugs to bind to DNA was historically the first effect to be described and is certainly the most thoroughly investigated. This binding is known to include intercalation as well as other modes of binding. The precise details of the intercalation remain to be defined, but the use of proton nuclear magnetic resonance and other techniques have recently helped to define the interaction of drug and DNA more clearly. The chromophore appears to insert itself between base pairs perpendicular to the long axis of the double helix, the major interaction coming between the B and C rings of the drugs and the bases above and below them. There is considerable uncertainty as to whether the anthracyclines show any preference for particular base sequences at their sites of intercalation.[4,5] The A and D rings protrude out of either side of the double helix, and the amino sugar is thought to interact ionically with the sugar phosphate backbone of DNA.[6,7] Intercalation results in a partial unwinding of the helix. Determination of the binding constant of these drugs with DNA has been the source of some controversy, primarily over which methods are appropriate. However, most estimates of the association constant range from $10^5 M^{-1}$ to $10^6 M^{-1}$.[8,9]

Much of the work on the DNA binding of these drugs has ignored the fact that mammalian DNA is organized into chromatin. In chromatin the DNA is wrapped around a series of histone core particles to create the effect of a "series of beads on a string." The linker DNA segments that connect one core particle with the next can be distinguished from the DNA segments wrapped around the core particles because the former is susceptible to digestion of micrococcal nuclease, whereas the latter is not. The chromatin condenses in preparation for mitosis by twisting into elaborate structures in which the organization into core and linker segments is critical. In this light, it is interesting to note that doxorubicin will condense chromatin and render it resistant to micrococcal nuclease digestion.[10]

The attempt to understand the biologic effects of doxorubicin and daunorubicin DNA binding is rendered difficult by the fact that, at certain concentrations, these drugs can affect every DNA function that has been examined, including DNA synthesis and RNA synthesis. As a result of intercalation, DNA template function for nucleic acid synthesis is impaired. Painter[11] found that the primary effect of doxorubicin was to inhibit chain elongation as opposed to initiation of DNA synthesis. In order to gain perspective, it is helpful to examine the effects of these agents on the cell cycle. Particularly pertinent is the finding that cells exposed to a lethal but not excessive concentration of doxorubicin in G_1 will proceed through S phase at a normal velocity, and then stop and die in G_2. At higher concentrations, an S-phase block will develop.[12] These results suggest that inhibition of DNA-directed DNA synthesis is not essential for cell kill, particularly at lower concentrations.

Currently, there are a number of possible explanations for the above observation. Daskal and co-workers[13] have shown that doxorubicin affects preribosomal RNA synthesis as well as DNA synthesis, and also that agents such as aclacinomycin A selectively inhibit preribosomal RNA synthesis as opposed to DNA synthesis. The fact that aclacinomycin A is also cytotoxic for tumor cells suggests that effects on RNA synthesis may be more important than inhibition of DNA synthesis.

In addition to these effects on DNA function, doxorubicin has been shown to damage DNA. Single- and double-stranded breaks have been observed[14,15] as well as sister chromatid exchanges. In addition, several authors have reported alkylation of DNA by doxorubicin.[16,17] In light of these observations, it is hardly surprising that doxorubicin is both mutagenic and carcinogenic. Ross et al.[15] have examined whether DNA damage produced by doxorubicin is responsible for the cytotoxicity of these agents. Surprisingly, they found that agents that block DNA repair, such as caffeine, lessened cytotoxicity while increasing DNA damage. The mechanism of this DNA damage is discussed below under Free Radical Formation.

In summary, doxorubicin and daunorubicin are known to intercalate DNA. Although this intercalation has been shown to be associated with effects on DNA synthesis and RNA synthesis, and to result in DNA damage, experiments to date seem to rule out blockade of DNA synthesis and DNA damage as mechanisms of cytotoxicity. The ability of these agents to effect preribosomal RNA synthesis seems to be, by virtue of elimination, the best candidate for the antitumor action.

Free Radical Formation

Free radicals are defined as compounds that possess an unpaired electron. Drug free radical intermediates are of interest because they are often highly reactive toward such biologically important macromolecules as cell membranes and DNA. For a general overview of drug-induced free radical damage, the reader is referred to the excellent review by Mason.[18]

Handa, Sato, and co-workers[19-21] were the first to report formation of free radicals during metabolism of doxorubicin and daunorubicin. These workers showed that microsomal enzyme P450 reductase in the presence of NADPH was able to catalyze the reduction of these anthracyclines to a semiquinone radical intermediate. This radical was in turn shown to react with oxygen to produce the superoxide radical with regeneration of the parent doxorubicin or daunorubicin. Nuclear membrane P450 reductase can also accomplish this reduction. In addition, both mitochondria and submitochondrial particles can catalyze an NADH-dependent one-electron reduction of doxorubicin, probably at an early step in the electron transport chain.

This work has been confirmed and extended by Bachur et al.,[22, 23] Goodman and Hochstein,[24] Kalyanaraman,[25] and others. The picture that has emerged is that in the presence of oxygen (Fig. 20–4) the doxorubicin or daunorubicin semiquinone radical rapidly reacts with oxygen to yield superoxide. The superoxide radical, regardless of its source in tumors, is known to engage in a series of reactions that result in oxidative damage to cell membranes and cleavage of DNA.[26] Although the details of these reactions remain controversial, they include dismutation of superoxide to form hydrogen peroxide and the subsequent reaction of superoxide and hydrogen peroxide to form the hydroxyl radical (OH ·). Both hydrogen peroxide and the hydroxyl radical are able to damage cells. The latter, in particular, is one of the most reactive substances known and is able to attack a variety of biologic substances, including pyrimidine and purine bases, thiols, and amines, with a reaction velocity

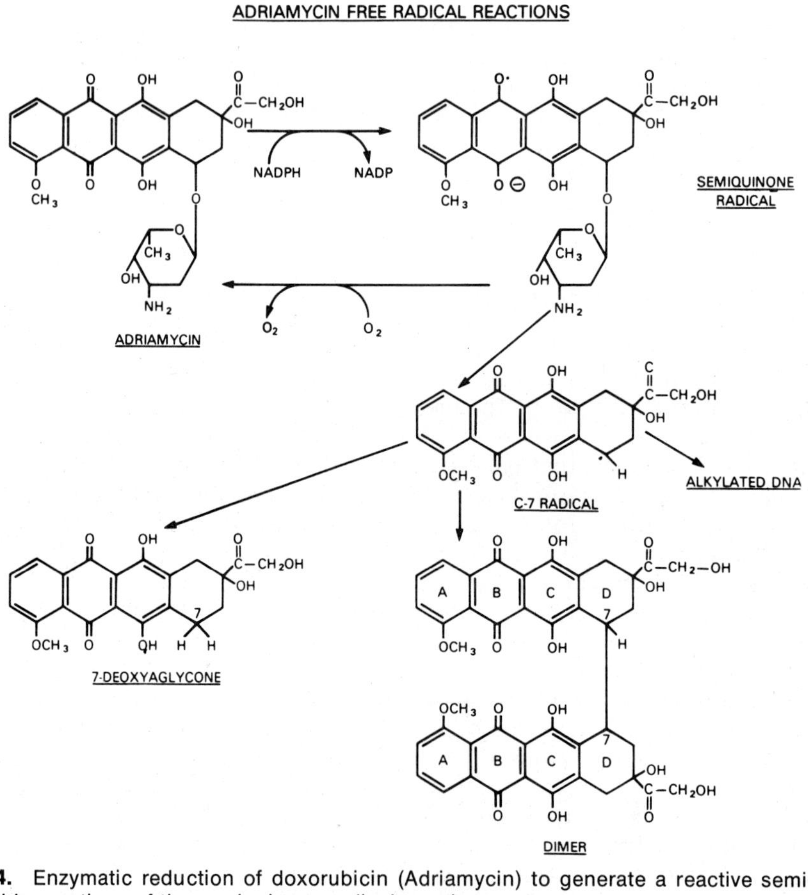

ADRIAMYCIN FREE RADICAL REACTIONS

Figure 20–4. Enzymatic reduction of doxorubicin (Adriamycin) to generate a reactive semiquinone. Subsequent possible reactions of the semiquinone radical are shown.

that is essentially diffusion-controlled. These reactions may be summarized as follows:

$$(1)\ 2\ O_2^- + 2H^+ \rightarrow H_2O_2 + O_2$$

$$(2)\ O_2^- + H_2O_2 \rightarrow OH\cdot + OH^- + O_2$$

Reaction 2, otherwise known as the Haber-Weiss reaction, is almost certainly more complex than illustrated here and is very slow in the absence of catalysts such as iron or its chelates. This iron catalysis is conventionally thought to proceed via the following mechanism:

$$(1)\ O_2^- + Fe^{+3} \rightarrow O_2 + Fe^{+2}$$

$$(2)\ Fe^{+2} + H_2O_2 \rightarrow OH\cdot + OH^- + Fe^{+3}$$

In the absence of oxygen (Fig. 20–3), the semiquinone radical can rearrange slowly ($t\frac{1}{2} > \frac{1}{2}$-sec). The unpaired electron shifts to the C-7 carbon and the bond to the sugar cleaves. The result is an aglycone free radical. This radical can abstract a hydride (proton plus one electron) to yield the 7-deoxyglycone. It is also possible for two aglycone radicals to react to form a dimer. At present, this dimer has been described only for aclacinomycin A. Finally, the aglycone radical would be expected to have the capacity to alkylate DNA. This may be the basis for the alkylation of DNA by doxorubicin recently reported by Sinha et al.[16-17] However, it must be stressed that our knowledge of the chemistry and biologic role of the aglycone radical is at present incomplete.

One of the most interesting aspects of the enzymatic activation of doxorubicin to its semiquinone radical is that the enzymes capable of catalyzing this reaction are flavin-dependent oxidoreductases. Examples include P450 reductase, xanthine oxidase, and NADH dehydrogenase. Interest, therefore, has focused on the interaction between flavins and doxorubicin. It has been shown[27] that doxorubicin and flavin mononucleotides interact directly to form a complex via ring–ring stacking. This close contact could provide conditions that favor electron transfer from the flavin to doxorubicin. In a similar vein, it has been demonstrated that the reduction potential of a variety of quinones correlates well with the reduction of these quinones by a variety of flavoproteins.[28] It would be of great interest to see whether a correlation existed between the reduction potential of a variety of anthracyclines and their biologic activity, in terms of either tumor response or cardiac toxicity.

There is now direct proof that doxorubicin free radical formation can occur in a variety of cell types, including tumor cells; there is also circumstantial evidence that these radicals can lead, under certain conditions, to cell damage. Electron spin resonance represents the least ambiguous evidence for the existence of a free radical. Handa, Sato, and co-workers[19-21] have shown that the classic electron spin resonance signal of the appropriate semiquinone radical can be detected in Ehrlich ascites tumor cells after exposure to an anthracycline. Doroshow et al.[29] in turn have shown superoxide radical production from Ehrlich ascites tumor cells following incubation in doxorubicin. The studies, however, have not linked free radical generation to cytotoxicity in these tumor cells. Evidence for oxygen radical generation has also been obtained for human red blood cells and platelets incubated in the presence of doxorubicin. In the case of the platelets, this was associated with an increase in platelet agglutination that could be blocked by the free radical scavenger alpha-tocopherol.[30, 31]

The heart is the only tissue for which a linkage has been developed between free radical formation and toxicity. This linkage was first pointed out by Myers et al.,[32] who detected evidence of lipid peroxidation in mouse hearts after administration of doxorubicin. They also noted that the free radical scavenger alpha-tocopherol lessened both lipid peroxidation and pathologic evidence of damage. These observations have since been confirmed in multiple species.[28-37] There is increasing evidence that there are at least two sites of doxorubicin free radical generation in the heart. Several workers[22, 38-40] have now confirmed that doxorubicin triggers superoxide generation from cardiac mitochondria and that this results in peroxidation of mitochondrial lipids. In this regard, it is important to note that mitochondria represent more than 40 per cent of the heart muscle by weight and are the major source for the ATP needed for myocardial contraction. Mitochondria also play a role in the release and uptake of calcium needed for electrical excitation–mechanical contraction coupling. Thus, mitochondrial free radical formation is likely to have profound effects on cardiac function. Bachur et al.[22] have also reported that doxorubicin stimulates superoxide production from cardiac sarcosomes.

In spite of the above evidence, questions remain as to why these agents exhibit selective cardiac toxicity. The enzymes known to activate doxorubicin to a free radical are widely distributed: xanthine oxidase and P450 reductase, for example, are present in liver in high concentration, but liver damage is not a major problem with doxorubicin. Most mammalian cells have elaborate mechanisms for the detoxification of oxygen radicals. This leads naturally to the question whether cardiac tissue has some defect in its defenses against oxygen radicals. It is now apparent that cardiac tissue in many species lacks catalase.[38, 41, 42] Furthermore, glutathione peroxidase, another enzyme able to dispose of hydrogen peroxide, is destroyed by doxorubicin.[41, 42] Thus, after doxorubicin treatment, cardiac tissue is deficient in the two major enzymes known to be involved in the detoxification of hydrogen peroxide at the same time that superoxide and hydrogen peroxide production is stimulated by the drug. The result is likely to be an increase in cardiac hydrogen peroxide concentration. This combined effect has been postulated as the basis for the selective cardiac toxicity of doxorubin.[41, 42]

In summary, doxorubicin and daunorubicin can be enzymatically reduced to semiquinone free radicals, which in turn can trigger oxygen radical generation or alkylation. Free radical formation in living cells has been demonstrated, and circumstantial evidence has accumulated to suggest a role for free radical formation in the cardiac toxicity of these compounds. In contrast, there is no evidence at present that free radical formation plays a role in the antitumor effect of these agents.

OTHER BIOCHEMICAL ACTIONS OF DOXORUBICIN

Membrane Effects

There is now abundant evidence that doxorubicin and other anthracyclines exert direct effects on the cell membrane. Murphree et al.[43] showed that exposure of sarcoma 180 cells to doxorubicin concentrations as low as 0.1 μM affected the clustering of concanavalin A–capped receptors. Solie and Yunker[44] found that doxorubicin induced changes in the transmembrane flux of sodium in the frog epithelium. Villani et al.[45] examined the effects of doxorubicin on the exchangeability of calcium in isolated guinea pig atria, and showed that a rapidly exchangeable calcium pool, presumably membrane-bound, shifted to a slowly exchanging, presumably intracellular, pool. Goldman et al.[46] and Mikkelsen et al.[47] have demonstrated that a variety of anthracyclines bind to red cell membranes and cause altered membrane morphology and lysis. Kessel[48] showed that doxorubicin exposure led to a rapid increase in the electronegativity and alterations in membrane glycoproteins.

The binding of doxorubicin has been studied in greater detail by Duarte-Karim et al.,[49] Tritton et al.,[50] and Goormaghtigh et al.[51, 52] These authors all found that doxorubicin binds most tightly to cardiolipin, of all the cell membrane phospholipids. Estimates of the affinity of doxorubicin for cardiolipin are in the range of $K_a = 1 \times 10^6 M^{-1}$. This is of the same range as the affinity of doxorubicin for DNA and serves to underline the potential biologic importance of this interaction. Cardiolipin concentrations are highest in the mitochondrial membrane, but are generally low in cell membranes. Tritton et al.[50] pointed out that cardiolipin content is also increased in cell membranes of transformed cells. Based on this, these authors suggested that this is why anthracyclines cause tumor cell death and cardiac toxicity.

Interesting as this evidence of direct membrane binding is, it fails to provide any reason why this binding should have toxic consequences. Changes in membrane fluidity and morphology have been observed, but there is a real need for a hypothesis based on these observations that explains the cytotoxicity in specific chemical or biochemical terms. This author believes that membrane-bound doxorubicin is likely still to be available for free radical activation and that redox cycling at the membrane surface will prove to be of pathologic significance. This proposal has a number of attractive aspects. First, the hydroxyl radical is so reactive that its diffusion distance from its site of generation must average only a few angstroms. Generation of the hydroxyl radical by a membrane-bound drug should optimize the probability of a toxic consequence. Second, many of the consequences of membrane binding can be explained on this basis. Free radical–induced lipid peroxidation can be expected to alter membrane permeability by damaging the unsaturated fatty acids in the membrane phospholipids. This can also alter the function of a variety of membrane-bound proteins. Sarcotubular ATPase-dependent calcium pumping, for example, has been shown to require enzyme-bound phosphatidyl ethanolamine.[53] This phospholipid has the highest concentration of unsaturated fatty acids of any of the common phospholipids and is notoriously sensitive to peroxidative damage.

Metal Ion Chelation

Anthraquinones as a group are known to chelate metal ions. For doxorubicin specifically, chelation of a variety of metal ions has been observed.[54, 55] Although doxorubicin can bind metal ions of the alkaline earth series, such as calcium or magnesium, its affinity is greater for the transition metals such as copper, zinc, and iron. There is a tendency for some of these chelates to precipitate. Thus, the preparative scale isolation of doxorubicin and daunorubicin from *Streptomyces* culture can be accomplished via precipitation as the copper chelate. Of these metal ions, the tightest complex seems to be of doxorubicin to ferric ion. May et al.[56] have reported that three doxorubicins will bind to one ferric ion with step association constants of 10^{18}, 10^{11}, and $10^{4.4}$.

This binding of metal ions should, in fact, have been expected. The B and C rings of doxorubicin show considerable analogy with alizarin and other classic "metal lake" dyes (Fig. 20–3), which bind to cloth via metal ions that serve to chelate both the cloth on one hand and the quinone and hydroxyl of the dye on the other hand.

The biologic significance of metal chelation has been examined only superficially. Copper has been shown to facilitate the binding of daunorubicin aglycone to DNA, and evidence has been presented that copper may also be involved in the binding of doxorubicin and daunorubicin to DNA.[57] This may be via a "metal-lake"–type bond. Doxorubicin is also known to bind to bone matrix,[58] presumably because of its ability to chelate calcium.

Not all the metal chelates of doxorubicin are chemically inert. Myers et al. have found that the doxorubicin-iron chelate can act as a redox catalyst for the transfer of electrons from glutathione to oxygen.[59] This leads to the production of oxygen radicals that can rapidly lyse a red cell ghost target. As mentioned previously, iron chelates may also catalyze hydroxyl radical production from hydrogen peroxide and superoxide.

From the above, it should be apparent that the ability of anthracyclines to bind metal ions has possible biologic significance. Unfortunately, our knowledge of this area is fragmentary at best, and additional study is clearly warranted.

Overview on the Mechanisms of Action

From the above discussions, it should be apparent that the biologic effects of these compounds are certain to be complex. The evidence presented to date indicates that DNA binding, free radical formation, membrane binding, and metal ion chelation are all likely to occur *in vivo*. The determination of which of these biochemical events is/are important for any one cell or tissue is likely to remain experimentally difficult. Furthermore, these biochemical effects are not necessarily independent. Thus, metal chelation and DNA binding are not mutually exclusive, nor are free radical production and membrane binding. There is a real need to study how these biochemical actions might act in sequence to yield the observed biologic effects, including normal tissue toxicity and antitumor effect.

ANALOGUES

The clinical utility of doxorubicin and daunorubicin has led to the development of a wide range of analogues. Since it is impossible to review all the analogues produced, a selection has been made of those analogue classes that seem most promising. For a more general and comprehensive review, the reader is referred to Henry.[60]

Alterations in the Quinone-Hydroquinone Functionalities

The quinone-hydroquinone functionalities are of theoretical interest because such analogues would be expected to differ from doxorubicin in both metal chelation properties and free radical biochemistry. Aclacinomycin A,[2] the most extensively developed of this series, incorporates the aklavinone aglycone (Fig. 20–1). Presumably because it lacks the 11 position hydroxyl, this compound is only about one tenth as active as doxorubicin as regards free radical formation in the P450 reductase system. It also is not precipitated as the copper chelate, whereas doxorubicin and daunorubicin *are*. This allows facile separation of aclacinomycin A from a *Streptomyces* culture containing doxorubicin. It also does not bind to DNA as well as does doxorubicin.[61] Perhaps as a result of these differences, aclacinomycin is not mutagenic in a variety of test systems in which doxorubicin *is*; it is also less cardiotoxic than doxorubicin and it does not cause as much local tissue damage when extravasated.

Based on the above considerations, one would anticipate that other anthracyclines containing the aklavinone or citromycinone aglycone should also be less active as metal chelates and in free radical reactions. It would be very instructive to see if these aclacinomycin-like antibiotics are also less cardiotoxic and mutagenic.

The synthetic anthracycline 5-iminodaunorubicin also fits into this group.[62] Here, the 5 position quinone carbonyl is replaced with an imino group. As might be expected, this compound is less reactive as a free radical than is doxorubicin; even when chemically reduced, it produces less DNA damage than does doxorubicin.[63]

Although further study of B and C ring changes is of interest, there are practical limits to the alterations possible on the B and C rings. In intercalation, these two rings are buried within the DNA double helix. Intercalation becomes difficult if the planar nature of the ring system is changed or if bulky substituents are added.

Multiple Sugars

The conventional anthracyclines such as doxorubicin and daunorubicin have only one sugar, daunosamine, but others may have two or three. Crooke and co-workers[64] have pointed out that anthracyclines with multiple sugars selectively inhibit preribosomal RNA synthesis, whereas those with only one sugar also inhibit DNA synthesis.

Other Alterations in the Amino Sugars

Tong et al.[65] prepared a series of derivatives in which alkyl groups were added to the daunosamine amino group. These authors found that when the alkyl groups became very large (dibenzyl, for example), the cardiac toxicity lessened significantly. These compounds also preserved antitumor efficacy. The Farmatalia group has also found that removal of the 4′ hydroxyl group markedly lessened the cardiac toxicity of these compounds without eliminating the antitumor effects. AD32 also fits this pattern and is less cardiotoxic than doxorubicin.

These results suggest that the structure of the sugar at or in the immediate vicinity of the amino group is a critical determinant of the cardiac toxicity of the anthracyclines. The antitumor effect is also sensitive to alterations in this region — the aglycones are generally quite inactive — but obviously the requirements for cardiac toxicity and antitumor effect differ.

Aminoethylaminoanthraquinones

The aminoethylaminoanthraquinones are not in fact anthracyclines and are not naturally occurring, but instead derive from studies in dye chemistry. The first active agent in this series, 1,4-bis[(2-dimethylaminoethyl)-amino]anthraquinone, was discovered in the drug screening program of the National Cancer Institute. This has led to a wide-ranging synthetic effort[66, 67] resulting in development of a number of interesting drugs. Because of the planar quinoid chromophore common to these agents, they possess as a group the capacity to intercalate DNA. The basic aminoalkyl side chain is thought to stabilize the intercalation in a manner similar to that of the amino sugar of the anthracyclines. It is also of interest that a number of these agents appear to possess the cardiotoxicity of the anthracyclines[68] in several animal models. One of these drugs, 1,4 - dihydroxy - 5,8 - bis[(2 - hydroxyethyl) - amino]-9,10-anthracenedione dihydrochloride (dihydroxyanthracenedione) (Fig. 20–3) has seen extensive human testing. It seems likely that a careful structure-activity relationship study of this drug class would be of value to an understanding of both the antitumor and the cardiotoxic actions of the anthracyclines.

A related, nonquinoidal anthracene, bisantrene, is also shown in Figure 20–3 and is currently undergoing early clinical trials.

CELLULAR PHARMACOLOGY

Study of the membrane transport of the anthracyclines is rendered difficult by the capacity of these drugs to bind to cell membranes, proteins, DNA, and metal ions. In addition, their metabolism to a variety of compounds creates further problems. This author considers that none of the published studies properly controls for these problems, and that they therefore must be interpreted with caution.

The work of Skovsgaard,[69, 70] Dano,[71] and others[72] has suggested that doxorubicin and daunorubicin enter via a passive, carrier-mediated transport process. This picture has recently been challenged by Dalmark and Strom,[73] who have claimed that drug uptake is dependent on a fickian diffusion process of the electrically neutral molecule through the lipid domain of the cell membrane.

Efflux, on the other hand, appears to be an active, energy-requiring process that is blocked by metabolic inhibitors such as 2,4-dinitrophenol. In murine cells, the primary mode of drug resistance appears to be an increase in the activity of this efflux pump; mutants resistant to vinblastine and other antibiotic-type compounds may be cross-resistant to the anthracyclines on the basis of altered membrane transport properties. The major change appears to be the development of a more active efflux pump for these drugs. Cells resistant to multiple antibiotics have been found to contain increased quantities of a membrane glycoprotein[74] and to have additional genetic material in the form of double minute chromosomes,[75] indicating that gene amplification for a membrane constituent may underlie this form of resistance.

Once in the cells, doxorubicin and daunorubicin are rapidly concentrated in the nucleus. As much as 80 per cent of the drug will be found in that location. It has generally been assumed that this occurs as a result of DNA binding of the drug. However, fluorescent microscopy reveals intense nuclear fluorescence. This finding must be viewed in light of the observation that DNA binding results in a marked loss in doxorubicin fluorescence, and suggests that a significant proportion of the nuclear drug might be free rather than bound. This indicates a possible concentration gradient for free drug across the nuclear membrane, and thus suggests the possibility of nuclear membrane transport. This possibility remains to be tested.

There are two major pathways of drug metabolism in mammalian cells. The best described is the conversion of doxorubicin to doxorubicinol. This conversion is accomplished by at least two broad classes of NADPH-requiring reductases, each class in turn being composed of multiple isoenzymes.[76] The true identity of these enzymes remains an open question. Doxorubicinol and daunorubicinol appear to be somewhat less toxic than the parent drugs,[77, 78] so this conversion is possibly a mechanism that reduces drug toxicity.

The second metabolic pathway is one that has already been discussed, namely, free radical formation leading to both oxygen radical formation and generation of the C-7 radical. The latter may cause DNA alkylation and 7-deoxy aglycone formation. The biologic consequences of this free radical formation are not clear, but it is difficult to imagine this change as a detoxification reaction.

Assay Methods

Doxorubicin, daunorubicin, and most of their analogues are intensely fluorescent, a property that has formed the basis for most of the existing assay techniques. The first and simplest approach[79] was merely to measure the total fluorescence of an extract of tissue or plasma. This technique, however, does not provide any means for distinguishing parent drug from metabolite. The first practical technique for separating parent from metabolite was thin-layer chromatography, in which the drug was detected on the thin-layer plate by fluorescence scanning. This technique reached its maximal development in the hands of Chan and Wong;[80] however, this approach has, by and large, been abandoned because it is laborious and time-consuming, and requires great care to obtain consistent results. Chan and Watson[81] have also developed a GLC–mass spectroscopic method that is sensitive and applicable to a range of anthracyclines. In general, however, the technique of choice is based on high-performance liquid chromatography (HPLC).[82-84] The major advantages of this approach over GLC–mass spectroscopy are that sample preparation is less laborious and the equipment used less expensive and easier to maintain. The best separations at present result from the use of reverse-phase chromatography, with the nonpolar groups on the solid phase being either phenyl or C_{18}. Fluorescent detection is again used. The major limitation in sensitivity is the intensity of the light source; maximal sensitivity is obtained with an argon laser.[85]

The major problem with most of the above techniques is that nonfluorescent metabolites would not be detected. Such products might be expected as the result of the free radical reactions of these compounds and also their metal-binding properties.

Pharmacokinetics

As might be expected, doxorubicin and daunorubicin exhibit significant plasma protein binding (0.5–0.9).[86] In addition, binding to tissue sites such as DNA is probably quantitatively significant, with tissue-to-plasma concentration ratios ranging from 20 to 550. As a consequence of this intracellular binding, there is a complex relationship between plasma doxorubicin concentration and that at various sites of action.

Following intravenous bolus administration, plasma clearance curves are triphasic, with half-lives of 8–25 minutes, 1.50–10 hours, and 24–48 hours, respectively.[86, 87] The initial phase is dominated by distribution, the second by metabolism, and the final phase by release of the drug from sites of binding such as spectrin, DNA, and cardiolipin.

The predominant metabolite is doxorubicinol or daunomycinol for doxorubicin and daunorubicin, respectively. Although this metabolic conversion may occur in a range of tissues, liver seems to be the major site. As mentioned previously, deoxydoxorubicin aglycone is also formed as an end product of free radical formation. A range of other metabolites has been described,[88] but their quantitative significance is not clear.

Renal clearance appears to be quantitatively insignificant in man, and dose modification is not required for renal failure. The overall importance of the liver is less clear. One study suggests that liver extraction may reach 45 to 50 per cent.[89] However, nearly normal plasma pharmacokinetics have been observed in patients with advanced hepatoma.[90] Thus, although dose modification has been recommended for those with hepatic dysfunction, there is no convincing quantitative relationship among any given test of liver function, doxorubicin clearance, and toxicity.

TABLE 20–1. Steps in the Use of HPLC for Measurement of Doxorubicin in Plasma Samples*

1. Add daunorubicin as an internal standard
2. Bring to pH 9.8 with sodium borate buffer
3. Extract with chloroform:methanol (4:1, v/v)
4. Evaporate organic layer to dryness under nitrogen
5. Redissolve in 100 μl methanol and inject into HPLC using a phenyl reverse-phase column on acetonitrile:water mobile phase and fluorescent detection

*Modified from the assay proposed by Israel et al.: J. Liquid Chromatogr. 1:795, 1978.

Drug Interactions

Perhaps the most important drug interaction of the anthracyclines is their binding to sulfated mucopolysaccharides such as heparin and chondroitin sulfate.[91] The binding to heparin can lead to precipitation of doxorubicin in intravenous preparations. The interaction can even prevent the measurement of doxorubicin in heparinized blood samples. There is no direct evidence that this interaction will occur *in vivo*, but coadministration of both agents seems ill-advised.

Given the important role of microsomal enzymes in anthracycline metabolism, it is hardly surprising that administration of phenobarbital, a known inducer of microsomal metabolism, led to more rapid clearance of doxorubicin from plasma and an increase in drug toxicity.[92] A similar interaction in man has not been documented; however, it is rarely necessary to administer the two agents at the same time. The one exception might be for seizures secondary to tumor involvement of the central nervous system.

A third possible interaction is with the intercalator actinomycin D. Krugh and Young[93] showed that doxorubicin and daunorubicin more effectively intercalate DNA that has already been pretreated with actinomycin D. This has been rationalized on the basis of partial DNA unwinding after actinomycin D treatment. This interaction has apparent therapeutic advantages, but these remain to be evaluated.

Finally, membrane-active agents such as amphotericin B are able to increase tumor cell uptake of doxorubicin, presumably because of increased membrane permeability.[94] As a result, amphotericin B has been shown to partially reverse doxorubicin resistance in tumor cells thought to be resistant via altered membrane transport properties.

TOXICITY

Cardiac Toxicity

The clinical use of the anthracyclines is associated with both an acute and a chronic cumulative cardiomyopathy that is not infrequently fatal. The importance of this problem is increased by the potential value of this agent in the adjuvant treatment of soft tissue sarcomas and breast cancer.

Natural History. The cardiac toxicity of these agents can manifest itself as either an acute or a chronic syndrome. The most common manifestations of the acute syndrome are arrhythmias and conduction abnormalities,[95, 96] which occur minutes to hours after drug infusion. These arrhythmias can range from benign supraventricular tachycardias to complete heart block and ventricular tachycardia. Perhaps this explains the cases of sudden death reported to occur within a few days following administration of doxorubicin.[97] In addition to these arrhythmias, patients may develop what has been termed the "pericarditis-myocarditis syndrome."[98] This has been characterized by the onset of florid congestive heart failure associated with pericarditis, and typically begins a few days after the patient receives doxorubicin. Evidence suggests that this may represent an exaggerated manifestation of acute myocardial damage that usually produces a clinically inapparent acute drop in left ventricular function.[99] One of the current controversies revolves around the relationship of the acute and chronic cardiomyopathies. It has been clearly shown that the severity of the transient arrhythmias discussed above does not correlate with the probability of the patient subsequently developing chronic cardiomyopathy.[96, 97] However, the acute alterations in myocardial contractility exemplified in an extreme form by the pericarditis-myocarditis syndrome and its variants may reflect the same process that leads to chronic cardiomyopathy. Patients who survive the acute syndrome may be left with a persistent defect in myocardial function and pathologic evidence of severe damage. In addition, endocardial biopsies done in asymptomatic patients have shown a linear correlation between pathologic damage and total dose of drug administered. This latter observation implies that a constant amount of permanent damage occurs with each dose of doxorubicin. All this evidence suggests that the cumulative chronic cardiac toxicity may be the net result of repeated episodes of subclinical acute cardiac damage. The alternative concept, that the chronic toxicity is a separate entity without any organic relationship to the acute syndrome, at present lacks supporting evidence.

The natural history of the chronic cardiomyopathy has been the subject of a number of studies. As mentioned earlier, endocardial biopsies have shown that there is a linear correlation between biopsy score and total dose of doxorubicin.[100] A similar relationship has also been described between ejection fraction as measured by radionuclide angiocardiography and total doxorubicin dose.[101] In these studies, as well as in the retrospective study by Von Hoff and Layard,[102] few patients survived for long periods after doxorubicin treatment. This problem has recently been corrected in a study by Gottdiener et al.,[103] who were able to evaluate the long-term consequences of doxorubicin administration in a group of patients who received the drug as adjuvant therapy for soft tissue sarcoma. Using radionuclide cineangiography as a measurement technique, these authors found that, of the asymptomatic patients who received a total dose of 480 to 550 mg per m^2, 63 per cent had an abnormal scan. Furthermore, the incidence of abnormal scans remained the same in these patients from less than nine months to more than 21 months after their last dose of doxorubicin. It thus seems that the damage, once produced, does not undergo significant repair. Inspection of the above reports suggests that in most patients the degree of myocardial damage rapidly stabilizes after the last dose of doxorubicin. However, a few patients in the studies of both Alexander et al.[101] and Gottdiener et al.[103] had dramatic improvement or decline in myocardial function over time. Certainly, this author has seen patients enter congestive heart failure one year or longer after the last dose of doxorubicin.

Once clinically overt cardiomyopathy is present, the prognosis is grave, with mortality rates reported to be as high as 48 per cent.[104] A fatal outcome appears more likely if the onset of congestive heart failure occurs less than one month after the last dose of doxorubicin.[105]

Pathophysiology. In both skeletal and cardiac muscle, contraction begins with a wave of membrane depolarization. This electrical event causes rapid release of free calcium within the myocyte. In turn, this increase in free calcium leads to increased calcium binding to the actin–myosin complex, triggering contraction. Following contraction, muscle relaxation occurs as calcium dissociates from the actin–myosin complex and is bound to a variety of intracellular storage sites. This entire process has been called "excitation contraction coupling" because it serves to link electrical events at the membrane with the mechanical events of contraction.[106]

Skeletal and cardiac muscle differ, however, in the way in which the above mechanism is used to regulate the force of contraction. In skeletal muscle, the myocytes are organized into motor units, each with its own nerve supply, and each motor unit is capable of firing independently. The force of contraction is controlled by the number of motor units activated, with each motor unit either firing at full force or remaining at rest. In contrast, cardiac muscle is a syncytium in which every myocyte contracts with each heart beat. In the heart, the force of contraction is controlled by the amount of calcium bound in the actin–myosin complex. This gives calcium a central role in the regulation of the force of myocardial contraction that it does not have for skeletal muscle. It is, therefore, interesting to note that doxorubicin has a major impact on the myocardial calcium pools.

The two most important sites of intracellular calcium binding are the sarcoplasmic reticulum and mitochondria. Marked dilation and distortion of the sarcoplasmic reticulum is a hallmark of doxorubicin cardiac toxicity and gives rise to the vacuolization so characteristic of the chronic cardiomyopathy. In addition, several workers have now demonstrated marked alterations in mitochondrial calcium handling, including the rate of uptake and release of this ion after doxorubicin exposure.[107, 108] As might be expected, a number of laboratories have also documented that there are significant changes in myocardial calcium handling, including shifts of calcium from a rapidly exchanging, membrane-bound pool to a slowly exchanging pool whose anatomic location remains to be established.[109] In addition to the alterations in calcium handling, actual myocyte destruction occurs that may be secondary to the increased intracellular calcium[110] or to other toxic effects of doxorubicin reviewed previously in this chapter. In view of the role that calcium plays in myocardial contraction, these observations must be accounted for by any hypothesis that seeks to explain the pathogenesis of this cardiomyopathy. The manner in which the various biochemical actions of doxorubicin might explain these alterations is detailed above under Mechanisms of Action.

Monitoring Cardiac Function. Table 20–2 illustrates the range of physiologic tests used to assess cardiac damage after doxorubicin administration.[111] Of those listed, the only ones to have proved satisfactory are cardiac catheterization and radionuclide cineangiography. For clinical monitoring, cineangiography appears to have convincing advantages: it is noninvasive and allows cardiac function to be stressed through exercise. In addition, cardiac catheterization requires certain assumptions to be made about the geometry of the ventricular cavity (usually assumed to be a prolate ellipse) that may or may not be accurate. Cineangiography makes no such assumptons but rather counts the total ventricular blood pool radioactivity. Electrocardiography, systolic time intervals, and echocardiography are all less sensitive and less accurate than the other two. In addition, echocardiography can be performed on only 60 per cent of adults.

TABLE 20–2. Physiologic Tests of Cardiac Function

Modality Used	*Pertinent Measurement*	*Value Considered to Indicate Cardiomyopathy*	*Advantages*	*Disadvantages*
Systolic time intervals	PEP/LVET	a. Greater than 0.42–0.45 b. Increase of over 0.07 from control	Simple to perform; inexpensive	Large standard error; affected severely by load factors
Echocardiography	Fractional shortening	Less than 30%	Equipment widely available; personnel trained to perform tests widely available; inexpensive	30–40% of adults cannot be studied; measurement of ventricular volumes subject to errors
ECG	QRS voltage	A drop in QRS voltage of 30% or greater	Simple to perform; inexpensive	Lacks adequate sensitivity; detects abnormalities associated with cardiomyopathy rather than predicting changes
Cardiac catheterization	Ejection fraction; cardiac output; pressure measurement	Resting cardiac index of under 2.5 liters/min; exercise increase under 5; pulmonary wedge pressure over 12 mm Hg; resting right ventricular end-diastolic pressure over 12 mm Hg	Allows comprehensive assessment of cardiac function	Invasive, with the risks that this entails; expensive
Radionuclide cardiography	Ejection fraction; dV/dt during diastole and systole	A drop of greater than 15% from pretreatment; ejection fraction of less than 45%; failure to increase EF by greater than 5% with exercise	Accurate measure of ventricular volumes; noninvasive; easy to obtain values at rest and with exercise	Expensive equipment

In contrast with these physiologic methods of cardiac assessment, endocardial biopsy gives a direct pathologic assessment of cardiac damage.[112] There appears to be a clear relationship between the total dose of doxorubicin administered and the pathologic score. In addition, the pathologic score has proved an excellent predictor of the risk of congestive heart failure, at least in the hands of Bristow and colleagues at Stanford University.[112] There are several limitations to, and criticisms to be made of, this technique. First, special training is required to learn the biopsy technique and how to evaluate the biopsy pathologically. Second, the biopsy yields small, 1-mm samples of cardiac tissue that may lead to sampling error in a focal lesion such as doxorubicin cardiomyopathy. Nevertheless, this technique is a valuable research tool in the study of anthracycline cardiomyopathy, and its use may become more widespread with time.

Risk Factors. Certain risk factors have been identified that are associated with a definite increased incidence of anthracycline-induced cardiomyopathy. Of these, the best defined is mediastinal radiation therapy.[113] Exposure of the heart to 2000 rads or more appears to accelerate markedly the development of cardiomyopathy, so that after a total doxorubicin dose of 350 mg per m^2 the cardiac damage is equivalent to that seen after greater than 500 mg per m^2 of doxorubicin alone. This effect has some very unusual properties. For example, several years may separate the administration of x-rays and doxorubicin and yet the combination still yields increased toxicity.[113] For these reasons, it is better to avoid doxorubicin administration in patients who have had mediastinal radiation therapy.

Patients with documented essential hypertension appear also to have an increased risk of congestive heart failure after receiving doxorubicin.[114] There is no evidence that hypertension increases the rate at which doxorubicin-induced cardiac damage develops. Rather, the cardiac damage is more likely to be clinically manifested in symptoms of congestive heart failure. This seems likely to be due to the poor tolerance for the afterload imposed by hypertension, which is so characteristic of the cardiomyopathies.

In view of the steady drop in myocardial physiologic reserve that follows doxorubicin therapy, there are other medical circumstances in which this drug should be used with caution. These include severe coronary artery disease, angina pectoris, and a history of myocardial infarction.

Prevention of Cardiac Toxicity. Various strategies have been developed to lessen the cardiac toxicity of these agents. None are sufficiently well established to warrant recommendation to the practicing oncologist, but several are of scientific interest and may prove to be of clinical value. The simplest approach has been one of schedule modification. Thus, it has been reported that weekly or infusional doxorubicin is less cardiotoxic than monthly doxorubicin.[114, 115] It remains to be seen whether such drug dosage schedules are as effective as the monthly schedule in terms of antitumor response.

The second strategy that has been proposed is the synthesis of anthracyclines that, although they are active anticancer agents, are not cardiotoxic. Several drugs have been produced that do appear to have less cardiotoxicity. These include 5-iminodaunorubicin, aclacinomycin A, AD32, N,N-dibenzyl daunorubicin, and 4′-deoxydaunorubicin. The extent to which any of these agents can match doxorubicin and daunorubicin in terms of antitumor effect remains to be seen.

The third approach has been through the development of antidotal agents. Free radical scavengers such as tocopherol[30, 31] and N-acetyl cysteine[116] have been reported to show activity in animals and are currently undergoing clinical trial. The chelating agent ICRF-187 also has shown activity in a range of animal models.[117] Finally, ubiquinone, a member of the mitochondrial electron transport chain, has lessened cardiac toxicity in mice and rabbits. The activity of ubiquinone may be based on several mechanisms. Iwamoto and co-workers[118] have proposed that ubiquinone and doxorubicin compete for key ubiquinone-requiring enzymes in mitochondria. However, ubiquinone can potentially act as a free radical scavenger by picking up unpaired electrons from a variety of free radicals and transferring them to the mitochondrial electron transport chain. This would have a double benefit: the free radical is detoxified and ATP is generated.

Extravasation

Extravasation of doxorubicin and daunorubicin results in progressive inflammation and necrosis. The result can be an ulcer that can erode down to underlying bone, tendon, or muscle, and that heals very poorly. It has been shown that these drugs fix to the tissues locally and persist in high concentration for months. Although the biochemical mechanism of this damage remains unclear, the recent demonstration that a combination of DMSO (a hydroxyl radical scavenger) and alpha-tocopherol (a general radical scavenger) significantly lessens the damage when injected locally[119] suggests that free radical generation may play a role in this syndrome. In this regard, it should be noted that aclacinomycin A, which is less active than doxorubicin as a cardiotoxin and less active in terms of free radical generation in the P450 reductase system, causes much less damage when extravasated.

More conventional treatment of this complication has included ice, local steroids, bicarbonate, and surgical excision of the involved area followed by skin grafting. No randomized trials are available to test which of these are really effective. Experience at the National Cancer Institute has suggested that surgical excision is rarely necessary, and excellent results may be had with the more conservative measures outlined above.

Other Toxicities

Doxorubicin and daunorubicin also cause myelosuppression, gastrointestinal toxicity, and alopecia. The myelosuppression is usually the dose-limiting toxicity, whether the drugs are given by intravenous bolus monthly, weekly, or by continuous infusion. Myelosuppression reaches its nadir seven to ten days after treatment and reverses within three weeks.

Doxorubicin also causes a recall reaction in previously irradiated sites and increases tissue sensitivity to subsequent x-ray therapy. This effect appears to be tissue-specific and has been noted for skin, lung, esophagus, gastrointestinal mucosa, and heart.[120-122] The results extend to both the early and late effects of radiation: doxorubicin recall reaction in the skin and heart parallels that seen in acute radiation injury, and in the lung it can increase late radiation fibrosis. Pathologic examination suggests that the predominant interaction occurs in the vascular endothelium, with doxorubicin causing an increase in the classic radiation-induced damage to the endothelial cells.

The biochemical basis for this interaction remains obscure. It should be pointed out, however, that other drugs that cause radiation recall, namely, bleomycin and actinomycin D, also share with the anthracyclines the ability both to bind DNA and to elicit the production of free radicals.[123, 124]

References

1. Brockmann H: Anthracyclinone und Anthracycline. Fortschr. Chem. Org. Naturst. 50:121, 1973.
2. Oki T: New anthracycline antibiotics. Jpn. J. Antibiot. 30:S70, 1977.

2A. Brown JP: A review of the genetic effects of naturally occurring flavonoids, anthraquinones and related compounds. Mutat. Res. 75:243, 1980.

3. El Ezaby MS, Salem TM, Zewail AH, et al.: Spectral studies of some hydroxy-derivatives of anthraquinones. J. Chem. Soc. 8:1293, 1976.
4. Phillips R, Di Marco A, and Zunino F: The interaction of daunomycin with polydeoxynucleotides. Eur. J. Biochem. 85:487, 1978.
5. Krugh TR, and Young MA: Daunomycin and Adriamycin facilitate actinomycin D binding to poly(dA-dT) · poly (dA-dT). Nature (Lond.) 269:627, 1977.
6. Patel DJ, and Canuel LL: Anthracycline antitumor antibiotic nucleic acid interactions. Structural aspects of the daunomycin–DNA complex in solution. Eur. J. Biochem. 90:247, 1978.
7. Grant M, and Phillips DR: Dissociation of polydeoxynucleotide–daunomycin complexes. Mol. Pharmacol. 16:357, 1979.
8. Pigram WJ, Fuller W, and Hamilton LD: Stereochemistry of intercalation: interaction of daunomycin with DNA. Nature 235:17, 1972.
9. Neidle S, and Taylor GL: Nucleic acid binding drugs. Some conformational properties of the anticancer drug daunomycin and several of its derivatives. FEBS Lett. 107:348, 1979.
10. Waldes H, and Center MS: The interaction of Adriamycin with nuclear DNA: evidence for a drug-induced compaction of isolated chromatin. Biochem. Biophys. Res. Commun. 98:95, 1981.
11. Painter RB: Inhibition of DNA replicon initiation by 4-nitroquinoline 1-oxide, Adriamycin and ethyleneimine. Cancer Res. 38:4445, 1978.
12. Ritch PS, Occhipinti SJ, Cunningham RE, and Shackney SE: Schedule-dependent synergism of combinations of hydroxyurea with Adriamycin and 1-beta-D-arabinofuranosylcytosine with Adriamycin. Cancer Res. 41:3881, 1981.
13. Daskal G, Woodard C, Crooke ST, et al.: Comparative ultrastructural studies on nucleoli of tumor cells treated with Adriamycin and the newer anthracyclines, carminomycin and marcellomycin. Cancer Res. 38:467, 1978.
14. Schwartz HS: DNA breaks in P288 tumor cells in mice after treatment with daunomycin and Adriamycin. Res. Commun. Chem. Pathol. Pharmacol. 10:51, 1975.
15. Ross WE, Zwelling LA, and Kohn KW: Relationship between cytotoxicity and DNA strand breakage produced by Adriamycin and other intercalating agents. Int. J. Radiat. Oncol. Biol. Phys. 5:1221, 1979.
16. Sinha BK, and Chignell CF: Binding made of chemically activated semiquinone free radicals from quinone anticancer agents to DNA. Chem. Biol. Interact. 28:301, 1979.
17. Sinha B, and Sik RH: Binding of Adriamycin to cellular macromolecules *in vivo*. Biochem. Pharmacol. 29:1867, 1980.
18. Mason RP: Free radical metabolites of foreign compounds and their toxicological significance. Rev. Biochem. Toxicol. 2:151, 1979.
19. Handa K, and Sato S: Generation of free radicals of quinone group containing anticancer chemicals in NADPH-microsome system as evidenced by initiation of sulfate oxidation. Gann 66:43, 1975.
20. Handa K, and Sato S: Stimulation of microsomal NADPH oxidation by quinone group containing anticancer chemicals. Gann 67:523, 1976.
21. Sato S, Iwaizumi M, Handa K, et al.: Electron spin resonance study on the mode of generation of free radicals of daunomycin, Adriamycin and carboquine in NADPH microsomal system. Gann 68:603, 1977.
22. Bachur NR, Gordon SL, and Gee MV: Anthracycline antibiotic augmentation of microsomal electron transport and free radical formation. Mol. Pharmacol. 13:901, 1977.
23. Bachur NR, Gordon SL, and Gee MV: A general mechanism for microsomal activation of quinone anticancer agents to free radicals. Cancer Res. 38:1745, 1977.
24. Goodman, J, and Hochstein P: Generation of free radicals and lipid peroxidation by redox cycling of Adriamycin and daunomycin. Biochem. Biophys. Res. Commun. 77:797, 1977.
25. Kalyanaraman B, Perez-Reyes E, and Mason PR: Spin-

trapping and direct electron spin resonance investigations of the redox metabolism of quinone anticancer drugs. Biochim. Biophys. Acta 630:119, 1980.

26. Fridovich I: The biology of oxygen radicals. Science 201:875, 1978.
27. Kharasch ED, and Novals RF: Ring current effects in Adriamycin–flavin mononucleotide complexation as observed by H-FT NMR spectroscopy. Biochem. Biophys. Res. Commun. 92:1320, 1980.
28. Powis G, and Appel PL: Relationship of the single-electron reduction potential of quinones to their reduction by flavoproteins. Biochem. Pharmacol. 29:2567, 1980.
29. Doroshow J: Effect of doxorubicin on oxygen radical metabolism in Ehrlich ascites tumor cells. Proc. Am. Assoc. Cancer Res. 22:805, 1981. (Abstr.)
30. Henderson CA, Metz EN, Balcerzak SP, et al.: Adriamycin and daunomycin generate reactive oxygen compounds in erythrocytes. Blood 52:878, 1978.
31. Stuart MJ, deAlarcon PA, and Barvinchak MK: Inhibition of Adriamycin-induced human platelet lipid peroxidation by vitamin E. Am. J. Hematol. 5:297, 1978.
32. Myers CE, McGuire WP, Liss RH, et al.: Adriamycin: the role of lipid peroxidation in cardiac toxicity and tumor response. Science 197:165, 1977.
33. Sonneveld P: Effect of alpha-tocopherol on the cardiac toxicity of Adriamycin in the rat. Cancer Treat. Rep. 62:1033, 1978.
34. Auerbach S, and Singer O: Adriamycin: cellular electrophysiologic changes. Fed Proc. 38:3998, 1979. (Abstr.)
35. Poggi A, Delaini F, and Donati MB: Lipid peroxidation and cardiotoxicity of Adriamycin in experimental animals: a protective role of vitamin E? *In* Internal Medicine, Part I, Excerpta Medica Internatl. Cong. Series 502, 1980, p. 386.
36. Wang YM, Madanat FF, and Kimball JC: Effect of vitamin E against Adriamycin-induced toxicity in rabbits. Cancer Res. 40:1022, 1980.
37. Olson RD, MacDonald JS, vanBoxtel CJ, et al.: Regulatory role of glutathione and soluble sulfhydryl groups in the toxicity of Adriamycin. J. Pharmacol. Exp. Ther. 215:450, 1980.
38. Thayer WS: Adriamycin-stimulated superoxide formation in submitochondrial particles. Chem. Biol. Interact. 19:265, 1977.
39. Ogura R, Toyama H, Shimada T, et al.: The role of ubiquinone in preventing Adriamycin-induced mitochondrial disorders in rat heart. J. Appl. Biochem. 1:325, 1979.
40. Doroshow JH: Mitomycin C–enhanced superoxide and hydrogen peroxide formation in rat heart. J. Pharmacol. Exp. Ther. 218:206, 1981.
41. Doroshow JH, Locker GY, and Myers CE: Enzymatic defenses of the mouse heart against reactive oxygen metabolites. J. Clin. Invest. 65:128, 1980.
42. Revis NW, and Marusic N: Glutathione peroxidase activity and selenium concentration in the hearts of doxorubicin-treated rabbtis. J. Mol. Cell. Cardiol. 10:945, 1978.
43. Murphree SA, Cunningham LS, Hwang KM, et al.: Effects of Adriamycin on surface properties of sarcoma 180 ascites cells. Biochem. Pharmacol. 25:1227, 1976.
44. Solie TN, and Yunker C: Adriamycin-induced changes in translocation of sodium ions in transporting epithelial cells. Life Sci. 22:1907, 1978.
45. Villani F, Piccinini F, Merelli P, et al.: Influence of Adriamycin on calcium exchangeability in cardiac muscle and its modification by ouabain. Biochem. Pharmacol. 27:985, 1978.
46. Goldman, R, Facchinetti T, Bach D, et al.: A differential interaction of daunomycin, Adriamycin and their derivatives with human erythrocytes and phospholipid bilayers. Biochim. Biophys. Acta 512:254, 1978.
47. Mikkelsen RB, Lin PS, and Wallach DF: Interaction of Adriamycin with human red blood cells: a biochemical and morphological study. J. Mol. Med. 2:33, 1977.
48. Kessel D: Enhanced glycosylation induced by Adriamycin. Mol. Pharmacol. 16:306, 1979.
49. Duarte-Karim M, Ruysschaert JM, and Hildebrand J: Affinity of Adriamycin to phospholipids — a possible explanation for cardiac mitochondrial lesions. Biochem. Biophys. Res. Commun. 71:658, 1976.
50. Tritton TR, Murphree SA, and Sartorelli AC: Adriamycin: a proposal on the specificity of drug action. Biochem. Biophys. Res. Commun. 84:802, 1978.
51. Goormaghtigh E, Chatelain P, Caspers J, et al.: Evidence of a specific complex between Adriamycin and negatively charged phospholipids. Biochim. Biophys. Acta 597:1, 1980.
52. Goormaghtigh E, Chatelain P, Caspers J, et al.: Evidence of a complex between Adriamycin derivatives and cardiolipin: possible role in cardiotoxicity. Biochem. Pharmacol. 29:3003, 1980.
53. Knowles AF, Eytan E, and Racker E: Phospholipid-protein interactions in the calcium-adenosine triphosphatase of sarcoplasmic reticulum. J. Biol. Chem. 251:5161, 1976.
54. Sugioka K, Nakano H, Noguchi I, et al.: Decomposition of unsaturated phospholipid by iron–ADP–Adriamycin coordination complex. Biochem. Biophys. Res. Commun. 100:1251, 1981.
55. Calendi E, DiMarco A, Reggiani M, et al.: On physicochemical interactions between daunomycin and nucleic acids. Biochim. Biophys. Acta 103:25, 1965.
56. May PM, Williams GK, and Williams DR: Solution chemistry studies of Adriamycin–iron complexes present *in vivo*. Eur. J. Cancer 16:1275, 1980.
57. Mikelens P, and Levinson W: Metal ion participation in binding of daunomycinol, daunomycin and Adriamycin to nucleic acids. Bioinorg. Chem. 9:441, 1978.
58. Young DM: Pathologic effects of Adriamycin in experimental systems. Cancer Chemother. Rep. 6:159, 1975.
59. Myers C, Simone C, Gianni L, et al.: The role of doxorubicin–iron complex in superoxide production and membrane damage. Proc. Am. Assoc. Cancer Res. 22:112, 1981.
60. Henry DW: Structure-activity relationships among daunorubicin and Adriamycin analogs. Cancer Treat. Rep. 63:845, 1979.
61. Egorin MJ, Clawson RE, Ross LA, et al.: Cellular accumulation and disposition of aclacinomycin A. Cancer Res. 39:4396, 1979.
62. Tong GL, Henry DW, and Acton EM: 5-Iminodaunorubicin. Reduced cardiotoxic properties in an antitumor anthracycline. J. Med. Chem. 22:36, 1979.
63. Lown JW, Chen HH, Plambeck JA, et al.: Diminished superoxide anion generation by reduced 5-iminodaunorubicin relative to daunorubicin and the anthracycline antitumor agents. Biochem. Pharmacol. 28:2563, 1979.
64. Crooke ST, DuVernay VH, Galvan L, et al.: Structure-activity relationships of anthracyclines relative to effects on macromolecular syntheses. Mol. Pharmacol. 14:290, 1978.
65. Tong GL, Wu HY, Smith TH, et al.: Synthesis of N-alkylated anthracyclines with enhanced efficacy and reduced cardiotoxicity. J. Med. Chem. 22:912, 1979.
66. Zee-Cheng RKY, and Cheng CC: Antineoplastic agents. Structure-activity relationship study of bis (substituted aminoalkylamino) anthraquinones. J. Med. Chem. 21:291, 1978.
67. Double JL, and Brown JR: Evaluation of some substituted anthraquinones and naphthacarboquinones of DNA. J. Pharm. Pharmacol. 28:166, 1976.
68. Cheng CC, Zbinder G, and Zee-Cheng RKY: Comparison of antineoplastic activity of aminoethylaminoanthraquinones and anthracycline antibiotics. J. Pharm. Sci. 68:393, 1979.
69. Skovsgaard T: Carrier-mediated transport of daunorubicin, Adriamycin and rubidazone in Ehrlich ascites tumor cells. Biochem. Pharmacol. 27:1221, 1978.
70. Skovsgaard T: Transport and binding of daunorubicin, Adriamycin and rubidazone in Ehrlich ascites tumor cells. Biochem. Pharmacol. 26:215, 1977.
71. Dano K: Active outward transport of daunomycin in resistant Ehrlich ascites tumor cells. Biochim. Biophys. Acta 323:466, 1973.
72. Inaba M, Kobayashi H, Sakurai Y, et al.: Active efflux of

daunorubicin and Adriamycin in sensitive and resistant sublines to P388 leukemia. Cancer Res. 39:2200, 1979.
73. Dalmark M, and Strom HH: A fickian diffusion transport process with feature of transport catalysis. J. Gen. Physiol. 78:349, 1981.
74. Juliano RL, and Ling V: A surface glycoprotein modulating drug permeability in Chinese hamster ovary cell mutant. Biochem. Biophys. Acta 455:152, 1976.
75. Baskin F, Rosenbery R, and Dev V: Correlation of double-minute chromosomes with unstable multidrug cross-resistance in uptake mutants of neuroblastoma cells. Proc. Natl. Acad. Sci. USA 78:3654, 1981.
76. Ahmed NK, Felsted RL, and Bachur NR: Heterogeneity of anthracycline antibiotic carbamyl reductases in mammalian liver. Biochem. Pharmacol. 27:2713, 1978.
77. Beran M, Andersson B, Eksborg S, et al.: Comparative studies on the *in vitro* killing of human normal and leukemic clonogenic cells by daunorubicin, daunorubicinol and daunorubicin–DNA complex. Cancer Chemother. Pharmacol. 2:19, 1979.
78. Ozols RF, Willson JKV, Weltz MD, et al.: Inhibition of human ovarian cancer colony formation by Adriamycin and its major metabolites. Cancer Res. 40:4109, 1980.
79. Schwartz HS: A fluorometric assay for daunomycin and Adriamycin in animal tissues. Biochem. Med. 7:396, 1973.
80. Chan KK, and Wong CD: Quantitative thin-layer chromatography: thin film fluorescence scanning analysis of Adriamycin and metabolites in tissue. J. Chromatogr. 172:343, 1979.
81. Chan KK, and Watson E: GLC–mass spectrometry of several important anticancer drugs. II. Doxorubicin and daunorubicin aglycone analogs. J. Pharm. Sci. 67:1748, 1978.
82. Israel M, Pegg WJ, Wilkinson PM, et al.: Liquid chromatographic analysis of Adriamycin and metabolites in biological fluids. J. Liquid Chromatogr. 1:795, 1978.
83. Eksborg S, Ehronson H, and Andersson I: Reversed-phase liquid chromatographic determination of plasma levels of Adriamycin and adriamycinol. J. Chromatogr. 164:479, 1979.
84. Andrews PA, Brennen DE, Chou FTE, et al.: Facile and definitive determination of Adriamycin and daunorubicin metabolites. Drug Metab. Dispos. 8:152, 1980.
85. Sepanick MJ, and Yeung ES: Determination of Adriamycin and daunorubicin in urine by HPLC with laser fluorometric detection. J. Chromatogr. 190:377, 1980.
86. Chan KK, Cohen JL, Gross JF, et al.: Prediction of Adriamycin disposition in cancer patients using a physiologic pharmacokinetic model. Cancer Treat. Rep. 62:1161, 1978.
87. Reich SD: Clinical correlations of Adriamycin pharmacology. Pharmacol. Ther. 2:239, 1978.
88. Takanashi S, and Bachur NR: Adriamycin metabolism in man. Drug Metab. Dispos. 4:79, 1976.
89. Garnick MB, Ensminger WD, and Israel M: A clinical-pharmacological evaluation of hepatic arterial infusion of Adriamycin. Cancer Res. 34:4105, 1979.
90. Chan KK, Chlebowski RT, Tong M, et al.: Clinical pharmacokinetics of Adriamycin in hepatoma patients with cirrhosis. Cancer Res 40:1263, 1980.
91. Menozzi M, and Arcamone F: Binding of Adriamycin to sulphated mucopolysaccharides. Biochem. Biophys. Res. Commun. 80:313, 1978.
92. Wright SD, and Bachur MT: Alterations in Adriamycin efficacy by phenobarbital. Cancer Res. 36:3803, 1976.
93. Krugh TR, and Young MA: Daunomycin and Adriamycin facilitate actinomycin D binding to poly(dA-dT) poly(dA-dT). Nature (Lond.) 269:627, 1977.
94. Nishimura T, Muto K, and Tanaka N: Drug sensitivity of an Adriamycin-resistant mutant subline of mouse lymphoblastoma L5178Y cells. J. Antibiot. 31:493, 1978.
95. Tan L, Etubanas E, Wollner W, et al.: Adriamycin — an antitumor antibiotic in the treatment of neoplastic diseases. Cancer 32:9, 1973.
96. Cortes EP, Lutman G, Wanka J, et al.: Adriamycin cardiotoxicity: a clinicopathologic correlation. Cancer Chemother. Rep. (Pt. 3) 6:215, 1975.
97. O'Bryan R, Luce J, Talley R, et al.: Phase II evaluation of Adriamycin in human neoplasia. Cancer 32:1, 1973.
98. Bristow MR, Thompson PD, and Martin RP: Early anthracycline cardiotoxicity. Am. J. Med. 65:823, 1978.
99. Singer JW, Narahara KA, Ritchie JL, et al.: Time- and dose-dependent changes in ejection fraction determined by radionuclide angiography after anthracycline therapy. Cancer Treat. Rep. 62:945, 1978.
100. Bristow MR, Mason JW, Billingham ME, et al.: Adriamycin cardiomyopathy: evaluation by phonography, endomyocardial biopsy and cardiac catheterization. Ann. Intern. Med. 88:168, 1978.
101. Alexander J, Daniels N, Berger HJ, et al: Serial assessment of doxorubicin cardiotoxicity with quantitative radionuclide angiocardiography. N. Engl. J. Med. 300:278, 1979.
102. Von Hoff DD, and Layard MW: Risk factors for doxorubicin-induced congestive heart failure. Ann. Intern. Med. 91:710, 1979.
103. Gottdiener JS, Mathisen DJ, Borer JS, et al.: Doxorubicin cardiotoxicity: assessment of late left ventricular dysfunction by radionuclide cineangiography. Ann. Intern. Med. 94:430, 1981.
104. Pratt CB, Ransom JL, and Evans WE: Age-related Adriamycin cardiotoxicity in Children. Cancer Treat. Rep. 62:1381, 1978.
105. Minow RA, Benjamin RS, and Lee ET: Adriamycin cardiomyopathy — risk factors. Cancer 39:1397, 1977.
106. Braunwald E, and Ross J: Control of cardiac performance. *In* Berne R, Sperelakis N, and Geiger S (eds.): Handbook of Physiology. Sec. 2, The Cardiovascular System, Vol 1. The Heart. American Physiology Society, Bethesda, 1979.
107. Brockmann E, and Zbinden G: Effect of doxorubicin and rubidazone on respiratory function and calcium transport in rat heart mitochondria. Toxicol. Lett. 3:29, 1979.
108. Revis N, and Marusic N: Sequestration of calcium 45 by mitochondria from rabbit heart, liver and kidney after doxorubicin or digoxin, daunorubicin treatment. Exp. Mol. Pathol. 31:440, 1979.
109. Olson HM, Young DM, Prieun DJ, et al.: Electrolyte and morphologic alterations of myocardium in Adriamycin-treated rabbits. Am. J. Pathol. 77:439, 1974.
110. Toyo-Oka T, and Masaki T: Calcium-activated neutral protease from bovine ventricular muscle: isolation and some of its properties. J. Mol. Cell. Cardiol. 11:769, 1979.
111. Myers CE: Cardiac toxicity. *In* DeVita VT, Hellman S, and Rosenberg SA (eds.): Cancer: Principles and Practice of Oncology. J.B. Lippincott Co. Philadelphia, 1982.
112. Bristow MR, Mason JW, Billingham ME, et al.: Doxorubicin cardiomyopathy: evaluation by phonocardiography, endocardial biopsy and cardiac catheterization. Ann. Intern. Med. 88:168, 1978.
113. Billingham ME, Mason JW, Bristow MR, et al.: Anthracycline cardiomyopathy monitored by morphologic changes. Cancer Treat. Rep. 62:865, 1978.
114. Weiss AJ, and Manthel RW: Experience with the use of Adriamycin in combination with other anticancer agents using a weekly schedule, with particular reference to lack of cardiac toxicity. Cancer 40:2046, 1977.
115. Legha SS, Benjamin RS, Mackay B, et al.: Reduction of doxorubicin cardiotoxicity by prolonged continuous intravenous infusion. Ann. Intern. Med. 96:113, 1982.
116. Doroshow JH, Locker CY, Ifrim I, et al.: Prevention of doxorubicin cardiac toxicity in the mouse by N-acetylcysteine. J. Clin. Invest. 68:1053, 1981.
117. Herman E, Ardalan D, Bier C, et al.: Reduction of daunorubicin lethality and myocardial cellular alterations by pretreatment with ICRF-187 in Syrian golden hamsters. Cancer Treat. Rep. 63:89, 1979.
118. Iwamoto, Y, Hassen IL, Porter TH, et al.: Inhibition of coenzyme Q10 enzymes, succinoidase and NADH-oxidase by Adriamycin and other quinones having antitumor activity. Biochem. Biophys. Res. Commun. 58:633, 1974.
119. Svingen BA, Powis G, Appel PL, et al.: Protection against

Adriamycin-induced skin necrosis in the rat by dimethylsulfoxide and alpha-tocopherol. Cancer Res. 41:3395, 1981.

120. Aristizabal SA, Miller RC, Schlichtemeier AL, et al.: Adriamycin-irradiation cutaneous complications. Int. J. Radiat. Oncol. Biol. Phys. 2:325, 1977.

121. Billingham, ME, Mason GW, Bristow MR, et al.: Anthracycline cardiomyopathy monitored by morphologic changes. Cancer Treat. Rep. 62:865, 1978.

122. McInery DP, and Bullimore J: Reactivation of radiation pneumonitis by Adriamycin. Br. J. Radiol. 50:224, 1977.

123. Sausville EA, Stein RW, Pleisach J, et al.: Properties and products of the degradation of DNA by bleomycin and iron. Biochemistry 17:2746, 1978.

124. Bachur NR, Gee M, and Gordon L: Enzymatic activation of actinomycin D to a free radical state. Proc. Am. Assoc. Cancer Res. 19:78, 1978. (Abstr.)

ENZYME THERAPY: L-ASPARAGINASE

21

Yung-Pin Liu
Bruce A. Chabner

INTRODUCTION

The growth of malignant as well as normal cells depends on the availability of specific nutrients used in the synthesis of protein, nucleic acids, and lipids. Some of these nutrients can be synthesized within the cell, but others are required from external sources such as another organ (liver) or from food sources (essential amino acids). Nutritional therapy of cancer has been directed at identifying differences between the host and malignant cells that might be exploited in treatment; these attempts have been largely unsuccessful owing to difficulties in producing a deficiency state by dietary means, and a lack of clear differences between the rapidly proliferating host cells and the tumor. The only exception has been the use of L-asparaginase in the treatment of childhood acute leukemia.

L-Asparagine is a non-essential amino acid that is synthesized by transamination of L-aspartic acid (Fig. 21–1). The amine group in this reaction is donated by glutamine, and the reaction is catalyzed by the enzyme L-asparagine synthetase. This enzyme is constitutive in many tissues, thus accounting for the lack of toxicity of asparagine depletion, but is present in very low concentrations in certain human malignancies, particularly those of T-lymphocyte derivation. In tumor cells lacking L-asparagine synthetase, such as L5178Y murine leukemia cells,[1] the amino acid can be obtained only from a culture medium, or *in vivo*, from the circulating pool of amino acids.

L-Asparaginase (L-asparagine amidohydrolase, E.C. 3.5.1.1), which catalyzes the hydrolysis of asparagine to aspartic acid and ammonia as end products, is widely distributed in many plants, animals, and microorganisms. General interest in L-asparaginase as a therapeutic agent was the result of an early, unexplained observation by Kidd,[2] who in 1953 reported that the growth of transplantable lymphomas of rat and mouse was inhibited by guinea pig serum but not by rabbit, horse, or human sera. Ten years later, Broome and co-workers demonstrated that the responsible factor was the enzyme L-asparaginase.[3] Subsequently, highly purified preparations of enzyme from *Escherichia coli*[4] and *Erwinia carotovora*[5] have shown significant activity against childhood acute lymphocytic leukemia and have become standard components of induction regimens in this disease. The clinical and biochemical features of L-asparaginase chemotherapy have been summarized in several comprehensive reviews by important investigators in this field.[6-8]

PROPERTIES AND MECHANISM OF ACTION

L-Asparaginase purified from *E. coli*[9] has been utilized most widely in both basic and clinical research, although L-asparaginase obtained from other sources, including *Erwinia carotovora*, *Serratia marcescens*, guinea pig serum, and the serum from a variety of other members of the species *Caviodea* also possess antitumor activity. The purified bacterial enzyme has a molecular weight of 133,000 to 141,000 daltons and is composed of four subunits, each having one

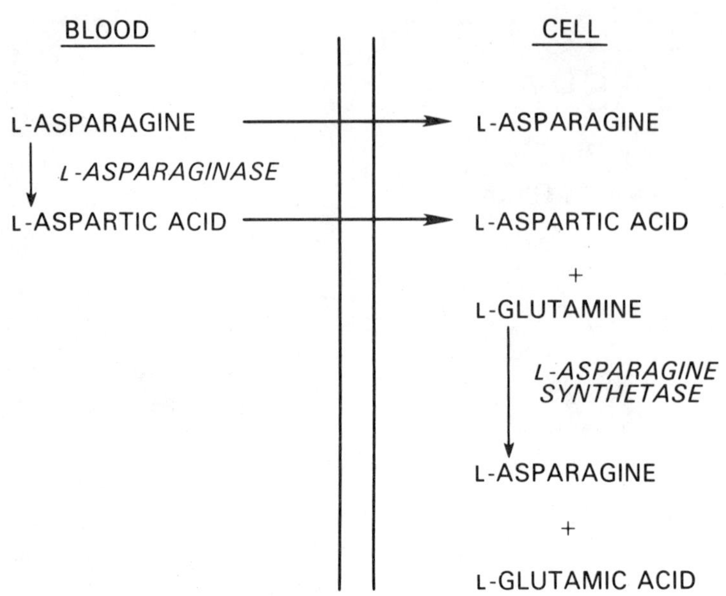

Figure 21–1. Sources of L-asparagine for peripheral tissues. The amino acid may be obtained directly from the circulating blood pool of L-asparagine, or may be synthesized by transamination of L-aspartic acid, L-glutamine acting as the NH_3 donor in a reaction catalyzed by L-asparagine synthetase.

active site.[10, 11] Preparations of enzyme from different bacterial strains and by different purification methods have slight differences in enzyme characteristics. For the bacterial enzymes, the specific activity of purified enzyme is usually 300 to 400 μmol per min per mg protein, the isoelectric point lies between pH 4.6 and 5.5, and the K_m for asparagine is usually 1×10^{-5}M.[10-12] The *E. coli* enzyme contains 321 amino acids in each subunit (molecular weight 34,080).[11] The complete amino acid sequence of this enzyme is shown in Figure 21–2.

The *E. coli* enzyme is highly specific for L-asparagine as substrate and has less than 10 per cent activity for the D-isomer, for N-acylated derivatives, or for L-asparagine in peptide linkage. In contrast, the enzyme from *Saccharomyces cerevisiae* has equal or greater activity with D-asparagine and with N-substituted substrates.[13]

The hydrolysis of L-asparagine proceeds according to a reaction mechanism that involves an initial displacement of the amino acid NH_2 group during the formation of an enzyme-aspartyl intermediate, followed by hydrolytic cleavage of the latter bond to generate free L-aspartate and active enzyme. The reaction may be summarized:

$$E + Asn \underset{+NH_3}{\overset{-NH_3}{\rightleftharpoons}} E \cdot Asp \longrightarrow E + Asp$$

where E · Asp represents the enzyme-aspartyl intermediate.[13, 14] The reaction is irreversibly inhibited by the L-asparagine analogue 5-diazo-4-oxo-L-norvaline, which binds covalently to the enzyme's active site.[15]

CHEMICAL MODIFICATION

In an attempt to reduce the immunogenicity of L-asparaginase, to eliminate L-glutaminase activity, and to prolong its plasma half-life, the *E. coli* enzyme has been subjected to various modifications. Most bacterial L-asparaginase preparations contain significant L-glutaminase activity (about 3 to 5 per cent of the L-asparaginase activity). The enzyme from mammalian sources or from certain bacteria (*Vibrio succinogenes* in particular) lacks L-glutaminase activity, but unfortunately has lesser affinity for L-asparaginase[16] and thus is less desirable for clinical purposes. There is evidence that the immunosuppressive properties of *E. coli* enzyme may result from L-glutamine depletion[17, 18] and that cerebral dysfunction observed clinically may be the result of L-glutamine degradation. Attempts have been made to modify the *E. coli* enzyme in order to eliminate the L-glutaminase activity[19]; the nitrated enzyme has little L-glutaminase, but also has reduced L-asparaginase action.

The addition of multiple poly-DL-alanine side chains varying in length from 14 to 34 amino acids markedly decreases the ability of the enzyme to elicit an antibody response

10 20 30
Leu-Pro-Asn-Ile-Thr-Ile-Leu-Ala-Thr-Gly-Gly-Thr-Ile-Ala-Gly-Gly-Gly-Asp-Ser-Ala-Thr-Lys-Ser-Asn-Tyr-Thr-Ala-Gly-Lys-Val-

40 50 60
Gly-Val-Glu-Asn-Leu-Val-Asn-Ala-Val-Pro-Gln-Leu-Lys-Asp-Ile-Ala-Asn-Val-Lys-Gly-Glu-Gln-Val-Val-Asn-Ile-Gly-Ser-Gln-Asp-

70 80 90
Met-Asn-Asp-Asp-Val-Trp-Leu-Thr-Leu-Ala-Lys-Lys-Ile-Asn-Thr-Asp-Cys-Asp-Lys-Thr-Asp-Gly-Phe-Val-Ile-Thr-His-Gly-Thr-Asp-

100 110 120
Thr-Met-Glu-Glu-Thr-Ala-Tyr-Phe-Leu-Asp-Leu-Thr-Val-Lys-Cys-Asp-Lys-Pro-Val-Met-Val-Gly-Ala-Met-Arg-Pro-Ser-Thr-Ser-Met-

130 140 150
Ser-Ala-Asp-Gly-Pro-Phe-Asn-Leu-Tyr-Asn-Ala-Val-Thr-Ala-Ala-Asp-Lys-Ala-Ser-Ala-Asn-Arg-Gly-Val-Leu-Val-Met-Asn-Asp-Thr-

160 170 180
Val-Leu-Asp-Gly-Arg-Asp-Val-Thr-Lys-Thr-Asn-Thr-Thr-Asp-Val-Ala-Thr-Phe-Lys-Ser-Val-Asn-Tyr-Gly-Pro-Leu-Gly-Tyr-Ile-His-

190 200 210
Asp-Gly-Lys-Ile-Asp-Tyr-Gln-Arg-Thr-Pro-Ala-Arg-Lys-His-Thr-Ser-Asp-Thr-Pro-Phe-Asp-Val-Ser-Lys-Leu-Asn-Glu-Leu-Pro-Lys-

220 230 240
Val-Gly-Ile-Val-Tyr-Asn-Tyr-Ala-Asn-Ala-Ser-Asp-Leu-Pro-Ala-Lys-Ala-Leu-Val-Asp-Ala-Gly-Tyr-Asp-Gly-Ile-Val-Ser-Ala-Gly-

250 260 270
Val-Gly-Asp-Gly-Asn-Leu-Tyr-Lys-Thr-Val-Phe-Asp-Thr-Leu-Ala-Thr-Ala-Ala-Lys-Asp-Gly-Thr-Ala-Val-Arg-Ser-Ser-Arg-Val-Pro-

280 290 300
Thr-Gly-Ala-Thr-Thr-Gln-Asp-Ala-Glu-Val-Asp-Asp-Ala-Lys-Tyr-Gly-Phe-Val-Ala-Ser-Gly-Thr-Leu-Asn-Pro-Gln-Lys-Ala-Arg-Val-

310 320
Leu-Leu-Gln-Ala-Leu-Thr-Gln-Thr-Lys-Asp-Pro-Gln-Gln-Ile-Gln-Gln-Ile-Phe-Asn-Gln-Tyr

Figure 21–2. Complete amino acid sequence of the subunit of *E. coli* L-asparaginase. (Reproduced with permission from Maita T, and Matsuda G: The primary structure of L-asparaginase from *Escherichia coli.* Hoppe Seylers Z. Physiol. Chem. 361:105, 1980.)

in mice, and produces a 3000-fold decrease in reactivity with anti-L-asparaginase antibody, without substantially changing the enzymatic activity or its affinity for L-asparagine.[20] The modified enzyme is markedly resistant to tryptic degradation and has a sevenfold prolonged plasma half-life as compared with the native preparation. The poly-alanyl side chains appear to prevent access of antigen-processing cells, antibody, and digestive enzymes to L-asparaginase. The enzyme, modified by conjugation with monomethoxypolyethylene glycol, displays a similar decrease in immunogenicity and an increase in plasma half-life, but retains only 8 per cent of its initial activity.[21] A copolymer formed with albumin has markedly reduced immunoreactivity and "satisfactory" activity in mice.[22] However, since allergic reactions can be reduced in clinical use by intramuscular administration, and combination treatment with 6-mercaptopurine, the decreased immunogenicity of these preparations has not proved sufficiently advantageous to justify the increased cost of their production.

In addition to chemical modification, the enzyme has been attached to the external surface of hollow fiber dialysis tubing with the aim of hydrolyzing the filtered amino acid during hemodialysis, thus avoiding patient exposure to the immunogenic enzyme.[23, 24] The approach has the significant drawback of requiring prolonged periods of dialysis and is likely to achieve only temporary depletion of plasma L-asparagine since the amino acid levels are rapidly replenished by release of L-asparagine from the liver.[25]

MODE OF ACTION

The antitumor effects of L-asparaginase result from the rapid and complete depletion of circulating pools of L-asparagine, while resistance to treatment arises through an increase in L-asparagine synthetase activity in tumor cells.[26, 27] This increase occurs either through selection of a subpopulation of cells containing the synthetase, or by derepression of the synthetase as the result of a fall in intracellular L-asparagine levels. Plasma L-asparagine levels (usually in the range of 4×10^{-5}M) are more than sufficient to supply the amino acid for L-asparagine–requiring tumor cells, which can be maintained in tissue culture by concentrations of

1×10^{-6}M.[28] Since the K_m of the *E. coli* enzyme for L-asparagine is 1×10^{-5}M, considerable excess L-asparaginase is required in plasma to degrade L-asparagine to sufficiently low concentrations to halt tumor growth.

CELLULAR EFFECTS

The cellular effects of L-asparaginase result from inhibition of protein synthesis. Cytotoxicity correlates well with the enzyme's effects on the incorporation of an amino acid such as ^{3}H-valine into protein. Inhibition of nucleic acid synthesis is also observed in sensitive cells, but is believed to be secondary to the block in protein synthesis. Cells insensitive to asparagine depletion from growth medium *in vitro* are also insensitive to L-asparaginase, and show little inhibition of RNA or protein synthesis in the presence of the enzyme. As might be expected, these resistant cells have high endogenous activity of asparagine synthetase.[26, 27]

PHARMACOLOGIC CONSIDERATIONS

The *in vivo* clearance rate of the enzyme and its Michaelis constant (K_m) are two important factors that may play roles in determining the efficacy of asparaginase as an antitumor agent. L-Asparaginases isolated from *Bacillus coagulans, Fusarium tricinctum,* and *Candida albicans* are devoid of antitumor activity and are almost completely cleared from the circulation in 30 minutes to one hour after intravenous administration into mice. On the other hand, enzymes derived from guinea pig serum and from *E. coli* exhibited antitumor activity and have a much longer half-life.[29, 30] The affinity of the enzyme for L-asparagine might be another important factor responsible for the antitumor activity of L-asparaginase.[31] *E. coli* and *Erwinia carotovora* L-asparaginase, which possess strong antitumor activity, have K_m values of 1 to 1.25×10^{-5}M,[32] whereas L-asparaginase derived from agouti or guinea pig serum has only moderate antitumor activity and a K_m of 4.1 and 7.2×10^{-5}M, respectively.[33] In addition, enzymes from *Erwinia aroideae* ($K_m = 3 \times 10^{-3}$M)[34] or *Bacillus coagulans* ($K_m = 4.7 \times 10^{-3}$M)[35] have low substrate affinity and have no tumor-inhibitory activity.

Drug Assay and Pharmacokinetics

L-Asparaginase is easily measured in biologic fluids by assays that detect ammonia release[36] or by a coupled enzymic assay.[37] The drug is given intravenously or intramuscularly; the latter route produces peak blood levels 50 per cent lower than the former. The usual doses are 6000 International Units (IU) per m^2 every other day for three to four weeks, or daily doses of 1000 to 2000 IU per m^2 for 10 to 20 days. A comparison of the clinical effectiveness of various doses of L-asparaginase given three times per week demonstrated a higher complete remission rate for doses of 6000 IU per m^2 or higher as compared with 3000 IU per m^2 or less[38] (Fig. 21–3). Although blood levels of L-asparaginase are detectable for one to three weeks after these doses, and L-asparagine is absent from serum for similar time intervals, widely spaced schedules of administration are infrequently used because of lesser therapeutic effectiveness and the increased risk of anaphylaxis.[39] Blood concentrations of L-asparagine fall below 1 μM within minutes of enzyme injection, and remain unmeasurable for seven to ten days after completion of therapy.[40]

L-Asparaginase concentration in plasma is proportional to dose for doses up to 200,000 IU per m^2, and falls with a primary half-life of 14 to 22 hours. The Merck preparation of L-asparaginase has a somewhat longer half-life than the Bayer preparation. In patients who develop hypersensitivity to the enzyme, plasma clearance is greatly accelerated and enzyme activity may be undetectable in plasma as soon as four hours after administration.[41] The enzyme distributes primarily within the intravascular space. However, the cerebrospinal fluid concentration of asparagine falls rapidly, and an antileukemic effect is exerted in this sanctuary, despite the poor penetration of enzyme into the CSF. The drug can be given directly into the CSF, but exits rapidly from this site, and there appears to be no clear therapeutic advantage for this route.

TOXICITY

The primary toxicities of L-asparaginase, listed in Table 21–1,[40] fall into two main groups: those related to immunologic sensi-

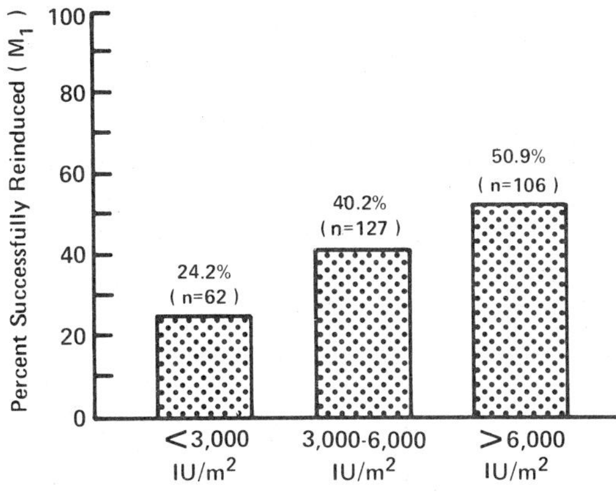

Figure 21–3. Relationship between dose of L-asparaginase and response in the treatment of acute lymphoblastic leukemia. Patients received the indicated doses every other day, three doses per week for a maximum of six weeks. Successful induction is judged by achievement of an M-1 bone marrow status. (Reproduced with permission from Ertel et al.: Effective dose of L-asparaginase for induction of remission in previously treated children with acute lymphocytic leukemia: a report from Children's Cancer Study Group. Cancer Res. 39:3893, 1979.)

tization to the foreign protein, and those resulting from depletion of asparagine pools and inhibition of protein synthesis. Hypersensitivity reactions to L-asparaginase are a common complication of therapy, particularly when the drug is used as a single agent.[41, 42] Up to 43 per cent of patients receiving single-agent treatment develop some evidence of sensitization.[42, 43] Possibly because of the immunosuppressive effect of corticosteroids, 6-mercaptopurine, and other antileukemic agents, the incidence of hypersensitivity reactions falls to less than 10 per cent in patients receiving combination chemotherapy.[42] Other factors that increase the incidence of reactions include doses above 6000 IU per m^2,[42, 44] intravenous as opposed to intramuscular administration,[44] and repeated courses of treatment. Reactions to an initial dose rarely occur; more commonly, hypersensitivity phenomena appear during the second week of treatment or later.[45]

The clinical manifestations of hypersensitivity vary from urticaria (approximately two thirds of reported reactions)[42] to true anaphylactic reactions (hypotension, laryngospasm, cardiac arrest). Rarely, serum sickness–type responses — with arthralgias, proteinuria, and fever — may follow an extended course of treatment.[42, 45] Fatal reactions occur in less than 1 per cent of patients treated,[45, 46] but evidence of hypersensitivity should prompt a change in treatment to L-asparaginase derived from *Erwinia carotovora*,[47] which does not share antigenic cross-reactivity with the *E. coli* preparation and thus can safely be given to patients hypersensitive to the latter agent. The *E. carotovora* drug is not sold commercially, but, for treatment of acute lymphocytic leukemia, can be obtained from the Investigational Drug Branch, National Cancer Institute, Bethesda, MD 20205. Allergic reactions to *Erwinia* L-asparaginase may occur as an independent phenomenon in patients who have not previously received *E. coli* enzyme.[48]

Because of the frequency and severity of allergic reactions to L-asparaginase, some investigators have sought to use skin testing for prediction of these reactions, but allergic reactions may occur in patients with negative skin tests,[49] and positive skin tests are not invariably predictive of reactions. Hypersensitive patients usually have both IgE and IgG antibodies to L-asparaginase in serum,[50, 51] but more than half the patients with such antibodies will not display an allergic reaction to the drug clinically. Thus, the antibody tests have limited value for

TABLE 21–1. Toxicity of L-Asparaginase*

Immediate Reaction	(70%)
Nausea, vomiting, fever, chills	
Hypersensitivity Reactions	(<10%)
Urticaria	
Bronchospasm	
Hypotension	
Decreased Protein Synthesis	(100%)
Albumin	
Insulin	
Clotting factors II, V, VII, VIII, IX, X	
Serum lipoproteins	
Antithrombin III	
Cerebral Dysfunction	(33%)
Disorientation	
Coma	
Seizures	
Organ Toxicities	
Pancreatitis	(15%)
Liver function test abnormalities	(100%)
Azotemia (? increased nitrogen load)	(68%)

*Reproduced with permission from Ohnuma T, Holland JF, and Sinks LF: Biochemical and pharmacological studies with L-asparaginase in man. Cancer Res. 30:2297, 1970.

predicting which patient will have an allergic reaction.

Other toxic effects result from inhibition of protein synthesis and include hypoalbuminemia, decrease in clotting factors, decreased serum insulin with hyperglycemia, and decreased serum lipoproteins. Abnormalities in clotting function are regularly observed in association with L-asparaginase therapy and include prolongation of the prothrombin time, partial thromboplastin time, and thrombin time[43, 52, 53]; a marked fall in plasma fibrinogen[54]; and decrease in factors IX and XI.[42, 55] In addition, platelets from L-asparaginase–treated subjects display deficient aggregation in response to collagen, but not to adenosine diphosphate, arachidonic acid, or epinephrine.[56] Bleeding episodes have been infrequent in patients treated with the enzyme; when such episodes do occur, they have been difficult to attribute to L-asparaginase because of the presence of thrombocytopenia in leukemic patients. Two instances have been reported[57] of a spontaneous intracranial hemorrhage in children with marked hypofibrinogenemia.

Although the above defects tend to prevent clotting, L-asparaginase also decreases the synthesis of antithrombin III, a physiologic anticoagulant and protease inhibitor. Circulating levels of this factor fall to 50 per cent or less as compared with controls during daily or thrice-weekly treatment with L-asparaginase.[58] Two cases of venous thrombosis associated with depressed antithrombin III levels have been reported,[59, 60] but again it is difficult to be certain of a causal relationship.

Other toxicities are not as easily explained by the drug's mode of action. In 25 per cent of patients, cerebral dysfunction with confusion, stupor, or frank coma may develop.[40] The latter syndrome resembles ammonia toxicity, but is not clearly correlated with serum ammonia levels and may be the result of low concentrations of either L-asparagine or L-glutamine in the brain. Probable or definite improvement in cerebral dysfunction has been observed in three patients treated with infusions of L-asparagine, 1 to 2 mmoles per kg per day for up to 44 days.[40]

Acute pancreatitis is an infrequent complication, occurring in fewer than 15 per cent of patients, but it may progress to severe hemorrhagic pancreatitis. L-Asparaginase is frequently the cause of abnormal liver function tests, including increased serum bilirubin, SGOT, and alkaline phosphatase. Liver biopsy reveals fatty metamorphosis that is probably due to decreased mobilization of lipids.

Approximately two thirds of patients receiving L-asparaginase experience nausea, vomiting, and chills as an immediate reaction, but these side effects can be mitigated by antiemetics, antihistamines, or, in extreme cases, corticosteroids.

L-Asparaginase has no known toxicity to gastrointestinal mucosa or bone marrow, and is thus a favorable agent for use in combination chemotherapy. The only well-established drug interaction is its ability to terminate methotrexate action.[61] The antagonism of L-asparaginase given prior to methotrexate is likely the result of inhibition of protein synthesis, with consequent prevention of cell entry into the vulnerable S phase of the cell cycle. Following a single intravenous dose of L-asparaginase, inhibition of DNA synthesis lasts for approximately ten days, a period during which cells are refractory to methotrexate. This interval is followed by a period of increased DNA synthetic activity as cells recover from the block in protein synthesis; during this recovery period, cells are thought to be particularly vulnerable to methotrexate.[62] These considerations form the rationale for the clinical trials that employ an initial dose of L-asparaginase, followed in 10 to 14 days by methotrexate.

A second feature of L-asparaginase–

TABLE 21–2. Regimen for Combined Methotrexate–L-Asparaginase Treatment of Refractory Acute Leukemia*

Day:	0	13	14	27	28
R_x:					
L-Asparaginase 500 IU/kg	x		x		x
Methotrexate		100 mg/m²		↑ or ↓ per toxicity	

*Reproduced with permission from Lobel et al.: Methotrexate and asparaginase combination chemotherapy in refractory acute leukemia of childhood. Cancer 43:1089, 1979.

methotrexate interaction is important in combination chemotherapy. If the enzyme is given 24 hours after methotrexate, the action of the antifolate is abbreviated at that point. Thus, large doses of methotrexate are well tolerated if followed in 24 hours by L-asparaginase. Capizzi has devised a regimen, shown in Table 21–2, which begins with L-asparaginase, followed in 10 days by methotrexate and 24 hours later by L-asparaginase rescue.[61, 62] Cycles of methotrexate–L-asparaginase are repeated thereafter at 14-day intervals. The combination seems to be particularly effective in acute leukemia refractory to conventional methotrexate doses, with complete remission rates between 33 and 67 per cent in acute lymphocytic leukemia of childhood, and 35 per cent in acute nonlymphocytic leukemia.[63, 64] The complete response rate is highest in patients who have not been treated previously with L-asparaginase,[62] indicating that the success of the regimen depends at least in part on the antitumor effects of the enzyme.

OTHER FORMS OF ENZYME THERAPY AND AMINO ACID ANTAGONISTS

A number of other enzymes, primarily of bacterial origin, have antitumor activity in animal systems and may undergo clinical trial in the future. The most prominent of these are listed in Table 21–3. The reader is referred to reviews for a more detailed consideration of this subject.[6-8]

L-Glutaminase–L-asparaginase from *Acinetobacter glutaminasificans*[65] and a succinylated derivative of the same enzyme that has a longer plasma half-life have both received preliminary trials in acute leukemia.[66] With the nonsuccinylated enzyme, more than 10,000 IU per m^2 per day are required to produce continuous depletion of

TABLE 21–3. Amino Acid–Directed Antitumor Therapy*

I. Amino Acid Degrading Enzymes With Antitumor Activity

ENZYME	SOURCE	SUBSTRATE	COMMENT	REF.
A. L-glutaminase	*Acinetobacter glutaminasificans*	L-glutamine L-asparagine	Antitumor activity in man	67,68
B. L-threonine deaminase	Sheep liver	L-threonine	Active vs. murine leukemia	69
C. L-methionase	*Clostridium sporogenes*	L-methionine	Active vs. cultured human lymphoblasts	70
D. L-tyrosine phenol-lyase	*Erwinia herbicola*	L-tyrosine L-phenylalanine	Active vs. murine B_{16} melanoma	71
E. L-phenylalanine ammonia-lyase	*Rhodotorula glutinis*	L-phenylalanine	Active vs. murine leukemia	72
F. L-tryptophan hydroxylase	*Rhodotorula glutinis*	L-tryptophan	Active vs. murine leukemia	73

II. Amino Acid Analogues

	COMPOUND	MECHANISM OF ACTION	ANTITUMOR ACTIVITY IN MAN
A. L-glutamine analogues[74]	1. 6-diazo-5-oxo-L-norleucine (DON)	Inhibits glutamine-dependent transaminases	Breast, lung, choriocarcinoma
	2. Azaserine	Inhibits glutamine-dependent transaminases	Childhood acute leukemia, Hodgkin's disease
	3. Azotomycin	Precursor of DON	Colorectal carcinomas; soft tissue sarcoma
B. L-aspartate analogues[75, 76]	1. L-alanosine	Inhibitis purine biosynthesis	Unknown
	2. N-phosphonacetyl-L-aspartic acid (PALA)	Inhibits *de novo* pyrimidine synthesis	Breast, colon carcinoma; soft tissue sarcoma

*Reproduced with permission from Uren R, and Handschumacher RE: Enzyme therapy. *In* Becker FF: Cancer: A Comprehensive Treatise. Plenum Press, New York, 1977, pp. 457–487.

serum L-glutamine and L-asparagine. The succinylated enzyme used in doses of less than 1000 IU per m^2 per day produces rapid depletion of L-glutamine that lasts for at least 24 hours.[67, 68] A lowering of peripheral lymphoblast count was reported in seven of 14 patients resistant to L-asparaginase,[67] but severe neurotoxicity with coma was observed in five patients in association with a marked anomalous elevation of CSF L-glutamine levels that was noted in all patients tested. The more common toxicities associated with L-asparaginase are also seen in patients treated with L-glutaminase, including decreases in various serum proteins, hyperglycemia, fever, and allergic reactions.

L-Glutamine analogues (see Table 21–3) have also received limited clinical trial, but with little success. The strong activity of DON against human xenografts in nude mice has prompted a re-examination of this drug. Inhibitors of the L-asparagine synthetase reaction have also been described and may have a use in combination with L-asparaginase.

References

1. Haley EE, Fischer GA, and Welch AD: The requirement for L-asparagine of mouse leukemic cells L5178Y in culture. Cancer Res 21:532, 1961.
2. Kidd JG: Regression of transplanted lymphomas induced *in vivo* by means of normal guinea pig serum. I. Course of transplanted cancers of various kinds in mice and rats given guinea pig serum, horse serum, or rabbit serum. J. Exp. Med.98:565, 1953.
3. Broome JD: Evidence that the L-asparaginase of guinea pig serum is responsible for its antilymphoma effects. I. Properties of the L-asparaginase of guinea pig serum in relation to those of the antilymphoma substance. J. Exp. Med. 118:99, 1963.
4. Hill JM, Loeb E, MacLellan A, et al.: Response to highly purified L-asparaginase during therapy of acute leukemia. Cancer Res. 29:1574, 1969.
5. Ohnuma T, Holland JF, and Meyer P: *Erwinia carotovora* asparaginase in patients with prior anaphylaxis to asparaginase from *E. coli*. Cancer 30:376, 1972.
6. Holcenberg JS, and Roberts J: Enzymes as drugs. Annu. Rev. Pharmacol. 17:97, 1977.
7. Cooney DA, and Rosenbluth RJ: Enzymes as therapeutic agents. Adv. Pharmacol. Chemother. 12:185, 1975.
8. Capizzi RL, Bertino JR, and Handschumacher RE: L-Asparaginase. Annu. Rev. Med. 21:433, 1970.
9. Ho PK, Milikin EB, Bobbitt JL, et al.: Crystalline L-asparaginase from *E. coli* B. Purification and chemical characterization. J. Biol. Chem. 245:3703, 1970.
10. Jackson RC, and Handschumacher RE: *Escherichia coli* L-asparaginase. Catalytic activity and subunit nature. Biochemistry 9:3585, 1970.
11. Maita T, and Matsuda G: The primary structure of L-asparaginase from *Escherichia coli*. Hoppe Seylers Z. Physiol. Chem. 361:105, 1980.
12. Howard JB, and Carpenter FH: L-Asparaginase from *Erwinia carotovora*. Substrate specificity and enzymatic properties. J. Biol. Chem. 247:1020, 1972.
13. Dunlop PC, Meyer GM, and Roon RJ: Reactions of asparaginase II of *Saccharomyces cerevisiae*. A mechanistic analysis of hydrolysis and hydroxylaminolysis. J. Biol. Chem. 255:1542, 1980.
14. Ehrman M, Cedar H, and Schwartz JH: L-Asparaginase II of *E. coli*. Studies on the enzymatic mechanism of action. J. Biol. Chem. 246:88, 1971.
15. Lachman LB, and Handschumacher RE: The active site of L-asparaginase: dimethylsulfoxide effect of 5-diazo-4-oxo-L-norvaline interactions. Biochem. Biophys. Res. Commun. 73:1094, 1976.
16. Distasio JA, Niederman RA, Kafkewitz D, et al.: Purification and characterization of L-asparaginase with antilymphoma activity from *Vibrio succinogenes*. J. Biol. Chem. 251:6929, 1976.
17. Haw T, and Ohnuma T: L-Asparaginase: *in vitro* inhibition of blastogenesis by enzyme from *Erwinia carotovora*. Nature (Lond.) New Biol. 239:50, 1972.
18. Durden DL, and Distasio JA: Comparison of the immunosuppressive effects of asparaginases from *Escherichia coli* and *Vibrio succinogenes*. Cancer Res. 40:1125, 1980.
19. Liu YP, and Handschumacher RE: Nitroasparaginase: subunit cross-linkage and altered substrate specificity. J. Biol. Chem. 247:66–69, 1972.
20. Uren JR, and Ragin RC: Improvement in the therapeutic, immunological, and clearance properties of *E. coli* and *Erwinia carotovora* L-asparaginases by attachment of poly-DL-alanyl peptides. Cancer Res. 39:1927, 1979.
21. Kamisaki Y, Wada H, Yasura T, et al.: Reduction in immunogenicity and clearance rate of *E. coli* L-asparaginase by modification with monomethoxypolyethylene glycol. J. Pharmacol. Exp. Ther. 216:410, 1981.
22. Yasura T, Kamisaki Y, Wada H, et al.: Immunological studies on modified enzymes. I. Soluble L-asparaginase/mouse albumin copolymer with enzyme activity and substantial loss of immunosensitivity. Int. Arch. Allergy Appl. Immunol. 64:11, 1981.
23. Mazzola G, and Vecchio G: Immobilization and characterization of L-asparaginase on hollow fibers. Int. J. Artif. Organs 3:120, 1980.
24. Jackson JA, Halvorson HR, Furlons JW, et al.: A new extracorporeal reactor-dialyzer for enzyme therapy using immobilized L-asparaginase. J. Pharmacol. Exp. Ther. 209:271, 1979.
25. Woods JS, and Handschumacher RE: Hepatic regulation of plasma L-asparaginase. Am. J. Physiol. 224:740, 1973.
26. Haskell CM, and Canellos GP: L-Asparaginase resistance in human leukemia–asparagine synthetase. Biochem. Pharmacol. 18:2578, 1969.
27. Horowitz B, Madras BK, Meister A, et al.: Asparagine synthetase activity of mouse leukemia. Science 160:533, 1968.
28. Haley EE, Fischer GA, and Welch AD: The requirement for L-asparagine of mouse leukemia cells L5178Y in culture. Cancer Res. 21:532, 1961.
29. Campbell HA, Mashburn LT, Boyse SE, et al.: Two L-asparaginases from *E. coli* B: their separation, purification, and antitumor activity. Biochemistry 6:721, 1967.
30. Mashburn LT, and Landin LM: Some physiochemical aspects of L-asparaginase therapy. Recent Results Cancer Res. 33:48, 1970.
31. Broome JD: Factors which may influence the effectiveness of L-asparaginases as tumor inhibitors. Br. J. Cancer 22:595, 1968.
32. Howard JB, and Carpenter FH: L-Asparaginase from *Erwinia carotovora*. Substrate specificity and enzymatic properties. J. Biol. Chem. 247:1020, 1972.
33. Yellin TO, and Wriston JC Jr: Purification and properties of guinea pig serum asparaginase. Biochemistry 5:1605, 1966.
34. Peterson RE, and Ciegler A: L-Asparaginase production by *Erwinia aroideae*. Appl. Microbiol. 18:64, 1969.
35. Law AS, and Wriston JC Jr: Purification and properties of *Bacillus coagulans* L-asparaginase. Arch. Biochem. Biophys. 147:744, 1971.
36. Meister A, Levintow L, Greenfield RE, et al.: Hydrolysis and transfer reactions catalyzed by amidase preparations. J. Biol. Chem. 215:441, 1955.
37. Cooney DA, Capizzi RL, and Handschumacher RE: Evalua-

tion of L-asparagine metabolism in animals and man. Cancer Res. 30:929, 1970.

38. Ertel IJ, Nesbit ME, Hammond D, et al.: Effective dose of L-asparaginase for induction of remission in previously treated children with acute lymphocytic leukemia: a report from Children's Cancer Study Group. Cancer Res. 39:3893, 1979.
39. Nesbitt M, Chard R, Evans A, et al.: Intermittent L-asparaginase therapy for acute childhood leukemia. Proc. 10th International Cancer Congress, 1970, p. 477.
40. Ohnuma T, Holland JF, and Sinks LF: Biochemical and pharmacological studies with L-asparaginase in man. Cancer Res. 30:2297, 1970.
41. Peterson RC, Handschumacher RF, and Mitchell MS: Immunological responses to L-asparaginase. J. Clin. Invest. 50:1080, 1971.
42. Oettgen HF, Stephenson PA, Schwartz MK, et al.: Toxicity of *E. coli* L-asparaginase in man. Cancer 25:253, 1970.
43. Haskell CM, Canellos GP, Leventhal BG, et al.: L-Asparaginase: therapeutic and toxic effects in patients with neoplastic disease. N. Engl. J. Med. 281:1028, 1969.
44. Nesbit ME, Ertel I, and Hammond GD: L-Asparaginase as a single agent in acute lymphocyte leukemia: survey of studies from Children's Cancer Study Group. Cancer Treat. Rep., in press.
45. Jones B, Holland JF, Glidewell O, et al.: Optimal use of L-asparaginase (NSC-109229) in acute lymphocytic leukemia. Med. Pediatr. Oncol. 3:387, 1977.
46. Rausen AR, Glidewell O, Holland JF, et al.: Superiority of L-asparaginase combination chemotherapy in advanced acute lymphocytic leukemia of childhood. Randomized comparative trial of combination versus solo therapy. Cancer Clin. Trials, in press.
47. Ohnuma T, Holland JF, and Meyer P: *Erwinia carotovora* asparaginase in patients with prior anaphylaxis to asparaginase from *E. coli*. Cancer 30:376, 1972.
48. Rutter DA: Toxicity of asparaginases. Lancet 1:1293, 1975.
49. Land VJ, Sutow WW, Fernbach DJ, et al.: Toxicity of L-asparaginase in children with advanced leukemia. Cancer 40:339, 1972.
50. Khan A, and Hill JM: Atopic hypersensitivity to L-asparaginase. Int. Arch. Allergy 40:463, 1971.
51. Killander D, Dohlwitz A, Engstedt L, et al.: Hypersensitive reactions and antibody formation during L-asparaginase treatment of children and adults with acute leukemia. Cancer 37:220, 1976.
52. Land VJ, Sutow WW, Fernbach DJ, et al.: Toxicity of L-asparaginase in children with advanced leukemia. Cancer 30:339, 1972.
53. Sills RH, Nelson DA, Stockman JA III: L-Asparaginase-induced coagulopathy during therapy of acute lymphocytic leukemia. Med. Pediatr. Oncol. 4:311, 1978.
54. Gralnick HR, and Henderson E: Hypofibrinogenemia and coagulation factor deficiencies with L-asparaginase treatment. Cancer 27:1313, 1970.
55. Ramsay NKC, Coccia PF, Krivit W, et al.: The effect of L-asparaginase on plasma coagulation factors in acute lymphoblastic leukemia. Cancer 40:1398, 1977.
56. Shapiro RS, Gerrard JM, Ramsay NK, et al.: Selective deficiency in collagen-induced platelet aggregation during L-asparaginase therapy. Am. J. Pediatr. Hematol. Oncol. 2:207, 1980.
57. Cairo MS, Lazarus K, Gilmore RL, et al.: Intracranial hemorrhage and focal seizures secondary to use of L-asparaginase during induction therapy of acute lymphocytic leukemia. J. Pediatr. 97:829, 1980.
58. Buchanan GR, and Holtkamp CA: Reduced antithrombin III levels during L-asparaginase therapy. Med. Pediatr. Oncol. 8:7, 1980.
59. Pitney WR, Phadke KP, and Dean S: Antithrombin III deficiency during asparaginase therapy (letter). Lancet 1:493, 1980.
60. Vellenga E, Mulder NH, and Nieweg HO: Antithrombin III deficiency during asparaginase therapy (letter). Lancet 1:649, 1980.
61. Capizzi R: Improvement in the therapeutic index of L-asparaginase by methotrexate. Cancer Chemother. Rep. (3) 6:37, 1975.
62. Lobel JS, O'Brien RT, McIntosh S, et al.: Methotrexate and asparaginase combination chemotherapy in refractory acute lymphoblastic leukemia of childhood. Cancer 43:1089, 1979.
63. Amadori S, Tribalto M, Pacilli L, et al.: Sequential combination of methotrexate and L-asparaginase in the treatment of refractory acute leukemia. Cancer Treat. Rep. 64:939, 1980.
64. Harris RE, McAllister JA, Provisor DS, et al.: Methotrexate/L-asparaginase combination chemotherapy for patients with acute leukemia in relapse: a study of 36 children. Cancer 46:2004, 1980.
65. Spiers ASD, and Wade HE: *Achromobacter* L-glutaminase–L-asparaginase: human pharmacology, toxicology, and activity in acute leukemia. Cancer Treat. Rep. 63:1019, 1979.
66. Holcenberg JS, Camitta BM, Borella LD, et al.: Phase I study of succinylated *Acinetobacter* L-glutaminase–L-asparaginase. Cancer Treat. Rep. 63:1025, 1979.
67. Holcenberg JS, Borella LD, Camitta BM, et al.: Human pharmacology and toxicology of succinylated *Acinetobacter* glutaminase-asparaginase. Cancer Res. 39:3145, 1979.
68. Warrell RP Jr, Chou TC, Gordon C, et al.: Phase I evaluation of succinylated *Acinetobacter* glutaminase-asparaginase in adults. Cancer Res. 40:4546, 1980.
69. Wellner D, and Greenfield RS: L-Threonine deaminase as a possible antitumor agent. Cancer Treat. Rep. 63:1089, 1979.
70. Kreis W: Tumor therapy by deprivation of L-methionine: rationale and results. Cancer Treat Rep. 63:1069, 1979.
71. Elmer GW, Linden C, and Meadows GG: Influence of L-tyrosine phenol-lyase on the growth and metabolism of B_{16} melanoma. Cancer Treat. Rep. 63:1055, 1979.
72. Abell CW, Smith WJ, and Hodgkins DS: An *in vivo* evaluation of the chemotherapeutic potency of phenylalanine ammonia-lyase. Cancer Res. 33:2529, 1973.
73. Schmer G, and Roberts J: Molecular engineering of the L-tryptophan–depleting enzyme indolyl-3 alkane alpha-hydroxylase. Cancer Treat. Rep. 63:1123, 1979.
74. Catane R, Von Hoff DD, Glaubiger DL, et al.: Azaserine, DON, and azotomycin: three diazo analogs of L-glutamine with clinical antitumor activity. Cancer Treat. Rep. 63:1033, 1979.
75. Jayaram HN, and Cooney DA: Analogs of L-aspartic acid in chemotherapy for cancer. Cancer Treat. Rep. 63:1095, 1979.
76. Erlichman C, Strong JM, Wiernik PH, et al.: Phase I trial of N-(phosphonacetyl)-L-aspartate. Cancer Res. 39:3992, 1979.
77. Uren R, and Handschumacher RE: Enzyme therapy. *In* Becker FF (ed.): Cancer: A Comprehensive Treatise. Plenum Press, New York, 1977, pp. 457–487. *A detailed discussion of therapies directed at amino acid depletion or analogue development.*

APPENDIX

SUGGESTED DOSE MODIFICATIONS FOR ANTICANCER DRUGS IN PATIENTS WITH ORGAN DYSFUNCTION

Agent	*Organ Dysfunction*	*Suggested Dose Modification*
Methotrexate Hydroxyurea	Renal failure or creatinine clearance	In proportion to creatinine clearance (normal, 60 ml/min/m^2)
cis-Platinum	Renal failure	In proportion to creatinine clearance
Cyclophosphamide	Renal failure (creatinine clearance below 25 ml/min)	50% decrease
Bleomycin	Renal failure (creatinine clearance below 25 ml/min)	50–75% decrease
Streptozotocin	Renal failure (creatinine clearance below 25 ml/min)	50–75% decrease
		Approximate Guidelines
Doxorubicin Daunorubicin Vincristine Vinblastine VP-16 VM-26	Hepatic dysfunction	1. For bilirubin of > 1.5 mg/dl, reduce dose by 50% 2. For bilirubin of > 3.0 mg/dl, reduce dose by 75%

INDEX

Page numbers in *italics* indicate illustrations; *t* indicates table.